foundations of nursing practice

Third Edition

Foundations of
Nursing
Practice

LEADING THE WAY

EDITED BY

RICHARD HOGSTON AND
BARBARA A. MARJORAM

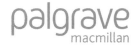

First edition 1999
Reprinted three times
Second edition 2002
Reprinted six times
Third edition 2007

Published by
PALGRAVE MACMILLAN
Houndmills, Basingstoke, Hampshire RG21 6XS and
175 Fifth Avenue, New York, N.Y. 10010
Companies and representatives throughout the world

PALGRAVE MACMILLAN is the global academic imprint of the Palgrave
Macmillan division of St. Martin's Press, LLC and of Palgrave Macmillan Ltd.
Macmillan® is a registered trademark in the United States, United Kingdom
and other countries. Palgrave is a registered trademark in the European
Union and other countries.

ISBN–13: 978–1–4039–8780–8
ISBN–10: 1–4039–8780–7

This book is printed on paper suitable for recycling and made from fully
managed and sustained forest sources.

A catalogue record for this book is available from the British Library.

10 9 8 7 6 5 4 3 2 1
16 15 14 13 12 11 10 09 08 07

Printed in China

Contents

Part 3 Professional Issues

List of Figures

List of Tables

List of Charts

Notes on Contributors

CATHY ALLEN MSc, BSc(Hons), DipNEd, RNT, RN(Adult) gained an honours degree in Psychology in Portsmouth and an MSc in Health Psychology at City University, London. Her clinical background is in the care of older people, specialising in dementia care. She was employed as the training coordinator for adult protection in Cambridgeshire and Peterborough, and, until recently, was Senior Lecturer with the BSc(Hons) Nursing programme at the University of Lincoln, with a responsibility for practice placement.

WAYNE ARNETT BN(Hons), RGN, CertMan is Lecturer at the University of Southampton. Wayne is the Lead for Moving and Handling in the School of Nursing and Midwifery and teaches the topic within the School of Healthcare Professions. He also leads the orthopaedic module, and teaches in the spinal injuries and physical assessment modules.

SID CARTER MSc, BA, RN(LD), PGCEA, AdvCert(Human Sexuality) is Lecturer (Clinical) in Learning Disabilities at the European Institute of Health and Medical Sciences, University of Surrey. His clinical work centres on the empowerment of people with cognitive impairments. Sid's research interests include the skills of professionals working with people with learning disabilities, and the psychophysiology of emotion as it relates to learning.

NADIA CHAMBERS RGN, BSc(Hons), PgDipEd, MA, PhD is Consultant Nurse for Older People at Southampton University Hospitals NHS Trust. She was previously a Senior Lecturer at the University of Portsmouth, heading up the Clinical Governance and Clinical Leadership Education at the School of Postgraduate Medicine.

IAN DOUGLAS RGN, DPSN, RCNT, RNT, BA(Hons), MSc is Lecturer and Preregistration Deputy Award Leader at Southampton University. His area of speciality is accident and emergency nursing, and his research interest remains the epidemiological distribution of accidents related to A&E services.

DEBRA ELLIOTT MSc, BSc(Hons), RNT, CertEd(FE), CertEd, RGN is Head of Nursing and Midwifery Education in Portsmouth Hospitals NHS Trust. Debra has considerable experience within the Trust, having worked in workforce design, PFI and been a Matron in Medicine. She has also spent 10 years in the military, and six and a half years in higher education as a Nurse Teacher and Senior Lecturer for preregistration nursing and continuing education. Debra's main clinical background has been critical care medicine and, more latterly, emergency medicine.

ANITA J. GREEN PhD, MA, BA(Hons), RCNT, RGN, RMN is Lecturer (Clinical) in the European Institute of Health and Medical Sciences, University of Surrey. She has worked in both acute mental health and drug and alcohol services. She is presently working with the staff of the Drug and Alcohol Service for Sussex Weald and Downs NHS Trust. Anita's research interest focuses on the client's experience of the drug and alcohol service, in particular methadone prescribing. She has a consultancy relationship with the drug and alcohol services and a nursing college in St Petersburg, Russia and is currently completing an evaluation of that project.

SUE M. GREEN RN, BSc, MMedSci, PhD, PGCert gained BSc and Masters degrees in science subjects and a PhD in Biopsychology, qualified as a nurse in London and has worked in a variety of clinical areas including cardiothoracics, acute medical and care of the older adult. Sue is currently Senior Lecturer at the School of Nursing and Midwifery, University of Southampton.

RICHARD HOGSTON MSc(Nurs), PGDipEd, BA(Hons), RN is Dean of the Faculty of Health at Leeds Metropolitan University and Head of the School of Health and Community Care. Prior to that, Richard was at Hull University, joining from the Department of Health where he had been Nursing Officer for Education and Training. Richard held teaching posts at the University of Portsmouth, where his main teaching and research interests concentrated on quality and management. Before entering education, Richard followed a clinical career in Portsmouth.

PAM JACKSON MPhil, BSc(Hons), RGN, RHV, RNT is Senior Lecturer, with research interests in wound care, nutrition and evidence-based practice. Pam is Faculty Lead for curriculum development in Common Learning in Interprofessional Education at the Faculty of Medicine, Health and Life Sciences, University of Southampton.

MELANIE JASPER PhD, MSc, BNurs, BA, PGCEA, RGN, RHV, RM, NDNCert is Head of Health and Social Welfare Studies, Canterbury Christ Church University. Following a professional career in midwifery and health visiting, Melanie entered nursing education in 1990 at the University of Portsmouth, where her abiding interest became the development of reflective strategies as tools for learning within professional practice. She is committed to the concepts of enabling students to develop skills for lifelong learning, and facilitating independent, reflective practitioners who can hold their own in an increasingly technical and accountable profession. Melanie is Editor of the *Journal of Nursing Management*.

ADAM KEEN MSc, MEd, DipHE, MBCS, RN currently works as Senior Lecturer within the School of Health and Social Care at the School of Nursing and Midwifery, Chester College of Higher Education. He is involved in research relating to the potential for medical information systems to lead to dehumanisation. His current teaching interests relate to clinical skills and critical care.

JANET McCRAY PhD, MSc, BSc(Hons), RNT, RN(LD), CertEd is Principal Lecturer in Health and Social Care Management at the University College, Chichester. While working in practice, Janet has had a wide range of experiences supporting people with learning disabilities in community settings. More recently, her research and educational role has been in the interprofessional field, exploring the practice of nurses and social workers. Janet is now working in the field of management in health and social care.

BARBARA A. MARJORAM TD, MA, RN(A), CertEd is Senior Lecturer and Award Leader for the BN(Hons) preregistration programme and Lead for the Academic Development Group for Public Health and Health Promotion at the School of Nursing and Midwifery, University of Southampton. Her previous publications have covered the use of IT in nursing, enquiry-based learning, and elimination.

SUSAN MOORE MSc, MBA, PGDipEd, PGDipCritMan, BA(Hons), DipN(Lond), RMN, RGN is Senior Lecturer in the Mental Health of Older People at the School of Nursing and Midwifery, City University, London. Her main interests are health-care policy, health management and the nursing care of older people. She is currently Programme Leader for the Postgraduate Diploma in Mental Health Nursing. She is currently engaged in research to evaluate 'client attachment' in mental health nurse education.

SOMDUTH PARBOTEEAH PhD, MSc, SRN, RCNT, CertEd, DipN(Lond) is Programme Leader for the MSc in Nursing at DeMontfort University, Leicester and currently teaches physiology and critical care nursing. His research interests include investigating malodorous wounds, and student-centred learning.

DELIA POGSON RN(LD), FETC, CertEd, RNT, MSc, MPhil is Senior Lecturer in the School of Nursing and Midwifery, University of Southampton. Her interests are within genetics and the implications of the developing genetic knowledge base for health and social care, and the education of the workforce required to meet the needs of people arising from these developments in genetics. She is a member of the network of educators for the NHS Genetics Education and Development

Centre. She is undertaking PhD studies focused on breast and ovarian cancer and the needs of individuals arising from the genetic knowledge base of cancer.

ELIZABETH M. J. PORTER BA, MPhil, PGCEA, RN, RM, RHV, FWT practised as a health visitor for ten years, worked as a community tutor for two years and is currently Lecturer at the University of Southampton where she is Award Leader for the MSc and BSc(Hons) public health practice degrees. Her particular interests are health visiting and public health. She is a member and past chair of the United Kingdom Standing Conference on Health Visitor Education.

PHIL RUSSELL MSc, MA, BA(Hons), DipEd is Lecturer Practitioner and Bereavement Service Coordinator at The Rowans Hospice and an Associate Lecturer at the University of Portsmouth. He has over 30 years' experience as a nurse and is now a practising counsellor and teacher, with a particular interest in death, loss and palliative care.

PENELOPE M. SIMPSON MSc, DipEd, CertEd, DN(Lond), RCNT, RN is a freelance nurse educator and artist and supplied many illustrations for this text. Her published work covers the nutritional impact of alcohol on elderly people, surgical nursing and client profiles in nursing.

RUTH SADIK MSc, BA(Hons), RNT, RCNT, RSCN, RGN, CertEd(FE) currently teaches applied physiology related to respiratory disorders in both children and adults. She is Senior Lecturer in Child Health at the School of Nursing and Midwifery, Chester College of Higher Education.

CHRIS WALKER MSc, BSc(Hons), DipHE, RN is Senior Nurse for Majors, Accident and Emergency Department, Queen Alexandra Hospital, Portsmouth. His role includes assessing, diagnosing and managing a wide range of major conditions, such as MIs, exacerbations of COPD and abdominal obstruction. He also helps to coordinate the department's strategy for majors' patients, line managing the cardiac nurse practitioners and other major nurse practitioners, and is involved in teaching, audit and research, and deputises for the modern matron in her absence. His MSc in Autonomous Health Care Practice included his dissertation topic of ECG changes secondary to PEs.

GRAHAM WATKINSON RN, PGCE, MA, MIHPE, ILTM, ACMI served in nuclear submarines, undertaking health physics before training as a nurse in the Royal Navy. He specialised in coronary and intensive care nursing and managed an intensive care unit before becoming a lecturer in nursing. Graham has held a number of senior positions in the NHS and universities and is currently the Assistant Director of Public Health in a PCT and Honorary Senior Lecturer at the University of Southampton.

Acknowledgements

Many thanks to Penny Simpson who was the co-editor, with Richard Hogston, of the first two editions of this popular text. Thanks also to the authors and publishers for their support in the production of this third edition.

BARBARA A. MARJORAM

List of Acronyms

AIDS   acquired immune deficiency syndrome

AMHP   approved mental health professional

ASW   approved social worker

BSE   bovine spongiform encephalitis

CBI   Confederation of British Industry

CJD   Creutszfeldt–Jakob disease

CPA   care programme approach

ECR   electronic care record

FSA   Food Standards Agency

GMS   general medical services

HCAI   health-care associated infection

HIV   human immunodeficiency virus

HPA   Health Protection Agency

HPU   health-promoting university

HSE   Health and Safety Executive

LSAs   local supervising authorities

LSCBs   local safeguarding children boards

LSPs   local strategic partnerships

MHAC   Mental Health Act Commission

MRSA   methicillin-resistant staphylococcus aureus

NGOs   non-governmental organisations

NMC   Nursing and Midwifery Council

NSFs   National Service Frameworks

PCT   primary care trust

PHCT   primary health-care team

RNLD   registered nurse for people with learning difficulties

SHA   strategic health authorities

vCJD   new-variant CJD

WHO   World Health Organization

Introduction

This text is designed to be used as a study guide to support many aspects of your learning throughout the common foundation programme. Students on other programmes have also found the text useful, for example those undertaking the Return to Practice foundation degree programmes.

Each chapter has been written by subject specialists and we hope that their enthusiasm for their topic areas is evident when you read them. The chapters are not designed to be read in any particular order and should be tackled when you feel they are relevant to your learning. The interactive style of the chapters is intended to make you think, explore further and reflect on your learning. The learning outcomes give you an idea of what you can achieve when you are working through the chapters, and a glossary of terms used, within each chapter, will enhance your understanding and vocabulary. The cross-referencing between each chapter increases the coherence of the text. Client case studies, drawing on all four branches of nursing as well as featuring a range of settings, are designed to encourage reflection on your reading and its application to clients. Each chapter includes activities that will allow you to explore the topics further. At the end of each chapter, there are a number of Test Yourself! questions so that you can check your knowledge. As well as the references at the end of each chapter, many chapters have suggestions for further reading and also useful websites.

This third edition of *Foundations of Nursing Practice* presents the text in three parts, wherein each chapter discusses a particular topic. Part 1, Nursing in Context, has three chapters. In Chapter 1, the five stages of the problem-solving approach to care known as the nursing process will be used to help you to focus on the example of a client in pain. You will be able to map your own concept of health and, through Chapter 2 on health promotion, identify the concept of health gain. Chapter 3 encourages you to understand the climate in which current developments were conceived.

Part 2, Nursing Interventions, has eight chapters. As nurses tend to deal with uniquely vulnerable clients, and nursing carries its own risks, Chapter 4 will identify some of the safeguards, legal and otherwise, available to protect you and your clients. Eating and drinking can pose particular problems for clients, so you will be encouraged in Chapter 5 to review your own knowledge and habits, aiming to help clients to achieve optimum nourishment for their changing needs. Logically, elimination follows and so Chapter 6 will help to dispel some taboos and myths, with a healthy emphasis on achieving and attaining relative normality across a life span. Chapter 7, on respiration and circulation, explores the nurse's role in assessing and implementing the care of clients with difficulties of breathing and maintenance of the circulation. Chapter 8 explores body image and sexuality, which can be markedly affected by problems of diminished health; this area demands sensitive and thoughtful care. Mobility and immobility affects not only the client, across many areas of care, but also has an impact on the moving and handling of your clients, issues which are explored in Chapter 9. Nurses cover the life span of clients, from the cradle to the grave, and so Chapter 10 explores how loss and changes to health status can make clients question or confirm their beliefs, particularly when life is limited. Thus this chapter examines spirituality, dying and death. Chapter 11 explores issues related to wound management and how our client's lifestyles can have an impact on the healing process.

Part 3, Professional Issues, contains seven chapters; Chapters 17 and 18 being topics new to this third edition. Knowing yourself better, the topic of Chapter 12, will enable you to give yourself to clients and colleagues without being diminished. The image of nursing that you started out with is likely to change as you progress throughout your career, and reflective practice, which is explained in Chapter 13, will be one tool to help you with this. Working in a team is a key part of nursing, and social behaviour and professional interactions will enhance your skill in therapeutic and other communications and therefore Chapter 14 clearly covers this topic. Chapter 15 will be a clear focus for the future, as will challenges to professional practice, outlined in Chapter 16. Chapter 17 uses the topic of genetics to pose some thoughts for future health care within a legal framework. Informatics is affecting our everyday life and no more so than in health care, and Chapter 18 explores how this impacts across all health-care provision.

Finally, Chapter 19 contains the answers and feedback to the Test Yourself! questions posed in all 18 chapters.

We hope you enjoy this enlarged third edition and find it helpful, stimulating and thought-provoking. We wish you well in your nursing career.

RICHARD HOGSTON AND BARBARA A. MARJORAM

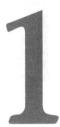

Nursing in Context

1

Managing Nursing Care

Contents

Learning Outcomes

The purpose of this chapter is to explore how nurses manage care; it will take you through a five-stage problem-solving approach known as the nursing process. At the end of the chapter, you should be able to:

- Define the stages of the nursing process
- Undertake a nursing assessment
- Identify nursing diagnoses from the assessment data
- Devise and implement a plan of care
- Evaluate your actions
- Consider the link between evaluation and quality of care.

Throughout the chapter, a working example using a client who is experiencing pain will be used to demonstrate how each of the stages of the nursing process is applied. The chapter also provides an opportunity for you to undertake some exercises that will assist you with your care-planning skills.

■ What is the Nursing Process?

The **nursing process** is a problem-solving framework that enables the nurse to plan care for a client on an individual basis. The nursing process is not undertaken once only, because the client's needs frequently change and the nurse must respond appropriately. It is thus a cyclical process consisting of the five stages shown in Figure 1.1. The nursing process originated in the USA and was formally introduced into the UK in 1977 when the then General Nursing Council introduced its revision of the nursing syllabus. It was an attempt to move nursing away from its traditional 'task-oriented' approach to a more scientific and individualised one.

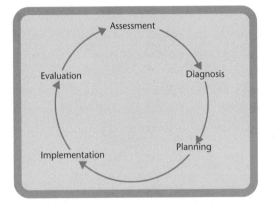

Figure 1.1 ● The nursing process

> nursing process
>
> a five-stage problem-solving framework enabling the nurse to plan individualised care for a client

The nurse is an autonomous practitioner whose responsibilities are now governed by the Nursing and Midwifery Council's (NMC) Code of Professional Conduct (NMC, 2004). This requires nurses to be accountable for the care that they prescribe and deliver with the nursing process, enabling them to document their actions in a logical and rational manner. Today, one's ability to use the nursing process is central to *Making a Difference* (DoH, 1999), *Fitness for Practice* (UKCC, 1999) and therefore *The NHS Plan* (DoH, 2000b), and is governed by the standards of proficiency for preregistration nursing education courses as outlined by the statutory body, the NMC, and embedded in parliamentary statute. This states that conditional to registration is the ability to:

Undertake and document a comprehensive, systematic and accurate nursing assessment of the physical, psychological, social, and spiritual needs of patients, clients and communities

Provide a rationale for the nursing care delivered which takes account of social, cultural, spiritual, legal, political and economic influences

Evaluate and document the outcomes of nursing and other interventions (DoH, 2000a)

Failure to keep a record of nursing care or use the nursing process can lead to a breakdown in the quality of care that is provided. The Clothier Report (DoH, 1994), which was published following the inquiry into Beverley Allitt (the nurse who was convicted of the murder of children in a hospital in Grantham, Lincolnshire), noted how:

Despite the availability of a nurse with responsibility for quality management, there were no explicit nursing standards set for ward four. In addition the nursing records were of poor quality and showed little understanding of the nursing process.

The Healthcare Commission (www.healthcarecommission.org.uk) is now responsible for encouraging improvement in public health and health care in England and Wales under statutory powers. In its guidance (HCC, 2004), it is stated that:

effective clinical governance should ensure a patient centred approach that includes treating patients courteously, involving them in decisions about their care and keeping them informed.

Thus, the importance of understanding and using a systematic patient-centred approach (such as the nursing process) to the provision of nursing care cannot be overestimated.

There has been some debate within the profession over the number of stages needed in the nursing process, some suggesting four and others five. With a four-stage approach, the nurse does not have time to reflect on the assessment data that have been collected and instead moves from assessment to planning. The five-stage process enables the nurse to identify the client's nursing diagnosis in order to plan the appropriate care.

The nursing process should not be seen as a linear process: it is a dynamic and ongoing cyclical process (Figure 1.1). Assessment, for example, is not a 'one-off' activity but a continuous one. Take the example of the individual who is in pain – it is not enough to make a pain assessment that may warrant an intervention; the nurse then needs to make a reassessment after having evaluated whether the pain-relieving intervention has been successful.

The nursing process is a problem-solving activity. Problem-solving approaches to decision-making are not unique to nursing. The medical profession uses a specific format based upon an assessment of the body's systems. A number of questions are asked in a systematic manner to enable the doctor to make a diagnosis based upon the information that has been collected. Problem-solving approaches are also taken outside the health-care field. Car mechanics undertake a sequence of activities in order to diagnose what is wrong with your car when you tell them that there is a squeak or a rattle.

■ Stage 1: Assessment

Sources of assessment data

Before beginning to consider what sort of information you might need to collect, we need to look at the skills that are necessary to ensure that the data analysed are comprehensive. Assessment is not an easy process as it includes collecting information from a variety of sources. The quality of the assessment will, however, depend on one's ability to put together all the sources at one's disposal. Spend a few minutes on Activity 1.1.

The sources that you have listed in Activity 1.1 have probably included the following:

> **Activity 1.1**
>
> Think about the client and other sources that you may be able to consult to assist you when conducting a comprehensive assessment. Write them down in a list.

- Your client
- Relatives, friends and significant others
- Current and previous nursing records
- The records of other health professionals such as doctors and physiotherapists
- Statements and information from the police, ambulance personnel, witnesses at an accident scene and others.

Your client

The first and most important source for data collection is obviously the individual whom you are assessing. It will not, however, always be possible to obtain all the information you require, for a number of reasons, so you will also need to consult other people.

Relatives, friends and significant others

If you are assessing a baby, most of the verbal information you require will be obtained from his or her parent(s) or guardian(s). With a child, you will need to qualify some of your information through the same source. In the case of an adult who is unconscious or having difficulty breathing, you will again need to obtain data from friends, relatives, ambulance personnel, the police and so on. The same applies if the client has difficulty understanding as a result of dementia or severe learning disabilities.

Nursing, medical and other records

Link

Chapter 18 has more information on the national IT programmes and electronic patient records.

It will not always be possible to have immediate access to existing records, especially in an emergency or with a first consultation, but these sources hold valuable information that you need to analyse. They provide details that may assist and prompt you. If the client has been admitted to a hospital, you may have a letter from the GP, district nurse, health visitor or community psychiatric nurse. Similarly, on discharge from hospital, you will provide discharge information if community-based professionals need to be involved. Telephone calls to these professionals, visits and case conferences may also feature. As the roll-out of the national programme for IT within the NHS occurs, the use of electronic patient records should enable much faster access to a range of data (www.connecting-forhealth.nhs.uk).

Activity 1.2

Spend a little while thinking about what kinds of skills you need in order to conduct your assessment. Write them down in list form.

Skills

Having considered some of the sources at your disposal, we now need to think about what other factors have a bearing on a successful assessment. Spend a few minutes on Activity 1.2.

As we are beginning to see, the process of assessment is a complex one. Although we have identified some of the sources of information, the quality of the information collected depends upon a number of other factors. In your list from Activity 1.2, you may have included:

Link

Chapter 14 contains a detailed examination of how the nurse can most effectively use some of these skills. You may wish to consult this before reading on.

- Listening
- Observing
- The use of verbal and non-verbal communication and open and closed questions
- Physical examination
- Measurements.

Listening

One of the most important features of an assessment interview is the nurse's ability to listen to the client. This means giving the client time to answer questions. You will appreciate from your own life experience that when you are asked a question, you want time to think and then answer without interruption. A premature interruption may lead to clients withholding information or not feeling that you are really interested in what they have to say. Although it is important for you to focus on the information you require and not digress, the fact that Mrs Jones has been admitted as an emergency and is meant to be on the school run in an hour will be the only thing of interest to her until you are able to contact someone who can collect her children.

Observation

Observation can in itself provide the nurse with a great deal of information. The bluish tinge (cyanosis) seen around the mouths, nailbeds and faces of some breathless patients may be indicative of respiratory distress and will be an indication of how little oxygen is circulating in their blood. A yellowish tinge to the skin (jaundice) may be indicative of biliary disease. Similarly, facial and other body expressions may give you an indication of pain.

> **Link**
> Chapter 7 explains some causes of cyanosis and identifies the difference between central and peripheral cyanosis.

Open and closed questioning

Both these methods of communication need to be used when collecting information. The use of **closed questions** allows the client who is, for example, breathless, anxious, in pain or depressed to answer with a simple 'yes' or 'no'. **Open questions**, however, will allow you to provide your clients with a full opportunity to tell you the history of their illness or pain.

> **closed questions**
> those designed to elicit a simple 'yes' or 'no' answer
>
> **open questions**
> those in which clients can express their answers in as many words as they choose

Physical examination

The physical examination of clients allows you to observe and make a judgement about their symptoms. You will be able to determine the integrity (state) of the skin, which is an important consideration in an immobile client. Physical damage such as wounds can be seen, as can even the small puncture marks left by an intravenous drug abuser. Skin that feels very warm and moist to the touch may be a sign of pyrexia.

> **Link**
> Chapter 9 briefly outlines the structure and function of the skin. Chapter 11 classifies wounds and has a section on wound assessment.

Measurements

Measurements come in many forms, for example the taking of a blood pressure, pulse or temperature. Also included here is the use of other assessment tools such as a nutritional analysis, a pressure sore risk calculator (for example Braden, Norton or Waterlow) or a pain chart.

> **Link**
> Chapter 7 explores blood pressure and explains how to take an arterial blood pressure reading.

Data collection

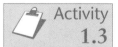

Activity 1.3

Select a friend or relative and ask them if you can spend about 20 minutes undertaking a health assessment. Now take a blank piece of paper and collect the information that you feel is important when making some decisions about your chosen person's health status.

As we have seen, nurses must, in order to be able to plan care for their clients, be able to gather information that will enable them to make informed decisions. But what information do nurses need to gather, what questions should they ask and how much do they need to know? The answer is determined on an individual basis, the nurse collecting both subjective and objective information. Before looking in detail at what information should be collected, undertake Activity 1.3.

From the activity, in addition to name, age and date of birth, you may have collected some of the following information:

Physical health information
- Current and past health problems
- Nutritional and dietary information
- Patterns of activity and rest
- Stamina
- Physical parameters
- Factors affecting health (cigarettes, alcohol and so on)
- Dental, hearing, vision and so on
- Elimination patterns
- Sexual history.

Psychological information
- How does the client react to stress, challenge and so on?
- What are the person's hopes, expectations, demands?
- Communication
- Values and beliefs.

Social health information
- What is the person's lifestyle?
- Employment/unemployment details
- Family or other responsibilities
- Leisure
- Exercise
- Social environment/networks.

How did you decide what you needed to ask, how did you decide to word the questions, and did you collect everything to enable you to feel that you had conducted a thorough assessment?

Framework for assessment

One way of organising the information that you need to collect is by using a nursing framework. The 'activities of living' framework devised by Roper et al. (2003) uses a list of the client's activities of living (Chart 1.1) as a framework for assessment, the nurse systematically collecting the physical, psychological, socio-cultural and economic aspects of these activities.

Breathing, one of the activities of living, will now be used as a framework to demonstrate the type of information that the nurse needs to collect during an assessment. At any given time during the assessment process, it may be necessary to concentrate more on one activity than another.

Chart 1.1 ● The activities of living

- Maintaining a safe environment
- Communicating
- Breathing
- Eating and drinking
- Eliminating
- Personal cleansing and dressing
- Controlling body temperature
- Mobilising
- Working and playing
- Expressing sexuality
- Sleeping
- Dying

Breathing

The information that the nurse needs to collect about this and any other activity of living depends on the answers to certain trigger questions. You may, for example, start off by asking your client whether she has any problems with breathing. Even though the answer may be 'no', you would, as a professional, need to investigate further. The client whom you are assessing may not feel that she has a problem with breathing, but consider the following questions:

> **Link**
> Chapter 7 provides methods of respiratory assessment.

1. 'Do you smoke?' The answer here may be 'yes', even though the client has said she has no problems with breathing. Indeed, she may still feel that she does not have any problems. This is, however, a trigger for further questioning.
2. 'Do you suffer from any breathlessness?' The answer at the outset may again be 'no', but if you ask about running up the stairs or running for a bus, the client may admit that, yes she does then, but this is because she does not usually do any exercise.
3. Taking this one step further allows the nurse to extract even more information about the status of the client's breathing: 'Do you cough?' The answer may be 'no', but when prompted the client may admit to coughing for a little while in the morning, although this clears rapidly and she thinks nothing of it.

If the client is a normal healthy young adult, the nurse may at this stage still perceive that the client does not actually have a problem with breathing in the short term even though she is partaking in health-damaging behaviour. In the long term, however, the consequences are obvious. At this stage in the assessment process, it may be sufficient to make a note of the information gathered so far; when it comes to planning care, the action that will be prescribed will then include health education about smoking. This will be expanded in the section on planning and implementation below.

Summary and worked example

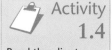

Activity 1.4

Read the client profiles in Casebox 1.1. Choose one of the profiles and, for any two of the activities of living, write down the information that you would need to collect during a nursing assessment.

This section has introduced you to the nursing process and looked in some detail at assessment. The activities should have enabled you to experience some of the issues that you need to consider when undertaking a nursing assessment. We have examined the skills that the nurse needs to use when assessing clients, and we have been introduced to one assessment framework that may assist the nurse during the process. By way of a summary of the information that needs to be gained when undertaking an assessment, the following section takes pain as an example and outlines the questions and methods that can be employed when assessing a client's pain. This will be revisited as we consider the other four stages of the nursing process later in the chapter. Having read this summary, you may like to return to the client profile that you chose and identify the information you feel would be important for your chosen profile. Alternatively, you might like to take the opportunity to participate in the assessment process during your practice placements in the common foundation programme.

Casebox 1.1

Joan Harris is a 69-year-old lady who tripped and fell over a protruding pavement slab this morning while out shopping. She has been admitted to the orthopaedic ward of her local NHS Trust hospital suffering from a fractured neck of femur. Mrs Harris is pale and is anxious about who will look after her cat while she is in hospital. She is complaining of severe pain in her hip and knee, and has grazes and cuts to her lower leg.

Amanda Cohen is 29 years old and has profound learning disabilities. She lives in staffed residential accommodation with two other young women. For two weeks, Amanda has been showing signs of distress – hitting her face, lifting her jumper and crying. At first it was thought that this might be because of premenstrual tension. After a while, however, someone thought to arrange a dental inspection under anaesthetic: the dentist found a particularly nasty dental abscess (adapted from NHSE, 1993).

Andrew Holly is five years old and has been admitted to the accident and emergency department of the local NHS

Trust hospital. He is complaining of a very sore and painful arm, is withdrawn and is sobbing. He is accompanied by his mother, his two-year-old sister and their newborn baby brother.

Alison Simpson, 21 years old, lives in a hostel for people with mental health problems. She has no close family, having left home at 18. She finds it difficult to develop relationships and is suspicious of people who try to befriend her. Alison is very withdrawn and has on two occasions attempted to take her own life through an unsuccessful paracetamol overdose. She was found this morning slumped in a corner, covered in blood and complaining of extreme pain in her left hand. On the floor nearby was a razor blade, and on examination she had severe lacerations to her left forearm.

■ Pain Assessment

The assessment of pain is a complex activity that involves a consideration of the physical, psychological and cultural aspects of the individual. Because pain is a subjective experience, the nurse needs to be able to summarise the information gained against some objective criteria. This is essential for diagnosis and for evaluating the effectiveness of interventions. Only the person experiencing the pain knows its nature, intensity, location and what it means to them. One of the most seminal, widely used and accepted definitions of pain was put forward by McCaffery (1979, p. 18), who suggests that pain is 'whatever the experiencing person says it is and exists whenever he says it does'.

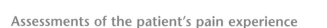

Link
Chapter 7 deals with pain arising from circulatory problems.

Assessments of the patient's pain experience

To begin with, it is essential to identify the characteristics of the client's pain. This means that the nurse should consider:

- *The type of pain:* is it crampy, stabbing, sharp? How the client describes the pain may help in diagnosing its cause. Myocardial (heart) pain is often described as stabbing, but biliary pain as cramping or aching
- *Its intensity:* is it mild, severe or excruciating? Pain assessment scales are helpful here. The nurse can ask the patient to rate the pain on a scale of 0 to 10, zero being no pain and 10 intolerable pain. With children, a range of pictures showing a child changing from happy to sad can be used. Colour 'mood' charts, with a series of colours from black through grey to yellow and orange, have also been used and are very useful for clients who have difficulty grasping numbers or articulating exactly what their pain is like

- *The onset:* was it sudden or gradual? Find out when it started and in what circumstances. What makes it worse? What makes it better? What was the patient doing immediately before it happened?
- *Its duration:* is it persistent, constant or intermittent?
- *Changes in the site:* there may be tenderness, swelling, discolouration, firmness or rigidity. With appendicitis, a classic sign is the movement of pain from the umbilicus to the right iliac fossa. In a myocardial infarction (a heart attack), pain classically radiates down the arm, and with biliary pain it can radiate to the shoulder
- *Its location:* ask the patient to be as specific as possible, for example indicating the site by pointing
- *Any associated symptoms:* Chart 1.2 shows some of the common symptoms of disease that can influence the response to pain
- Signs such as redness, swelling or heat.

Chart 1.2 ● Common symptoms of disease that influence the response to pain

- Anorexia
- Malaise and lassitude
- Constipation
- Diarrhoea
- Nausea and vomiting
- Cough
- Dyspnoea
- Inflammation
- Oedema
- Immobility
- Anxiety and fear
- Depression
- Dryness of the mouth

Table 1.1 Assessment of pain

Initial sympathetic responses to pain of low-to-moderate intensity	Parasympathetic responses to intense or chronic pain	Verbal responses	Muscular and postural responses
Increased blood pressure	Decreased blood pressure	Crying	Increased muscle tone
Increased heart rate	Decreased heart rate	Gasping	Immobilisation of the affected area
Increased respiratory rate	Weak pulse	Screaming	Rubbing movements
Decreased salivation and gastrointestinal activity	Increased gastrointestinal activity	Silence	Rocking movements
Dilated pupils	Nausea and vomiting		Drawing up of the knees
Increased perspiration	Weakness		Pacing the floor
Pallor	Decreased alertness		Thrashing and restlessness
Cool, clammy skin	Shock		Facial grimaces
Dry lips and mouth			Removal of the offending object

Table 1.1 provides a summary of some of the issues to consider when assessing pain. In essence, this section demonstrates how much detail the nurse needs to collect when making a full assessment of the client's pain. Consider your own experiences of pain, both personally and from clients you have nursed in clinical practice, and reflect on how comprehensive the assessment was then.

■ Stage 2: Nursing Diagnosis

The second stage of the nursing process is making a **nursing diagnosis**. This enables the nurse to translate the information gained during the assessment and identify the nursing problems. In order to avoid confusion, it is worth noting that 'diagnosis' is not a concept unique to medicine: car mechanics diagnose mechanical problems, teachers diagnose learning difficulties, and consequently nurses diagnose nursing problems. The language of nursing diagnosis originated in North America in an effort to move the art, science and theoretical basis of nursing forward and readers are advised to visit the informative website at http://www.nanda.org/.

> **nursing diagnosis**
> the second stage of the nursing process, often described as a 'nursing problem', for which the nurse can independently prescribe care

The benefits in a clinical setting have been positively described by Mills et al. (1997) and Hogston (1997). Nursing diagnosis is a critical step in the nursing process, depends on an accurate and comprehensive nursing assessment and forms the basis of nursing care-planning. Nursing diagnosis is the end-product of nursing assessment, a clear statement of the patient's problems as ascertained from the nursing assessment (Roper et al., 2000). The International Council of Nurses (ICN) identified the need for a nursing diagnosis before nursing interventions or outcomes can be achieved (ICN, 2005). A visit to the website at www.icn.ch is recommended for more detailed information and to appreciate that the collaborative work on nursing diagnosis and the International Classification for Nursing Practice is progressing.

The key components of what constitutes a nursing diagnosis are outlined in Chart 1.3.

Chart 1.3 ● Key components of a nursing diagnosis

A nursing diagnosis:
- Is a statement of a client's problem
- Refers to a health problem
- Is based on objective and subjective assessment data
- Is a statement of nursing judgement
- Is a short concise statement
- Consists of a two-part statement
- Is a condition for which a nurse can independently prescribe care
- Can be validated with the client

Source: Adapted from Shoemaker (1984); Bellack and Edlund (1992); Iyer et al. (1995).

Making a nursing diagnosis

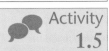

Link

Chapter 6 considers the causes, diagnosis and treatment of constipation.

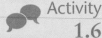

Activity 1.5

Return to the two activities of living that you assessed during Activity 1.4. Try to identify one actual and one potential nursing diagnosis. Use the guidelines in Chart 1.3 to ensure that your diagnoses meet the criteria.

goal

the intended outcome of a nursing intervention, sometimes referred to as an objective

Activity 1.6

For the diagnoses that you identified during Activity 1.4, try to identify one short-term and one long-term goal for your chosen client. Remember to ensure that they meet the MACROS criteria.

Nursing diagnoses can be actual or potential. Actual diagnoses are those which are evident from the assessment, for example pain caused by a fractured neck of femur. Potential diagnoses, on the other hand, are those which could or will arise as a consequence of the actual diagnoses. For example, an individual who is normally active but is confined to bed is at risk of becoming constipated or developing a pressure sore. In this instance, two potential diagnoses arise:

- a potential risk of constipation as a result of enforced bedrest
- a potential risk of pressure sore development from enforced bedrest.

Stage 3: Planning Nursing Care

There are two steps to the planning stage:

- Setting goals
- Identifying actions.

A **goal** is a statement of what the nurse expects the client to achieve and is sometimes referred to as an objective. In other words, goals are the intended outcomes and can be short or long term. Goals are client centred and must be realistic, being stated in objective and measurable language. They help both nurse and client to define how the nursing diagnosis will be addressed. Goals serve as the standard by which the nurse can evaluate the effectiveness of the nursing actions.

When writing goals, they need to conform to the MACROS criteria; they should be:

- Measurable and observable so that the outcome can be evaluated
- Achievable and time limited
- Client centred
- Realistic
- Outcome written
- Short.

Using the example of pain, the short-term goal will be that the client will state that he is comfortable and pain free within 20 minutes. The long-term goal, however, is that the client will state within 12 hours that he feels in control of his pain. (It is important to remember to take account of the non-verbal clues discussed earlier – is the client really pain free?) With the move to shorter hospital stays and the emphasis on care in the community, it may not always be necessary to formulate both long- and short-term goals for all problems. It is, however, always better to have a number of short-term goals that are reached so that new goals can be set, rather than having a long-term goal that takes weeks to achieve. With Mrs Harris (see Casebox 1.1 above), who will have surgery for her hip, this will be a series of goals that progress her towards full mobility following her operation, for example: 'Mrs Harris will walk one way to the toilet unaided by [enter date]. Mrs Harris will be able to climb one set of stairs by [enter date].' This avoids a long-term goal that reads 'Mrs Harris will be fully mobile by [enter date].'

Action planning

The next stage is to plan the nursing care that will ensure that clients achieve their goals. This is where the nurse prescribes nursing actions that can then be implemented and evaluated. In 'care-planning' language, these are the nursing actions – the prescribed interventions that are put into effect in order to solve the problem and reach the goal. It is against these actions that the nurse may, when evaluating care, have to make some adjustments if the actions have not been effective. In today's NHS, when we are seeing a decreasing number of registered nurses against an increase in those of bank and agency nurses and unqualified health-care support workers, documenting the prescribed nursing care ensures a degree of continuity. In this way, the care plan can be seen as the diary of the client's nursing care. When planning nursing care, use the REEPIG criteria, which will ensure that your plan of care is:

● *Realistic*: it is important that the care can be given within the available resources, otherwise it will not be achievable
● *Explicit*: ensure that statements are qualified. If you suggest that a dressing needs changing, state exactly when. This will ensure that there is no room for misinterpretation
● *Evidence based*: nursing is a research-based profession. When planning nursing care, the research findings that underpin the rationale for care must be considered
● *Prioritised*: start with the most pressing diagnosis. Given that time is of the essence, the first priority may be, for example, to plan care for the client's pain
● *Involved*: the plan of care should involve not only the client, so that he or she is aware of why such care is needed, but also the other members of the health-care team who have a stake in helping the client back to health, for example physiotherapists and dietitians
● *Goal centred*: ensure that the care planned meets the set goals.

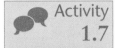

Activity 1.7

Return to the client for whom you chose to identify nursing diagnoses and goals. Consider what nursing care you would need to plan in order to achieve those goals.

Link

Chapter 11 examines pressure ulcer grading and risk assessment.

Returning now to the example of pain, the nurse needs to make decisions about what sorts of intervention will most effectively relieve Mrs Harris's pain. This involves not only decisions about prescribed medications, but also other considerations such as how often the pain assessment tool should be used and what alternative non-pharmacological methods, such as comfort through pillows, the use of skin traction for the leg and distraction therapy, can be implemented. The nursing care plan for Mrs Harris may therefore detail the following nursing actions:

- Give the prescribed analgesic and monitor its effects. Record them on the pain chart
- Apply skin traction (if appropriate)
- Nurse on a bed equipped with a pressure-reduction mattress
- Ensure two-hourly changes of position by attaching a trapeze pole to the bed, and encourage Mrs Harris to change her position regularly
- Ensure that Mrs Harris has a supply of chosen reading/writing materials and access to the television and radio.

■ Stage 4: Implementation

Implementation is the 'doing' phase of the nursing process. This is where the nurse puts into action the nursing care that will be delivered and addresses each of the diagnoses and their goals. The nurse will undertake the instructions written in the care plan in order to assist the client in reaching these goal(s). This will involve a process of teaching and helping clients to make decisions about their health. It also involves deciding upon the most appropriate method for providing nursing care, and the liaison and involvement of other health professionals. Look at the list of health professionals in Chart 1.4. Do you know what their primary roles and functions are and when you might need to involve them?

Chart 1.4 ● Other members of the health-care team

- Physiotherapist
- Community psychiatric nurse
- Speech therapist
- Health visitor
- District nurse
- Podiatrist
- Social worker
- Occupational therapist
- Dietitian
- Key worker
- School nurse
- GP

■ Managing Nursing Care in the Clinical Environment

A number of different approaches to the delivery of nursing care are available to nurses. These include task allocation, patient allocation, team nursing, primary nursing, the key worker and caseload management. The benefits or otherwise of each of these methods need to be considered in the light of the skill mix of available staff (that is, the number and grade of qualified and unqualified staff) and what it is that the nursing team wants to achieve. It is difficult to evaluate the right approach without considering the benefits or drawbacks of each of these methods. The published reports of clinical governance reviews by the Healthcare Commission (see above) will also consider the management and organisation of nursing care.

Task allocation

Task allocation (also known as functional nursing) is a highly ritualistic method of organising care that centres on nurses and support workers being assigned tasks. With this system, one nurse will be assigned to undertake the observations of temperature, pulse, blood pressure and respiration. Another nurse undertakes all the dressings, whereas another takes care of the drugs. This is a fragmented method of providing nursing care that will ensure that the client receives aspects of care from a multiplicity of nurses and support workers, akin to a production line process. The emphasis on tasks naturally removes the notion of individualised client care and as such is incompatible with the nursing process.

task allocation
the provision of nursing care that centres on a range of tasks allocated to nurses/support workers

Client allocation

One step removed from task allocation is client allocation. Here, total care for a number of clients is undertaken by one nurse, often assisted by a support worker. Although this system means that there is an emphasis on total client care being delivered by an individual nurse for a designated period of time, continuity of care may become compromised if the same clients are not cared for on a regular basis by the same nurse. With this system, extra attention needs to be paid to the detail in the nursing care plan because of the number of nurses who may have contact with a client.

client allocation
individualised care provided by a named nurse, often assisted by a support worker

Team nursing

Team nursing occurs where a designated group of clients is cared for by a team of two or more nurses (at least one of whom is a registered nurse) who accept collective responsibility for the assessment, planning, implementation and evalu-

team nursing
care provided by a team of nurses/support workers led by a 'team leader'

ation of the clients' care. Although each team will be headed by a team leader, each registered nurse is accountable for his or her actions in accordance with the Code of Professional Conduct (NMC, 2004). This is important to remember in an effort to counteract any criticism surrounding who is ultimately responsible under a system of collective responsibility.

Walsh and Ford (1989) have described how team nursing and client allocation evolved as the successor to task allocation on the premise that being cared for by a team rather than an array of nurses led to more holistic care. They suggested that team nursing really resembles a small-scale version of task allocation, especially if there is a lack of continuity between shifts when the same team may not be on duty, leading to fragmentation of care. Consequently, there has to be a commitment to ensure that tasks are not assigned to each team member.

Team nursing has received a positive press from student nurses. Lidbetter's (1990) small-scale study describes how students working in a hospital ward practising team nursing spent more time working alongside a qualified nurse and rated their skill acquisition and their evaluation of the effectiveness of client care higher than did those from a ward practising primary nursing. Students were also, as a learning experience, afforded the opportunity to assume the role of team leader, under supervision.

Primary nursing

primary nursing

care provided on an individual basis by a named nurse who, in its purest form, holds 24-hour accountability for the package of care

Primary nursing has been described as a professional patient-centred practice (Manley, 1990). In this approach, the primary nurse accepts full responsibility and accountability for his or her clients during their stay. In its purest form, the implication is that the primary nurse has 24-hour responsibility, seven days a week (Manthey, 1992). In reality, a team of associate nurses continues to provide nursing care under the direction of the primary nurse and in his or her absence. Again, accountability and autonomy rest with the individual registered nurse under the Code of Professional Conduct (NMC, 2004). Positive effects of a move to primary nursing can be seen in the literature (Laakso and Routasalo, 2001; Drach-Zahavy, 2004).

Person-centred planning

Popular in the field of learning disabilities, a person-centred approach to planning care is advocated in the White Paper *Valuing People* (DoH, 2001). Person-centred planning starts with the individual, is seen as 'a mechanism for reflecting the needs and preferences of a person with learning disability and covers issues such as housing, education employment and leisure' (DoH, 2001).

Caseload management

This is the most popular method of organising nursing care in the community setting. It revolves around the designated named nurse with extended qualifications in health visiting/district nursing who acts as the caseload manager. Caseloads are normally organised either geographically or by GP attachment, each caseload manager leading a team of qualified nurses and health-care support workers. Continuity of care is maintained because the teams are organised to ensure that a member of the team is available every day of the week; as such, it is less affected by the demands of the shift system. Each registered nurse is accountable for his or her own actions (NMC, 2004), the caseload manager being responsible for ensuring that the skill mix and resources are adequate. Given the shift of care from the secondary to primary setting, keeping patients out of hospital by managing long-term conditions in the community will see this method of managing care increase (DoH, 2005).

■ Stage 5: Evaluation

At the beginning of this chapter, it was noted that the stages of the nursing process need to be seen as ongoing rather than as once-only activities. This means that the final stage, evaluation, is in reality the end of the beginning and where the process in essence restarts. One of the key components of quality nursing practice is the nurse's ability to make a clinical judgement based upon a sound knowledge base. Evaluation is about reviewing the effectiveness of the care that has been given, and it serves two purposes. First, the nurse is able to ascertain whether the desired outcomes for the client have been achieved. Second, evaluation acts as an opportunity to review the entire process and determine whether the assessment was accurate and complete, the diagnosis correct, the goals realistic and achievable, and the prescribed actions appropriate. The nursing process provides nurses with a tool by which client outcomes are regularly monitored, and can be seen as a vehicle for improving the quality of nursing care and ultimately benefiting the client (Fitzpatrick et al., 1992).

Increased health-care costs require managers throughout the professions to reduce expenditure and seek the most cost-effective options. The population at large are also more informed about health-care matters and are arguably less passive recipients of health care, demanding a detailed and open explanation for their care (Hogston, 1997). It is therefore the responsibility of each nurse to ensure that the prescribed care takes account of these issues. Given that nursing records are legal documents that could be used in a court of law, extreme care and accuracy are essential when completing the care plan to which the registered nurse puts her signature.

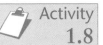

Link

Chapter 2 has more information on how teams interface between hospital, home and other community settings.

Activity 1.8

From your own experiences in clinical practice, what method(s) of care organisation have you experienced? Write down two positive aspects and then consider whether one of the other methods described above would have been suitable and why.

In order to raise standards of care, and in keeping with the clincial gover-nance agenda, the government has published benchmarks in eight fundamental aspects of care (DoH, 2003), one of which focuses on record-keeping. Readers should familiarise themselves with this particular benchmark. It is important to note that the document stresses that the 'eight aspects are by no means an exhaustive account of every fundamental aspect of care, but it represents those elements identified by patients and professionals as crucial to the quality of a patient's care experience' (DoH, 2003).

Methods of evaluating nursing care

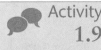

Activity 1.9

How do you think that nursing care is evaluated? You may have witnessed some methods in your own clinical placements; write them down as a list. If you have not, try to think generally about how you evaluate any service you have received – buying a meal or an item from a shop, for example.

Having discussed the importance of evaluation and the place it has in main-taining quality, it is important to consider some of the methods that nurses can use. First of all, undertake Activity 1.9.

Your list from Activity 1.9 may have included some of the following:

● Nursing handover
● Reflection
● Patient satisfaction or complaint
● Reviewing the nursing care plan.

Nursing handover

You may have had experience of a nursing handover, which is where a team of nurses hand over information about the nursing care of clients to another group of nurses, usually at the end of a shift, for example from daycare to night care. Using the nursing care plan as the focus, nurses share information about the clients and their planned care. This serves as a valuable forum for evaluating care through a discussion of its effectiveness. The variety of experiences and professional expertise held by a number of nurses allows a sharing of that infor-mation. The importance of nursing handover was stated by the Audit Commis-sion (1992) as being critical for maintaining continuity of client care.

Reflection

Link

Chapter 13 reviews types of reflection, thoughtful practice and reflection in practice settings.

The role of reflection in quality and evaluation has been discussed in some detail in the literature, and Chapter 13 discusses the concept in more detail. Reflection can, however, be both formal and informal. You probably reflect on your expe-riences both socially with other friends who are nurses and more formally in lecturer-led tutorials. This leads to an analysis of your actions and some of the ways in which you could have done things differently or which you would want to repeat. The use of critical incident analysis, for example, enables nurses to evaluate a given situation or event; this is a tool that is used by qualified nurses in their personal portfolios, which must be kept in order for the nurses to be eligible for triennial re-registration.

Patient satisfaction

The appreciation that is sometimes offered by clients through, for example, a letter is an indicator of how satisfied individuals have been with their nursing care. In contrast, a letter of complaint may lead to an investigation into the reasons why a client has not been satisfied with the care received. Although the number of letters of complaint appears to be on the increase, this is probably the result of a culture comprising a more informed public. In many ways, such letters lead to an analysis of what went wrong; this may not necessarily be a result of poor nursing care but of other environmental factors. Hopefully, however, such publicity allows those who have control over resources to evaluate the priorities.

Health-care providers are now required to publish statistics on indicators of quality ranging from, for example, how long clients have to wait in accident and emergency departments to the number of clients who receive a visit from the community nurse within the two-hour appointment time. In the same vein, letters and cards of satisfaction should be closely monitored.

Reviewing the nursing care plan

This is where the nurse evaluates the effectiveness of the care that has been given against the set goals and writes an evaluation statement. When evaluating care, it is useful to ask yourself a series of questions about each of the stages of the nursing process, which will provide you with answers about your plan of care:

- Have the short-term goals been met?
- If the answer is 'yes', has the diagnosis been resolved? If so, it no longer needs to be addressed
- If the answer is 'no', why have the goals not been met? Did they meet the MACROS criteria?
- Was the planned care realistic? Did it meet the REEPIG criteria?
- Has a new diagnosis arisen or a potential diagnosis become an actual one?
- Was the method of care delivery appropriate?
- Was there effective communication within and between the nursing staff and other members of the multidisciplinary team?
- How satisfied was the client with the care?

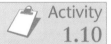

Activity 1.10

Review the assessment, nursing diagnosis, goal(s), planned care and method of implementation for your chosen client and then write an evaluation statement. Remember to ask the questions outlined in the text.

Finally, take a look at the completed care plan for Mrs Harris outlined in Table 1.2 and compare it with your own completed care plan.

Table 1.2 Worked example of a care plan for Mrs Harris

Nursing diagnosis	Pain due to fractured femur
Short-term goal	Mrs Harris states that she is comfortable with a pain scale rating below 2 within 15 minutes
Long-term goal	Mrs Harris feels that she is in control of her pain and that it is no longer a major concern for her within 24 hours
Nursing actions	Give the prescribed analgesic and monitor its effects Apply skin traction Nurse on a bed equipped with a pressure-relieving mattress Ensure two-hourly changes of position by attaching a trapeze pole to the bed, and encourage Mrs Harris to change her position regularly Ensure that Mrs Harris has a supply of chosen reading/writing materials and access to the television and radio
Evaluation	Mrs Harris states that she is comfortable and her pain scale rating remains below 2.

■ Information Technology and Care-planning

Link

Chapter 18 has more information on computerised care planning and the use of IT in health care.

The input of information technology to health care is having a significant impact on the NHS as advanced computerised information systems record and evaluate everything from finance to personal records. From your own experiences, you may already have seen laptop/palm-top and office-based computers that can record client details and an analysis of nurses' workload. As the NHS network expands, all health-care workers are able to access electronic records, email and increasingly the World Wide Web. This will provide nurses with rapid access to client data such as previous nursing records. There are also currently a number of care-planning computer packages used by different NHS Trusts.

Computerised care-planning offers the nurse a number of advantages. It is quick, because there are a number of templates for common nursing diagnoses. Although these are sometimes criticised for moving towards a more communal rather than an individualised approach to nursing care, each of the templates has a menu of options that can be tailored to the individual client. The ability to raise at the click of a mouse a client's previous records is also an advantage and generally allows a more rapid search than does a paper-based system.

Computerised care-planning is, however, only as effective as the person who operates the system and generates the care plan. The skills of assessment, identifying nursing diagnoses and goal-setting, and the required nursing actions can only be effective if the nurse has a sound knowledge base and uses the skills outlined within this chapter. The profession should, and indeed does, welcome the move to more electronic-based systems, if only because the approach is fast and usually efficient. The government has published its national programme for IT; a visit to its interactive website at www.connectingforhealth.nhs.uk is recommended in order to view the implementation plan and appreciate the rapid advances in this area.

■ Chapter Summary

This chapter has introduced you to a systematic method for delivering nursing care through the framework known as the nursing process. You have been introduced to the five basic stages of assessment, diagnosis, planning, implementation and evaluation. Using the vehicle of structured activities, you have been offered the opportunity to develop a care plan for a chosen client.

At this stage, you may feel that the nursing process is a complex activity that demands a great deal of thought and practice, but your skills and experiences will continue to grow and develop as your professional career continues. Working through a structured chapter such as this is no substitute for practice and experience, but the principles of care-planning and the issues you need to consider are offered as the basis of accountable nursing practice. You may, for example, have been surprised at how complex and comprehensive the process of assessment is. The depth of material that you needed to collate when undertaking your assessment may have led you to reflect on the importance of probing and accurate questioning. As you progress in your chosen professional career, you will find that your ability to plan care will become greater. The important point to remember is that the whole practice and process of nursing is ever changing, new strategies, treatments and knowledge arriving almost daily. New research informs nursing practice and must be incorporated into one's professional repertoire. The process of nursing, like the process of learning, is an ongoing rather than a once-only activity.

Test Yourself!

1. Name the stages of the nursing process.
2. Give two reasons for using the nursing process.
3. What sort of information needs to be collected during a nursing assessment?
4. How many types of nursing diagnosis are there?
5. What are the two stages of the planning phase?
6. What criteria should goals conform to?
7. How can the nursing care plan be evaluated?

References

Audit Commission (1992) *Making Time for Patients: A Handbook for Ward Sisters*. HMSO, London.

Bellack, J.P. and Edlund, B.J. (1992) *Nursing Assessment and Diagnosis*, 2nd edn. Jones & Bartlett, London.

DoH (Department of Health) (1994) *The Allitt Inquiry. Independent Inquiry Relating to Deaths and Injuries on the Children's Ward at Grantham and Kesteven Hospital During the Period February–April 1991* (Clothier Report). HMSO, London.

DoH (Department of Health) (1999) *Making a Difference: Strengthening the Nursing, Midwifery and Health Visiting Contribution to Health and Healthcare*. DoH, London.

DoH (Department of Health) (2000a) *Nurses, Midwives and Health Visitors (Training) Ammendment Rules Approval Order 2000*. Stationery Office, London.

DoH (Department of Health) (2000b) *The NHS Plan*. Stationery Office, London.

DoH (Department of Health) (2001) *Valuing People: A New Stratgy for Learning Disability for the 21st Century*. Stationery Office, London.

DoH (Department of Health) (2003) *Essence of Care: Patient-focused Benchmarking for Health Care Practitioners*. DoH, London. http://www.cgsupport.nhs.uk/PDFs/articles/Essence_of_Care_2003.pdf

DoH (2005) *National Service Framework for Long Term Conditions*. DoH. London

Drach-Zahavy, A. (2004) Primary nurses' performance: role of supportive management. *Journal of Advanced Nursing* **45**(1): 7–16.

Fitzpatrick, J.M., While, A.E. and Roberts, J.D. (1992) The role of the nurse in high quality patient care: a review of the literature. *Journal of Advanced Nursing* **17**: 1210–19.

HCC (Healthcare Commission) (2004) *Manual of Clinical Governance Review/Inspection Practices*, edn 4(web). www.healthcarecommission.org.uk/InformationForServiceProviders/ReviewsAndInspections/Reviews/fs/en.

Hogston, R. (1997) Nursing diagnosis: a position paper. *Journal of Advanced Nursing* **26**: 496–500.

ICN (International Council of Nurses) (2005) *International Classification for Nursing Practice*. ICN, Geneva.

Iyer, P.W., Taptich, B.J. and Bernocchi-losey, D. (1995) *Nursing Process and Nursing Diagnosis*, 3rd edn. W.B. Saunders, Philadelphia.

Laakso S. and Routasalo P. (2001) Changing to primary nursing in a nursing home in Finland: experiences of residents, their family members, and nurses. *Journal of Advanced Nursing* **33**: 475–83.

Lidbetter, J. (1990) A better way to learn? *Nursing Times* **86**(29): 61–4.

McCaffery, M. (1979) *Nursing Management of the Patient with Pain*. J.B. Lippincott, Philadelphia.

Manley, K. (1990) Intensive care nursing. *Nursing Times* **86**(19): 67–9.

Manthey, M. (1992) *The Practice of Primary Nursing*. King's Fund, London.

NHSE (National Health Service Executive) (1993) *Learning Disabilities*. DoH, London.

Mills, C., Howie, A. and Mone, F. (1997) Nursing diagnosis: use and potential in critical care. *Nursing in Critical Care* **2**(1): 11–6.

NMC (Nursing and Midwifery Council) (2004) *The NMC Code of Professional Conduct: Standards for Conduct, Performance and Ethics.* NMC, London. www.nmc-uk. org/cms/content/publications.

Roper, N., Logan., W. and Tierney., A. (2000) *The Roper-Logan-Tierney Model of Nursing based on Activities of Living.* Churchill Livingstone, Edinburgh.

Shoemaker, J. (1984) Essential features of a nursing diagnosis. In Kim, M.J., McFarland, G. and Mclane, A. (eds) *Classification of Nursing Diagnoses.* C.V. Mosby, St Louis.

UKCC (United Kingdom Central Council for Nursing, Midwifery and Health Visiting) (1999) *Fitness for Practice.* UKCC, London.

Walsh, M. and Ford, P. (1989) *Nursing Rituals: Research and Rational Actions.* Butterworth Heinemann, Oxford.

■ Useful Websites

www.healthcarecommission.org.uk Charity dedicated to promoting improvement of care across the NHS and independent sectors

www.connectingforhealth.nhs.uk An agency of the Department of Health, created to deliver the National Programme for IT, and to maintain the national critical business systems previously provided by the former NHS Information Authority

www.nanda.org NANDA International
A member-driven, grassroots organization committed to the development of nursing diagnostic terminology

www.icn.ch International Council of Nurses
A federation of national nurses' associations, representing nurses in more than 128 countries

www.dh.gov.uk Department of Health
Dedicated to improving the health and well-being of people in England

www.cgsupport.nhs.uk/programmes/essence_of_care_programme Essence of Care is a framework created by the Clinical Governance Support Programme that aims to improve patients' experiences and outcomes during care

Chapter   ELIZABETH M. J. PORTER AND GRAHAM WATKINSON

2

Promoting Health

Contents

- Promoting Health
- Health Protection
- Promoting Health and Preventing Ill-health
- The Role of the Nurse as a Health Promoter

- Chapter Summary
- Test Yourself!
- Further Reading
- References

Learning Outcomes

This chapter aims to provide analysis and discussion of the nursing contribution to the promotion of health. In order to achieve this, it will dissect and appraise different aspects of this role as part of public health activity. The chapter will draw on scenarios and activities as a way of providing illustration of this. At the end of the chapter, you should be able to:

- Describe the key aspects of public health, health promotion and health protection

- Identify public health issues and why these are important for the nurse

- Identify six aspects of health promotion in addressing the health of the population

- Define the knowledge and skills of reflection as part of promoting health.

■ Promoting Health

Enabling people to achieve better health is a fundamental part of good nursing practice, whatever the context of care (for example in the community, primary health care setting, the home or an acute hospital setting). Whether involved in primary prevention, secondary health care, tertiary rehabilitation or palliative care, a nurse who thinks critically about those whom they seek to help may be able to promote health, prevent ill-health and alleviate suffering by preventing conditions from deteriorating further.

In introducing *Choosing Health* (DoH, 2004, p. 5), the health secretary reminds us that:

> a founding principle for the National Health Service (NHS) in 1948 was that it should improve health and prevent disease, not just provide treatment for those who are ill.

At a superficial level this seems obvious, so why is it so difficult to achieve continually in practice? Perhaps we need to be more critical and define what we mean by public health and in particular health and examine why nurses should strive to improve the public's health and prevent disease.

What is public health?

> Public Health is the science and art of preventing disease, prolonging life, and promoting health through the organised efforts and informed choices of society, organisations, public and private communities and individuals. (Wanless, 2004, p. 27)

Within this definition, public health can be described as the overarching term for enabling activities that involve interactions around the health of populations, communities, groups of people, families and individuals.

What is health?

There is a substantial amount of literature about people's perceptions of health and over the last 60 years health as a concept has been defined in a number of different ways (WHO, 1946; Field, 1976; Seedhouse, 1986; Aggleton, 1991; Blaxter and Patterson, 1996; Naidoo and Wills, 2001). Health is inextricably linked to the way people live their lives and the opportunities available for choosing health in the communities where they live. Although on average we are living healthier and longer lives, health and life expectancy are not shared equally across the population.

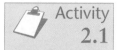

Activity 2.1

Write definitions of what being healthy means for you as:

- A student nurse
- A mother/ daughter
- A father/son
- A partner/sister/ brother
- Male/female
- A member of the community in which you live.

In conceptualising health, Raymond (2005) suggests that definitions can be viewed from the following four perspectives:

1. *Biomedical* – emphasising medical interventions as a way of preventing and treating disease and concerned with an individual's capacity to function.
2. *Behavioural* – emphasising the individual's responsibility for health-influencing behaviour.
3. *Social* – with a focus on the political and social determinants of health and emphasising social justice.
4. *Postmodernist* – in which the adequacy of perspectives 1–3 suggests that no one theory can sufficiently explain the health experience.

If no one theory can sufficiently explain the health experience for an individual, then it can be whatever it means to the individual at any one time, so, as Pearson (2002, p. 45) suggests, it is 'a number of ideas, which operate in different people's minds at different times'.

Experts agree that it is difficult to define precisely what health is but it is the definition identified in the World Health Organization (WHO) constitution of 1946 that many have used as a substructure to build upon:

> Health is a state of complete physical, mental and social well-being and not merely the absence of disease and infirmity. (Cowley, 2002, p. 45)

This definition is useful in that it identifies the factors that must be considered in assessing health, although it does not explain the criteria for recognising health as a positive human experience, or identify and acknowledge the levels of health that individuals may experience during their life span.

The definition has been widely criticised as presenting an unobtainable goal but it shows the distinction between negative and positive aspects of health: negative in respect of involving the absence of disease or infirmity and positive in respect of entailing the presence of the positive quality of well-being. Downie et al. (1996) suggest that positive health in this definition can be divided into the components of well-being and fitness.

The definition suggests that how people feel about themselves is more impor-tant than impairment or a disease process. So health is, as Pearson (2002, p. 45) suggests, 'not one but a number of ideas, which operate in different people's minds at different times'. It is more than the physical aspects and more than just the absence of disease. It is a multidimensional (holistic) phenomenon, that is, the focus is on the total person and health is viewed in the context of both internal and external environments.

The WHO (1946) definition is also exclusive in that it excludes so many people from ever achieving or hoping to achieve this elusive state of perfection. Dubos (1959) likened health to a mirage: unobtainable but arguably worth pursuing. He suggests that health and disease cannot be defined merely in terms of anatomical, physiological or mental attributes. The real measure of health is seen in the ability of the individual to function in a manner acceptable to himself and to the group of which he is part (Dubos, 1979).

Pike and Forster (1995) complement Dubos' statement by arguing that it is important to take into account people's own perceptions and views on health and that different people will see and express these in different ways. Furthermore, Seedhouse (1986) describes health as the 'foundations for achievement'. The idea that health as a particular, precisely determined, fully informed 'structure' to which each individual can strive is, he argues, absurd. It is as nonsensical as the supposition that there can be a faultless person.

Seedhouse (1997) has developed these ideas further into what he calls the foundations theory of health promotion. Fundamental to this is the extent to which a person's autonomy reflects their health status. As long as the foundations for health are complete in the context for that individual, they may be in a position to attain optimal health. A simplified version of this theory is included in Figure 2.1, but readers are strongly advised to consult the original text.

According to the foundations theory, a person will have a high level of health providing he or she can stand upon the four central boxes (with support from the fifth when, and as, required). Movement towards X will require additional provision or maintenance. Consequently, if any of these boxes is damaged or missing, only a lower level of health can be achieved.

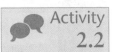

Activity 2.2

With reference to Figure 2.1, read the following three anonymised, real-life scenarios in Casebox 2.1 and justify whether these people are healthy.

Basic needs fulfilled	Key information available	Ability to understand and 'do'	Community integration	+	Bonus or supportive box
1	2	3	4		5

→ X

Figure 2.1 ● The foundations theory of health promotion (adapted from Seedhouse, 1997)

Casebox 2.1

Tanya, a student nurse, was on a four-week placement to a special school for children with health problems. The school cared for and educated a whole range of children whose needs were different from those who passed through what can be called the mainstream state education system. Many children were playing in the school playground when a six-year-old girl named Samantha caught Tanya's attention. Bending down to listen to the child's breathless voice, Tanya picked Samantha up and sat her on her knee. She had seen the child playing joyfully a few moments earlier as though she had not a care in the world. After a few minutes of conversation, Samantha stated that she needed a heart transplant. 'There is nothing wrong with my heart', she pointed out. 'The loving part works just fine, it's the pumping part that has a problem.' In the medical sense, this child was clearly very sick, yet having watched her at play and talked with her, Tanya was taken aback by the composed, almost matter-of-fact way in which the six-

year-old child had come to terms with a life-threatening illness. Indeed, she had a positive outlook on her potentially negative condition.

Yvette is 42 years old and has been married to Jim for 20 years. Unfortunately, shortly after they were married, Yvette had a road traffic accident, which resulted in her being hospitalised and undergoing an exploratory laparotomy for abdominal pain. During surgery, the surgeon discovered that Yvette had an ovarian cancer that had been asymptomatic until the accident. The diseased organ was successfully removed, and there were no other signs of injury. Was Yvette healthy before her accident? It appears not, but as far as Yvette was concerned, she certainly was.

Sophie, a 21-year-old married woman, had been looking forward to the birth of her first child. Her pregnancy had been relatively straightforward as far as she was concerned, with some morning sickness during the first trimester (third) of her pregnancy. A

routine ultrasound scan had demonstrated that all was progressing well, and there were no specific concerns for either mother or child. When Tom was born at full term (40 weeks) weighing over 3.6 kg (8 lb), Sophie went through an unexpectedly difficult labour, the prime reason being that Tom had a larger than normal head. A diagnosis of hydrocephalus was made. This condition resulted in Tom having many epileptic fits during the first few months of his life. Sophie coped well with Tom, but during his first Christmas, Tom's fits became more severe, progressing to status **epilepticus**. The consequence was that Tom sustained some brain damage due to a prolonged period of **apnoea**. He is now not expected ever to walk or indeed feed himself. Would you consider Sophie to be healthy in her present circumstances, looking forward to perhaps many years caring for her son? What about Tom and the potential he has for develop-ment? How does he fit into your definition of health? Or perhaps he doesn't.

epilepticus	apnoea
one of the classifications of epileptic seizures	temporary cessation of breathing

A consideration of these three different examples, involving four individuals, will demonstrate that health takes on many different forms. You may, of course, argue that these examples all involve a great deviation from the 'normal', whatever that is. Is someone who has a headache healthy? Is a hangover the residue of having had a great time or is it a transitory unhealthy state?

Check back to Activity 2.1 and review your statement about what health means to you. You may wish to revise this.

■ Health Protection

Health protection is about the surveillance and control of communicable diseases, the protection of the public from health risks caused by environmental hazards and the response to emergencies and disasters.

For all of us, health is in a dynamic state of continuity and change, constantly being challenged, stressed, abused and even enhanced by our genetic make-up and lifestyle, and our wider ecological environment.

It is truly amazing that, for the majority of people, health seems to be in a stable state most of the time. At the beginning of this new millennium, our ideas about health and illness are changing as research is identifying increasing risks to our health, for example tuberculosis (TB) (Chief Medical Officer, 2004) and methicillin-resistant staphylococcus aureus (MRSA) (Marshall et al., 2004). Conquered infectious diseases of the past are ridiculing modern antibiotic therapy through developed resistance.

Each time the media is informed of a case of **necrotising fasciitis**, or when antibiotic-resistant bacteria, for example MRSA, close down yet another hospital ward, it propagates the notion that 'superbugs' with flesh-eating powers lurk within our hospitals. Data on levels of MRSA bloodstream infections as a proportion of all *Staphylococcus aureus* bloodstream infections show that England is among those with the highest levels in Europe (DoH, 2003a), even though Emmerson et al. (1996) suggest that there is no evidence of an increase in infection rates from MRSA since 1980 in England.

necrotising fasciitis
death of areas of fascia surrounded by healthy parts

Other organisms that are routinely killed by simple hygiene methods are now reasserting their influence, perhaps because of our complacency. It only takes a few *Clostridium difficile* spore-forming bacteria in the wrong place at the wrong time to cause acute, even life-threatening illness. *C. difficile* are types of bacteria that produce resistant spores that are able to persist in the hospital environment longer than other bacteria. Infection can spread from person to person via spores in the faeces. Spores can survive for a long time in the environment and can be transported on the hands of the nurse who has direct contact with infected patients or with environmental surfaces (bedpans, toilets and so on) contaminated with *C. difficile*. The latest epidemiological data identify an increase in the number of reported cases across England, from 8,905 in 1995 to 40,180 in 2004. One such outbreak has recently been identified at Stoke Mandeville Hospital (HPA, 2005a).

The elderly are most at risk, with over 80 per cent of cases reported in the over 65 age group. For example, antibiotics may alter the normal gut flora and increase the risk of developing *C. difficile*. Immunocompromised patients are at risk, as are those who receive repeated enemas and/or gastrointestinal surgery.

Alcohol gel will not kill the *C. difficile* but they can be removed with soap and water. Hygiene can thus be seen to be an important aspect of caring for sick and vulnerable people to ensure safety in practice.

Health may be affected in a more insidious way as a result of intensive farming methods, perhaps where animals are fed contaminated or the wrong types of food, resulting in, for example, the foot-and-mouth disease crisis of 2001 or the bovine spongiform encephalitis (BSE) epidemic. The number of confirmed BSE cases fell from over 23,000 in 1994 to around 1,300 in 2000. Since its establishment on 1 April 2000, the Food Standards Agency (FSA) has been fully involved in the protection of public health, with responsibility for BSE controls relating to the food chain (DEFRA, 2001).

Creutzfeldt–Jakob disease

a central nervous system disease that causes distinctive EEG changes, presenile dementia and myoclonus

BSE is considered by some 'experts' to be transmissible to man, resulting in **Creutzfeldt–Jakob disease** (CJD). The causative virus in BSE and CJD is a 'slow virus', an agent inducing slow, degenerative encephalopathy (cerebral dysfunction characterised by disorientation and excitability of the central nervous system). In humans, this progressive dementia is usually fatal within six months. The Health Protection Agency (HPA) publishes monthly updates on the number of deaths and probable cases of CJD in the UK (http://www.hpa.org.uk).

spongiform encephalopathies

diseases characterised by the brain having the appearance of a sponge

New-variant CJD, known as variant CJD (vCJD), the hitherto unrecognised variant of CJD, is a rare and ultimately fatal progressive degenerative brain disease. It is one of a group of diseases called transmissible **spongiform encephalopathies** (TSEs) that affect humans and animals. It has been shown to account for 150 definite or probable cases up to 3 June 2005 (HPA, 2005b). Precisely defining the number of cases is difficult because of the complexities of data collection and the different varieties of CJD. No test is currently available to detect those who may be infected with vCJD at the preclinical stage. Sporadic cases appear to occur spontaneously, with no identifiable cause, and, according to HPA statistics (2005b), accounted for 52 of the total deaths from CJD in 2004. In contrast, only two deaths in 2004 were from **iatrogenic** infection (as the result of medical intervention, for example from contaminated neurosurgical instruments, dural grafts and treatment with human growth hormone).

iatrogenic

any adverse physical or mental condition that has been induced by the effects of a treatment

Challenges to health may occur in a crude cyclical fashion, whereby diseases pose no real threat until safeguards are removed or 'fail-safe' conditions are disrupted, often through complacency or neglect. This may be true for TB where the incidence of TB has increased by 27 per cent over the last 10 years, with 13 cases for every 100,000 people in the UK (Chief Medical Officer, 2004).

TB has re-emerged in the UK primarily due to immigration, poverty, loss of public health controls, diagnostic and clinical skills, drug resistance and HIV infection, even though it was never completely eradicated (Gandy and Zumala, 2004). An opportunistic infection, TB seems to be almost endemic where the most vulnerable are at risk because of poor or inadequate housing and diet or substance misuse, or as a result of migration from areas of the world where TB is endemic. These socially excluded groups consist of the disempowered, the frail, the young, the elderly, single parents with no real chance of escaping welfare under the present system and the long-term unemployed. The inequalities in health within these communities squeeze health and vitality out of the everyday lives of people. Health, life expectancy and social circumstances are inextricably linked, and TB kills, albeit slowly. Yet if you have a healthy immune system and are adequately nourished and housed, your body will rebuff these disease-causing pathogens. The vicious cycle of ill-health, unemployment and poverty is self-reinforcing and must be tackled.

■ Promoting Health and Preventing Ill-health

Promoting health and preventing ill-health can, even from the few illustrations given above, be seen as a complex business. The BSE problem involves the interests of commercial organisations and agriculture, as well as having a political element, with potential global repercussions. The jobs and livelihoods of some farmers and those within the beef and livestock industry are at stake. There is, of course, the possibility of widespread trans-species infection. Tuberculosis has its roots in poverty, involving the homeless and the vulnerable. *C. difficile*, like so many other bacterial infections, is preventable if scrupulous hygiene standards and thorough handwashing with soap and water are implemented.

Definitions of health promotion

Until recently health promotion was rarely defined within nursing practice but was seen as an accepted aim of it. It is generally taken to include activities intended to prevent disease, improve health and enhance well-being (Naidoo and Wills, 2001). It focuses on positive measures, such as education for healthy living and promotion of health-inducing environments and periodic selective screening. Following the Ottowa Charter (WHO, 1986) and other subsequent documents, health promotion is seen as any measure or planned activity that seeks to improve health, or prevent disease (WHO, 1986). This definition allows for a broader approach to health promotion, which should include policy, legislative and fiscal initiatives that facilitate the promotion of public health, and suggests that health promotion can be viewed as closely related to the new public health (Macdonald, 2003).

Recent government documents (DoH, 2000a, 2003b) reiterate the important role nurses can play in positively promoting health and preventing disease. Nurses have a good understanding of the health needs of individuals, families and communities with whom they have regular contact. The health topics identified in *Choosing Health* (DoH, 2004) are relevant to many nurses in their daily work but may not be a priority with every interaction with a patient, family member, elderly person or group (Chart 2.1).

Chart 2.1 ● Promotion of public health

- Health inequalities
- Supporting children and young people
- Healthy schools
- Improving health – community action, physical activity, smoke-free public places
- Health as a way of life
- Improving the health of adults

with social care needs, people in prison, support for mental health and well-being
- Transforming sexual health services
- Promoting health in the workplace
- Employment for health
- Government and public sector leading by example

Promoting public health

The essence of promoting public health for the nurse is to work in partnership with the patient and their family to keep the individual healthy, detect signs of abnormality or illness and facilitate the management of chronic disease.

The major settings for action in England include the hospital, home and other community groupings such as Sure Start (directly aimed at disadvantaged or socially excluded groups, with particular emphasis on teaching parenting skills in order to enhance all aspects of children's lives), health centres and health action zones (introduced in England to develop local, innovative, public health strategies to tackle health inequalities, and use the language of partnership and empowerment in relation to developing the health of communities and individuals).

Public health nurses (NMC, 2004a) make a specific contribution to the prevention of illness and the promotion of health but all nurses contribute to *Choosing Health* (DoH, 2004) objectives, ensuring that healthy alliances are developed in partnership with key players such as local authority departments (for example housing, environmental health and social services) and voluntary services. However, Adams et al. (2002, p. 1) argue that promoting public health goes beyond encouraging healthy lifestyles, improving health care services or developing healthy partnerships. It involves encouraging social changes which lead to ways of living which are sustainable, equitable and socially just.

Developing a partnership approach may be the first step in this process, where decisions can be made that affect the lifestyle and environmental factors influencing an individual's health, thus encouraging social change.

Some key aspects of health promotion are thus beginning to emerge (Figure 2.2):

- Social health
- Environmental health
- Organisational health
- Political health
- Spiritual health
- Individual health.

Kelly et al. (1993) argue forcibly that health cannot be effectively promoted unless the social, environmental, organisational and individual aspects of health are combined in an integrated approach. Their main objection is that many health-promoting activities focus lower than these four levels without the key element of integration.

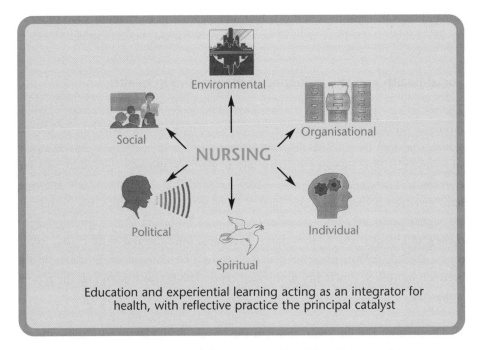

Figure 2.2 ● The integration of six aspects of health within nursing

Two further aspects of health promotion are the political and the spiritual. This is not to say that these aspects have to be overtly integrated to achieve health, but unless they are accounted for in a thoughtful manner, intolerance and non-receptiveness will result in at worst failure and at best partial success. Thus, nurses need to carefully consider not only the client's political values and spiritual beliefs, but also be aware of their own. Nurses and others involved in the promotion of health should take a more critical stance. Seedhouse (1997, p. 147) views health promotion as an 'endeavour to help individuals ... ultimately as a task for governments'. It is they who can ensure that everyone's chances for health are maximised throughout an individual's life span. The spiritual aspect of health is rarely referred to within general health promotion texts, but within nursing this aspect may be a most important part of the patient's health. It especially comes to the fore when an individual crisis occurs, be it acute or chronic, or indeed in the terminal stages of life.

According to Peterson and Lupton (1996) and supported by Wanless (2004), everyone is being called upon to play their part in creating a healthier, more ecologically sustainable environment through attention to 'lifestyle' and an involvement in various collective and collaborative endeavours to improve the health of the nation. All these concerns, expectations and projects are being articulated through the area of expert knowledge and action that is 'the new public health'. This takes as its foci the categories of 'population' and 'environment', conceived in their widest sense to include the social, environmental, organisational, political, spiritual and individual. Let us attempt to examine each of these six key components; there will, of necessity, be some overlap and integration.

Social health and the influence of inequalities in health

The social group into which we are born, or subsequently move, may have an influence on our health for better or worse. It may shape, constrain or indeed enable health to be realised. Factors such as class, gender, ethnicity and age may sway an individual's genetic predisposition. Biology, lifestyle behaviour and the environment all influence health. Much research has focused on the growing links between social class and health inequalities. Sir Donald Black and his colleagues were asked to consider differences in health status among social classes and identify the factors that might contribute to these differences. In his report (DHSS, 1980), Black provided a modern benchmark of the relationship between mortality, morbidity and social class. The major findings of the report were that:

1. Throughout the life span, those in the lower social classes had higher death rates than those above them.

2. At birth, children born into a lower social class were of a lower weight, often because of poor maternal diet.
3. The ill-effects of major diseases were more profound in the lower social classes than in those at the top of the social scale.

The economy of the late 1990s and this millennium adds a different slant worthy of mention as new dimensions to health, other than social class and morbidity, are identified and measured. These include the quality of life and indicators of wealth (housing tenure, car ownership, employment, gender and ethnicity). In his report on inequalities in health, Acheson (1998) made 39 recommendations covering inequalities in health, socioeconomic determinants of health and inequalities in health related to gender and ethnicity.

The middle classes are now feeling the effect of financial stress that may affect their health and well-being. International competition for work results in the 'downsizing' of companies and the further casualisation of labour. Middle and senior management are now experiencing what once lay within the realm of the working classes: short-term contracts and insecurity. A job for life is becoming a thing of the past, today's emphasis being on flexibility of skills and diversity. But not everyone can cope with managing the enormity of this type of change, often resulting in stresses and strains within seemingly secure families. As Graham (2001) suggests, the social and material circumstances in which people live are strongly linked to their individual behaviour.

The continual existence of widespread inequalities in health nearly 60 years after the foundation of the NHS is an indication of its inability to tackle inequalities. The NHS is geared to respond to identified need, dealing with illness; that is what it is good at. But the expectation in the twenty-first century is that it will have to shift its focus towards anticipated need and how the identified need can promote health by building on effective health maintenance strategies and primary prevention. It is not simply a matter of pouring more and more money into the NHS, thereby perpetuating a growing demand as technology caters for what were once unrealised needs. A strong governmental stand is now required to redirect money from the high-tech, often tertiary, care sector to be invested in long-term health maintenance and health promotion. A sustainable health strategy cannot be realised if medium- and long-term strategies are not resourced. The old adage that prevention is better than cure holds true.

In his final report on securing good health for the whole population, Wanless (2004) provides a review of the cost-effectiveness of action that can be taken to improve the health of the whole population and to reduce health inequalities. He suggests that 'our health services must evolve from dealing with acute problems through more effective control of chronic conditions to promoting the maintenance of good health' (p. 10). It has been argued that health care focuses on acute problems to the detriment of managing and indeed preventing chronic illness, which now affects around one in three people in the UK (Long-term Medical Conditions Alliance Conference, 2001). Such an approach to managing and preventing chronic disease is already underway with the roll-out of National Service Frameworks (NSFs) (see Chart 2.2). These target risk in the population and provide a structural basis on which to tackle inequalities in health and chronic disease and improve health in priority areas.

Chart 2.2 ● National Service Frameworks

● Mental Health (DoH, 1999)
● Coronary Heart Disease (DoH, 2000)
● The Cancer Plan: A Plan for Investment, A Plan for Reform (DoH, 2000)
● Older People (DoH, 2001)
● Diabetes Services (DoH, 1999)
● Diabetes Services (Standards) (DoH, 2001)
● The Diabetes Service Delivery Strategy (DoH, 2002)
● The Renal Framework (DoH, 2005)
● Acute Children's Framework (DoH, 2002)
● Children, Young People and Maternity Service Framework (DoH, 2004)

Link

Chapter 18 has further information on NSFs.

The NSF for coronary heart disease (DoH, 2000a) is on target to produce a 40 per cent reduction in the death rate from circulatory disease by 2006 (Robinson, 2004). The introduction of public health initiatives that are influencing these figures are the ban on tobacco advertising, a major smoking cessation programme and the introduction of the school fruit and vegetable scheme. The report *Winning the War on Heart Disease* states that deaths from cardiovascular disease have fallen by more than 23 per cent since 1995 and the treatment of heart attack patients has been revolutionised (Reid, 2004).

The diabetes NSF (DoH, 2001a) is also key in developing and managing this chronic disease. Soper (2004) has identified that people with diabetes are twice as likely to be admitted to hospital as the general population and once admitted are likely to stay twice as long as the average patient. Standard 8 of the NSF states that all those admitted to hospital with diabetes will, wherever possible, continue to be involved in decisions concerning the management of their diabetes.

Economic efficiency is something that most national governments aspire to create for the benefit of society, but Kickbusch (1996) illustrates the point that economic efficiency is not the same as a caring society. Key players such as Rupert Murdoch and Bill Gates, for example, who respectively have a vast global telecommunications network and a software empire, are building a global marketplace. But building a caring society is much more than linking health gain with profit margins. Just think about the type of work undertaken by the Missionaries of Charity, founded by Mother Teresa of Calcutta. More recently, in 2001, the world witnessed the terrorist destruction of the twin World Trade Center towers in New York. Thousands of people were killed and many more lives were damaged, yet the resolve of the business community to carry on gave a sense of coherence to their grieving and purpose to their work while surrounded by destruction.

Socially determined deprivation damages health. The poor can be socially isolated and lack the support that is necessary to achieve health. Social cohesion and the sense of solidarity that this brings are perhaps the most important influences on health status. For example, the two world wars of the twentieth century caused unprecedented suffering and disruption in Europe, but the social solidarity, elimination of unemployment and diminishing differences of living standards rapidly increased postwar life expectancy (Bradshaw, 1994). The notions of equal opportunity, social justice and egalitarian principles are required both across and throughout society to enable social health to be fully achieved.

Environmental health and sustainability

The environment in which we live, work and play has a direct impact upon the state of our health. Consider how the production and transportation of what we eat has changed over recent years. Many of our shops and supermarkets are located so far from our homes or workplaces that they require special trips to get there. The use of cars inevitably results in a lack of exercise, which contributes internally to the deposition of fatty tissue within our arteries and externally to the burning of non-renewable fossil fuels, which contributes to air pollution (Lang, 1997). This last fact has, according to the UK government (HM Government, 1993), been further compounded by the fact that the distance over which food is transported rose by over 50 per cent between 1979 and 1993. The growth in road freight transport conveying the commodities of food, drink and tobacco increased by more than one-third during this same period (MAFF, 1994).

In relation to the impact of climatic changes on our health, Peterson and Lupton (1996) state that the shortage of rain, ozone depletion and the greenhouse effect place public health in a global dimension. International air travel has created what has been termed the 'global village', whereby a traveller can literally have breakfast in one continent, lunch in another and dinner in yet another, and if the aircraft's cabin has not been spray-disinfested, so might some insects.

Public health experts and environmentalists have thus turned their attention to 'saving the sick planet'. Within this, the modern city has become the focal point for intervention because of its distortion of true nature. Its spaces and places have become sites for controlling pathology. There has been a rapid increase in the growth of modern megacities, with high population densities and often inadequate safe water and sanitation. The link between urban conditions and health status has a nineteenth-century ring to it. In the UK, we take it for granted that our water supply is safe. Yet a simple accidental mistake, as occurred for example in Camelford, Cornwall, when a very high level of aluminium entered the water supply, allegedly caused long-term health problems for scores of people.

At the Earth Summit in Rio de Janeiro in June 1992, many world leaders signed a global environment and development action plan known as Agenda 21. The aim of this plan was to ensure that development to meet the needs of the present does not compromise the ability of future generations to meet their own needs. The WHO suggested that ecologically sustainable development should include the prevention and control of environmental health risks while ensuring equitable access to healthy environments (WHO, 1992).

Five key areas of agreement covered a wide range of issues from climate change, biodiversity and sharing resources more equitably, to managing forests, economic growth and overseas aid. At the New York Earth Summit, Irwin (1997) reported that these five main agreements had not been fulfilled. The freezing, at the 1990 level, of carbon dioxide emissions, mainly from exhaust fumes and industry, may be achieved by only Britain and Germany within the next few years, whereas most G8 (Group of 8) countries will fail to meet this objective. In the USA, emissions have actually increased by 13 per cent since 1995. The protection of endangered species to ensure biodiversity has had some modest success, but this is being achieved as deforestation destroys approximately three species every hour. Overseas aid for sustainable development has, instead of increasing, actually decreased. As national governments across the world change, a few powerful politicians seem to continue to delay environmental protection measures, perhaps heaping untold consequences on future generations.

So why is Agenda 21 important and relevant for the world and in particular for us in the UK? Over two-thirds of the Agenda 21 plan cannot be delivered without the commitment and cooperation of local government, in which a lead role is played by local authorities. It calls for new planning approaches in order to achieve sustainable development. Specifically, it emphasises the integration of environmental and developmental concerns, the integration of the social sector, including health, into the process of development planning, and the development of plans for priority actions based on cooperative planning between the various levels of government, non-governmental organisations (NGOs) and local communities.

In 2001, local strategic partnerships (LSPs) were introduced into neighbourhood renewal areas in England and drew together members of statutory, voluntary and business sectors with local community representation in order to provide solutions to the complexities of deprivation. Today, monies under the neighbourhood renewal fund have meant that many new pockets of housing development and improvement have been set up in run-down and derelict former industrial areas. This type of approach to tackling problems through mainstream services and funding within disadvantaged areas, supported by neighbourhood renewal funds, could be rolled out to communities beyond these boundaries (Porter, 2005).

In England, health improvement plans have been identified and money sought from central government funding to enable local authorities to tackle the regeneration of cities and large towns and bring people and life back into the centre from the suburban fringes whither they had moved. Development strategies for cities and large towns now mean that these are safer areas for people to come into, especially at night. Policing, CCTV and pedestrian-only zones have meant that personal safety after dark has also been improved.

So, to recapitulate, the focus of LSPs is to bring together voluntary, statutory and business sectors with community representatives to provide an action plan to tackle deprivation. The focus of activity is to deliver services to meet the needs of the local population.

Organisational health: investing in the workforce

Most employers stress that their workforce is their greatest asset. Employees spend as much as half of their adult lives at work, so the working environment and the nature of the work will clearly have a significant impact on health.

Figures produced by the Confederation of British Industry (CBI) in 1999 on sickness absence during the previous year indicated that 200 million days were lost, an average of 8.5 days per employee. The cost of this loss of working time to British business was estimated to be around £10.2 billion for 1998. The Health and Safety Executive (HSE) has estimated that at least half of all lost work days related to stress (Cooper et al., 1996). It seems that managers are not blind to stress in the workplace. In a survey by the Institute of Directors, 40 per cent of responding members stated that stress was a big problem, 90 per cent of them believing that working practices could be a factor affecting the level of reported stress.

Further work reported by Cooper (1997), in a study examining working practices, indicated that the most highly rated causes of workplace stress are:

- 60 per cent time pressures to meet deadlines
- 54 per cent work overload

- 52 per cent threat of job losses
- 51 per cent lack of consultation or poor communication
- 46 per cent understaffing.

Kasl and Cooper stated in 1987 that the chance of the word 'stress' fading from our vocabulary is as high as that of the Communist state withering away from Russia! Stress has not only outlived Communism, but has also found a firm place in our modern lexicon of work, even though it remains an emotionally charged term.

To be stressed, or to suffer stress, means different things to different people (Selye, 1983). In recent years, the word 'stress' has been casually tossed around to describe a wide range of 'discomforts' resulting from our hectic pace of work and domestic life. From an organisational perspective, Sheridan and Radmacher (1992) argue that we are in the midst of an epidemic of stress that is causing illness and even death, but there is no agreed definition of stress. You may already have found that dealing with people in the daily context of nursing can be stressful and that stress is a personal experience. Hospital nurses take more days off sick than any other group in the public services (Healthcare Commission, 2005). The benefits of a healthier workforce should be viewed not purely in financial terms but as an integral part of good management. Health promotion at work is an investment in people.

Organisational health is complex and multifaceted. As an example involving a large organisation, health in the university will be examined as this is a place where nursing students work, so it should provide readers with a familiar setting. Approximately 10 universities in England and Scotland currently describe themselves as health promoting, although there is no official criteria or external accreditation against which they are judged. Issues tackled range from mental and sexual health to drink and drugs misuse and the design of buildings. A national planning group, established in 2002, aims to encourage more widespread use of the concept (Hampshire, 2003).

A health-promoting university (HPU) is much more than a place where people go to be educated (although this is its main business): it is concerned with introducing a new culture, rather than just a few health promotion projects, into our educational settings. Its goal is a commitment to health promotion as a core value of its mission and the development of its organisation in total. Within this setting, health is viewed as being everyone's business. The following are some reasons why universities should be involved in health-promoting activities:

- Most universities are large employers, forming a significant part of the local community

- Both students and staff spend a large percentage of their time within the university environment
- Young adult students are at university at a time when they are forming attitudes, behaviours and beliefs that may stay with them throughout their adult life
- Students will themselves play a major part in influencing the health of others, as policy-makers, educators, parents, partners, employers and members of our future society
- There are potentially huge resource savings to be made by becoming more efficient and effective
- Preventing communicable diseases like meningitis is a priority.

In 1995, the University of Portsmouth and the local health authority made a joint appointment of a health promotion adviser to coordinate a university-wide health promotion initiative. A health needs assessment was performed with both students and staff, which resulted in a report being published and a prioritised three-year action plan developed. But although an assessment can identify problems, only doing something about them makes the exercise succeed. The health promotion adviser is made available for students and staff by being situated in the students' advice centre. A short summary of the work already completed is set out in Chart 2.3.

Chart 2.3 ● Portsmouth University Health Initiative (1995)

Work with a primary focus on student health

- Access to primary health care – ensuring that all new students register with a GP and dentist, student induction talks being supported by displays to increase the uptake of registration. This information is also available on the World Wide Web under health on the university's home page, accessed outside the university at http://www.port.ac.uk/departments/healthpro
- Peer education project on mental health
- World Aids Day education and clubbing events
- Development of a sexual health peer education project
- Women's health issues
- Men's health issues
- Guidelines for drugs, alcohol and tobacco
- Meningitis awareness campaigns – especially during the first weeks of each new academic year
- Sensible drinking promotion
- Physical activity, sport and exercise promotion
- Non-smoking as the norm in parts of the students' union
- Exam-time summer health fair.

Work with a primary focus on staff health
- Lunch-time sessions for stress management
- Stress management workshops for departments
- Drugs education and development of a framework for residential staff
- Sexual health
- Smoking cessation
- Increasing physical activity.

The aims of these initiatives are to enable students and staff to fulfil their potential through:

- Reduced levels of absenteeism
- Achieving personal organisational goals
- Improving morale, especially the staff's – whereas stress is an individual experience, organisational stress affects groups of staff in similar ways
- Better social relationships throughout the university
- Increased networking across faculties and departments
- Reduced utilisation of clinical services (through awareness).

The HPU initiative works closely with a variety of local and national organisations, creating new networks with key partners including the WHO. At a local level, the HPU is part of the district-wide health improvement programme taken up by the local primary care Trust (PCT). There is much more still to be done to achieve a healthier potential for everyone who experiences university life, but at least a start has been made, as has an organisational commitment to accomplish this.

Political health: developing policies that influence health outcome

Since the creation of the NHS nearly 60 years ago, arguably the greatest politically egalitarian act in recent times, successive governments have sought to make it more effective and efficient. The past two decades have witnessed a drive to make it perform like a business (Griffiths, 1983; DoH, 1989a, 1989b, 1997, 2000b, 2001, 2003c).

The White Paper *Our Healthier Nation* (DoH, 1998) set out the government's strategy for improving health for those in England, laying out a set of priority health targets. The notion of 'health gain' is built upon, first, the reduction of premature mortality, thus increasing life expectancy, and second, the addition of 'life to years', ameliorating morbidity. These ideas originated from the Health for All initiative (WHO, 1985), are reiterated in *Health 21* (WHO, 1998) and have three basic values:

- Health as a fundamental human right
- Equity in health and solidarity in action between and within all countries and their inhabitants
- Participation and accountability of individuals, groups, institutions and communities for continued health development.

The one constant goal is to achieve full health potential for all and the two main aims are:

- To promote and protect people's health throughout their lives
- To reduce the incidence of the main diseases and injuries, and alleviate the suffering they cause (WHO, 1998).

In response to this, modern health care in England is now focused on a primary care-led NHS. Since the publication of *Our Healthier Nation* (DoH, 1998), the pattern of health promotion and health education is shifting away from an illness model to one that seeks to underpin health from a much wider perspective. The opportunities to help and advise individuals, families and communities are unparalleled and are becoming the focus and challenge for the delivery of health services today.

The areas of risk to be targeted are identified within the NSFs (see Chart 2.2), which provide a structural basis from which to tackle inequalities in health and improve health in priority areas. They do so by setting national standards, defining service models and putting in place strategies to support implementation and establishing performance measures against which progress is measured.

A brief description of four key areas identified in *Our Healthier Nation* (DoH, 1998) and the reasons for concern will be given, before illustrating how health authorities and PCTs can build on these targets for specific local needs. The four areas are coronary heart disease and stroke, cancers, mental health and accidents. Each local health authority is also required to set local targets, including those related to health inequalities, specifically tailored to meet local needs, for example teenage pregnancy. Because HIV and AIDS were targets in the earlier White Paper *The Health of the Nation* (DoH, 1992) and present a significant threat, they will also be briefly discussed here.

The government's role has been to facilitate action at a high level, providing networks for health across all ministerial departments (DoH, 1999b). For example, the Department for Education and Employment (DfEE) and the Department of Health jointly fund the National Healthy School Standard (DfEE, 1999). This standard provides a process of quality, ensuring that local services provided to schools support whole-school practice and are therefore more likely to impact on the health of pupils, learning opportunities and achievement (see the healthy

> **Link**
>
> *Chapter 3 discusses health policies and the government's role further.*

schools website http://www.wiredforhealth.gov.uk). Translating this activity into practice to promote health at a local level will be the responsibility of health authorities working with local education authorities, local authorities and others.

Coronary heart disease and stroke

Coronary heart disease and stroke account for one-third of all deaths in men and one-fifth of all deaths in women. Major risk factors include cigarette smoking (DoH, 1998), a raised plasma cholesterol level, elevated blood pressure and a lack of physical activity. The potential for reducing both morbidity and mortality through modifying these risk factors seems obvious.

Cancers

aetiology

the cause of a condition; also the study of all the factors involved in the development of a disease

Although there are many types of cancer, each with a different **aetiology**, the potential to prevent, treat and cure them varies considerably. The *Our Healthier Nation* (DoH, 1998) overall target is to reduce the death rate from cancer in people under 75 years by at least a fifth by 2010. A national cancer action team will drive progress to achieve this reduction in mortality. More specifically:

- *Breast cancer:* around 14,000 women die from breast cancer each year. Breast cancer screening is likely to be extended to include the routine screening of women up to 69 years of age to provide earlier diagnosis and treatment
- *Colorectal cancer:* this is the second most common cancer in England, about 30,000 new cases being recorded each year, with a lifetime risk of 1 in 25. Pilot screening studies have commenced, using faecal occult blood as an indicator for further investigation, and a national screening programme is to be rolled out in the second half of 2006
- About 1,000 women die from *cervical cancer* each year, a figure that seems to be falling by around 7 per cent per year. The NHS cervical screening programme set up in 1988 is based on a computer call and recall system for all women aged 20–64 years
- *Skin cancer:* the aim is to halt the year-on-year increase
- *Lung cancer:* the target of *Our Healthier Nation* is to reduce the mortality rate by 30 per cent in men and 15 per cent in women under 75 years of age by 2010.

Mental health

Poor mental health is a leading cause of disability and ill-health, resulting in approximately 14 per cent of certified cases of sickness in England. It is also estimated to account for 14 per cent of NHS inpatient costs. Depression and anxiety have a prevalence of between 2 and 7 per cent in the adult population, with a lifetime risk of over 20 per cent. Psychotic illnesses, like affective psychosis and schizophrenia, are less common albeit more severe. The aim is for a significant improvement in the health of those with mental illness, with a reduction of 15 per cent in the overall suicide rate and of 33 per cent for those with severe mental illness.

Accidents

Accidents cause death and a high incidence of morbidity, especially among people under 30 years of age. The number of deaths of children under 15 years, young adults aged 15–24 years and people aged over 65 have been separately targeted, with reductions of 33 per cent, 25 per cent and 33 per cent respectively (DoH, 1999). The UK government has based its strategy on a better coordination of agencies to prevent accidents, for example local authority involvement in planning, building control, highways, housing, social services, education, environmental health and the emergency services, as well as public health promotion in terms of accident prevention to enable people to be better informed, taking action on specific types of accident and considering vulnerable groups.

HIV/AIDS and sexual health

The human immunodeficiency virus (HIV) causes the acquired immune deficiency syndrome (AIDS). This key area, targeted in an earlier White Paper (DoH, 1992), also deals with sexually transmitted diseases, encompassing family planning and unplanned pregnancy. The government acknowledges that reliable statistics are difficult to obtain in this complex area: no one really knows the size of the problem in England, although, as we learn more about the disease process, the epidemiology is becoming more sophisticated.

The main objectives are to:

- Reduce the incidence of HIV and other sexually transmitted infections
- Provide for their effective prevention, diagnosis and treatment
- Develop surveillance and monitoring systems
- Provide effective family planning services
- Reduce the number of unplanned pregnancies.

> **Link**
> Chapter 8 explores sexual health, relationships and body image.

Safer sexual practices, together with the use of condoms to reduce the risk of infection, are stressed. Those who inject drugs and share equipment are noted to be at significant risk of HIV as well as hepatitis B and C.

Health promotion receives a relatively small proportion of the entirety of the UK health budget, and the prevailing political philosophy towards societal health needs will affect the relationship between national and local government. *Tackling Health Inequalities: A Programme for Action* (DoH, 2003c) recommends that local people should help to plan and develop local services and set priorities within national plans and targets. Under Section 11 of the Health and Social Care Act 2001, a duty is placed on NHS Trusts, PCTs and strategic health authorities (SHAs) to involve and consult patients and the public in the planning of services and any proposals for change. This will involve setting out to tackle the inequalities that give rise to ill-health alongside the service that provides treatment and care. By tackling the wider influences that detract from health, such as poverty, poor housing, unemployment and polluted environments, government can make an impact on health inequalities.

Smoking has been recognised as the greatest single cause of preventable illness and premature death in the UK, yet the powerful tobacco lobby has managed to convince politicians that totally banning tobacco advertising is not in their political interest. Many people still smoke, the largest increase in smoking rates being seen in teenagers, especially girls. Maternal smoking during pregnancy has consistently shown a significant statistical relationship to the risk of sudden infant death syndrome. A total ban on tobacco advertising and the consequent removal of tobacco sports sponsorship in the UK is undoubtedly a courageous and long overdue political step. Meanwhile, a total ban on smoking in enclosed public spaces comes into effect in 2007 in England, something that Scotland achieved early in 2006, and is probably the greatest health-promoting measure in the past 40 years. The NHS in England will become smoke free by the end of 2006, some acute and primary care Trusts have already achieved this.

To help the public, patients and staff to quit smoking, the NHS smoking cessation services are available across the NHS in England, and provide counselling and support to smokers wanting to quit, complementing the use of stop smoking aids nicotine replacement therapy (NRT) and bupropion (Zyban). These services are provided in group sessions or one to one, depending on the local circumstances and client's preferences. Most stop smoking advisers are nurses or pharmacists, and all have received training for their role. A total of £138 million was made available to the services in the period 2003–06 (DoH, 2006).

Spiritual health: maintaining equilibrium

Link

Chapter 10 deals with issues of spirituality.

Talk of spirituality and health means in essence to look beyond the physical body. Health in a spiritual perspective is concerned with both the physical, emotional, mental and spiritual aspects of our being. An approach where spirituality and health are seen as two sides of the same coin is holistic by nature and looks at the whole being to understand and correct that which is not in balance.

A person's spiritual dimension enables them to move from self-interest to care for another, as well as allowing a greater enjoyment in the fullness of life. Although the word 'spirituality' has an association with religious activity, Langford (1993) suggests that it is that state in which a person finds his view of life (spiritual life) to be matched by his experience within it. The spiritual dimension perhaps acts as a means of integrating the other dimensions of life. It is ultimately concerned with issues and life principles, and is often seen as a search for meaning. Spirituality, it may therefore be argued, permeates every aspect and moment of living. It involves eating, drinking, working, creating, showing love, sharing laughter and tears, worshipping and dying. Langford (1993) goes on to suggest that all these activities are equally 'spiritual' occasions.

Nursing can be both physically and emotionally draining, as dealing with life-and-death situations can be both rewarding and exhausting. Nurses perhaps need four things to assist them in assisting others:

1. A *confidant*, a friend, preferably someone outside the family, with whom they can share deeply issues concerning work and their emotional reactions to them. A confidant enables a person to be aware of him- or herself and keep a balance by being alert to possible problems.
2. *Peer support* offers mutual support and the chance to talk through issues that others can understand because they share the same experience. A student cohort provides a variety of characters, each person then being able to relate to someone who is right to help them.
3. *Doing something completely different* – taking time out, developing a hobby or going on holiday – can help to recharge nurses' spiritual batteries.
4. *Developing their spiritual base* to withstand a multitude of questions, pressures and changes as they progress through their nursing careers.

Individual health: the lottery of life

An individual's life chances for health will be dependent on the five other aspects of health (social, environmental, organisational, political and spiritual) and how they interrelate. The basic essentials in maintaining health for all are: no wars, threat of terrorism or civil disturbance; assured personal safety; good housing; safe clean water and sewage disposal; and nutritious uncontaminated food.

Our current health status is not fixed but is instead highly dependent upon what has gone before and, to some extent, what the future holds. Although we cannot predict the future with absolute accuracy, a future without hope would be severely detrimental. Conversely, when individuals are given hope for their future, they can overcome enormous threats and challenges to their health: think back to Yvette with the ovarian cancer or young Samantha waiting for her heart transplant (Casebox 2.1).

The past history of an individual may show a balance in their personal life or there may be a negative health course, as in the case of baby Tom (Casebox 2.1). The current health balance depends on the six aspects contributing to well-being and functioning as determined by the individuals concerned and those who share life with them. Future health potential is dependent upon a strong integration of these six aspects of health, supporting and enabling a positive self-concept, having developed coping skills as part of the health resource repertoire of the individual.

Let us take an everyday example of a life skill and relate this to individual health and the potential to maintain or improve it. In a study undertaken on behalf of the National Food Alliance by MORI (1993), fewer than half the national sample of children could boil an egg or bake a potato. We are all consumers of food, but individuals are being deskilled or underskilled when it comes to preparing and cooking. Conversely, however, there is an abundance of advice within the media, from television programmes to magazines, on how to cook. Convenience and fast foods have played a part in the deskilling process, but fast food can be nutritious. Fast Food Fit (http://www.port.ac.uk/departments/healthpro) is a campaign developed by Portsmouth City Council to help families on low budgets to cook nutritious food. It has a number of healthy recipes that can be prepared quickly and at a low cost. This scheme now covers university students, many of whom find cooking boring, cannot afford decent wholesome food or prefer a 'liquid diet', with all the threats to health that this may bring. Another example of such an initiative can be seen in the Kids Cookery School in Acton, London (Gaze, 2002), where disadvantaged children, including those with special needs, are learning about healthy eating and how to put their knowledge into practice at the school.

■ The Role of the Nurse as a Health Promoter

Investment in the health sector is rapidly becoming an amalgam of public and private partnerships, some key individuals being involved in joint societal efforts. Although it is evident that the responsibility for health promotion does not lie with the health sector alone, nurses nevertheless have an unequal contribution to make to alliances created in the pursuit of health. Within the UK, this is especially true as nurses form the largest body of health-care professionals orchestrated by the NHS, with an immeasurable number of client and patient interactions.

The Nursing and Midwifery Council Code of Professional Conduct (NMC, 2004b) has set standards within a professional framework to regulate the conduct of members. Eight core statements make up the code, which is founded upon the practitioner being personally accountable in safeguarding and promoting the interests of individual patients and clients within the context of society. These core values and characteristics of acceptable practice act in a way to protect the public. Specifically, practitioners must:

Promote and protect the interests and dignity of patients, irrespective of gender, age, race, ability, sexuality, economic status, lifestyle, culture and religious or political beliefs (clause 2.2).

Recognise and respect the role of patients as partners in their care and the contribution they can make to it. This involves identifying their preferences regarding care and respecting these within the limits of professional practice, existing legislation, resources and the goals of the therapeutic relationship (clause 2.1) (NMC, 2004b).

Health promotion is not simply something that is done to the patient, as in changing a dressing, giving drugs to prevent auditory hallucinations or taking a blood pressure, but instead informs and pervades all aspects of nursing care in enhancing health through:

- Assessment of health need
- Planning health gain
- Evaluating interventions and strategies for effectiveness and efficiency.

Knowing those whom we seek to support within our professional capacity as nurses will help us to understand their health needs. 'Knowing the patient' has become a buzz phrase within contemporary nursing, but understanding the individual's status in terms of health, beliefs, values and attitudes, along with the structural determinants of health and outside influences, will form a starting point for an assessment of health needs.

Within the acute illness setting, a nurse's professionalism may be the sustaining presence in the facilitation of the patient's own coping abilities. This contrasts with the episodic and often **interventionist** nature of the medical relationship. In planning health gain, the power that nursing possesses is often very subtle. For health promotion to be effective, the nurse must move from a nurse-controlled model of care to an **egalitarian** relationship that promotes patient input and **autonomy** (Whitehead, 2000). Care must be offered in such a way that it engages people in their own care and encourages and supports them as they commit to fostering their own health gains (Caelli et al., 2003). It is, or should be, the nature of nursing care that empowers the patient, and Campbell (1993) suggests that nursing is a form of health promotion. The notion of health gain lies at the centre of health promotion as a core value.

Brown and Piper (1997) suggest that giving power back to patients and working with them to meet their needs must lie at the very heart of nursing, as it represents the aggrandisement of human care by enabling potential to be fulfilled. Robinson and Hill (1998, p. 236) suggest that nurses' health promotion goals

interventionist
act of intervening

egalitarian
the doctrine of equality of mankind

autonomy
freedom to determine one's own actions

must enable them to 'raise awareness about health, provide information, promote self-awareness, improve self-esteem, encourage decision making, change attitudes and behaviour, or change the physical and social environment'.

Within nursing practice, an awareness of the nuances of the patient is essential, especially if the observant nurse is to pick up on these cues to potentiate health. Because awareness makes demands upon us, usually in the form of some action, but also equally by just providing a listening ear, it costs us in terms of our time. Continually responding to the demands of others requires effort, patience and a degree of self-denial. It can be painful, especially when you are busy and this is the umpteenth time that Mrs Moon has had a commode, or in the community, when you are dressing Miss Patel's leg ulcer and her cat walks across your sterile field. Nurses may lapse into deaf or partially sighted mode as a coping mechanism.

It is important that nurses are realistic in terms of what they can achieve within their professional role. One way is through the use of praxis (reflective practice and action) to prevent the adoption of second-rate or diminished care by lowering standards through a lack of awareness or inaction. Professional dialogue in terms of a discussion with qualified staff and peers often helps to clarify issues before they become problematic.

> **Link**
> *Chapter 13 discusses reflection further.*

How do nurses promote health?

The present-day practice of nursing is effected by the skills and activities of the individual, which develop from the principles underpinning the development of knowledge and skills that are nursing. In turn, these skills and activities are based on knowledge derived from social and behavioural sciences as well as the social aspects of health and disease. The conceptual relationship between the principles of nursing, skills of nursing and subject knowledge serves as a framework for understanding and developing health promotion activity with patient groups.

Manifest in professional statements about the nature of health promotion within nursing (NMC, 2004b, clause 2.2), nursing knowledge forms the basis of management, decision-making and professional judgements. Searching for health needs and assisting the patient in meeting them is a legitimate activity of nursing, where the primary aim is to promote personal health by searching for needs and helping patients, families and carers to provide them. Responsible for the assessment of need and prescription of a plan to care for patients, the nurse is intimately concerned with the delivery of that care and evaluation of the care given (Porter, 1999). In preventing disease and promoting health, nurses act as facilitators, innovators and change agents in the fostering of decision-making for achieving optimum well-being for the patient. The trigger for assessment, action or intervention stems from the analysis of the patient care plan and the needs assessment identified in partnership with the patient and their carers.

Using one of the many reflective tools (Palmer et al., 1994) assists nurses in working in this way by providing a framework for action, which enables them to recognise their knowledge of health promotion, evaluate the research findings and guide their practice as follows:

- Explore the process through which reflection takes place
- Analyse and interpret an aspect of health promotion activity
- Consider the dilemmas posed by the incident/therapeutic intervention
- Develop a critical understanding of how nursing judgement and clinical reasoning influence and improve the health promotion activity of the nurse.

Reviewing practice is something that all nurses need to do (see Table 2.1). It is particularly valuable for students of nursing as it links very closely with the identification of their learning needs. Within a supervised capacity, students should develop ways and means of involving patients and clients in strategies to make health gains. These strategies may be individualised (designed specifically for the patient) and form part of their overall care. Planning for health through raising awareness in an enabling way is crucial. There should be no place for 'victim-blaming', in which often rushed and ill-informed judgements are made based on stereotypical and partial information. Health promotion strategies will need to be assessed for effectiveness and evaluated in terms of how well they meet the needs of patients and the normative needs of the health professionals involved.

Table 2.1 What to include in a reflection on a health promotion activity

• Introduction	• Reason for selection of the health promotion intervention
• About the health promotion intervention	• Describe the intervention • The relationship between the intervention and yourself as either the participant or observer • The theories that support the concepts you have identified from the intervention (referenced to recent literature) • Relate the concepts and theories back to the intervention and show how these might enhance or alter the intervention • How the intervention relates to the wider organisation, that is, the ward, patient's home, community or society at large • Any ethical or legal implications that can be drawn from the incident
• Analysis of the reflective process	• Did I present the intervention clearly? • Was my reflection on practice supported with evidence from the literature? • Did I offer evidence in support of the incident? • Did I identify issues in the analysis of the situation? • Did I structure my conclusion/summary?

▨ Chapter Summary

This chapter has examined the concept of health and definitions of health before exploring aspects of public health, health protection and health promotion. Six key aspects of health promotion are used to provide a framework from which to identify the role of the nurse in promoting health. A plan for using reflection as an aid to the evaluation of health promotion activity is offered.

Test Yourself!

1. Define health and identify three strengths of the definition and three limitations of it.

2. Describe the components of health protection and identify three health protection issues for the nurse and the patient and strategies for dealing with them.

3. What do we mean by promoting public health? List six possible aspects of health promotion.

4. Why are health inequalities so important for the nurse to understand?

5. How do government policies influence the development of public health activity for you?

6. How can the nurse promote health?

▨ Further Reading

DfES (Department for Education and Skills) (2006) *School Nurse: Practice Development Resource Pack*, HMSO, London.

▨ References

Acheson, D. (1998) *The Independent Inquiry into Inequalities in Health Report*. Stationery Office, London.

Adams, L., Amos, M. and Munro, J. (2002) *Promoting Health: Politics and Practice*. Sage, London.

Aggleton, P. (1991) *Health*. Routledge, London.

Blaxter, M. and Patterson, E. (1996) Mothers and daughters. A three generational study of health attitudes and behaviour. In Twinn, S., Roberts, B. and Andrews, S. (eds) *Community Health Care Nursing*. Butterworth Heinemann, Oxford.

Bradshaw, P. (1994) The conceptualisation and measurement of need. In Popay, J. and Williams, G. (eds) *Researching the People's Health*. Routledge. London.

Brown, P.A. and Piper, S.M. (1997) Nursing and the health of the nation: schism or symbiosis? *Journal of Advanced Nursing* **25**: 297–301.

Caelli, K., Downie, J. and Caelli, P. (2003) Towards a decision support system for health promotion in nursing. *Journal of Advanced Nursing* **43**(2): 170—80.

Campbell, A.V. (1993) The ethics of health education. In Wilson-Barnett, J. and Macleod Clark, J. (eds) *Research in Health Promotion and Nursing*. Macmillan – now Palgrave Macmillan, Basingstoke.

Chief Medical Officer (2004) *Stopping Tuberculosis in England. An Action Plan from the Chief Medical Officer*. DoH, London.

Cooper, C.L. (1997) Crisis talks. In Arnold, H. *Personnel Today*, 2 October, pp. 29–32.

Cooper, C.L., Liukkonen, P. and Cartwright, S. (1996) *Stress Prevention in the Workplace: Assessing the Costs and Benefits to Organisations*. European Foundation for the Improvement of Living and Working Conditions, Dublin.

Cowley, S. (ed.) (2002) *Public Health in Policy and Practice*. Baillière Tindall, London.

DEFRA (Department of Environment, Food and Rural Affairs) (2001) *Bovine Spongiform Encephalopathy in Great Britain: A Progress Report*. http://www.defra.gov.uk/animalh/bse/bse-publications/progress/jun01/report.pdf.

DfEE (Department for Education and Employment) (1999) *Healthy Schools: National Healthy Schools Standard*. DfEE, Nottingham.

DHSS (Department of Health and Social Security) (1980) *Inequalities in Health* (Black Report). DHSS, London.

DoH (Department of Health) (1989a) *Working for Patients*. HMSO, London.

DoH (Department of Health) (1989b) *Caring for Patients*. HMSO, London.

DoH (Department of Health) (1992) *The Health of the Nation: A Strategy for England*. HMSO, London.

DoH (Department of Health) (1997) *The New NHS: Modern and Dependable*. Stationery Office, London.

DoH (Department of Health) (1998) *Our Healthier Nation*. Stationery Office, London.

DoH (Department of Health) (1999a) *Diabetes National Service Framework*. Stationery Office, London.

DoH (Department of Health) (1999b) *Saving Lives: Our Healthier Nation*. Stationery Office, London.

DoH (Department of Health) (2000a) *Coronary Heart Disease National Service Framework*. Stationery Office, London.

DoH (Department of Health) (2000b) *The NHS Plan: A Plan for Investment, a Plan for Action*. DoH, London.

DoH (Department of Health) (2001) *Shifting the Balance of Power within the NHS: Securing Delivery*. DoH, London.

DoH (Department of Health) (2003a) *Winning Ways: Working Together to Reduce Healthcare-associated Infection in England*. Report of the Chief Medical Officer. DoH, London.

DoH (Department of Health) (2003b) *Liberating the Talents of Community Practitioners and Health Visitors*. DoH, London.

DoH (Department of Health) (2003c) *Tackling Health Inequalities: A Programme for Action*. DoH, London.

DoH (Department of Health) (2004) *Choosing Health: Making Healthier Choices Easier Choices*. HMSO, London.

DoH (Department of Health) (2006) http://www.dh.gov.uk/PolicyAndGuidance/ HealthAndSocialCareTopics/Tobacco/TobaccoGeneralinformation/ TobaccoGeneralArticle/fs/en?CONTENT_ID=4002192&chk=5Xx9q6.

Downie, R.S., Tannahill, C. and Tannahill, A. (1996) *Health Promotion: Models and Values*, 2nd edn. Oxford University Press, Oxford.

Dubos, R. (1959) *The Mirage of Health*. Harper & Row, New York.

Dubos, R. (1979) Mirage of health. In Black, N., Boswell, D., Gray, A., Murphy, S. and Popjay, J. (eds) *Health and Disease: A Reader*. Open University Press, Milton Keynes.

Emerson, A., Enstone, J., Griffin, M., Kelsey, M. and Smyth, E. (1996) The second national prevalence survey of infection in hospitals: overview of the results. *Journal of Hospital Infection* **32**: 175–90.

Field, D. (1976) The social definition of illness. In Tuckett, D. (ed.) *An Introduction to Medical Sociology*. Tavistock, London.

Gandy, M. and Zumala, A. (2004) *The Return of the Great White Plague*. Verso, London.

Gaze, H. (2002) The right mix. *Health Development Today* **7**: 14–15.

Graham, H. (2001) *Understanding Health Inequalities*. Open University Press, Buckingham.

Griffiths, R. (1983) *NHS Management Inquiry*. DHSS, London.

Hampshire, M. (2003) To a healthy degree. *Health Development Today* **13**: 17–19.

Healthcare Commission (2005) *Acute Hospital Portfolio Review: Ward Staffing*. Stationery Office, London.

HPA (Health Protection Agency) (2005a) *Reports of Clostridium difficile*. http:// www.hpa.org.uk/infections/topics_az/clostridium_difficile/vol_data.htm.

HPA (Health Protection Agency) (2005b) *Variant Creutzfeldt-Jakob Disease (vCJD) Statistics*. http://www.cjd.ed.ac.uk/figures.htm.

HM Government (1993) *MM20 Overseas statistics*. HMSO, London.

Irwin, J. (1997) The five failures. *Daily Telegraph* 24 June, p. 13.

Kasl, S.V. and Cooper, C.L. (eds) (1987) *Research Methods in Stress and Health Psychology*. John Wiley & Sons, Chichester.

Kelly, M., Charlton, B. and Hanlon, P. (1993) The four levels of health promotion: An integrated approach. *Public Health* **107**(5): 320.

Kickbusch, I. (1996) New players for a new era: How up to date is health promotion? *Health Promotion International* **11**(4) editorial.

Lang, T. (1997) Food policy for the 21st century: Can it be both radical and reasonable? Discussion paper number 4. Thames Valley University, London.

Langford, D. (1993) *Where is God in all this?* 2nd edn. Countess Mountbatten House, Moorgreen Hospital, Southampton.

Long-term Medical Conditions Alliance Conference, Royal College of Physicians (2001). http://www.doh.gov.uk/healthinequalities.

Macdonald, G. (2003) Promoting public health. In Watkins, D., Edwards, J. and Gastrell, P. (eds) *Community Health Nursing: Frameworks for Practice*. Baillière Tindall, London.

MAFF (Ministry of Food and Agriculture) (1994) *Agriculture in the UK in 1993*. HMSO, London.

Marshall, C., Wesselingh, S., McDonald, S. and Spelman, D. (2004) Control of endemic MRSA – what is the evidence? A personal view. *Journal of Hospital Infection* **56**(4): 253–68.

MORI (1993) *Poll for Get Cooking Project*. National Food Alliance, London.

Naidoo, J. and Wills, J. (2001) *Practising Health Promotion*. Baillière Tindall, London.

NMC (Nursing and Midwifery Council) (2004a) *Standards of Proficiency for Specialist Community Public Health Nurses*. NMC, London.

NMC (Nursing and Midwifery Council) (2004b) *The NMC Code of Professional Conduct: Standards for Conduct, Performance and Ethics*. NMC, London.

Palmer, A., Burns, S. and Bulman, C. (1994) *Reflective Practice in Nursing*. Blackwell Science, Oxford.

Pearson, P. (2002) Public health and health promotion. In Cowley, S. (ed.) *Public Health in Policy and Practice*. Baillière Tindall, London.

Peterson, A. and Lupton, D. (1996) *The New Public Health*. Sage, London.

Pike, S. and Forster, D. (eds) (1995) *Health Promotion for All*. Churchill Livingstone, London.

Porter, E. (1999) How health visitors perceive/use their knowledge and skills in relation to teaching Project 2000 nurse students. Unpublished MPhil, University of Southampton.

Porter, E. (2005) Public health and health visiting. In Robotham, A. and Frost, M. (eds) *Health Visiting*. Elsevier, Edinburgh.

Raymond, B. (2005) Health needs assessment. In Sines, D., Appleby, F. and Frost, M. (eds) *Community Health Care Nursing*. Blackwell, Oxford.

Reid, J. (2004) *Winning the War on Heart Disease*. Progress Report. www.dh.gov.uk.

Robinson, F. (2004) Treating heart disease in primary care. *Community Practitioner* **77**(6): 211–12.

Robinson, S. and Hill, Y. (1998) The health promoting nurse. *Journal of Clinical Nursing* **7**: 232–8.

Seedhouse, D. (1986) *Health: The Foundations for Achievement*. John Wiley & Sons, Chichester.

Seedhouse, D. (1997) *Health Promotion: Philosophy, Prejudice and Practice*. John Wiley & Sons, Chichester.

Selye, H. (ed.) (1983) *Seyle's Guide to Stress Research*, vol 2. Van Nostrand Reinhold, New York.

Sheridan, C. and Radmacher, S. (1992) *Health Psychology: Challenging the Bio-Medical Model*. John Wiley & Sons, Chichester.

Soper C. (2004) Standard 8: Hospital Admission. *Primary Health Care* **14**(8): 37–9.

University of Portsmouth (1995) *Health Initiative*. University of Portsmouth.

Wanless, D. (2004) *Securing Good Health for the Whole Population*. Final Report, Treasury, London.

Whitehead, D. (2000) What is the role of health promotion in nursing? *Professional Nurse* **15**: 257–9.

WHO (World Health Organization) (1946) *Constitution*. WHO, Geneva.

WHO (World Health Organization) (1985) *Targets for Health for All by the Year 2000*. WHO, Copenhagen.

WHO (World Health Organization) (1986) *Ottawa Charter for Health Promotion: an International Conference on Health Promotion*. WHO, Copenhagen.

WHO (World Health Organization) (1992) *Agenda 21*. WHO, Geneva.

WHO (World Health Organization) (1998) *Health 21: An Introduction to the Health for All Policy Framework for the WHO European Region*. WHO, Geneva.

■ Useful Websites

www.dh.gov.uk Department of Health

www.5aday.nhs.uk Website supporting the NHS five portions of fruit or vegetables per day campaign

www.eatwell.gov.uk Food Standards Agency guidelines to healthy eating

www.foodinschools.org Provides information about the Department of Health and Department for Education and Skills Food in Schools programme

www.wiredforhealth.gov.uk A series of websites developed by the Department of Health and the Department for Education and Skills to provide health information that relates to the National Curriculum and the National Healthy Schools Programme

www.raisingkids.co.uk Advice on parenting

www.nelh.nhs.uk National Electronic Library for Health Programme
Works with NHS Libraries to develop a digital library for NHS staff, patients and the public

www.givingupsmoking.co.uk Advice and support on stopping smoking

www.publichealth.nice.org.uk National Institute for Health and Clinical Excellence
An independent organisation responsible for providing national guidance on promoting good health and preventing and treating ill health

www.hpa.org.uk Health Protection Agency
Aims to provide an integrated approach to protecting UK public health through the provision of support and advice to public bodies

SUSAN MOORE

Chapter

The Politics of Health Care

3

Contents

- The Political Process
- Social Policy and Nursing Practice
- Chapter Summary
- Test Yourself!
- Further Reading
- References

Learning Outcomes

This chapter explores the wider context of health care, looking at how health-care policy is made. The first section describes the British political system and the parts of the process that contribute to the formation of health policy. The second section examines some health policies and legislation that affect nursing and midwifery practice today. First, the whole structure of the NHS is described. Next, we turn to an outline of the legal structures that govern the professions of nursing, midwifery and health visiting. Finally, specific branches of practice are discussed in relation to the legislation that provides a framework for practice. At the end of this chapter, you should be able to:

- Outline the key political institutions involved in the development of social policy

- Justify the need for nurses to have a knowledge of social policy

- Describe the key features of policy relating to midwifery, children's nursing and mental health and learning disability practice

- Discuss the development of the statutory regulation of nursing, midwifery and health visiting.

■ The Political Process

Why study politics?

This is surely a legitimate question to pose. Why do nurses need to know about political institutions and how social policy is devised, enacted and implemented? How will this affect the way in which they deliver effective care to their clients? What will it matter to a client, who is in severe pain or hallucinating, how politically astute the nurse is who offers him help? The immediate answer is that, at this stage in an illness, a client will not be interested in any other skills that a nurse has but those which help to ease the pain or distract him from the hallucinations. Later on, however, a significant proportion of acute illnesses become long-term conditions that affect significant areas of a person's life. It is possible in this situation, where service users and nurses alike are motivated by a need, to influence and improve the service. They are facilitated in doing this if they understand the social and political systems that created it.

It can be argued then that several justifications can be put forward for nurses to understand the process of policy formation in health care. First of all, the nurse is a citizen, and it could be argued that all citizens should have an understanding of the systems and processes by which decisions are made that affect their lives. Second, nurses who begin their career at 18 years old may work within the health-care system for 40 years or more, during which they will have the potential to effect care for a significant number of people. Nurses will be more effective if they understand the history, development, values and beliefs of the health-care delivery system and its institutions within which they operate. Third, when nurses are acting as advocates for clients or client groups, it may be helpful to assist them to understand the system and why care is delivered in the way it is. In addition, as care is increasingly delivered outside the hospital setting and in the community, care packages have to be put together with contributions from a range of agencies such as social services, housing and education. Nurses who aim to deliver effective care to clients need to have an understanding of these agencies and the legal frameworks within which they operate. Finally, having gained an understanding of the system, the nurse may seek, either individually or as part of a pressure group, to change or improve health-care policies. For example, the Royal College of Nursing, the Royal College of Midwives and the Community Psychiatric Nurses Association are organisations that seek to influence **health policy** on behalf of their members.

Political values and beliefs

It is important, when considering health policy, to have an understanding of the values and beliefs that shape it. Ranade (1994) argues that the philosophy that

Link

Pain is discussed further in Chapter 1.

health policy

the principles that govern public actions to deliver health services

provided an impetus for the formation of the NHS in 1948 was rooted in the principles of **socialism**. Before 1948, people were aware of the significant inequalities in health care. Beveridge, the author of the report that provided the blueprint for the NHS (Ministry of Health, 1942), was also concerned with the economic benefits that would result for society if health were improved. These values of shared social responsibility for welfare provision and extensive state economic intervention continued to dominate during the 1950s and 60s and are now referred to as the **Old Left**. They were based upon the optimistic view that resources invested in health and welfare would support economic growth by improving the quality of the workforce and contributing to full employment.

socialism
a political doctrine that seeks to organise society on the basis of fairness and equity

In the 1970s, academic writing challenged the view that public welfare services were an equalising force in society. It was suggested by the Black Report (DHSS, 1980) that, despite 30 years of a **welfare state**, there were still significant inequalities in health. The medical dominance of health care was also challenged (Illich, 1976; McKeown, 1976). It was argued that medicine focused too much on science and the promotion of the profession and not enough on meeting clients' needs.

Old Left
socialism in its fullest sense: nationalisation of industry, redistribution of wealth, high taxes for the rich, state knows best in all circumstances

welfare state
a collective term to describe all the government provision, for example education, health or social security, that offers aid to those who need it

The values and beliefs that underpinned the policies of the Conservative administrations from 1979 to 1997 have been summarised by the term 'New Right'. At that time, the welfare state seemed to be failing, and a 'crisis of welfare' was described, in which the growth in the population of older people would coincide with a reduction in the population of wage-earners, combined with slow economic growth. This would result in economic disaster. The New Right solution to this problem was to reduce the level of state intervention in the economy. It was argued that market forces were distorted by too much economic planning and regulation. Furthermore, citizens had to fund welfare from taxation, and this resulted in a tax burden that stunted free enterprise. Last, economic decline resulted from having a large public sector that did not contribute to wealth creation.

The New Right believed that professionals tended to promote their own interests above those of the service, which resulted in inefficiency. In addition, they felt that because welfare was provided by state monopolies, the service was inefficient and wasteful, which would not be tolerated in organisations that were motivated by competition. It was argued from a moral stance that citizens were being coerced in two ways by the welfare state: first, by having to pay more tax because the service was wasteful; and second, because, as a prospective consumer, the citizen was offered no choice.

In 1997, a new Labour government was elected, the values and beliefs that characterise its health policy having been termed the 'Third Way'. This approach calls for economic growth founded on free-market policies. Emphasis is placed on shifting the balance from financing pensions and cash benefits towards the

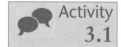

Activity 3.1

Compare the three approaches to policy – the Old Left, the New Right and the Third Way. Decide which you think is the most convincing and say why.

provision of better public services, particularly education and health. Those to be targeted are disabled people, single parents and, by being offered retraining, unemployed people. Another characteristic of the Third Way is stakeholder involvement, the aim of the whole policy being for stakeholders to have a say in the development of services (Leathard, 2000).

There are significant differences between the Old Left, New Right and Third Way philosophies. These have been the driving force behind the development of social policy, and it is essential, when evaluating the effectiveness of policies, that the underpinning values and beliefs are understood.

Central government and the political decision-making process

It is important to be aware that social policies start with governments. Social policies are the expression of that government's values and beliefs. In order for nurses to understand, analyse and criticise social policies, they must first have some understanding of the political system that produces them and the process of government that enacts them.

In Britain, there is a system of democratic representative government, whereby approximately 650 representatives are elected every five years by a 'first past the post' or simple majority voting system. After a general election, the monarch formally requests the leader of the majority party to form a government. The majority party leader then becomes the prime minister. When forming a government, there are over 100 positions to be filled, which will be taken up by members of the winning party. The most important positions are those of

the Cabinet

the executive decision-making body of government, made up of ministers of state, led by the prime minister

members of **the Cabinet**, the executive body of government, which is made up of between 15 and 25 members. These are mainly ministers who lead government departments, but there may in addition be members without departmental responsibilities who have political or coordinating roles, for example the deputy prime minister.

The Cabinet is a key body in the decision-making process. Any new policy proposal or change to legislation is discussed, argued through and negotiated within the Cabinet forum. When such proposals need detailed work, Cabinet committees are set up to complete this. These then refer work back to the Cabinet for a final decision.

Within the UK, some powers have now been devolved to the Scottish Parliament and the Welsh and Northern Ireland Assemblies. These bodies have locally elected members and leaders who can make local decisions about a range of matters that include health and social policy.

Government ministers

A **government minister** has the role of and responsibility for leading a government department, such as **the Treasury** or the Department of Health (DoH). A department consists of a large staff of permanent civil servants who administer it and put policy into effect. Ministers accept responsibility for work carried out in their name and are accountable to Parliament. Government ministers can find themselves in some conflict, as they have to contribute to developing and coordinating central policy and strategy for the government, while having a partisan commitment to their own department to advance and protect its interests.

There are four main aspects to the role of government ministers. First, they put forward legislation. Second, they have to attend to a high workload of departmental administration, perhaps the development of policy that does not require legislation. Third, ministers have to respond to questions put to them in the House of Commons. These might be probing questions posed by opposition Members of Parliament (MPs), designed to embarrass or challenge the government. Equally, they may be questions asked by members of their own party that are designed to offer the opportunity to announce new policy or report favourable statistics. The final aspect of a minister's role is public relations. This will involve a programme of formal visits, media interviews, speeches and meetings aimed to publicise the work of the department.

The House of Commons

In the UK, the seat of government is the Houses of Parliament. This is situated in Westminster in London and comprises two chambers. The House of Commons is the chamber within which government policy is presented, debated, negotiated and finally voted upon by MPs. Policy starts as an Act of Parliament. Proposals for change are set out in the form of a **Bill**, which requires skilled presentation and wording, carried out by civil servants, who are permanent government employees. They are engaged in a wide variety of administrative roles within each of the government departments.

Bills have to pass through four stages in both the House of Commons and the House of Lords. Stage one is the 'first reading', which occurs when the Bill is formally presented to the House. The 'second reading' is when the main principles of the Bill are debated by all parties within the House. The third stage, called the 'committee stage', involves an examination of the Bill in detail by a small standing committee. This is the stage during which changes or amendments can be made. The final stage is known as the 'third reading' or 'report stage': the revised Bill, having been examined by the committee, is referred back to the House, where it can be amended yet again.

government minister
a person with responsibility for running a government department

the Treasury
the government department with the responsibility of receiving the government's financial income, distributing it to other departments and setting the annual budget. Its chief minister is the chancellor of the exchequer

Bill
a draft of proposed legislation. It is work in progress until it becomes an Act of Parliament

The House of Lords

This is the second chamber of government, made up of non-elected representatives. The purpose of the House is to offer a second opinion on the Bills that appear before it. It works as a check and a balance to the House of Commons. Bills go through the same four stages in the House of Lords. This second House can recommend amendments to Bills, but the House of Commons does not have to accept them. The final stage for a Bill to become an 'Act of Parliament' is for it to receive royal assent from the monarch.

The work performed by the ministry

The secretaries of states or ministers are the statutory heads of the departments. They have a number of junior ministers, themselves elected MPs, who support the secretary in his or her function. The junior ministers are appointed by the prime minister, and they are in turn supported in administering the work of the department by a staff of civil servants. It is important to note the differences between these two groups. The ministers may be at the department for a relatively short period of time, during which they may well wish to make their mark and achieve significant policy change. Civil servants, however, are likely to work in one department for the whole of their career. They tend, therefore, to see policy change in the longer term. This can cause some difficulties and disharmony in the promotion of policy change. The most significant civil service role in this context is that of the permanent secretary, the most senior civil servant within a department. This person is in daily contact with the minister and is the minister's source of communication and information about the department.

Financing policy

An important part of any policy relates to how it will be funded. Where will the money come from? How will it be distributed? How much money is there? The NHS provides a good example of how a budget is agreed and subsequently distributed. Money to finance the NHS derives from three sources: central government tax revenues, national insurance contributions and charges to service users. Ham (2004) points out that in 2003/4, central taxation rendered approximately 75 per cent of NHS funding. Almost 20 per cent came from national insurance contributions. The remainder came from land sales and service user charges. The allocation of funding for public services is regulated by the Treasury and is dictated by the economic policy of the current government, which, for either economic or social reasons, may decide to restrict or develop spending on public services.

The Department of Health negotiates with the public services division of the Treasury, submitting to it revised annual plans for spending. The result of the joint work of these two government departments is to produce the Public Expenditure Survey Committee Report. This is subsequently presented to the Treasury ministers and is studied in the light of the current economic climate and the government's overall strategy. The allocation of funding between various departments is finally decided at Cabinet level, the eventual decisions being set out in the White Paper on Public Expenditure. The end result is that Parliament votes on the money for the year ahead for all public expenditure, including the NHS.

How is policy effected?

The previous sections have described how policy is made at governmental level and the political institutions that support that process. It is equally important, however, to understand how that policy is effected at the level of the workforce. Hill (2003) suggests that policy-making and policy implementation are not discrete operations but in fact merge: the implementation process influences policy design from an early stage and continues throughout it.

Policy implementation involves several sets of relationships. Initially, there is the relationship between central government agencies, in the case of health policy, for example, the Department of Health, and local agencies such as strategic health authorities (SHAs) or NHS Trusts. The relationships underlying policy implementation become more complex when the effective realisation of the legislation involves the collaboration and cooperation of several organisations, each with its own discrete culture and operating system.

Policy implementation will also be influenced by the values and beliefs of the practitioners who put the policy into effect. Because there is such a distance between the central controlling agency and the individual who is delivering the service, there can be much room for discretion in how he or she acts. This can result in a considerable gap between the original principles and objectives of the policy and the actuality of the implementation.

Another important feature that influences policy implementation is finance. For change to take place, extra resources are sometimes required to make a change effective, perhaps to provide new environments or train staff for new roles. Policy implementation is a complex, interactive process that shapes the nature of service delivery and also provides the feedback that ultimately results in policy change.

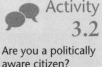

Activity 3.2

Are you a politically aware citizen? Which constituency do you live in? What is the name of its MP? Which political party does he or she represent? Does your MP hold a government office? Where and when does he or she hold constituency 'clinics' to obtain feedback and meet constituency residents?

■ Social Policy and Nursing Practice

In this second section, the structure and function of the NHS will be outlined, before describing how nursing is regulated. The final part of the chapter examines specific legislation that governs everyday nursing and midwifery practice.

The National Health Service

The NHS came into existence on 5 July 1948. It represented a significant social reform, the underpinning idea being that all members of society are entitled to health care, whatever their ability to pay. The service is paid for from the taxation of the whole population, and the organisation of the service is taken on by the government. Patients are able to receive treatment whenever they need it without having to negotiate payment. It is argued that this is the most cost-effective way of delivering health care to a population. Furthermore, it contributes to the overall health potential of that population and is fair and equitable. In 1948, hospitals and community services that had been run and financed by charities or on a commercial basis were all brought under the public umbrella of the NHS.

The NHS experienced funding difficulties almost from its inception. Delivery costs escalated, and successive governments have since struggled to deliver an effective service when faced by economic recession, an old and crumbling infrastructure and an ageing population. Both Conservative and Labour governments have tried to make the NHS more effective by reorganising its structure. In 1974, an attempt was made to solve the problem by including more layers of bureaucracy to control its operations. Health service management had three layers of administration – regional, area and district – but this quickly became untenable as decision-making had to fight its way through several layers of red tape.

In 1982, the Conservative government attempted to control the NHS by introducing a new kind of management system called 'general management'. In this system, a new breed of manager was introduced who might or might not have a professional training. The important feature was that the manager had the skills to manage human and material resources.

A further attempt was made in 1990 to control the overwhelming public expenditure on health and social welfare by introducing systems based on the 'internal market'. In this approach, various parts of the health system competed for contracts in a similar way to that seen in commercial enterprise. Different parts of the system were termed 'purchasers' and 'providers', with health authorities and some general practitioners purchasing health care from NHS Trusts. Operating like a commercial business in a competitive internal market was designed to reduce costs and increase quality.

None of these reforms has, however, entirely worked. The NHS still struggled to fund the renewal of antiquated buildings, keep up with the constant growth of technology and manage a huge workforce. In 1997, the country elected a new Labour government that made the reform of the NHS its foremost priority. This government has also reorganised and restructured the NHS with the objective of delivering an effective service.

Throughout all these changes, what has remained constant is the belief of the British people that the NHS is the best way to deliver health care to the whole population.

The new NHS: modern and dependable

In December 1997, the Labour government published a White Paper *The New NHS: Modern, Dependable* (DoH, 1997). This set out the government's strategy to reform the NHS using the values and beliefs of the Third Way. This Third Way lies between the central control approach of the 1970's NHS and the inequity of the internal market of the 1990s. Underlying this social policy are the principles of partnership and collaboration. The policy was further developed and presented as *The NHS Plan* (DoH, 2000).

> **Link**
> *Chapter 15 outlines other relevant legislation.*

The NHS structure

The current blueprint for the NHS aims to give local citizens and local health providers more power to decide upon and deliver health services locally. This is set out in the document *Shifting the Balance of Power within the NHS* (DoH, 2001b).

Department of Health

Ultimate management and control rests with the Department of Health, which is led by the secretary of state for health, who is a full member of the Cabinet. He or she also holds responsibility for social care. The secretary of state ensures the delivery of health services through a range of NHS bodies. These are SHAs, NHS Trusts, primary care Trusts (PCTs) and special health authorities. There are four regional directorates of health and social care in the Department of Health.

England has 10 SHAs whose main role is to lead the strategic development of the local health service and manage the performance of PCTs and NHS Trusts. This level of management relates to a geographical area that has a population of around 1.5 million people. It is the SHAs' job to focus upon the overall needs of the health economy. They are charged with the responsibility of ensuring that all the NHS organisations work together, managing performance by how they negotiate targets and ensure that these are achieved.

> **Link**
> *Chapters 1 and 15 provide more information about clinical teams.*

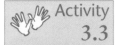

Activity 3.3

To investigate structures in your locality, identify the members of your local NHS Trust or PCT, who they have contracts with and the Trust's annual income. A good source of information is the annual report available from the Trust's headquarters, copies of which may be available in clinical departments or on its website.

The local delivery of care is managed by PCTs, which have two functions. First, they assess local health need and then negotiate and commission services for an improvement in the health of the local population. Second, they manage and deliver primary and community service. Working through local strategic partnerships, PCTs coordinate planning and community engagement and the influence of the wider government agenda. They also have a responsibility to work with local authorities to integrate health and social care. From April 2004, PCTs receive 75 per cent of NHS funds directly from the Department of Health. This gives them significant powers as they will then determine how those funds will be distributed.

NHS Trusts differ in that they have only a responsibility to provide specialist health services, for example district general services, mental health services and ambulance services. The intention, expressed in the Third Way, is to ensure patient-centredness by devolving power to clinical teams able to make decisions about patient care.

National Service Frameworks

Link

Chapters 2 and 18 also discuss NSFs.

One way that the government has devised to ensure an acceptable and equitable standard of service is National Service Frameworks (NSF), which offer a blueprint to service providers of how services should be organised and the standard of performance that is required. These are constructed by consultation with social policy experts, health professionals and service users. For example, there are now NSFs outlining service planning and provision for mental health, older people, children, diabetes, cancer, renal services and coronary heart disease.

Regulating the profession

The profession of nursing itself is also subject to social policy and legislation. After a protracted campaign at the beginning of the twentieth century, nurses eventually persuaded the government to create a professional register. This was finally achieved in 1919, when the Nurses Registration Act was passed, creating registers for different parts of the profession. The aim of the register was to protect the public as only those who had trained to be nurses would be admitted to it. Equally, those nurses who did not uphold the required standard of professional conduct would be removed from the register and would not be able to practise as registered practitioners.

The Act also created the General Nursing Council, a governing body for the profession whose role was to set the standards of education necessary to prepare nurses, examine nurses and maintain the register. Members were appointed to the Council by the minister of health, and a similar one was created for midwives.

This system remained in place for 60 years. In 1979, the systems for regulating the profession were reorganised by the Nurses, Midwives and Health Visitors Act, creating a new body, the United Kingdom Central Council for Nursing, Midwifery and Health Visiting (UKCC). This brought together all the separate organisations and councils of the four kingdoms under one administration, so that all the parts of the profession – nursing, midwifery and health visiting – were regulated by the same body. The principal functions of the UKCC were to establish and improve standards of training and professional conduct.

Since April 2002, the regulatory body has been the Nursing and Midwifery Council (NMC). It is composed of a smaller number of elected nurses, midwives and health visitors and appointed lay members and includes representation from all four countries of the UK (DoH, 2001c). The Health Act 1999 defines its functions as:

- Keeping the register of members admitted to practice
- Determining standards of education and training for admission to practice
- Giving guidance about standards of conduct and performance
- Administering procedures (including making rules) relating to misconduct, lack of fitness to practise and similar matters.

Midwifery services

The practice of midwifery has always been considered to be distinct from that of nursing, and it developed its own set of policy provisions over the twentieth century. There were several attempts to introduce legislation to regulate the profession of midwifery during the nineteenth century, the main driver behind this being the Matrons Aid Society, founded in 1881. The Society comprised a small group of educated midwives who wanted to improve standards of care and the professional status of midwives. In the late nineteenth century, eight Bills proposing a midwives' register were introduced to Parliament, but all failed. As this had been partly because the government did not give it priority, the proposed legislation was then advanced by the use of a Private Member's Bill. The Bill was opposed by members of the medical profession because it trespassed upon their professional territory, but equally there was opposition from the developing nursing profession, led by Ethel Bedford Fenwick, who wished to see the professions united and regulated jointly.

A Midwives Act was eventually passed in 1902, its main provision being to establish a Central Midwives Board (CMB), initially for England and Wales, provision later also being made for Scotland and Ireland. The CMB was charged with maintaining a roll of certificated midwives, and it also set up local supervising authorities (LSAs) to supervise the practice of midwives. The Central

Midwives Board set out rules governing midwifery practice, provided for the education of midwives and set up structures to maintain professional discipline.

In the first half of the twentieth century, the practice of midwifery took place largely in the client's home. Women had to pay a fee to the midwife, and to the GP if he was required. As many clients could not afford the doctor, midwives would often pay the fee, so the Midwives Act 1918 provided for the LSA to pay the fees of doctors who were called to obstetric emergencies. The later Midwives Act of 1936 made it compulsory for LSAs to provide a salaried domiciliary midwifery service; the fact that midwives could now receive a salary allowed them to provide a fuller service, which included antenatal care.

The Second World War had an effect upon the organisation of obstetric care. As a result of the war effort, there were fewer friends and family available to support a woman through a delivery, so women were drawn to having their babies delivered in hospital. The advent of the NHS in 1948 again changed the nature of obstetric care. As the service was now free, women took it up more readily and were more prepared to have their babies in hospital.

The Nurses, Midwives and Health Visitors Act 1979 created a statutory committee for midwives, important in the regulation of practice. The committee is required to make midwives' rules, which relate to the LSAs and midwives' practice. The recent reform of nursing regulation (DoH, 2001c) proposes to maintain this policy. The Nursing and Midwifery Council will still have a midwifery committee, and the council will make midwives' rules. Supervision of midwifery will continue under LSAs, which will still require midwives to attend educational courses to update their practice.

> **Activity 3.4**
>
> Based upon your reading of this section and your observations in obstetric practice, make a list of the ways in which the regulation of midwifery differs from that of nursing.

Mental health care

Care for people with mental health problems in the nineteenth and the first half of the twentieth century was based in large asylums, later to be termed 'psychiatric hospitals'. More recently, however, there has been a movement to assist service users to live independently in the community, and policy and legislation have been developed to support this movement.

Caring for people who have mental health problems sometimes involves the use of powers that infringe civil liberties, so this area of client care is subject to significantly more legal involvement. In their daily practice, mental health nurses have to be knowledgeable about the law that regulates mental health practice.

Mental Health Act 1959

A significant change occurred in mental health care in the late 1950s. Before this, the delivery of care had occurred through the large psychiatric hospitals built in the nineteenth century. Admission to hospital was by a system of certification, all clients who were admitted being legally committed into the care of the hospital and detained against their will. During the 1950s, however, there was considerable social change, which created the climate for the development of legislation that was revolutionary in its approach.

The Mental Health Act 1959 repealed all previous mental health legislation, introduced a single code for all types of mental disorder and set out new definitions of mental disorder. Clients could be admitted for treatment on a voluntary basis, as with any other hospital. Provision was made for compulsory admission to hospital only for those who were a danger to themselves or others because of mental illness. A new body, the Mental Health Review Tribunal, consisting of legal, medical and lay members, was created to safeguard clients' civil rights. This allowed clients who were detained to have a right of appeal. The Tribunal also has the power to discharge clients from hospital following a successful appeal. The effect of the Act was to reduce the number of clients who were compulsorily detained as clients could be admitted to hospital before they became severely ill. The stigma associated with mental illness was significantly reduced, discharging clients from hospital became much easier, and staff could contemplate the concept of the client living in the community.

Hospital closure

In 1961, Enoch Powell, then minister of health, announced a new policy – a programme of closure of the mental hospitals. He recognised that a huge proportion of the NHS budget was spent on maintaining mental hospitals and envisaged that this programme would lead to a reduction in spending on the NHS. Powell wanted to see the development of mental illness units within general hospitals, so a trend was started to decrease institutional care and increase community services, although this did not happen with anything like the speed that Powell had anticipated.

Better services for the mentally ill

The Department of Health and Social Security (DHSS) published a report in 1975, which showed that although the client population of mental hospitals had been reduced, not one hospital had been closed and the volume of work was in fact increasing. The report drew a picture of how future services would be centred on general hospitals, provision also being made for hostels for recovering clients, outclient clinics and daycare.

Mental Health Act 1983

As services developed in the community and more effective drug therapies were discovered, the nature of mental health care changed. Once again, the legal framework required amendment, a Mental Health Amendment Act being passed in 1983. The main tenets of the 1959 Act were upheld but new provisions were added. Clients who are detained under treatment orders may be treated without their consent for the first three months after admission, after which a second opinion has to be sought to continue treatment. This second opinion is supplied by a qualified psychiatrist appointed by the Mental Health Act Commission (MHAC). Treatment in this case is most often electroconvulsive therapy (ECT) or drug therapy.

The MHAC, created by the 1983 Act, is a special health authority whose role is to be an independent inspectorate, its powers being limited to detained clients. MHAC members are charged with the duty of visiting and interviewing detained clients and investigating their complaints. In addition, the MHAC makes an annual report to Parliament.

The Act also makes provision for social care. Social services departments are required to appoint approved social workers (ASW), who have to be competent in the care of mentally ill people. The ASW has the duty to apply to the hospital for a client to be detained. Before doing this, however, he or she must interview the client and ensure that there is no means of providing care other than compulsory admission. Health and social services are charged with a duty to provide aftercare for clients who have been detained on a treatment order.

Care programme approach

care programme approach

a systematic framework for mental health practice, which ensures that the service user has an assessment, a care plan and a key worker, and ensures that the client is fully involved

In 1991, the government responded to several incidents that had caused public concern by developing a system for the organisation of mental health care for people with severe mental illness living in the community. The approach is to be followed by all health practitioners who deliver care to people with mental health problems. The first essential element of this **care programme approach** (CPA) is a systematic assessment of health and social care needs, based on which the client possesses an agreed care plan. A key worker is appointed to coordinate the care plan and liaise with all the agencies that contribute to the package of care. The client's progress is subject to regular review, and he or she is involved in care decisions at every stage.

The care programme approach is still the framework that is employed to structure the care of people with mental health problems, especially those who are seriously mentally ill.

Further reform to the mental health legal framework

Even a cursory review of the history of mental illness and the law would show that devising an effective, just and workable mental health legal framework has proved an almost insurmountable task for lawyers, politicians and practitioners over the past 200 years. Consequently, significant change happens relatively infrequently. Reform of the 1983 Mental Health Act was initially proposed in 1998 (DoH, 2004a). After a prolonged public debate, which included a range of government proposals, many of which were challenged and rejected by service users, practitioners and civil rights lobbyists, a version of the framework has been devised that is likely to be acceptable to all stakeholders, will protect the civil rights of patients and maintain public safety.

In 2005, a Bill was included in the government's schedule to be placed before Parliament. The most significant proposed changes are that the new Act will replace the Mental Health Act 1983. There are proposed changes to procedures, defined terms, clinical roles and institutions. It is proposed that the definition of mental disorder will be changed to place emphasis on the presence of psychological dysfunction and its effect on the person rather than its cause.

The Act still provides for compulsory detention, however there is a change to the system of checks and balances. There is provision for compulsory treatment to take place when the patient is resident or non-resident in hospital. It is proposed that there is a significant broadening of formal roles with members of the multidisciplinary clinical team. The role of ASW is to be broadened to approved mental health professional (AMHP). The first stage of a decision to detain someone compulsorily will be termed 'examination', and two doctors and the AMHP are required to be involved in the examination stage decision-making to ensure a holistic review of the person's circumstances.

The second stage of the procedure is termed 'assessment', which can be carried out from 72 hours to 28 days, according to the circumstances. The patient is liable to formal assessment under the Act. Several new roles come into play. The AMHP is responsible for registering the patient with the hospital and for appointing a 'nominated person'. The role of this person, who can be a relative, significant other or advocate preferred by the patient, is to speak with or for them. The hospital managers appoint a 'clinical supervisor'. This person may be a psychiatrist or other senior mental health practitioner, and their role is to take responsibility for the care of the detained person and to produce a 'care plan' within five days.

To be able to continue assessment or treatment beyond 28 days, the clinical supervisor is required to make an application to the Mental Health Review Tribunal. The Tribunal can make one of the following four decisions:

1. Patient not liable to assessment or treatment under formal powers of compulsion.

2. Confirm need for assessment but change patient's residency status.
3. Make an order for a further 28-day assessment.
4. Make a treatment order that can be for up to six months and may change the patient's residency status.

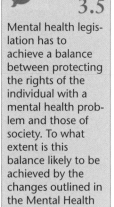

Activity 3.5

Mental health legislation has to achieve a balance between protecting the rights of the individual with a mental health problem and those of society. To what extent is this balance likely to be achieved by the changes outlined in the Mental Health Bill 2005?

The Mental Health Act Commission would be abolished and its functions and powers transferred to the Commission for Healthcare Audit and Inspection. Separate Codes of Conduct will be published for England and Wales. The guiding principles of the proposed legislation and code are that:

1. Wherever possible, patients will be involved in decision-making events and processes.
2. Decisions will be open and fair.
3. The least restrictive and intrusive method of treatment will be adopted.

In the case of mentally disordered offenders, in general terms, courts will maintain the same powers available to them as under the 1983 Act. The proposed framework will, however, offer them the option of assessing or treating a 'non-dangerous offender' in the community.

Learning disability nursing

The legal framework that supports learning disability practice is the Mental Health Act 1983. Practitioners use this legal framework to detain clients, give compulsory treatment and offer protection of rights.

In 2001, the government published the White Paper *Valuing People: A New Strategy for Learning Disability for the 21st Century* (DoH, 2001a). This document offers a blueprint for the way in which services are to be planned and delivered for people with a learning disability. It is presented as an action plan that will be rolled out over the five years from 2001 to 2006. The White Paper outlines a considerable amount of funding that is to be allocated to learning disability services, specifically to be spent on supporting people with a learning disability in a move from long-stay hospital facilities to more appropriate supported accommodation, modernising day centres and improving services for children.

A key feature of the development is effective advocacy services, which will be carried out in conjunction with voluntary agencies. Significant funding, partly financial support to be offered through increased social security benefits, is allocated to increasing the support offered to carers. Support is also offered via a national information centre and helpline developed in partnership with the charity MENCAP.

A key deficiency in learning disability services has been that clients have found it difficult to gain equal access to the health services, so the White Paper proposes to develop systems able to cater for complex health needs. Equally, it sets out to enable people with a learning disability to have the same right of access to mainstream health services as any other citizen.

Significant factors in providing a high quality of life are the comfort of and the facilities available in one's housing accommodation. People with a learning disability are to be offered a greater choice and control over where and how they live. Similarly, services will be developed to enable a greater choice of employment and to meet the needs of people from a wide range of cultural and ethnic backgrounds. This policy is supported by the four principles of rights, independence, choice and inclusion.

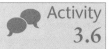

Activity 3.6

Discuss the argument that the principles of *Valuing People* (DoH, 2001a) arise from the values and beliefs of the Third Way.

Working with children and young people

Children and young people are a group who are vulnerable, especially when in need of health and social care. As with mental health care, there is a legal framework that supports and guides practitioners in their work with children.

The Children Act 1989

The legal framework that currently supports practice is the Children Act 1989 (DoH, 1992), which took effect in 1991. It is addressed mainly to the courts and local authority social services, but parts of it are important for nurses to understand.

The main principles of the Act are child and family focused: the welfare of the child is paramount, and the overall aim is that children should be brought up and cared for within their own family. If children are in danger, they should be protected by effective intervention. An important tenet is that children should be kept informed about what happens to them and be involved in the decision-making process. Care should also be designed to support parents, ensuring that **parental responsibility** is maintained and effective support is provided.

parental responsibility
a set of rights and duties against which parents can be assessed

The Act requires health practitioners to work with parents to enable them to care for their children to the best of their ability by enhancing their knowledge and understanding of childcare and development. Working in the spirit of the Act means listening to the child, providing appropriate information and taking account of his or her feelings and wishes. Health-care professionals are also required to cooperate with the social service and education departments to meet the health needs of the child. Most important is the identification of children in need and their referral to social services if that is appropriate.

Section 17(10) of the Act specifically defines a 'child in need' as one who:

> is unlikely to achieve or maintain, or to have the opportunity of achieving or maintaining, a reasonable standard of health or development without the provision for him of services by a local authority [or whose] health or development is likely to be significantly impaired, or further impaired, without the provision for him of such services [or who] is disabled.

The Act recognises the role of midwives, health visitors and school nurses in having contact with the child from birth. They are likely to be the first to recognise a child in need and are expected to refer the child to social services using agreed health authority protocols. They are also expected to cooperate with social workers to provide the health care needed to promote the child's welfare.

The Act outlines a new concept of 'parental responsibility', which has replaced the phrase 'parental rights', emphasis being placed on the ongoing obligations of the parents' role. This includes the duties, rights, powers, responsibilities and authority that a parent has in respect of a child and his or her property. Parental responsibility is not affected by parental separation or divorce.

The nurse may be involved in a case in which a court order may be applied, so it is important to be aware of the different types of order that might be granted. The following orders can be made by the court under public law:

- A *care order* is made if a court decides that a child is suffering or is likely to suffer significant harm through a lack of adequate parental care or control. The child is placed in the care of the local authority, which then has parental responsibility for the child that is shared with the parents. It does not take parental responsibility from the parents, but the local authority may decide how the parents exercise it
- A *supervision order* is made if the court decides that the local authority should observe a child closely and give guidance, the child then being under the supervision of a local authority or probation officer. Under this order, the local authority or the supervisor has parental responsibility
- A *child assessment order* is for use in situations in which there are reasonable grounds to suspect that the child is suffering significant harm but is not at immediate risk. The applicant may form the opinion that an assessment is needed but that the parents are unwilling to cooperate. Either the local authority or the National Society for the Prevention of Cruelty to Children may apply for this order. It has a maximum duration of seven days, and the court decides on the nature of the assessment
- An *emergency protection order* is reserved for extremely urgent cases in which the child's safety is immediately threatened. This order can be applied

for eight days, with a additional seven if necessary, but the order may be challenged by the parents after the first 72 hours of the order have elapsed. Parental responsibility is given to the applicant but only insofar as it is necessary to safeguard the child and promote his or her welfare.

In addition, there are a number of orders that are at the disposal of the courts but which are under private law proceedings relating to cases of divorce, domestic violence or adoption:

- A *residence order* states with whom the child will live. This order may be made while the child is in the care of the local authority. It can thus end any care order and give parental responsibility to the person with the benefit of the order
- A *contact order* requires the person with whom the child lives to permit the child to have contact with those named in the order
- A *prohibited steps order* prevents the child's parents or any other person taking steps as outlined in the order without first obtaining the permission of the court.

Nurses may be required to attend a child protection conference before an application is made for a court order; the conference has to be clear and certain about the evidence before applying for an order. Nurses must also be prepared to write reports for court proceedings. In a child protection case, the nurse is required to provide documentation describing the nature of the significant harm that the child has already suffered. In addition, a statement of the child's future risk is required.

Almost any nurse, midwife or health visitor may, at some time in his or her practice, encounter a child who is at risk, so having a working knowledge of the principles and powers of the Children Act is important for all practitioners.

The Children Act 2004

The main provisions and spirit of the 1989 Act were preserved but further measures were added to strengthen safeguarding children under the Children Act 2004. This act sets out the duties of local authorities and their key partners to cooperate effectively. Most importantly it sets up local safeguarding children boards (LSCBs). These are a key safeguarding mechanism for agreeing how organisations in each local area will cooperate. They have a duty to ensure that safeguarding and promoting the welfare of children is effected. Members of the board are drawn from all organisations that engage with services for children,

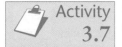

Activity 3.7

Make notes on how you think the Children Act 2004 protects and supports the rights of children.

including the police, probation services, PCTs and SHAs. Responsibility for coordinating the boards rests with the local authority (DoH, 2004b).

Every Child Matters

Government policy on services for children is drawn together under the banner of *Every Child Matters* (DoH, 2005). This is a programme of local and national action that aims to transform the whole system of children's services. It focuses upon effective interagency cooperation, safeguarding children, a skilled children's workforce, a common assessment framework and information-sharing.

The United Kingdom of Great Britain

Policy for England has been set out here to illustrate the political process in relation to making health policy. It should be noted that each of the other three countries in the UK may have its own policy. Usually the same principles underpin the policy but these are adapted to meet the individual needs and values of each country. Students can explore variations in policy by accessing the appropriate websites given at the end of the chapter.

■ Chapter Summary

This chapter has described the main institutions of government and the processes that are undertaken in order to enact social policy. It has outlined how the NHS came into being and its subsequent development, and has discussed the statutory regulation of the profession and the development of education. In addition, social policy relating specifically to midwifery, children's nursing and mental health practice has been described in some detail. Finally, it should be emphasised that nurses can often be a support and help to service users as much because of their knowledge of the wider social context of care as because of their clinical skills.

Test Yourself!

1. How many stages must a Bill pass through in the House of Commons?

2. In which year did the NHS begin?

3. What are the main functions of a primary care Trust?

4. In which year did midwives gain the power to establish a Central Midwives Board?

5. What is the name of the inspectorate created by the Mental Health Act 1983?

6. What is the name of the order in the Children Act in which the court decides that the local authority should observe a child closely and give guidance?

■ Further Reading

Dimond, B.C. and Barker, F.H. (1997) *Mental Health Law for Nurses*. Blackwell, Oxford.

Hanson, A.H. and Walles, M. (1990) *Governing Britain*, 5th edn. Fontana, London.

■ References

DHSS (Department of Health and Social Security) (1975) *Better Services for the Mentally Ill*. HMSO, London.

DHSS (Department of Health and Social Security) (1980) *Inequalities in Health* (Black Report). HMSO, London.

DoH (Department of Health) (1992) *The Children Act 1989: An Introductory Guide for the NHS*. HMSO, London.

DoH (Department of Health) (1997) *The New NHS: Modern, Dependable*. HMSO, London.

DoH (Department of Health) (2000) *The NHS Plan*. HMSO, London.

DoH (Department of Health) (2001a) *Valuing People: A New Strategy for Learning Disability for the 21st Century*. HMSO, London.

DoH (Department of Health) (2001b) *Shifting the Balance of Power within the NHS*. HMSO, London.

DoH (Department of Health) (2001c) *Shaping the Future*. HMSO, London.

DoH (Department of Health) (2004a) *Improving Mental Health Law: Towards a New Mental Health Act*. HMSO, London.

DoH (Department of Health) (2004b) *The Children Act 2004*. HMSO, London.

DoH (Department of Health) (2005) *Every Child Matters – Change for Children: An Overview of Cross Government Guidance*. HMSO, London.

Ham, C. (2004) *Health Policy in Britain: The Politics and Organisation of the National Health Service*, 5th edn. Palgrave Macmillan, Basingstoke.

Hill, M. (2003) *Understanding Social Policy*, 7th edn. Blackwell, Oxford.

Illich, I. (1976) *Limits to Medicine: Medical Nemesis*, 2nd edn. Marion Boyars, London.

Leathard, A. (2000) *Health Care Provision: Past Present and into the 21st Century*, 2nd edn. Stanley Thornes, Cheltenham.

McKeown, T. (1976) *The Modern Rise of Population and the Role of Medicine: Dream, Mirage or Nemesis?* Rock Carling Monograph. Nuffield Provincial Hospitals Trust, London.

Ministry of Health (1942) *Report of Committee on Social Insurance and Allied Services* (Beveridge Report). HMSO, London.

Ranade, W. (1994) *A Future for the NHS?: Health Care in the 1990s*. Longman, London.

Useful Websites

www.dh.gov.uk **Department of Health**

www.dhsspsni.gov.uk **Department of Health, Social Services and Public Safelty for Northern Ireland**

www.show.scot.nhs.uk **NHS Scotland**

www.wales.nhs.uk **NHS Wales**

www.nationalarchives.gov.uk **National Archives**

Nursing Interventions

Part **2**

SOMDUTH PARBOTEEAH

Chapter

4

Infection Control and Administration of Medications

Contents

- Control of Infection
- Administration of Medications
- Chapter Summary

- Test Yourself!
- Further Reading
- References

Learning Outcomes

This chapter describes the policies and procedures for the control of infection and the safe administration of medications. It is intended that this chapter will provide practitioners with evidence-based knowledge to carry out nursing practice in a manner that will safeguard them and the patients in their care. At the end of the chapter, you should be able to:

- Describe and explain the principles of infection control
- Describe the role of the nurse in infection control
- Develop safe practices in the administration of medications.

Throughout the chapter you will be given an opportunity to undertake some exercises that will assist you in further developing your knowledge, skills and competence. Some of these activities may initially be practised in a skills laboratory under supervision and may also require you to access and read additional policies relevant to your health-care setting and suggested textbooks listed at the end of the chapter.

■ Control of Infection

This section will describe the role of the nurse in the prevention of health-care associated infection (HCAI). By the end of this section, the nurse will be able to:

- Describe HCAI
- Identify the causes of HCAI
- Understand the need for universal precautions
- Describe the role of the infection control team
- Discuss local infection control policies.

Infections are caused by germs such as bacteria, viruses and fungi. They may remain localised, causing infection in certain parts of the body such as skin infections, for example ringworm infection. Germs may also spread systemically and affect other organs thus debilitating the patient. Patients can become infected in several ways when they are in health-care settings and it is vital that nurses take adequate precautions to prevent HCAI. Resistant strains of *Staphylococcus*, difficult to control and treat, have become a major problem in hospitals.

HCAI

A health-care associated infection (HCAI) is one that is neither present nor incubating at the time the patient is admitted to hospital and is caught from other patients during a hospital stay. The level of HCAI in England is 9 per cent and the National Audit Office estimates that the cost is £1 billion per year (DoH, 2005), with patients who acquire an HCAI staying an average of 2.5 times longer than a non-infected patient. A host of factors may contribute to the development of HCAI and these include:

- Critically ill patients with weakened immunity
- Increase in invasive procedures
- High turnover of patients
- Poor compliance of good practice
- Lack of cleanliness
- Inappropriate use of antibiotics (MRSA).

The development of modern-day health care, including complex invasive surgical interventions on critically ill patients with a greater susceptibility to infection, has increased the risk of acquiring an infection while in a health-care setting. Emmerson et al. (1996) reported that the commonest sites of HCAI are the:

- Urinary tract: 23 per cent (80 per cent caused by indwelling catheters)
- Lungs: 22 per cent (common in ventilated patients)
- Wound: 9 per cent (surgical site infections)
- Blood: 6 per cent (60 per cent caused by intravenous catheters).

For HCAI to occur, there has to be a source or reservoir of organisms that can cause the infection and a means by which the germs are transmitted. The most likely means of transmission of infectious organisms is by direct contact or the percutaneous inoculation of infected material. Measures to control HCAI are twofold: if possible, the source of infection should be eliminated and, second, the implementation of strategies to break the chain of infection (Figure 4.1).

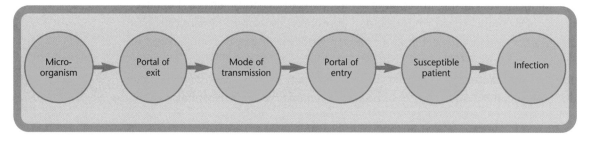

Figure 4.1 ● Chain of infection

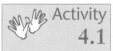

Activity 4.1

Identify local and national guidelines concerning the control of infection in hospitals and the community.

The most effective and efficient way of breaking the chain of infection is to follow the standard precautions in daily practice. As many patients are unaware or unwilling to disclose any infection that may be present, the only way to ensure that the risk of transmission is reduced is by following standard precautions across all patients. The standard precautions to be adhered to are discussed in the following sections.

Standard principles for preventing HCAI

Hand hygiene

Hand hygiene is essential in the prevention of HCAI. Many infections spread by contact and hands are a major vehicle in the transmission of infection (RCN, 1992). Normal skin has a resident population of microorganisms and additional transient organisms are picked up during contact in the delivery of nursing care. The aim of handwashing is to remove these microorganisms or reduce their numbers below that of an infective dose. Hands should be washed following the procedures shown in Chart 4.1.

Chart 4.1 ● Indications for handwashing

- Before direct contact with patient
- When hands are visibly soiled or potentially contaminated
- After handling contaminated items
- After handling body fluids
- Before serving meals
- After removing aprons and gloves
- At the beginning and end of duty
- If in any doubt about the cleanliness of hands

Hands can be decontaminated by applying an alcohol-based hand rub or washing hands with soap and running water from a tap. An effective handwashing technique involves three stages: preparation, washing and rinsing and drying. In the preparation phase, the hands are wet and an appropriate antimicrobial preparation applied. The solution must be applied to all the skin surfaces of the hands. The hands should be rubbed vigorously for about 10–15 seconds, ensuring that the tips of fingers, the thumb and the areas between the fingers have been attended to before rinsing thoroughly and drying using paper towels.

When using alcohol hand rub, it is important to ensure that hands are free of dirt or organic matter, otherwise handwashing using soap and water is recommended. The decontamination agent should come into contact with all surfaces of the hand and rubbed vigorously until all the alcohol has evaporated.

The skin should be intact and any cuts or abrasions should be covered with waterproof dressings. Staff should also avoid contact with clinical waste and refrain from undertaking invasive procedures.

Proper handling of equipment

When equipment is being used for a group of patients, it must be cleaned and disinfected after each use and between patients. If it is not possible to clean and disinfect the equipment, then single-use or disposable equipment should be considered.

Use of protective wear

Staff should wear protective equipment depending on the risks to themselves and other patients. Gloves should be worn in the following situations:

- Contact with open wounds
- Contact with sterile sites
- Contact with mucous membranes
- Contact with body fluids

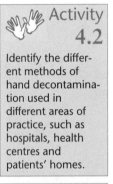

Activity 4.2

Identify the different methods of hand decontamination used in different areas of practice, such as hospitals, health centres and patients' homes.

Activity 4.3

Identify how the following types of linen are dealt with in your hospital/ community: used linen, soiled linen, infected linen, patients' personal clothing and duvets.

- Contact with body secretions and excretions
- When handling contaminated equipment.

Gloves should be used as single-use items and sterile gloves must be used for aseptic procedures. Gloves should be applied immediately before a procedure and removed when the course of action is complete. Gloves must be changed in between patients and in some instances when undertaking different activities for the same patient such as washing and aseptic dressing.

Plastic aprons must be worn as single-use items per patient when there is a risk of spillage of body fluids. Other protective clothing such as goggles, face masks and boots should be worn on the basis of an assessment of the risks of cross-infection.

Prevention of injury

The use of sharp items such as needles, scissors, blades and scalpels can result in injury and the inoculation of germs. It is essential that extreme care is taken in the use and disposal of sharps. The handling of sharps should be kept to a minimum. Needles and syringes must not be disassembled before disposal. Needles must not be resheathed and used sharps must be discarded into a sharps container conforming to BS standards.

Waste disposal

All waste must be handled and disposed of safely as it can potentially cause infection to another person coming into contact with it. The NHS has a legal responsibility for the safe disposal of clinical and hazardous waste. Furthermore, all employers have a legal obligation under the Health and Safety at Work Act 1974 to ensure that all their employees are appropriately trained and proficient in procedures for working safely. All clinical areas should also have a written policy on waste disposal.

All waste is categorised into household waste and clinical waste. Household waste includes items such as paper, cardboard, flowers and those of a non-hazardous, non-contaminated nature. It is disposed of in an appropriate bag.

Clinical waste

The legal definition of clinical waste is given in the Controlled Waste Regulations 1992 as:

> any waste which consists wholly or partly of human or animal tissue, blood or other bodily fluids, excretions, drugs or other pharmaceutical products,

swabs or dressings, or syringes, needles or other sharp instruments, being waste which unless rendered safe may prove hazardous to any person coming into contact with it; and any other waste arising from medical, nursing, dental, veterinary, pharmaceutical or similar practice, investigation, treatment, care, teaching or research, or in the collection of blood for transfusion, being waste which may cause infection to any person coming in contact with it.

Clinical waste is categorised into five groups as shown in Table 4.1.

Table 4.1 Safe disposal of clinical waste

Category of waste	Description	Method of disposal
Group A	Soiled dressings, swabs, and all other contaminated waste. Waste materials from cases of infectious diseases. All human tissues	Waste placed in yellow clinical waste bag (in accordance with local policy)
Group B	Used syringes, needles, cartridges, broken glass, glass ampoules, cannulae and any other sharp instruments	Sharps containers that comply with BS 7320 and of a type approved by the infection control team
Group C	Microbiological cultures and potentially infected waste from pathology departments, research laboratories and post mortem rooms	Yellow clinical waste bag
Group D	Pharmaceutical products that are unsuitable for use on safety grounds and chemical waste such as amalgam	Yellow clinical waste bag
Group E	Used disposable items such as bed pans, urinals, incontinence pads, stoma bags and any items that do not fall into Group A	Contents of disposable items can be disposed of via the toilets. If assessment indicates a risk, then follow instruction as for disposal of Group A waste

Source: Adapted from Health Services Advisory Committee (1999).

The following principles should be followed when handling waste:

- Bags should be filled no more than two-thirds full
- Bags should not be compressed when closing
- Bags must be secured using a plastic tie or by tying a knot at the top
- Avoid bodily contact with bags and handle them by the top end.

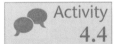

Activity
4.4

Describe the policy for the safe disposal of used needles, syringes, vials and glass ampoules.

The following principles should be followed when handling sharps:

- Only fill container up to three-quarters full
- Use the handles provided to handle the containers
- On no account should attempts be made to open a sealed sharps container
- Place sharp items at the point of use
- Do not resheath needles and syringes before disposal.

Effective infection control can only be achieved when each and every member of the health-care team accepts total responsibility for implementing preventive measures. Only then can the risk of infection be reduced in health-care settings.

This section has focused on the practical aspects of preventing the spread of infection in the day-to-day management of patient care. There should be an organisational strategy with the responsibility for preventing and managing infection. The infection control team should be able to advise staff with difficult cases or if there as an outbreak of infection on the ward.

■ Administration of Medications

This section will describe the role of the nurse in the practice of safe drug administration. By the end of this section, the nurse should be able to:

- Understand the legislation governing the administration of drugs by health-care professionals
- Safely administer drugs to patients by a variety of routes
- Be involved in the storage and preparation of drugs
- Understand how drugs work.

The administration of medicines is an important aspect of the professional practice of persons whose names are on the Nursing and Midwifery Council register (NMC, 2004). The nurse is responsible for assessing, planning, implementing and evaluating drug therapies as well as educating patients about their drug regimens. It is more than a mechanistic task, requiring thought and the exercise of professional judgement. To be effective, the nurse must have an understanding of the fundamental principles of drug action, the purposes of drug use and the nursing actions necessary to bring about beneficial outcomes. The student is advised to consult textbooks listed in the further reading section at the end of this chapter for more comprehensive information on drug actions and pharmacokinetics. The administration of medications via intravenous and epidural routes using electronic devices, for example pumps, is not described in this section as it requires further training at postregistration level.

In the UK, the range of substances intended for medicinal use must conform to standards specified in the *British Pharmacopoeia* or the *British Pharmaceutical Codex* and must satisfy the relevant government legislation listed in Chart 4.2. Those with a keen interest are recommended to consult a current copy of the *British National Formulary*. Failure to comply with legal requirements, and any ensuing errors, may result in criminal prosecution and professional suspension from practising as a nurse.

Chart 4.2 ● Statutes controlling substances intended for medicinal use

- The Misuse of Drugs Act 1971
- The Poisons Act 1972
- The Medicines Act 1968, 1983
- The Prescription by Nurses Act 1992

Before any medication is administered, it is important that the nurse carries out a detailed assessment of the patient, including:

- Medications that the patient is currently taking
- Their frequency and dosage
- Any home remedies being taken
- Other complementary therapies being used
- Allergies to any drugs
- Height, weight, blood pressure, temperature and respiration, as some drug dosages, for example dopamine infusion, are calculated on body mass, and side-effects can affect blood pressure
- General fitness and health, as such information can influence decisions about the routes and methods of drug administration, for example an emaciated patient may not be able to tolerate deep intramuscular injections
- Diet, because if foods such as cheese, yogurt, broad beans, marmite, red wine and beer are administered to a patient who is receiving monoamine oxidase inhibitors (MAOIs), dangerous side-effects may ensue.

Activity 4.5

Take the medication history of a client you have cared for and discuss any relevant issues with your mentor.

In hospitals, medicines should not be administered without a written prescription and all prescriptions should include information necessary for the safe administration of the drug. The prescription chart should detail the following:

- The name of the patient
- The date the prescription was written and the signature of the prescriber
- The medication and dosage
- The route for administering the drug
- The time of administration

● Any specific information, for example that it is to be taken with meals.

Prescriptions are normally written on a standard prescription sheet (usually produced locally and differing between hospitals and in the community). In a study of medication prescription orders, Winslow (1997) found that 78 per cent of signatures were illegible or legible only with effort, thus increasing the risk of medication errors and patient harm. **The nurse should not administer any drug if the prescription is illegible.** It is important that all records of prescribed medicines should be kept together to prevent drug interactions and overdosage and for monitoring purposes. The following criteria should be adhered to in order to prevent drug errors:

Activity 4.6

Examine a prescription chart for its legibility, accuracy and completeness as outlined above.

1. The prescription must be legible, and the approved or generic name should be used.
2. Details of the client's name and address, the dose required and the frequency and route of administration must be clearly stated. For certain drugs (for example antibiotics), the proposed duration of therapy should be stated.
3. **Controlled drugs**, that is, drugs that are subject to the prescription requirements of the Misuse of Drug Regulations 1985, should be clearly monitored.
4. A prescription should not be altered once it has been written and should be written out in full again if a change in dose or frequency is indicated.
5. When a prescription is to be cancelled, it should be crossed out and signed and dated by the doctor.
6. In emergencies, telephone orders for the administration of medicines can be accepted by a first-level registered nurse (providing there is local agreement) if the doctor is unable to attend the ward. The prescription must then be written and signed by the nurse, stating that it is a verbal prescription. The doctor's name should be recorded on the prescription sheet and the doctor should sign the prescription as soon as possible. No telephone orders should be repeated.

controlled drugs

those drugs, such as morphine, subject to the prescription requirements of the Misuse of Drug Regulations 1985

When administering medications, the nurse's first task is to check the prescription for completeness, then he or she can prepare to administer the drug. In preparing medications, it is important to ensure cleanliness of the hands, a clean surface and sterility of all the materials used. All the components must be assembled in a well-lit room and medicines prepared in a safe area away from distraction. A general guide to ensure patients' safety in the administration of medications is to check the 'five Rs':

1. The right medication.
2. The right amount.

3. The right time.
4. The right patient.
5. The right route.

Right medication

After checking the prescription, the nurse selects the right medication, carefully checking the labels on the containers. Medications from a container that is unlabelled, defaced or illegible must never be used. The nurse should read any instructions pertaining to the medication and check the expiry date. Nurses must never administer a drug prepared by someone else because the nurse administering the drug will still be held accountable for any errors made by others during preparation. Medications must never be decanted from one container to another. The nurse should be familiar with basic information about the drug, including its action, contraindications and side-effects, and current reference books, such as the *British National Formulary*, should be available at all times.

For the administration of controlled (Schedule 1–4) drugs, two nurses, one of whom must be a registered nurse, should be involved. Local guidelines may differ and it is important to adhere to protocols.

Right amount

To prepare the right amount of medication, the nurse must be familiar with the different measurement systems and common abbreviations used (Chart 4.3).

Chart 4.3 ● Common abbreviations used in prescriptions

p.o.	–	by mouth	e.c.	–	enteric coated
p.r.n.	–	given as necessary	b.i.d.	–	twice a day
caps	–	capsules	mcg	–	microgram
s.c.	–	subcutaneous	s.c.	–	sugar coated
q.d.	–	daily	a.c.	–	before meals
elix.	–	elixir	mg	–	milligram
s.l.	–	sublinginal	m.r.	–	modified release
q.h.	–	every hour	p.c.	–	after meals
I.U.	–	International Units	l	–	litre
i.m.	–	intramuscular	stat	–	given immediately
q.d.s.	–	four times a day	tr.	–	tincture
kg	–	kilograms	ml	–	millilitre
i.v.	–	intravenous	neb.	–	nebuliser
t.d.s.	–	three times a day	guttae	–	drops

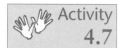

Activity 4.7

Scrutinise at least six prescription charts. Were you able to recognise the abbreviations used? Discuss your findings with your mentor.

When preparing liquid medications for oral administration, it is important to shake all suspensions and emulsions to ensure a proper distribution of the drug. A calibrated medicine pot or syringe may be used to draw up the right amount of medication. If the medication is poured from the container, the medicine pot should be placed on a flat surface. To check for accuracy, the pot should be raised to eye level and the measurement read at the lowest point of the meniscus.

Some medications, for example eye drops, are measured with a dropper. The dropper must be held vertically, and the bulb should be slowly squeezed and released until the required dosage is reached.

The administration of injections depends on the drugs prescribed. Some injectables, for example pethidine, are available in liquid form, and the required amount can easily be drawn up. Administering the correct amount also depends on the strength of the drug. For example, heparin is available in 5,000, 10,000 or 25,000 units/ml, so the amount injected will vary. Other injectables, such as penicillin, are produced in 'powder form' and require dilution before they can be administered. Where fluid is added, the solution displacement value must be taken into account. This can be found in the literature accompanying the vial and is usually 0.02 ml. If this value is not checked, it can result in erroneous doses being administered. When drugs are supplied at strengths different from the dosages that have been prescribed, the nurse must determine the quantity of drug that is to be administered. Special formulae are available, but it is also essential for the nurse to have a basic knowledge of arithmetic. The student who is experiencing difficulty should consult one of the many drug calculation textbooks now available (see further reading at end of chapter) or seek help from lecturers and clinical practice mentors.

Right time

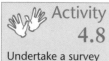

Activity 4.8

Undertake a survey of your patients to find out whether they receive their medications on time. Discuss your findings with your mentor. What effects will a delay have on the treatment programme?

In order to achieve maximum therapeutic effectiveness, the doctor will specify the number of times a day the drug is to be given. It is important to adhere to this regimen as closely as possible in order to maintain a relatively constant blood plasma level of the drug (Figure 4.2). If the plasma concentration of the drug falls below the minimum effective concentration, the action of the drug will be diminished. With antibiotics, this can lead to the development of resistant strains of bacteria. If the drug reaches the minimum toxic concentration, this may cause toxicity. Drugs often have to be given with or after meals, and it is important to ensure that the patient understands the reason for this.

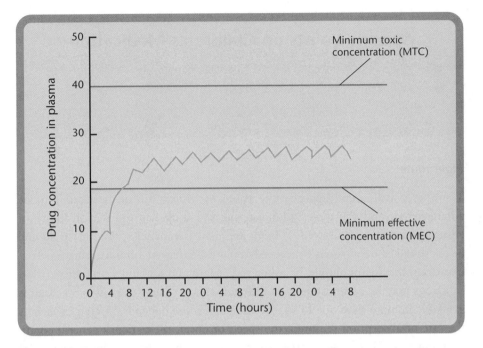

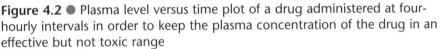

Figure 4.2 ● Plasma level versus time plot of a drug administered at four-hourly intervals in order to keep the plasma concentration of the drug in an effective but not toxic range

Right patient

It is vital to identify the right patient or client as drug errors can cause complications and may even become fatal. The following principles should be employed as a matter of routine regardless of the number of patients involved:

● In acute care settings, check the wrist identity bracelet and the name band on the bed
● If the patient is not confused, ask him to state his name but never prompt or say 'Are you Mr/Mrs ...?'
● If the patient questions the dosage, appearance or method of administration, always double-check the prescription and medication
● Never leave medicines for a patient who is not available during the drug round
● Never administer medications if you cannot confirm the identity of the patient.

Specific Points on Children's Medication

- ■ If the child is too young, ask the parents to confirm the child's identity
- ■ Children and parents have a right to know about the treatments and they should always be addressed by name.

Right route

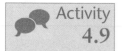

Activity
4.9

Discuss with your mentor the importance of administering medicines via the prescribed route. What information is given to the patients in anticipation of the procedure?

The doctor will usually specify the route by which the medication is to be administered, and the nurse administering the drug has the responsibility of ensuring that this is followed. If there are any discrepancies, the doctor should be consulted. If the nurse is concerned about the safety of administering a particular drug, the doctor should be asked to prepare and administer the drug.

Drugs may be administered via different routes (Chart 4.4). When a drug is available in more than one form, the choice of route depends on factors such as the rate of absorption required, the speed of onset, the patient's general condition and any side-effects. Nurses are not responsible for the administration of drugs by all these routes but may have to assist doctors, for example with intrathecal administration.

Chart 4.4 ● Routes of drug administration

- ● **Oral** – by mouth
- ● **Sublingual** – under the tongue
- ● **Injection** – intramuscular, subcutaneous, intradermal (into soft tissues)
- ● **Rectal** – into the rectum
- ● **Vaginal** – into the vagina
- ● **Topical** – on the skin or mucous membranes
- ● **Inhalation** – via the respiratory tract
- ● **Optic** – into the eye
- ● **Aural** – into the ear
- ● **Nasal** – into the nose
- ● **Intra-articular** – into the cavity of a joint
- ● **Intrathecal** – into the spinal fluid
- ● **Intravenous** – into a vein
- ● **Intracardiac** – into the heart

Oral medications

The **oral route** is the most frequently used route for drug administration. Oral medications are either in liquid (for example elixir) or solid (for example tablet) form. Some tablets (enteric coated) are covered with a substance that does not dissolve until the medication reaches the small intestine. These tablets should never be crushed or chewed because the medication will irritate the gastric mucosa. The administration of oral medication may be carried out by one or two registered nurses, depending on local policy.

oral route
via the mouth

Guidelines for oral drug administration

1. Wash your hands and wear gloves.
2. Check the prescription for completeness of date, time, drug to be given, dosage, route, frequency and duration of therapy. Check that the drug has not already been given and is due.
3. The nurse must have a basic understanding of the effects of the drug to be administered.
4. Select and check the required medication for discolouration, precipitation, contamination and expiry date.
5. Prepare the dosage as prescribed. Do not crush enteric-coated, sublingual or sustained-action tablets. Empty the required dose into a medicine pot. To prevent contamination, avoid touching the preparation. If dispensing liquid, the bottle should be held with the label towards the palm of the hand to prevent spillage obscuring the name of the drug.
6. Check the labels on containers again.
7. Take the medication and the prescription chart to the patient. Check the patient's identity (as described earlier) and the drug to be given.
8. Position the patient as upright as possible to aid swallowing, and instruct the patient accordingly. A glass of water or juice (50 ml or more) should be given to facilitate swallowing. The nurse must ensure that the patient has swallowed the medication. Infants and young children should be supported firmly to avoid spilling the medication.
9. Make the patient comfortable and ask her to stay upright for a few minutes.
10. Immediately complete all the necessary records.
11. Clear all the equipment.

Some patients with a nasogastric tube may have their oral medications administered through it. The procedure for administering a drug via this route is described in Chart 4.5. Liquid medications will flow easily down the tube; tablets and other solid medications should be avoided and alternative drugs

> **Link**
> Chapter 5 outlines the principles of managing a nasogastric tube.

Activity 4.10

Under direct supervision, help to administer oral drugs to clients.

used. Staff should avoid crushing tablets or opening capsules in order to administer the drug via the nasogastric tube as this process is in breach of the Medicines Act 1968 (Griffith, 2003).

The medication should not be added to the 'feed'. Instead, the continuous feeding should be interrupted and resumed after administration of the drug. The tube should be flushed with water prior to and after the administration of the drug.

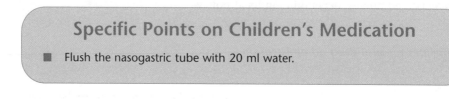

Specific Points on Children's Medication

■ Flush the nasogastric tube with 20 ml water.

Chart 4.5 ● Administering drugs via nasogastric tube

1. If possible, elevate the patient's head 30–45 degrees to avoid aspiration during and following administration

2. Check the placement of the nasogastric tube by aspirating a small quantity of gastric contents and testing for pH (Tremayne and Parboteeah, 2006). Acidity would indicate that the tube is in the stomach

3. Ensure the patency of the tube by flushing the tube with 30 ml of water for adults and 20 ml for children, using a 50 ml catheter tip syringe (Pickering, 2003)

4. Administer the medication* through a syringe barrel connected to the tubing, as shown in Figure 4.3. Hold the barrel of the syringe about 15 cms (6 inches) higher than the patient's nose and allow the fluid to flow into the stomach by gravity

5. Between medications, flush the tube with 5 ml of water

6. If the patient is on continuous feeding, the feeding is recommenced; otherwise the tube is clamped

* Follow the guidelines for preparing drugs as outlined above.

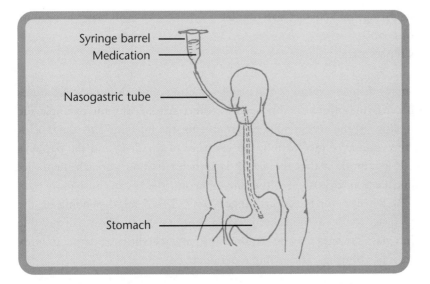

Figure 4.3 ● Administration of medication via a nasogastric tube. The fluid is allowed to flow into the stomach by gravity

Parenteral injections

The term **parenteral** refers to the act of administering medications by a route other than the alimentary tract. The term is most commonly used to indicate the injection routes such as intramuscular, subcutaneous and intravenous. (No details of intravenous administration are included, as this method requires additional training and competences that are outside the scope of this book.) Less common ways by which medications are administered include intrathecally, intra-articularly, intracardiac and intra-arterially, these more specialised procedures being performed by doctors. Drugs given parenterally have a more rapid effect as they achieve high plasma levels and therefore aid speedy treatment.

parenteral route
a route other than via the alimentary canal

Giving an injection is a procedure routinely undertaken by nurses and good technique is important as it can make the injection less painful and less traumatic for the patient. An injection is a procedure that introduces a substance into the body by piercing the skin or a mucosal membrane and depositing the medication in the right region; in the subcutaneous layer (subcutaneous injection), or in the muscle fascia (intramuscular injection).

When administering drugs by injection, it is important first to select and assemble the correct equipment:

● The patient's prescription
● The medication
● A clean tray

- A sterile syringe and correct size needles
- Alcohol swabs
- Gloves if necessary.

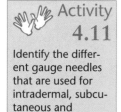

Activity 4.11

Identify the different gauge needles that are used for intradermal, subcutaneous and intramuscular injections, and for drawing up medications.

There are many different syringes and needles, suiting many different procedures (Table 4.2). It is important to choose the correct size needle, for example the length and gauge of the needle must be suitable for the injection site, the type of injection, the volume of medication, the viscosity of the drug and the patient's condition. It is important that the needle is sufficiently long to reach the target organ, as medications deposited in the subcutaneous tissues can cause more pain (Lenz, 1983). Syringes for injections range from 0.1 to 5 ml, depending on the volume of drug to be administered. Most hospitals use plastic disposable syringes, but glass syringes may be required for patients who are allergic to latex or for some types of drugs, for example paraldehyde.

Table 4.2 Selection of needles for different types of injection

Type of injection	Suggested needle gauge		Size of syringe
	Adult	Child	
Intradermal	26 G x ⅜" (0.45 x 10 mm)	26 G x ⅜" (0.45 x 10 mm)	1 ml calibrated in 0.1 ml divisions
Subcutaneous	25/26 G x ⅝" (0.45 x 16 mm)	26 G x ⅝" (0.45 x 16 mm)	1 ml calibrated in 0.1 ml divisions
Intramuscular	21 G x 1½" (0.8 x 40 mm)	23 G x 1¼" (0.6 x 30 mm)	5 ml calibrated in 0.2 ml divisions

Gloves should be worn to prevent cross-infection or if the drug is likely to cause skin sensitisation with frequent use. For example, dermatitis can be caused by frequent contact with drugs such as penicillin, streptomycin and chlorpromazine. When cytotoxic drugs are given, vinyl gloves should be worn; goggles and a mask may also be necessary.

Intramuscular injection

intramuscular route

into a muscle

The **intramuscular route** is used to administer medications that are irritating or painful. Skeletal muscles are well perfused with blood and have fewer pain receptors, so pain is minimal, causing less discomfort (Newton et al., 1992), and up to 5 ml of injectate may be given into the large muscles (1–2 ml into the deltoid muscle for example). To give an intramuscular injection:

1. Collect and check all the equipment to ensure sterility. If the outer packaging is damaged, replace the pack.
2. Wash your hands.
3. Prepare the needle(s) and syringe(s) on a tray. Check for any defects.
4. Check the patient's prescription(s) for completeness.
5. Select the drug and verify it against the prescription.
6. Prepare the drug, using gloves if necessary.
7. Administer the intramuscular injection.

Drawing medication from a single-dose ampoule

1. Check the ampoule for cracks, cloudiness and precipitation.
2. Gently tap the upper area of the ampoule to release any medication trapped at the top of the ampoule.
3. Cover the neck of the ampoule or use an 'ampoule breaker' when snapping it open.
4. Insert the needle into the ampoule and withdraw the required amount. Avoid contaminating the medication.
5. Change the needle and dispose of it as per hospital policy.
6. Tap the barrel to dislodge any air bubbles towards the needle and expel the air.

Drawing medication from a multidose vial solution

1. Remove the metal cover from the vial and inspect the medication as above.
2. Clean the rubber cap with antiseptic solution and let it dry.
3. Withdraw the prescribed amount of solution. Two methods can be used to draw the solution:
   – Method A. Insert a 19 G needle into the cap to vent the vial. Insert the assembled needle and syringe, and draw up the required amount.
   – Method B. Assemble the needle and syringe. Fill the syringe with the same volume of air as the medication that will be withdrawn. Insert the needle through the rubber stopper, holding the vial at an oblique angle, and inject the air into the vial. Keep the needle in the solution, invert the vial and allow the medication to enter the syringe. The volume can be adjusted by using the plunger, and the needle is removed when the required amount has been drawn up.
4. Change the needle as it may have become blunted/damaged.
5. Tap the barrel to dislodge any air bubbles towards the needle and expel the air.

It is preferable to use single-dose vials rather than multidose vials whenever possible, as these multidose vials remain prone to bacterial contamination (Phillips et al., 1989; Simon et al., 1993).

Reconstituting a powdered medication

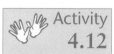

Activity 4.12

Under direct supervision in the skills laboratory or clinical area, prepare a powdered medication for injection.

1. Clean the rubber cap with an antiseptic and allow it to dry.
2. Add the required amount of diluent carefully down the wall of the vial, and allow an equal amount of air to escape into the syringe.
3. Check for the displacement value of the drug.
4. Remove the needle and syringe.
5. Shake the vial to dissolve the powder.
6. The reconstituted solution can now be withdrawn as described for removing solutions from a multidose vial.

Guidelines for intramuscular injection

1. Identify the patient and explain the procedure. It is important to gain the patient's cooperation. Bolander (1994) advocates engaging the patient in conversation to distract the patient from the procedure.
2. Position the patient for easy access to the injection site, comfort and privacy. Infants and children should be held firmly so that they do not move and thus receive injuries during the procedure.
3. Clean the site with antiseptic and allow the alcohol to evaporate.
4. Holding the needle at 90 degrees (Figure 4.4), quickly insert the needle into the muscle. Leave a third of the needle shaft exposed. If the needle breaks from the hub, it can thus be removed safely.

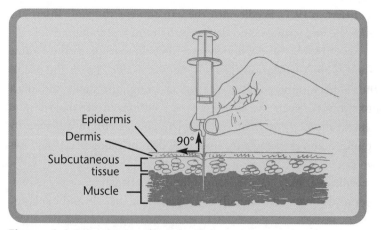

Figure 4.4 ● Intramuscular injection

5. Pull back the plunger for 5–10 seconds. If blood appears, withdraw the needle and repeat the procedure with a sterile needle in a different place. Explain to the patient what is happening.
6. If no blood appears, depress the plunger and inject the drug slowly.
7. Quickly withdraw the needle and apply gentle pressure over the puncture site.
8. Position the patient comfortably.
9. Dispose of the needle and syringe as per hospital policy.
10. Complete all the necessary records.

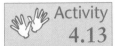

Activity 4.13

On a model, identify the sites for intramuscular injections. Did your patients have a preference for which sites were used? Observe patients during an intramuscular injection and discuss your findings with your supervisor.

Sites for intramuscular injection

Various sites on the human body may be used for giving an injection. When choosing a site, it is important to identify the anatomical landmarks in order to avoid injuring nerves, striking bones or puncturing blood vessels. The site must also be inspected for its suitability, for example:

● Is there sufficient muscle mass?
● Does the area to be injected have a good blood supply?
● Is there any skin damage?
● Is there evidence of fibrosis or infection?

When patients are receiving frequent intramuscular or subcutaneous injections, for example of insulin, it is important to rotate the injection site to obtain greater drug absorption, decrease tissue fibrosis and cause minimal discomfort to the patient. A rotation chart may be useful in implementing an effective rotation programme. The most frequently used sites for intramuscular injections are outlined below.

The deltoid muscle in the upper arm
The deltoid is used for small quantities of injectate, 1 ml or less, of clear, non-irritating medication such as vaccines. The muscle is located in the lateral aspect of the upper arm. The injection site (Figure 4. 5) is located 4–5 cm below the acromion process and above the deltoid groove in adults, and approximately 2 cm below the acromion process in older children.

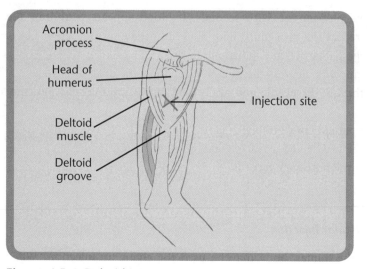

Figure 4.5 ● Deltoid injection site

The dorsogluteal site in the buttocks

If the dorsogluteal site (Figure 4.6) is chosen for the intramuscular injection, the nurse must have a full understanding of the anatomy of the site and surrounding anatomical structures, be able to accurately identify anatomical landmarks and site boundaries, and administer the injection with meticulous technique, as the sciatic nerve and the superior gluteal artery run close to this site. The injection site is identified by palpating the anatomical landmarks of the posterior superior iliac spine and the greater trochanter (at the head of the femur). A line is drawn between these two points and a safe injection site is in the area above and lateral

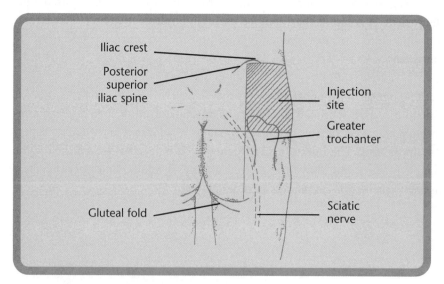

Figure 4.6 ● Dorsogluteal injection site

to this line. The area below this line should be avoided to prevent damage to the sciatic nerve.

The patient should be asked to lie prone with the toes pointing inwards to relax the buttocks. This site should not be used in infants or children who have not been walking for at least one year since this muscle is not developed.

The ventrogluteal site in the hip area

There is wide agreement in the literature that the ventrogluteal site is preferable to the dorsogluteal site for intramuscular injections as it is free of major nerves and blood vessels (Beecroft and Redick, 1990; Covington and Trattler, 1997). The injection is given in the gluteus medius and gluteus maximus muscles. The patient is placed on his side or can be allowed to stay in the supine or prone position. To find the injection site on the right hip (the most convenient site for right-handed practitioners), palpate the greater trochanter, the iliac crest and the anterior superior iliac spine. Place the palm of the left hand on the greater trochanter and the left index finger towards the anterior superior iliac spine (Figure 4.7). Move the middle finger away from the index finger to form a V between the fingers. The injection is given into the centre of the V. This is the preferred site for infants and children who have not been walking for a year (Beecroft, 1990; Whalley and Wong, 1995) because the pelvis is concave below the iliac crest and contains a relatively large muscle mass.

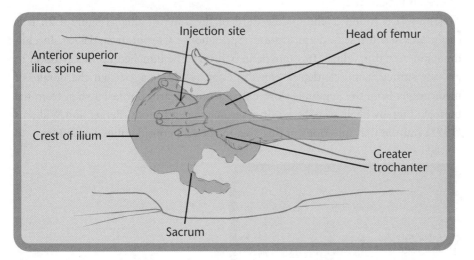

Figure 4.7 ● Ventrogluteal site on the right hip

The vastus lateralis in the thigh

This muscle is situated in the lateral thigh and can be used for both adults and children. This site (Figure 4.8) is preferable because there are no major blood vessels or nerves in the area. The patient is asked to lie in the supine position with the thigh well exposed, pointing the toe inwards to give a better exposure of the lateral aspects of the thigh. The injection site can be located by dividing the thigh horizontally and vertically into thirds by placing one hand's breadth below the greater trochanter at the top of the thigh and one hand's breadth from the knee. The thigh is then measured vertically, this time by placing one hand's breadth along the middle of the inner side of the thigh and one hand's breadth on the outer side of the thigh, thus creating a rectangle in the middle where it is safe to inject. This strip is 2–4 cm long in children and about 7 cm long in adults. The needle is directed into the tissues at a right angle.

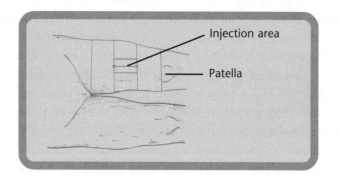

Figure 4.8 ● Vastus lateralis injection site

The rectus femoris site

This muscle is found in the middle third of the anterior thigh (Figure 4.9). It is easily accessed for self-administration (Springhouse Corporation, 1993). In children and very thin adults, this muscle may need to be bunched up in a handful to 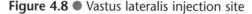 provide sufficient muscle depth. Newton et al. (1992) suggest that the uptake of medications from this region is slower than from the arm but faster than from the buttock, thereby facilitating better drug serum concentrations. Berger and Williams (1992) caution that injections in this area may cause considerable discomfort.

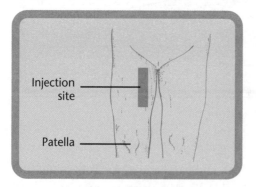

Figure 4.9 ● Rectus femoris site

Specific Points on Children's Injections

Injections can cause substantial distress to children and many view injections as the most traumatic experience of being in a hospital (Cummings et al., 1996; Cordoni and Cordoni, 2001). An important factor in helping children to cope with the procedure is to enable them to have some control of the situation, such as indicating their preferences with respect to time and events, positive reinforcements or even some form of reward.

■ Sites for intramuscular injection in infants and children who have not been walking for one year

　1.　Vastus lateralis in the middle third of femur (Figure 4.8)

　2.　Ventrogluteal (Figure 4.7).

■ Sites for intramuscular injection in older children who have been walking for more than one year

　1.　Vastus lateralis (Figure 4.8)

　2.　Dorsogluteal site in the gluteus medius muscle (Figure 4.6)

　3.　Deltoid muscle for older children (Figure 4.5).

Z-track intramuscular injection

This technique for intramuscular injection has been primarily reserved for use with medications such as iron preparations that are known to be particularly irritating and can permanently stain the subcutaneous tissue. During this procedure, there is lateral displacement of the cutaneous tissue prior to injection, and the tension is released immediately after injection. When utilising the Z-track technique, the nurse grasps the muscle and pulls it laterally about 2.5 cm until it is taut, holding the tissue in this position. The needle is inserted at a 90 degree angle. After ensuring the position of the needle, the medication is injected. Following withdrawal of the needle, the skin is immediately released.

Complications of intramuscular injections

The nurse should be aware of the possible complications of injections and make every effort to prevent them.

Infection

The introduction of infection via a needle may lead to local (abscesses) or systemic (septicaemia) complications. It is important to maintain strict asepsis during all invasive procedures. All equipment should be sterile, and good hand-washing is essential.

Muscle myopathy

Intramuscular injections, by their very nature, cause injury to tissues. Needle myopathy damage can be prevented by good injection technique using the optimum-sized needles. Focal myopathy can be caused by the injectates and by using injectorates of neutral pH.

Wrong route

Injectates may accidentally be given into a vein or an artery, resulting in a rapid physiological response. Depending on the drug used, severe complications and even death may occur. The syringe should be aspirated before the drug is injected. If blood appears in the barrel of the syringe, the needle is withdrawn and an alternative site used. The patient should be informed of the reasons for this. Drugs injected in an artery may cause thrombosis, with disruption of the blood supply.

Nerve damage

Nerve damage (to the sciatic nerve) in the dorsogluteal region should be avoided. The nurse should identify the landmarks, as shown in Figure 4.6 and select a safe area for injection. Sciatic nerve injury resulting from erroneous injection cause client discomfort, morbidity and lasting disability (Small, 2004).

Activity 4.14

Undertake an internet search to find out more about the complications of intramuscular injections and discuss your findings with your mentor.

Subcutaneous injections

subcutaneous route

under the skin

The sites for administering **subcutaneous** injections include the lateral aspects of the upper arm, the abdomen on either side of the umbilicus, the middle and outer area of the thigh and the back (Figure 4.10). It is important to allow diabetic patients to maintain their own subcutaneous injections while in hospital.

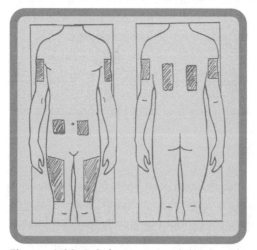

Figure 4.10 ● Subcutaneous injection site

Guidelines for administering a subcutaneous injection

1. Explain the procedure to the patient and gain his cooperation.
2. Select the site and assist the patient into position to maintain his comfort and dignity.
3. Expose the injection site; in a viable injection site the nurse should be able to pinch at least 2.5 cm of subcutaneous tissue. Check the rotation chart if one is in use.
4. Wash your hands thoroughly to prevent infection.
5. Prepare medication.
6. Ensure site is clean and safe for injecting medication.
7. Grasp the skin firmly between the thumb and forefinger, as shown in Figure 4.11.
8. Maintain the fold and insert the needle almost to its full length at an angle of 90 degrees.
9. Inject the medication and remove the needle.
10. Safely discard the syringe and needle.
11. Wash your hands.
12. Complete all the relevant records.

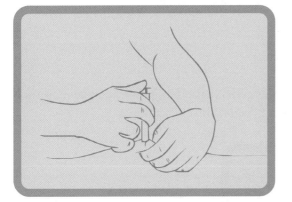

Figure 4.11 ● Current recommended method for injecting insulin at right angles with the skin pinched

Intradermal injections

Intradermal administration is frequently used for diagnostic purposes, the injectate being placed within the layers of the skin just below the epidermis (Figure 4.12). Small amounts of medication, usually not more than 0.5 ml, are administered. The site most often used is the central forearm, but other areas, such as the back and the chest, are acceptable.

intradermal
_____
within the layers of the skin

Guidelines for giving an intradermal injection

1. Wash your hands. Check the prescription for completeness as described earlier. Prepare the equipment (a 1 ml syringe with a 26 G × 16 mm needle).
2. Explain the procedure to the patient and gain his cooperation.
3. Select the site and assist the patient into position to maintain his comfort and dignity. Select a site with minimal, or preferably no, hair and skin blemishes.
4. Clean the area with antiseptic solution. Avoid using iodine solutions as the residual stain may interfere with interpreting the results of the skin test. If the skin is oily, cleanse the area with acetone to remove any fat deposits. Allow the skin to dry.
5. Support the patient's arm and stretch the skin taut.
6. Place the bevel of the needle almost flat against the patient's skin and insert the needle with the bevel side up at an angle of 10–15 degrees (Figure 4.12). The needle should be about 3 mm below the skin surface. The medication is slowly injected while watching for a wheal to develop, which verifies that the medication has entered the dermis (McConnell, 2000).
7. Once the wheal appears, withdraw the needle and circle the injection site.
8. The area should never be massaged as it may interfere with the test results.
9. If the test is carried out to determine sensitivity, follow the text instructions to determine, for example, signs of local reaction.
10. Discard the equipment.
11. Wash your hands.
12. Complete all the relevant records.

When testing for allergies, it is essential that resuscitation equipment is available in case the patient develops a hypersensitive reaction.

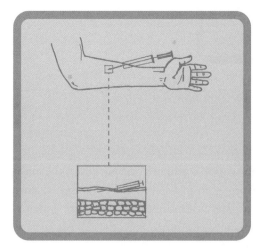

Figure 4.12 ● Intradermal injection

Topical medications

Topical administration refers to the application of medications to the skin or mucous membranes to achieve local or systemic effects. The medication may be incorporated into a base such as an oil, lotion or cream, which is rubbed into the skin (**inunction**), the area being cleaned with soap and water before application. The inunction can be applied with the fingers and hands, or using cotton wool balls or gauze swabs. If there is a risk of infection or application is to the mucous membranes, gloves should be worn.

topical
applied to the skin or mucous membranes

inunction
rubbing a drug mixed with a fatty base into the skin; also the name given to the mixture

Guidelines for the topical administration of drugs

1. Wash your hands. Check the prescription as discussed above before administering the drug.
2. Explain the procedure to the patient, who is positioned to expose the area and carry out any assessments. Observe for any changes. The patient's privacy and dignity should be maintained.
3. Prepare the equipment, and follow aseptic guidelines if there is risk of infection. Remove solid or semisolid medications with a sterile spatula.
4. Apply the medication to the site.
5. Inform the patient if the preparation is likely to cause skin staining or soiling of clothing.
6. Complete the appropriate records.

Guidelines for application of transdermal medications

More drugs are now becoming available that can be administered via the **transdermal route**, for example glyceryl trinitrate derivatives (Transiderm-Nitro), opiates and some analgesics (Amitop, Emla). Following application of the patch, the drug is absorbed through the hair follicles and sweat glands, entering the bloodstream.

transdermal route
application directly on to the skin, the substance applied then being absorbed via the skin

Before any patch can be applied, the previous application must be removed from the patient's skin. The prescription is checked to ensure the patient's safety. The new patch is then applied to a clean, non-hairy skin surface, the most frequently used sites being the chest wall, the upper arms, the backs of the hands and the antecubital fossae, depending on the intended use of the medication. The patches should have labels indicating the date and time of application and the signature of the practitioner.

To prevent inflammation and irritation, the site should be rotated and recorded on a rotation chart. If the patch has been properly applied, the patient is able to shower or bath.

Eye medication

Eye medications are available in two forms: eye ointment and eye drops. The administration of eye drops and eye ointment will initially be the responsibility of the nurse, but he or she may also be involved in instructing the patient as well as other members of the family how to administer the medication. It is important that the correct eye is treated. The prescription must be carefully checked and any abbreviations verified. The patient should be informed if her vision is going to be affected after the procedure. Although the eye is not sterile, it is important to use aseptic techniques when performing eye treatment. If infection is present in both eyes, the least affected eye is treated first to prevent cross-contamination. The following general guidelines should be used when administering eye drops and eye ointment.

1. Explain the procedure to the patient, emphasising that her nose may feel as if it is 'running', because the punctum of the eye drains into the nasal space. The patient may also get a taste of the drug at the back of her throat.
2. Ideally, the patient should be lying flat, with her head tilted backwards to allow easy access to the eyes. The nurse should stand behind the patient's head as it is easier to administer the drug from that position.
3. Prepare all the necessary equipment. Warm the eye drops and ointment to room temperature.
4. Wash your hands and put on gloves if necessary.
5. Check the eye and perform eye toilet as necessary.
6. Gently pull down the lower lid to form a pouch, as shown in Figure 4.13. Gently drop the required number of drops into the pouch. Ask the patient to close the eye gently and blink several times. The nurse must wait for two minutes before instilling another drug. For eye ointment, start from the angle near the nose (the inner canthus) and work towards the ear, gently squeezing the tube along the inner edge of the lower lid. Avoid touching the eye with the sharp nozzle. An eye pad may be applied if requested. Separate tubes/bottles should always be used for the left and right eyes.
7. The patient should be advised not to rub or squeeze the eye. Leave the patient comfortable.
8. Remove any gloves used. Wash your hands.
9. Complete all the necessary documentation.

Specific Points on Children's Medication

■ The nurse should get extra help so that the head can be held still during eye and ear treatments, to prevent the child rubbing his eyes or ears, and to provide comfort and reassurance.

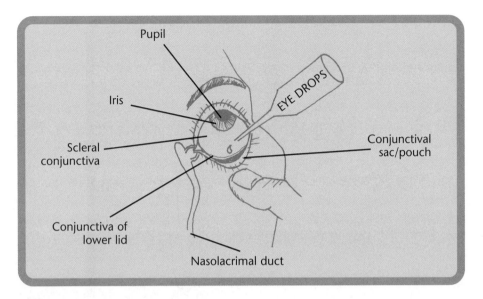

Figure 4.13 ● Instilling eye drops or ointment into the conjunctival sac/pouch

Ear medication

1. Wash your hands and put on gloves if necessary.
2. Prepare all the necessary equipment and check the prescription for completeness.
3. Warm the medication to room temperature.
4. Clean the outer canal if necessary. Normal saline may be used.
5. Ask the patient to lie on the side with the ear to be treated facing upwards.
6. In adults and children over three years old, gently pull the pinna upwards and backwards and instil the prescribed number of drops in the ear canal (Figure 4.14b). In children below three years of age, gently pull the pinna downwards and backwards and instil the prescribed number of drops (Figure 4.14a).
7. Advise the patient to remain in that position for five minutes.
8. When the patient is allowed to sit up, cleanse the external ear of any spillages or leakages, and make the patient comfortable.
9. Remove gloves and wash your hands.
10. Complete all the relevant records.

If both ears are to be treated, wait for 15 minutes between instillations.

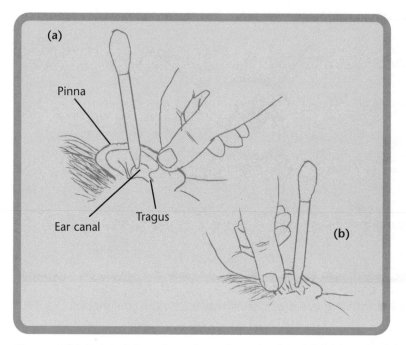

Figure 4.14 ● Administration of ear drops in the child (a) and adult (b)

Nasal medication

A number of drugs, for example nitroglycerine and ephedrine, are available for use as nasal sprays or nasal drops. The nasal drops and sprays should be used appropriately or the drug's effectiveness will be diminished.

Nasal drops may flood the sinuses or dribble down the throat and be ingested. The patient should be advised to expectorate any drug going down the throat rather than swallow it. The timing of these drugs is important, and they should be administered 20 minutes before meals so that the nasal passages will be clear during feeding.

1. Wash your hands and put on gloves if necessary.
2. Prepare all the necessary equipment and check the prescription for completeness.
3. Get the patient to clear his nasal passages; provide some tissues.
4. For a nasal spray, keep the head and spray container upright. Squeeze the container as instructed and, following each spray, ask the patient to take a deep sniff. Repeat with the other nostril. For nasal drops, it is better if the patient is lying down. Instil the required amount of medication, inserting the dropper approximately 0.5 cm into the nostril. The tip of the dropper should

not become contaminated. Young children may be held on the lap with the neck extended.

5. Provide the patient with tissues and make him comfortable.
6. Complete all the relevant documentation.

Administering medication via a nebuliser

A number of drugs are now available for administration via a nebuliser for their action in the respiratory system. Administering a drug via a nebuliser produces a mist, enabling the drug to be inhaled directly into the lungs (Porter-Jones, 2000). Before starting the procedure, it is important to ensure that the equipment is in good working order and, if a cylinder of gas is used, that there is sufficient gas to complete the treatment.

> **Link**
>
> *Chapter 7 discusses methods of delivering drugs by inhalation.*

1. The nurse should assemble oxygen supply or compressed air box machine/cylinder, mouthpiece or mask as preferred by the patient, a nebuliser system and tubing.
2. Sit the patient up to maximise lung expansion and record peak flow.
3. Inform patient of the noise generated by the system to allay anxiety.
4. Encourage the patient to adopt a normal pattern of breathing when receiving the nebuliser.
5. Prepare the medication as instructed.
6. Unscrew the nebuliser (in the middle) and pour the contents of the drug/solution into the nebuliser chamber.
7. Screw the nebuliser back together, attach the mouthpiece or mask to the nebuliser and connect the tubing to the nebuliser and attach to either the oxygen supply or compressed air box/cylinder.
8. Turn the flow rate on the oxygen/air cylinder to the required prescribed amount or switch on the compressed air box machine.
9. Once the mist begins to appear at the mouthpiece, ask the patient to insert mouthpiece into their mouth or to put the mask on.
10. Observe for any side-effects.
11. Record peak flow to monitor the effectiveness of the nebulised medication. Make patient comfortable at the end of the procedure.
12. Complete all documentation.

Rectal medications

The **rectal route** is frequently used for the administration of drugs in adults and children. The action of the drug can be local (for example lubricant suppositories) or systemic (for example aminophylline). These medications are in the form

rectal route
via the rectum

of a suppository, cream or solution. It is vital that children receiving such medication have been prepared for the procedure, using phrases that the child can understand.

Link

Chapter 6 also discusses the administration of suppositories.

1. Wash your hands.
2. Prepare all the equipment and check the prescription for completeness.
3. Explain the procedure to the patient and provide privacy.
4. Position the patient on his left side and only expose the buttocks.
5. Put gloves on.
6. The suppository is lubricated with a water-soluble lubricant (KY-Jelly).
7. The buttocks are separated to expose the anus.
8. Ask the patient to take a deep breath and insert the suppository past the anal sphincter. Clean away any excess lubricant.
9. Ask the patient to refrain from pushing the suppository out and make him comfortable. Children and infants may be held or cuddled to distract them. (A commode should be available to avoid any embarrassment.)
10. Dispose of all equipment and wash your hands.
11. Complete all the relevant records.

Specific Points on Children's Medication

■ When giving a suppository to an infant or toddler, he can lie on his back with his legs flexed. The suppository is inserted using the index finger for children over three years. In children of three years or less, the little finger may be used.

Vaginal medications

vaginal route
into the vagina

Medications intended for administration via the **vaginal route** are available in many forms – pessaries, creams and medicated douches – most of which can only be administered using special applicators.

The patient should be encouraged to empty her bladder as she is expected to remain lying down for 20 minutes after insertion of the medication.

1. Wash your hands.
2. Prepare all the equipment and check the prescription for completeness.
3. Explain the procedure to the patient and provide privacy. Select the appropriate position, either supine with the knees drawn up and legs parted, or left lateral with the knees drawn up.
4. Wash your hands and put on gloves.
5. Lubricate the pessary or applicator.

6. Insert the pessary along the posterior vaginal wall and into the top of the vagina. If using an applicator, insert the barrel of the applicator into the vagina as far as it will go. Squeeze the tube to insert the drug while holding the applicator steady. Withdraw the applicator, and make the patient comfortable.
7. Provide the patient with sanitary towels and advise her to remain in position for 20 minutes.
8. Discard the equipment or clean it for reuse.
9. Remove gloves and wash your hands.
10. Complete all the relevant documentation.

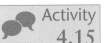

Activity 4.15

Discuss with your mentor the benefits of administering drugs rectally. What are the ethical issues when administering drugs via the rectal and vaginal routes? Identify which drugs are routinely given via these routes.

Patient education and compliance in drug administration

Drug therapy can only be effective when the patient cooperates with the drug regimen and correctly takes all the prescribed drugs. In hospitalised patients, drug treatment is closely supervised. In contrast, once discharged from hospital care, many patients fail to continue with their treatment for a number of reasons:

● Forgetfulness
● A lack of understanding of the illness and/or drugs
● Unclear instructions
● The cost of the medication
● Non-acceptance of the diagnosis
● Inconvenience, such as when at school
● A confusing cocktail of medications
● Side-effects of the drugs, including the fear of addiction.

The concept of concordance has been put forward, which describes the interaction between prescriber, patient and their medicines as being more of a shared process leading to an agreement of the overall aims of any medication and how these can be achieved. In this process, the patient is actively involved and ultimately influences the outcome.

General principles when administering medications to children

It is essential to provide safe and effective drug therapy to children. Because of anatomical and physiological differences, the drug's pharmacokinetic properties – absorption, distribution, metabolism and excretion – may be affected. For more details of drug pharmacokinetics in children and infants, the reader is advised to consult textbooks on paediatric pharmacology.

General guidelines for giving medications to children

1. It is important to establish a trusting relationship with the child and identify any preferences. Always be honest regarding painful injections or distasteful medications. Remain calm.
2. Adequate time should be allowed prior to and after the administration of drugs to comfort the child. It may take longer than expected to explain to the child and give any instructions that they must follow to enhance the effectiveness of therapy.
3. The nurse should be kind but firm when approaching the child.
4. Organise help to control and support children. Do not interrupt what the child is doing; make medicine-taking a part of it.
5. Identify the child correctly, checking with the parents. If possible, organise drug administration when the parents are present.
6. Explain the procedure to the child and parents. Parents may provide information on how the child likes to take her medication. Offer a choice, for example taking it from the parent or nurse.
7. Avoid mixing medications in milk or essential foods or the child may avoid those foods and develop malnutrition or dehydration.
8. If possible, allow children to participate, for example choosing the juice to be drunk with the medicine.
9. Reward children for taking their medication, but avoid punishing children who are uncooperative.
10. Do not anticipate difficulty: the child quickly picks up your anxiety.
11. Never make a promise you cannot keep.

Specific guidelines when giving injections to children

1. The aseptic and safe-checking procedures should be followed as discussed.
2. Prepare the equipment and check the prescription for completeness.
3. Explain the procedure to the child in a manner consistent with the child's age and understanding. Audiovisual aids such as booklets or dolls may be used to get the message across. Parents should be informed and involved in supporting the child.
4. Appropriate restraint, for example a blanket, may be required.
5. Select the injection site (see above).
6. The procedure should be undertaken quickly and gently.
7. Support is provided as necessary by the nurse and/or parents.

Giving medications to clients with learning disabilities

Clients with learning disabilities may have varying degrees of mental and physical disabilities, and it may be as difficult for the nurse to explain as for the patient to understand. Following the five Rs of drug administration should secure the client's safety. The client may also suffer from physical deformities, which may require adapting methods and in some cases changing the form of the drug and the route of administration. The pharmacist may be able to help with special preparations. Liquid preparations are safer than tablets or capsules. Swallowing may also be stimulated by gentle downward stroking motions over the larynx.

Giving medications to patients with mental illness

The principle of consent continues to apply to any medication for conditions not related to the mental disorder for which clients have been detained (UKCC, 2001). In relation to medication for the mental disorder for which the client has been detained, medicines can be given against patient's wishes during the first three months of a treatment order (UKCC, 2001).

The side-effects of some medications used to treat mental health problems may cause physical symptoms (Seymour, 2003) and it is important that regular reviews are in place to monitor for side-effects. Side-effects of antipsychotic drugs are listed in Chart 4.6.

Chart 4.6 ● Side-effects of antipsychotic drugs

- Unusual body movements
- Feeling drowsy and sedated
- Heart arrhythmia
- Weight gain (Clozapine, olanzapine)
- Diabetes
- Excess salivation
- Stroke
- Dizziness
- Blurred vision
- Hormonal changes: increased levels of prolactin causing osteoporosis, reduced libido, impotence

The National Institute for Mental Health (NIMH) and Mentality (2004) recommend that patients are closely monitored to assess the impact of medication on physical illness.

Medication errors

Finally, although medication errors should be avoided at all costs, it is possible that these may occur. Incidents should be immediately reported to the nurse in charge and the doctor. The patient should be monitored for any side-effects and be informed of what has happened. Preventive measures may be taken to control the effects of the drugs. The incident is usually investigated, and if the nurse has been found to be negligent, disciplinary action may be taken by the employing authority and the NMC. The patient can also take legal action against the nurse or the employer. Thus, the advice is to be a safe practitioner.

■ Chapter Summary

This chapter has described some of the key aspects of safe practice in preventing cross-infection and the administration of medicines. Every activity that the nurse undertakes carries considerable risk to the patient as well as to the nurse. By applying the principles described in this chapter, the nurse can ensure that nursing procedures are carried out safely, that patients are not harmed and that their care is optimised.

Test Yourself!

1. What does HCAI stand for?
2. What stages are involved in the chain of infection?
3. What are the commonest sites for HCAIs?
4. Describe the classification for clinical waste.
5. Name the five Rs in relation to drug administration.
6. Which five sites can be used for injections?
7. What side-effects can arise from using antipsychotic drugs?

■ Further Reading

Lapham, R. and Agar, H. (1995) *Drug Calculations for Nurses: A Step by Step Approach.* Arnold, London.

Greenstein, B. (2004) *Trounce's Clinical Pharmacology for Nurses*, 17th edn. Churchill Livingstone, Edinburgh.

■ References

Beecroft, P.C. (1990) Intramuscular injection practices of paediatric nurses: site selection. *Nurse Educator* **5**(4): 23–8.

Beecroft, P.C. and Redick, S.A. (1990) Intramuscular injection practices of paediatric nurses: site selection. *Nurse Educator* **15**: 23–8.

Berger, K.J. and Williams, M.S. (1992) *Fundamentals of Nursing: Collaborating for Optimal Health*. Appleton and Lange, Stamford, CT.

Bolander, V.R. (1994) A psychological approach. In Sorenson, K.C. and Luckmann, J. *Basic Nursing*, 3rd edn. WB Saunders, Philadelphia.

Cordoni, A. and Cordoni, L.E. (2001) Eutectic mixture of local anesthetics reduces pain during catheter insertion in paediatric patients. *Clinical Journal of Pain* **17**: 115–18.

Covington, T.P. and Tratler, M.R. (1997) Bull's eye! Finding the right target for IM injections. *Nursing* **27**: 62–3.

Cummings, E.A., Reid, C.J., Finley, G.A., McGrath, P.J. and Ritchie, J.A. (1996) Prevalence and source of pain in paediatric inpatients. *Pain* **68**: 25–31.

DoH (Department of Health) (2005) *Action on Health Care Associated Infection in England*. DoH, London.

Emmerson, A.M., Kelsey, M,C. and Smyth, S.T.M. (1996) The second national prevalence survey of infection in hospitals – overview of results. *Journal of Hospital Infection* **32**: 175–90.

Griffith, R. (2003) Covert administration of medicines. *The Pharmaceutical Journal* **271**(7258): 90–1.

Health Services Advisory Committee (1999) *Safe Disposal of Clinical Waste*. Health and Safety Executive, Norwich.

Lenz, C.L. (1983) Make your needle selection right to the point. *Nursing* **13**: 50–1.

McConnell, E.S. (2000) Administering an intradermal injection. *Nursing* **30**(3): 17.

NIMH/Mentality (2004) *Promoting Healthy Living for People who Experience Mental Distress*. NIMH/Mentality, London. http://kc.nimhe.orgn.uk.upload_HealthyBody-HealthyMind/-servicesusers.pdf.

Newton. M., Newton, D.W. and Fudin, J. (1992) Reviewing the three big injection routes. *Nursing* **22**: 34–42.

NMC (Nursing and Midwifery Council) (2004) *Guidelines for the Administration of Medicines*. NMC, London.

Phillips, G., Fleming, L.W. and Stewart, W.K. (1989) The potential hazard of using multiple-dose heparin and insulin vials in continuous ambulatory peritoneal dialysis. *Journal of Hospital Infection* **14**: 174–7.

Pickering, K. (2003) The administration of drugs via the enteral feeding tubes. *Nursing Times* **99**(46): 46–9.

Porter-Jones, G. (2000) Nebulisers – 1: Preparation. *Nursing Times* **96**(36): 45–6.

RCN (Royal College of Nursing) (1992) *Introduction to Methicillin Resistant Staphylococcus Aureus*. Safety Representatives Conference Committee, RCN, London.

Seymour, L. (2003) *Not all in the Mind – The Physical Health of Mental Health Users. Radical Mentalities*, briefing paper 2. Mentality, London.

Simon, P.A., Chen, R.T., Elliot, J.A. and Schwartz, B. (1993) Outbreak of pyogenic abscesses after diphtheria and tetanus toxoids and pertussis vaccination. *Pediatric Infectious Disease* **12**: 368–71.

Small, S.P. (2004) Preventing sciatic nerve injury from intramuscular injections: literature review. *Journal of Advanced Nursing* **47**(3): 287–96.

Springhouse Corporation (1993) *Medication Administration and IV Therapy Manual*, 2nd edn. Springhouse Corporation, Philadelphia, PA.

Tremayne, P. and Parboteeah, S. (2006) *Fundamental Aspects of Adult Nursing*, Quay Publishing, London.

UKCC (2001) *Position Statement on the Covert Administration of Medicines*. UKCC, London.

Whalley, L.F. and Wong, D.L. (1995) *Nursing Care of Infants and Children*, 4th edn. Mosby, London.

Winslow, E.H. (1997) Just how illegible are physicians' medical orders? *American Journal of Nursing* **97**(9): 66.

◼ Useful Websites

www.bnf.org British National Formulary
Provides information on the selection and clinical use of medicines

www.nhs.direct.nhs.uk NHS Direct
Online NHS help guide to aid diagnosis and treatment of illness

www.mentality.org.uk The Sainsbury Centre for Mental Health
Provides information about mental health promotion

www.nelh.nhs.uk/clinicalevidence National Electronic Library for Health
Provides information on clinical evidence

SUE M. GREEN AND PENELOPE M. SIMPSON

Chapter

Eating and Drinking

5

Contents

Learning Outcomes

The purpose of this chapter is to encourage you to apply the essentials of nutrition and hydration to your everyday life and that of your clients. At the end of the chapter, you should be able to:

- Describe and explain the principles of a healthy diet and fluid intake

- Enable others to make healthy changes to their food and fluid intake

- Screen clients' nutritional status

- Assist clients in achieving optimum nutrition and hydration

- Suggest a range of helpful strategies for use when assisting clients to eat and drink

- Extend your range of skills in promoting effective nutrition and hydration

- Promote the dignity of the client needing nutritional support.

There will be reflective activities, activities for you to undertake, reading activities, case histories and review questions to ensure that you interact with the material in a useful and practical way.

Food is fundamental to physical survival. It is needed for growth, repair and the manufacture of elements that protect us from disease. Humans will literally eat almost anything to satisfy extreme hunger. Once survival has been ensured, other factors, for example age, culture, history, religion, access, taste and preferences, come into play.

Food is composed of nutrients, which are required in appropriate amounts by the body to enable it to function effectively, not just today but next week and next year, and in order to stay healthy into later life. Clients' ability, motivation or knowledge to obtain appropriate amounts of nutrients may, however, be impaired, in which case it is the nurse's responsibility to assist, empower and educate. The United Kingdom Central Council for Nursing, Midwifery and Health Visiting (UKCC) reminded us in the 1997 'Feeding of Patients' letter that, even if this task is delegated to others, the responsibility remains with the nurse, who is accountable for all aspects of nursing care. This chapter reviews the concept of a healthy diet and what nutrients form foods, and then considers the role of the nurse in the nutritional care of patients or clients.

■ What is a Healthy Diet?

Concepts of a 'healthy diet' have steadily altered across time in response to beliefs and research, and at no other time in history have we had access to so much evidence of the impact of food on the human body. Despite considerable 'hype' from those with vested interests and frivolous speculation from irresponsible journalism, there is now a clear consensus about what a 'healthy diet' consists of, which has remained relatively consistent over the past few years. The Department of Health's guidelines (2003a) for a healthy diet are represented in the health promotion tool 'The plate model' (FSA, 2005), shown in Figure 5.1.

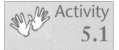

Activity 5.1

Give an example of your own food choices for each category. Try to identify why your choice has developed this way. Then do this activity with a client.

This shows the five major food groups and the proportion each should contribute to the dietary intake. This model outlines that the diet should consist of 33 per cent vegetables and fruit, 33 per cent complex carbohydrate, 12 per cent protein-containing foods, 15 per cent dairy products or similar foods and 8 per cent fat and sugar-containing foods. Additionally, it is recommended each individual should eat five or more portions of a variety of fruit and vegetables a day (DoH, 2003a). Chart 5.1 identifies tips for eating well produced by the Food Standards Agency (2005). However, people who are unwell often require a more energy-dense diet in order to obtain sufficient nutrients to meet their needs and therefore adherence to healthy eating guidelines may not be appropriate. In addition, some people are prescribed a therapeutic diet for a particular medical condition and are required to avoid certain types of food. The type of diet outlined above is not suitable for those under five years of age.

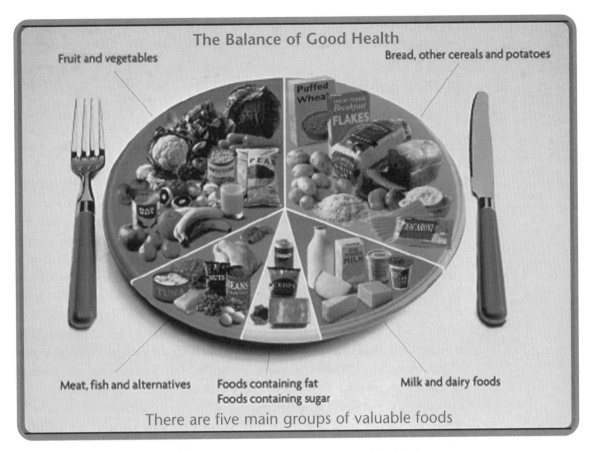

Figure 5.1 ● The plate model (reproduced with kind permission of the Food Standards Agency, 2005)

Chart 5.1 ● Tips for eating well

- Base your meals on starchy foods
- Eat lots of fruit and veg
- Eat more fish
- Cut down on saturated fat and sugar
- Try to eat less salt – no more than 6 g a day
- Get active and try to be a healthy weight
- Drink plenty of water
- Don't skip breakfast

Source: The FSA (2005)

Activity
5.2

Think about your dietary intake over the past seven days. Does it follow healthy eating guidelines? Are healthy eating guidelines easy to follow?

Food consists of various types of nutrients, which are used by the body in different ways. Nutrients can be classified into two broad categories: macronutrients and micronutrients. Macronutrients include carbohydrate, protein and fat and micronutrients include vitamins and minerals. These are described below.

■ Macronutrients

Carbohydrate

carbohydrate

organic compound containing carbon, hydrogen and oxygen that are the body's main source of energy

Foods rich in **carbohydrate** include bread, rice, breakfast cereals, pasta, potatoes, chapattis, poppadums and porridge. Other sources of carbohydrate include cakes, biscuits and pastry, but these also tend to have high levels of fat. Carbohydrates are used by the body for energy. Carbohydrates can be classified into three major groups: monosaccharides, oligosaccharides (which include disaccharides) and polysaccharides. The monosaccharides are also known as 'simple sugars' and include glucose and fructose. Carbohydrate is absorbed as monosaccharides for use by the body. Oligosaccharides include sucrose (table sugar), lactose (milk sugar) and maltose and are broken down to monosaccharides prior to absorption. Polysaccharides include starch and non-starch polysaccharides ('fibre') and are sometimes termed 'complex carbohydrates'. Starch is digested in the gastrointestinal tract so it can be absorbed. With the exception of non-starch polysaccharides, carbohydrate is used by the body for energy, with each gram of carbohydrate yielding about 17 kjoules/g (4 kcals/g). A healthy adult's diet should contain enough carbohydrate, mainly in the form of starch, to provide 45–60 per cent of food energy. Sucrose intake should be low and the intake of complex carbohydrates increased to compensate for this. A limited amount of carbohydrate can be stored in the body in the form of glycogen.

Protein

proteins

complex nitrogenous compounds, proteins are formed from amino acids and are essential for growth and repair

Rich sources of **protein** include meat, fish, eggs, pulses (peas, beans and lentils), nuts, tofu, soya and textured vegetable protein.

Protein is made from 20 or so different amino acids, which are classified into:

- *Essential*, which cannot be synthesised in the body
- *Non-essential*, which can be synthesised in the body.

It is possible to get all the essential amino acids from vegetable sources, providing that the right amount, combination and range of protein-containing foods are consumed, that is, proteins from different plant sources are eaten together. These include:

- Nuts and cereal: a peanut butter sandwich, or muesli with nuts

- Beans and rice: a casserole or salad
- Beans and cereal: for example hummus (chickpea spread) and bread
- Lentils and rice: as in soup.

These are known as complementary combinations. The major principle of a vegetarian diet, therefore, is that pulse dishes must be eaten with bread, rice or other cereal foods. For healthy adults, an intake of about 0.8 g protein per kg body weight (0.8 g/kg) per 24 hours is generally considered to be acceptable, requirements increasing during pregnancy and breastfeeding. About 10–20 per cent of dietary energy should derive from protein. There is some evidence that excessive dietary protein may contribute to demineralisation of bone and may have some effect on renal function. Protein is needed by the body for growth and defence and repair, such as wound healing and replacing blood loss. A small amount of protein is continually lost from the body throughout life in hair, shed skin scales, shed gut lining (a major constituent of faeces) and enzymes and other proteins secreted into the gut and incompletely digested. There is also a turnover of body proteins as tissue proteins are continuously broken down and replaced. Protein can be used by the body to provide energy if needed. One gram of protein provides 16 kJ (4 kcal) of energy.

> **Link**
>
> *Chapter 11 describes the factors needed for wound healing.*

Fat

The major form of **fat** in foods are triglycerides. Fat is found in solid fat and liquid oils in foods, for example in meat, nuts, cereals, vegetables and fruit (especially avocados). As well as the fat contained in food, fat, in the form of oils and butter, is used extensively in the processing and cooking of foods. There is a requirement for essential fatty acids, which play an important role in cell structure and function. These cannot be formed in the body so must be gained from the diet. The two essential fatty acids are linoleic acid (an omega-6 fat; see below) and alpha-linolenic acid (an omega-3 fat; see below). Vitamins A, D, E and K are fat soluble so are found in fatty or oily foods. Their absorption from the gut requires an adequate amount of fat in the diet since they are absorbed dissolved in this fat.

> **fats**
>
> organic substances that are insoluble in water but soluble in organic solvents. They include triacylglycerols, phospholipids, sterols and waxes

The fatty acids that make up the fats in our diet can be, in chemical terms, saturated or unsaturated. Saturated fatty acids have only single bonds between the carbon atoms that make up the molecule, whereas in unsaturated fatty acids there may be one (mono-unsaturated) or more (polyunsaturated) double bonds between carbon atoms. In general, fats that contain mainly saturated fatty acids are solid at room temperature, whereas those containing mainly unsaturated fatty acids are liquid at room temperature (although they usually solidify when chilled).

Saturated fatty acids are mainly of animal origin and a high intake of this type of fat is associated with high levels of low-density lipoprotein (LDL; see below) cholesterol, which in turn is associated with an increased risk of heart disease (reviewed by Gibney et al., 2005). Certain cancers, such as those of the bowel and breast, have been linked to a high intake of saturated fats (Field et al., 2001).

Polyunsaturated fatty acids lower the total blood cholesterol level by decreasing the concentration of LDL cholesterol and high-density lipoprotein (HDL) cholesterol (see below). The two main types of polyunsaturated fats are omega-3 and omega-6. Omega-3 fatty acids are associated with a reduction in inflammatory symptoms in diseases such as ulcerative colitis and rheumatoid arthritis (Gibney et al., 2005). They also make the blood less likely to clot (Gibney et al., 2005). The principle source of omega-3 fatty acids is fish oil and people living in the UK are advised to eat two servings of fish a week, one of which should be oily (FSA, 2004). Omega-6 sources include corn, sunflower, rapeseed and soya bean oils. It is recommended that individual consumption of polyunsaturated fats should be limited to no more than 10 per cent of total energy.

Mono-unsaturated fat is thought to have a lowering effect on LDL choles-terol but maintains or slightly increases HDL ('healthy') cholesterol. The main function of HDL is to transport excess cholesterol from tissues and other blood lipoproteins, ferrying it to the liver where it is broken down into bile. Foods rich in mono-unsaturated fat include olive and rapeseed oil.

Trans-fats are polyunsaturates that have been artificially hardened by adding extra hydrogen; this can occur in food processing and in frying. They are thought to be at least as unhealthy as saturated fat and have been linked to an increased risk of heart disease. Hydrogenated fats/oils can be noted on processed food labels.

Cholesterol is essential for life, being present in the membranes of animal and plant cells, and is also important in the formation of oestrogen and other sex hormones. Most cholesterol in the body is manufactured in the liver from satu-rated fatty acids contained in digested meat and dairy products. Once the fatty acids have been produced, globules of fat cling to proteins in the blood to form lipoproteins. These ferry the cholesterol around the bloodstream. It is only when the level of these is too high or too low that health is at risk; this is especially so for LDL cholesterol, which is related to the development of atherosclerosis and ischaemic heart disease.

Sources of cholesterol in the diet include eggs, offal and shellfish, but the main dietary factor that affects the concentration of cholesterol in the plasma is fat intake. Both the total amount of fat and the relative amounts of saturated and unsaturated fat affect the concentration of cholesterol in LDL cholesterol. A high intake of total fat, especially saturated fat, is associated with an undesirably high concentration of LDL cholesterol. A relatively low intake of fat, with a high proportion in the form of unsaturated fat, is associated with a desirable lower LDL concentration. Regular aerobic exercise appears to increase the HDL cholesterol level.

The flavour and lubrication of many foods come from the fat component, enhancing the pleasure of eating, the 'mouthfeel' of chocolate being an example.

One gram of fat provides 38 kJ (9 kcal) of energy. It is therefore the most energy-dense form of food. For adults and older children, it is recommended that no more than 35 per cent of food energy should come from fat. The guidelines suggest:

- no more than 10 per cent of total energy from saturated fatty acids, for example butter
- no more that 2 per cent from trans-fatty acids, for example in biscuits and pastry (as hydrogenated vegetable oil or fat)
- dietary cholesterol intake should not rise
- no further increase of polyunsaturated fat
- increase intake of omega-3 polyunsaturated fatty acids (minimum 0.2 g/day).

A restricted dietary fat intake is not recommended for those below the age of five years.

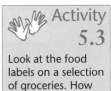

Activity 5.3

Look at the food labels on a selection of groceries. How easy is it to identify foods high in saturated and trans-fatty acids?

Energy

Energy output is measured in joules, but this is not practical when studying human nutrition, so kilojoules (kJ; 1,000 joules) and megajoules (MJ; 1,000,000 joules or 1,000 kJ) are used instead. In human nutrition, kilocalories (kcal) are also encountered. One calorie is the amount of heat needed to raise the temperature of 1 g of water by 1°C, and one kilocalorie – 1,000 calories – is the amount of heat needed to raise 1 kg of water by 1°C.

Conversion: 1 kcal = 4.184 kJ; 1 kJ = 0.239 kcal

The metabolic fuels are fat, carbohydrate, protein and alcohol. For people whose body weight lies within the healthy range, energy intake should be enough to maintain a reasonably constant body weight when an adequate amount of exercise is taken. Requirements are also related to age, gender and level of physical activity. Women, for example, often have a slower metabolism than men, people with well-developed muscles have a faster metabolism than sedentary people, older people have a slower metabolism than young people. A physically active body with lots of metabolically active muscle requires more energy than a relatively sedentary one with a higher percentage of body fat. A baby boy of 4–6 months of age needs about 2.89 MJ (690 kcal) per day and a

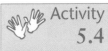

Activity 5.4

Look at the food levels of a high fat item and similar 'healthy eating' or lower fat item, for example biscuits. Compare the energy content.

girl of the same age 2.69 MJ (645 kcal). By the time the boy is 11–14 years old, he will need about 9.27 MJ (2,220 kcal), whereas the girl will need 7.92 MJ (1,845 kcal). The average daily energy requirement for adults aged 19–50 years is 10.60 MJ (2,550 kcal) per day for men and 8.10 MJ (1,940 kcal) per day for women. Breastfeeding may increase a woman's energy requirements by as much as 2.30 MJ (550 kcal) per day.

If a person does not consume enough energy, tissue breakdown will take place to make up the deficit. If too much energy is consumed, it is stored as glycogen or fat. Fifteen or more years ago, before the widespread use of mobile phones, remote controls and other labour-saving devices, you probably expended more energy than now. You may also have used the bus and walked or cycled more than at present.

Although we have a requirement for energy in our diet, in theory it does not matter how the requirement is met. There is no necessity as such for a dietary source of carbohydrate, for example: the body can make as much as it requires from proteins, albeit expensively. Similarly, there is no need for a dietary source of fat apart from the essential fatty acids. And a dietary source of alcohol is non-essential (see below). Some dietary elements are, however, needed for specific purposes, for example fibre, which used to be called roughage.

The terms 'roughage' and 'fibre' should be replaced by **non-starch polysaccharides** (NSPs). NSPs are a collection of indigestible substances found in plant cells, the main action of which is to aid the passage of food through the bowel and ease elimination. Sources include fruit and vegetables, whole grains, wholemeal bread, cereals, beans and pulses. There is no fibre in animal food sources such as milk, meat, cheese and eggs. For good health, it is recommended that adults consume 18 g of fibre a day, with the range being 12–18 g per day. There are two sorts of NSP:

- *Soluble NSP* dissolves in the gut and helps to maintain a healthy blood glucose level by a sort of slow-release effect. The richest sources are pulses, oats (for example porridge), barley (for example pearl barley in soups), rye (for example in bread), beans and lentils, but it is also found in fruits and vegetables. Soluble NSP is also thought to help to decrease a high blood cholesterol level by combining with bile acids and cholesterol in the intestine and preventing their absorption
- *Insoluble NSP* soaks up moisture as it travels through the digestive system, forming bulk that aids the easy passage of waste products. It is found in wheat-based breakfast cereals, bread, rice, maize, pasta, fruits and vegetables. Large amounts of insoluble NSP can reduce the absorption of some micronutrients.

non-starch polysaccharides

structural components of plant cell walls, soluble substances in cell sap. They are resistant to digestion by the human gastrointestinal tract. Commonly known as fibre

Link

Chapter 6 covers the effects of diet on faecal elimination.

Taking enough NSP in the diet means eating a *varied* selection of fruits and vegetables as whole and unpeeled as possible. A **minimum** of five different fruits and/or vegetables a day is recommended for most people. The diet should contain whole grains (rather than completely white, refined versions) such as wholemeal bread, rice and pasta.

Fluid

Water is the main constituent of the body, comprising about 60 per cent of adult body weight. The body gains some water from foods, but adults need to drink another 1.5–2.0 litres of fluid daily to ensure efficient functioning at all levels. People with cardiac or renal problems may need to drink less fluid a day due to their medical condition. The body needs more fluid if it is sweating, as a result of hot conditions or pyrexia, or if it is losing fluid through diarrhoea and vomiting.

Fluid intake should not consist solely of strongly flavoured, calorific or stimulating drinks such as coffee, tea, cola, sugar and alcohol. Children should be encouraged to drink plain water to avoid the problems associated with sugary, flavoured drinks, such as dental caries, obesity and the overconsumption of additives.

Body composition alters as it gets older, elderly people having a higher percentage of body fat to fluid, and younger people having more fluid.

> **Activity 5.5**
>
> Look up water and electrolyte balance in your preferred anatomy and physiology book. Why is a detailed know ledge of normal fluid and electrolyte balance necessary for nurses?

■ Micronutrients

Vitamins

Vitamins are relatively complex organic compounds that have essential functions in metabolic processes and are needed in very small amounts. There is a constant turnover of vitamins so they must be replaced. Vitamin C, for example, is water soluble, needing constant replenishment as there is limited storage in the body. For estimated average requirements, see the FSA website (www.food.gov.uk).

> **vitamins**
> complex chemical substances found in minute quantities in food. Essential to life.

The main vitamins are outlined below but for a more comprehensive review a nutrition textbook should be consulted.

Vitamin A (retinol, carotene)

Vitamin A is needed to promote vision and cell differentiation, for maintaining the health of epithelial tissues and skin and for a healthy immune system. In children, it helps to ensure correct bone development and growth. It is one of the **antioxidants**, which may help to protect against bowel cancer and heart

> **antioxidant**
> a substance that prevents deterioration by the activity of oxygen

disease. Vitamin A is fat soluble and is found in liver, fish oils, dairy products, fortified margarine and some green, yellow and orange fruits and vegetables. It is stored in the liver and released when needed.

Vitamin A can be obtained in two forms: retinol in animal foods, and carotenoid pigments from fruit and vegetables. Pregnant women should avoid supplements containing vitamin A (unless advised otherwise at antenatal clinic) and liver and liver products.

Vitamin B group

These are water-soluble vitamins.

Thiamine (B1)

Thiamine is important in some metabolic processes, particularly the release of energy from carbohydrate, fat and alcohol. It is found in most foods, particularly unrefined cereal grains, fortified flour, some breakfast cereals, meat, dairy products and legumes.

Riboflavin (B2)

Riboflavin is necessary for the production of energy by the body. It is found in many foods, particularly dairy products, eggs, fortified cereals, ice cream and liver.

Vitamin B3 (niacin, nicotinic acid, nicotinamide)

Vitamin B3 is an important component of one of the factors of the metabolic pathway, which produces energy in the body. It is found in red meat, wheat flour, maize, eggs and milk.

Vitamin B6 (pyridoxal, pyridoxamine)

Vitamin B6 is important in protein metabolism. It can be found in meats, fish, eggs, milk, wheat germ, brewers yeast, brown rice, soya beans, unrefined wheat grains and some nuts. Women may take large amounts (without medical advice) to relieve premenstrual syndrome symptoms. The FSA (2003) advises against taking more than 10 mg/day to avoid the development of neuropathy.

Vitamin B12 (cobalamin)

Vitamin B12 is essential for red blood cell production and a healthy nervous system. It is also needed for the synthesis of deoxyribonucleic acid (DNA) and ribonucleic acid (RNA). Vitamin B12 is made by microorganisms and incorporated into the food chain by animals. It is present in meats or foods of animal origin. Vitamin B12 is absorbed in the terminal ileum, deficiency most often being caused by a lack of absorption. Intrinsic factor, a glycoprotein produced by the parietal cells of the stomach, is needed for the absorption of vitamin B12.

Post-gastrectomy patients will require injections of B12.

Folate/folic acid

Folate/folic acid is important in the synthesis of DNA. It is widely distributed in foods, particularly liver, yeast extract, leafy green vegetables, fortified grains and breakfast cereals. A lack of folate/folic acid during the first few weeks of pregnancy has been associated with neural tube defects such as spina bifida. Women in the first trimester of pregnancy or those thinking of becoming pregnant should take a daily supplement of 400 mcg (FSA, 2003). A higher dose may be recommended by the doctor or midwife if there is a history of neural tube defect.

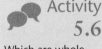

Activity 5.6

Which are whole-grain cereals? What foods are rich in folic acid? Why is this relevant?

Vitamin C (ascorbic acid)

Vitamin C is important in the development of connective tissue and promotes iron absorption. It is an antioxidant, is water soluble and can be found in fresh vegetables and fruit, particularly spinach, tomatoes, broccoli, strawberries and citrus fruits. It helps to increase iron absorption. Smokers have an increased requirement.

Vitamin C deficiency causes hair follicle eruption, petechial haemorrhage on limbs, bleeding gums, impairment of connective tissue formation in wound repair tissue, joint pains and fatigue. Deficiency disease is termed 'scurvy' and the symptoms result from the failure of the body to synthesise collagen. Those at risk of deficiency include smokers, and individuals with an absence of fruit and vegetables in the diet. Over 1,000–2,000 mg per day of vitamin C may cause gastric upset.

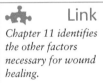

Link

Chapter 11 identifies the other factors necessary for wound healing.

Vitamin D (calciferol)

Vitamin D regulates calcium absorption and utilisation for healthy bones and teeth. Fat soluble, it is synthesised mostly from the action of sunlight on skin. Vitamin D food sources include fatty fish, liver, milk, eggs and fortified food such as margarine and breakfast cereals. Deficiency results in **rickets** in children, **osteomalacia**, muscle weakness and bone tenderness. Deficiency can be caused by inadequate exposure to sunlight (for example nursing home residents, and those with a dark skin colour who habitually cover their skin). Malabsorption can also cause vitamin D deficiency.

rickets

a condition in children where vitamin D deficiency results in poor bone development and softening and bending of long bones

osteomalacia

a condition in which adults experience bone softening due to vitamin D deficiency or deficiency of calcium and phosphate or excessive absorption from the bones

Vitamin E (tocopherols)

Vitamin E is needed for the protection of cell membranes and lipids against oxidative damage and can help to guard against heart attacks. Vitamin E is fat soluble and is synthesised by plants. Plant oils, nuts and seeds are a rich source.

Vitamin K (phylloquinone and menaquinones)

Vitamin K is essential for blood clotting and energy metabolism. A fat-soluble vitamin, it is found in green leafy vegetables and vegetable oils. It is also produced by bacteria in the intestine. In adults, deficiency is very rare and results in bleeding disorders. Vitamin K supplement is given **prophylactically** to prevent haemorrhagic disease of the newborn.

Minerals

In addition to metabolic fuels, protein and vitamins, the body has a requirement for a variety of mineral salts (**minerals**) in very small (trace) amounts. The requirements of a growing child will be greater than those of a healthy adult who simply has to replace body losses from mineral turnover. An ill person or pregnant or lactating mother will have an increased requirement of these micronutrients.

Calcium

Calcium (Ca) is needed for the growth and development of bones and teeth, the correct functioning of nerves and muscles, and blood clotting. It is found in milk, cheese, small fish (such as sardines), some green leafy vegetables, soya bean products, fortified wheat flour and breakfast cereals, and some nuts. The body requires an adequate level of vitamin D to absorb and regulate calcium. Absorption may be reduced by a high intake of phytates. There are widespread effects of deficiency, which include stunted growth and bone malformation in children and skeletal and tooth changes in adults.

Phosphorus

Phosphorus (P) is a component of all cells, necessary for energy storage, membrane function, growth and reproduction. It is found widely in foods. Rich sources include fish, poultry, red meat, dairy products and cereal grains. Effects of deficiency are widespread and include osteomalacia, myopathy and growth failure.

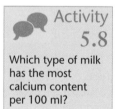

Activity 5.7

Why might a client confined to bed become deficient in vitamin D? What could be the long-term effects? (See also Chapter 9.)

prophylactically

an agent or therapy that contributes to the prevention of infection or disease

minerals

naturally occurring inorganic substances needed in trace amounts in the diet

Activity 5.8

Which type of milk has the most calcium content per 100 ml?

Sodium chloride

Sodium chloride (NaCl) is needed for the maintenance of a constant body water content and plays an important role in the conduction of nervous impulses. It is found in many foods. Young infants should not have salt added to food as renal excretion is limited. In adults, intake of no more than 6 g/day is recommended to promote health.

Potassium

Potassium (K) is necessary for the maintenance of a constant body water content, for acid–base balance and for nerve conduction. Rich sources include milk, fruit and vegetables, shellfish, red meat, white meat and liver. Deficiency is associated with the use of some diuretics and very low energy diets.

Iodine

Iodine (I) is needed for the functioning of the thyroid gland, which controls the metabolic rate of the body. Rich sources include marine fish, shellfish, sea salt and supplemented salt. Dietary deficiency is endemic in some areas of the world.

Iron

Iron (Fe) is essential for red blood cell formation, oxygen transport and transfer, enzyme activation and drug metabolism. There are two sorts: haem iron, found in meat, and non-haem iron gained from beans, nuts, dried fruit, fish, enriched cereals, soya bean flour and dark green leafy vegetables. Balti cooking is a good source because the food absorbs iron from the cooking pot. Haem iron is more accessible and more easily absorbed than non-haem iron. Vegetarians may, therefore, be at risk of deficiency. Iron is best absorbed with vitamin C, so the 2 mg of iron found in your fortified breakfast cereal is better absorbed with a glass of orange juice than a cup of tea. A lack of iron causes **iron deficiency anaemia**. Those at risk include infants over six months, toddlers, adolescents, pregnant women, menstruating women, older people, people with parasitic infestations and those with a high intake of inhibitors of absorption, for example tea.

iron deficiency anaemia
a reduced amount of haemoglobin in red blood cells, causing fatigue, glossitis and paraesthesia (sensation of numbness, prickling or tingling)

Zinc

Zinc (Zn) is needed for bone metabolism, enzyme activation, the release of vitamin A, growth, healing, healthy immune and reproductive systems, taste and insulin release. Sources include meat, unrefined cereals and fortified cereal products. Features of zinc deficiency include growth retardation and defects of rapidly dividing tissues such as skin, intestinal mucosa and the immune system.

Selenium

Selenium (Se) is necessary for part of an enzyme involved in the protection of membranes and lipids against oxidative damage. Rich sources include fish, offal, brazil nuts and cereals.

Mineral tailpieces

- *Phytates*, found in high levels in unprocessed wheat bran and soya, can lead to the malabsorption of minerals, especially calcium and zinc
- *Oxalates*, found in high levels in spinach and rhubarb, can reduce mineral availability.

■ Alcohol

Alcohol has a long history of bad and good press (Simpson, 1992). It is high in energy and usually carbohydrates, and, when taken in excess, can be a factor in obesity and vitamin deficiency, especially that of vitamin B1. It is dehydrating, so is unhelpful in maintaining the body's fluid balance: hangovers are largely the result of dehydration.

A moderate alcohol intake has been associated with a raised level of HDL cholesterol and inhibition of platelet aggregation, and thus can be a protective factor against heart disease. Red wine contains antioxidant polyphenols and has been suggested to offer greater protection against heart disease. Alcohol should be consumed with food in moderate amounts only. Current guidelines suggest that women can drink up to 2–3 units/day and men up to 3–4 units/day without significant risk to health (www.food.gov.uk, 2005) – one unit being half a pint of standard strength beer, lager or cider or a pub measure of spirit, and a glass of wine being 1.5 units.

An excessive alcohol intake leads to long-term problems, for example liver cirrhosis, increased risk of accidents, pancreatitis and cancer of the oesophagus. Binge drinking, common in the UK, is damaging to health. Liver disease caused by habitual excessive alcohol consumption is not uncommon in younger people. One gram of alcohol provides 29 kJ (7 kcal) of energy.

■ Nutrient Intake

Nutritional requirements will vary, depending on a person's size, gender, activity level, state of health and age. Infants and children require sufficient nutrients to develop and grow. People at certain stages in their life may require an increased intake of nutrients, for example pre-conception, during pregnancy and while breastfeeding (Barasi, 2003). In the UK, estimated nutritional requirements for different groups of people within the population have been established (DoH, 1991). These are termed 'dietary reference values'. It is important to recognise that these are not recommendations for intake by individuals but are estimates for healthy populations; within a clinical setting, the advice of a dietitian must be sought.

Appetite and choices

The psychology of eating is highly complex, so the reader is advised to consult a psychology or nutritional text (for example Barasi, 2003) in addition to reading this section. This is also an extremely important area because food and eating are essential parts of lifestyle.

There are four principal taste sensations, sweet, sour, bitter and salty being all that the tongue can detect. Monosodium glutamate (umami), which enhances flavours, may be considered. What adds to taste is the sense of smell. Taste and smell together make up the flavour system, which can evoke strong emotional responses.

Flavour also includes other characteristics of food, such as temperature and texture. Variety in food seems to stimulate the appetite, and flavour motivates eating by the pleasure derived from its taste, smell and 'mouthfeel'. For this reason, children often come to prefer foods with a high fat content. Social situations and other people also provide cues that stimulate the appetite for certain foods, the presence of other people also generally tending to induce one to eat more. In addition, changes in people's nutritional state can affect their motivation to consume certain foods.

The selection and preparation of food require a number of psychological processes, including choice, cognition, knowledge and attitudes. We classify food as edible or inedible, having developed attitudes about what makes an object appropriate and desirable as food.

Three factors account for food rejection and acceptance:

1. *Sensory-affective factors:* like and dislike are based on sensory attributes such as taste, smell and sometimes appearance. Good tastes are accepted; those which are unappealing are rejected as distasteful.

Activity 5.9

Look up metabolism in your preferred anatomy and physiology or nutrition text. What is the difference between **anabolism** and **catabolism**? Why is this relevant to eating and drinking?

anabolism
the building up of body substance; the constructive phase of metabolism

catabolism
the breakdown of body substance; the destructive phase of metabolism

2. *Anticipated consequences:* acceptance or rejection are based on beliefs about the consequences of ingestion. An elderly person may, for example, believe that 'eggs are binding' or that 'bread is fattening'. The rejection of an item because of perceived negative consequences is based on its 'dangerous' nature. Conversely, the acceptance of an item is based on its anticipated beneficial effects.

3. *Ideational factors:* items are accepted or rejected because of our knowledge of what they are, their origins and their symbolic meanings. Ideational factors are mostly concerned with food rejection.

Thus, in summary:

Activity 5.10

What food and drink selections have you made in the past 24 hours? Can you identify some of the factors influencing those selections?

- Psychological categories of rejection (strongly linked to the biological) include distaste, danger, inappropriateness and disgust
- Psychological categories of acceptance include good taste, benefits and appropriateness
- We consume food because of the perceived benefits or for its own sake, because it tastes good or for comfort
- We avoid foods because of their dangerous properties, because of our intolerance or allergy to them, or because of dislike or unfamiliarity.

Social factors are important in determining how we come to like or dislike certain foods. Parental choice can, for example, influence children one way or the other. People develop long-term food preferences that are stable over long periods of time and unaffected by changes in their mood or environment; these can be highly resistant to change if a more healthy diet is advised. Some food preferences change from day to day and are more likely to be affected by mood. For example, we may chose to eat a bar of chocolate to 'cheer ourselves up', or have a glass of champagne to celebrate an event.

Casebox 5.1

Miss Quinn, aged 82, has progressive dementia and has lived in a residential care home for two years. She wanders restlessly all round the clock and rarely spends more than a few minutes at anything. The staff are concerned that she appears to be losing weight.

What steps could be taken to ensure that this does not become a problem?

- Make every mouthful count, so avoid wasting eating and drinking time on low-energy fillers.

- Use the fact that she has

limited memory to encourage nutritious snacks around the clock instead of expecting her to concentrate for a full meal.

- Instead of a cup of coffee made with water, she could be offered a cup of

- coffee made entirely with full-cream milk, a little more sugar being added over time.

- Always present a cup of tea with a biscuit, small cake or sandwich.

- Food supplements may be prescribed for her and she should be encouraged to eat or drink them.

- Has she chocolates, fruit and crisps in her room for constant access?

- Meals can be enriched to enhance the energy count by adding butter, cream or sugar as appropriate.

Political, social and economic influences

Political, social and economic factors shape what we eat as they influence the types and amount of food available to us. Some people are, for social, economic, geographical and other reasons, unable to access the basics of a healthy diet without considerable difficulty. Some groups, such as elderly people, the homeless, the unemployed or those with children, may live on very little money and have reduced access to food services. They may, for example, live on large housing estates, where shopping for fresh food may involve a bus journey costing time and money. Local shops may be more expensive and have a more limited choice of foods than supermarkets. Some may not sell fresh fruit and vegetables. Children are particularly vulnerable to the effects of poor dietary intake and recently efforts have been made to address the poor dietary intake of children. Aspects of the government programme Sure Start (which aims to deliver the best start in life for every child) focus on nutrition. Further, the school fruit and vegetable scheme (part of the 5 a day programme) aims to increase fruit and vegetable consumption of all 4–6-year-old children in LEA-maintained infant, primary and special schools. According to this scheme, these children are entitled to a free piece of fruit or vegetable each school day. Examples of other government initiatives aimed at increasing the quality of nutritional intake can be seen on the Department of Health website. It is also important that nurses are aware of the Food Standards Agency, which is an independent government department set up in 2000 to protect the public's health and consumer interests in relation to food. The website for this agency (www.food.gov.uk) contains up-to-date information on diet and health issues.

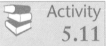

Link

Chapter 2 discusses Sure Start.

Activity 5.11

Examine a food chart completed for a patient in your clinical area. Is it accurate? How could it be made more accurate?

Casebox 5.2

Trevor, aged 47, is suffering from depression. He barely has the energy to get himself out of bed in the mornings, is off sick from his work as a storeman and goes to group therapy once a week.

What is likely to be the effect of this on his eating pattern and weight?

■ Trevor may suffer from early morning wakening but his activity level will be very low.

■ If he eats as much as he used to before he went off sick, and/or eats for comfort, with a high level of refined carbohydrate and fat, Trevor may put on weight.

■ It is also possible that he could lose interest in food, have no appetite and not bother to shop or cook for himself, ending up with weight loss, some of which will be loss of muscle mass from inactivity (see Chapter 9).

Cultural issues – ethnic and religious practices

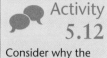

Activity 5.12

Consider why the fish and chip shop is busier on Fridays. Identify the food ideology of a client who comes from a different cultural, ethnic or religious group.

Cultural factors inform food ideology, that is, the collection of customs, attitudes, beliefs and taboos that affect the diet of a particular group. Some people, for example, may feel that their diet is incomplete without a hot meal at least once a day. For centuries, Roman Catholics consumed no meat on Fridays, and Mormons do not consume caffeine or alcohol.

Clients' food ideology is important because it influences their behaviour as well as their motivation to alter their food habits across time. These food habits are acquired as part of primary socialisation in childhood and may be difficult to change, which reinforces the necessity of initially developing good food habits (Fieldhouse, 1995). Secondary socialisation takes place through the school and workplace, and may contradict food habits learned at home. The attempts of health professionals to change people's eating habits in more healthy directions can be termed 'resocialisation'. This process can be helped or hindered by influences at local, regional and national levels, including such factors as advertising. People may regard foods as 'good' or 'bad', yin or yang, 'hot' or 'cold', reward or punishment. The social meanings of food are bound up with notions and traditions of hospitality, expressions of love, friendship, affection and status (Fieldhouse, 1995).

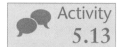

Activity 5.13

Identify one food that you regard as 'good' and one you regard as 'bad'. Why have these foods come to mean this to you? What is the basis for this belief? Is it rational?

Abstinence from meat is practised in many world religions, such as Buddhism, Hinduism and Rastafarianism. Fruitarians eat only fruit, vegans eat no animal products, lactovegetarians eat no eggs, meat, fish or poultry, and lacto-ovovegetarians don't eat meat, fish or poultry but do eat eggs.

Some religions advocate fasting at various times and although they usually absolve the sick from participating, the nurse must take into account the client's religion when planning nutritional care. It is important that food preferences and customary intake are identified. It is distressing for a person to be offered food that is not acceptable to them on religious grounds. All care settings should offer an appropriate menu for individuals from different religions.

Functional foods

Foods termed 'functional foods' have now started to appear on food shelves for purchase by the general public. A functional food is defined as a food which has health-promoting benefits and/or disease promoting properties in addition to usual nutritional value (Barasi, 2003). Examples of functional foods include omega-enriched eggs and sterol-enriched margarine.

■ Screening and Assessing Nutritional Status

The aim of screening and assessing nutritional status is to identify those with, or at risk of, malnutrition and to highlight potential causes. If an individual is screened and considered to be at risk of or have malnutrition, then a more detailed assessment should be undertaken. This will usually be undertaken by the dietitian but may be undertaken by another health-care professional, for example a speech and language therapist will be asked to see the patient if a swallow deficit is suspected. Screening and assessment enables the identification of nutritional needs, planning of nutritional interventions and setting of nutritional goals (McLaren and Green, 1998). Following this, interventions can be implemented that should be regularly evaluated and modified by assessment.

Casebox 5.3

Ms Cohen, a retired civil servant of 60, underwent hip surgery two weeks ago. She has little interest in food and was identified, on admission, as being underweight and malnourished.

How might this affect her surgery?

What advice would be needed for her convalescence to be an opportunity to improve her nutritional status?

■ Malnutrition will delay her recovery and increase the likelihood of complications. It interferes with respiratory function, partly by loss of muscle mass and strength, making Ms Cohen more likely to develop a chest infection (see also Chapter 7). Immune function is also depressed so she will be at high risk of wound infection. Ms Cohen's grip may be diminished, making it harder for her to be mobile on crutches (see Chapter 9 for effects of immobility). Malnutrition has psychological effects such as apathy, depression and loss of the will to recover (Rollins, 1997), making Ms Cohen less likely to cooperate with her rehabilitation regimen.

■ Ms Cohen needs to be encouraged to eat as a

matter of urgency or she is unlikely to get better. Nutritional support may need to be directed along the lines of food as medicine, and considerable effort should be employed to coax her to eat and drink, little and often, high-energy and nutrient-dense foodstuffs. Vitamin supplements may be an option. Her belief systems need to be identified: as she is an Orthodox Jew, is kosher food available? An education programme needs to be implemented to gain her interest in 'eating for convalescence'. Family, friends or neighbours could be encouraged to bring in her favourite foods. Her community nurse may be asked to monitor her nutritional status.

There are five principle methods of screening or assessing for nutritional status; assessment of dietary history and intake, clinical examination, functional tests, biochemical tests and anthropometric measures. Factors other than nutritional status can affect functional and biochemical tests of nutritional status and therefore analysis is not straightforward. For example, a low haemoglobin level can result from poor iron intake but can also be due to other factors such as blood loss. These ways of assessing nutritional status are not considered here.

Dietary intake

One way of checking whether someone is well nourished is to get him or her to keep a food diary and then rate it against the 'plate model' (Figure 5.1). One day's intake is not enough information on which to make a judgement, unless it is typical of a consistent intake, so the more information that can be gained, the more accurate the resulting baseline. Seven days is the ideal length of time. This type of recording can be useful to the nurse to highlight where changes in the diet can be made; however, this method of assessing dietary intake is more commonly used by the dietitian to accurately assess nutrient intake.

In order to monitor a client's food and fluid intake, food and fluid charts can be completed. It is important that they are completed with the highest degree of accuracy possible and that the intake is added up and related to the client's needs by someone with the knowledge and interest to ensure that findings are acted upon. A food chart should be completed if it is suspected that a person's food intake is poor and needs monitoring. In an acute setting, accurate completion of a food chart is essential information required by the dietitian in order for him or her to more accurately assess nutritional status.

Dietary history

Asking a person or their carer about their habitual food and fluid intake is an important method of assessing dietary quality. Reasons for their habitual diet should also be considered. Problems such as pain, nausea, constipation, breathlessness or **anorexia** will diminish a person's ability to take adequate food and fluids. People who are undergoing investigations or surgery may be required to fast for extended periods. The client's ability to access food and drink normally, in terms of shopping, storing, cooking or cutting up food, must also be considered. General lifestyle questions will include an assessment of their activity and exercise levels, how much time they spend out of doors, whether they smoke and what their alcohol consumption is. Clients must also be asked about the type of diet they prefer to eat, as it is the nurses' responsibility to ensure that they are provided with a diet appropriate to meet their cultural needs.

anorexia
loss of appetite

Clinical assessment

Observation of clients will include a clinical assessment to see whether they appear well nourished, and will include looking at the fit of their clothes, the condition of their skin, mouth, eyes, hair and nails, how they move and how alert or apathetic they appear.

Anthropometric measures

Anthropometry refers to the measurement of the human body. Simple anthropometric measures can be used by nurses to screen and assess nutritional status. It is important to weigh clients on admission to care to provide a baseline measure and weigh them at regular intervals subsequently to identify any losses or gains. If possible, the person should be weighed on the same scales at the same time each day, in similar clothes after voiding. As with all equipment, it is important that weighing machines are regularly checked for accuracy.

Percentage weight can be used to assess weight (wght) loss or gain and is calculated using the equation:

$$\% \text{ wght loss/gain} = \frac{\text{usual wght} - \text{current wght (kg)}}{\text{usual wght (kg)}} \times 100$$

A loss of 10 per cent in the previous three months is suggestive of malnutrition. It must be remembered though that weight changes for other reasons too, such as dehydration or oedema.

Weight in relation to height is a more accurate way of assessing the degree to

body mass index (BMI)

a figure derived from a person's height and weight, which indicates whether his or her weight is within a range that is considered best to promote health

which a person is under- or overweight. **Body mass index** (BMI) is commonly used for this reason. This can be calculated by dividing body weight in kilograms (kg) by the height in metres squared (m^2). If height cannot be measured, it can be estimated in other ways, for example by the use of ulna length (Elia, 2003). A BMI of <18.5 suggests that a person is underweight, a BMI of 18.5–24.9 is considered normal. A BMI of 25.0–29.9 suggests that a person is overweight and a BMI of >30 suggests that a person is obese (International Obesity Task Force, 2000). The use of BMI with old people may not be appropriate (BDA, 2003).

Chart 5.2 ● Body mass index (BMI)

BMI calculation = weight (kg)/height (m^2)

Reference ranges for desirable BMI =

- <18.5   underweight
- 18.5–24.9   normal range
- 25–29.9   overweight
- >30   obese

Source: International Obesity Task Force (2000).

Measuring waist circumference is increasingly being carried out to screen for cardiovascular risk in primary care. Men with a waist circumference of greater that 102 cm and women with a waist circumference of greater than 88 cm are at increased risk of cardiovascular disease and should consider losing weight (Lean, 2000).

Anthropometric measures that assess fat levels or muscle mass of the body are sometimes used, such as skinfold measures to estimate body fat and mid-arm muscle circumference to estimate skeletal muscle mass.

Casebox 5.4

Susan is 19 years old and lives with her parents and younger brother in a terraced house with a small garden in a large town. She drives to work and to various activities with her friends. Her BMI is 32. She has seen her GP, who has referred her to the practice nurse for some advice.

What would be the main principles of this advice?

- Activity levels must be increased, building up steadily over time.

- Susan can be encouraged to drink water, rather than cola, juice or carbonated drinks, when she is thirsty and with her meals.

- Energy-dense foods should be reserved for treats.

- Susan should be advised to follow healthy eating guidelines.

To try to identify those with malnutrition and at risk of malnutrition on admission to care, many nutritional screening and assessment tools have been developed (Green and Watson, 2005). Most have a series of questions to be answered, these being scored to identify the client's level of risk of malnutrition. A national valid and reliable tool has been developed for use recently by the British Association of Parenteral and Enteral Nutrition (BAPEN, 2005a). It is for use in all clinical areas.

As highlighted in recent national publications (Nursing and Midwifery Practice Development Unit, 2002; DoH, 2003b), it is important that clients are screened for malnutrition on admission to care. Only then can an appropriate plan of care be made. The plan of care may require referral to another member of the multidisciplinary team, for example the dietitian or doctor, for nutritional needs to be assessed fully and met. Or it may require the nurse to assist the client to meet their nutritional needs. The plan of care must be evaluated to ensure that it is effective. This can be done by returning to the process of screening and assessing. For example, if a person is provided with modified cutlery by the occupational therapist as a result of a problem being identified with handling normal cutlery on assessment, then the ability of the client to consume adequate amounts of food with the modified cutlery needs to be assessed to ensure that the intervention has been successful.

Casebox 5.5

Raul is 17 years old and has learning disabilities and many physical problems. He is moving to a new care home, and the opportunity is being taken to reassess his needs.

How can the team assess his nutritional status and identify what assistance Raul requires?

■ Measure his height and weight, and calculate his BMI.

■ Use a nutritional screening tool.

■ Keep a food record over a week to check for likes, dislikes and overall balance.

■ Is Raul getting enough fluid? What are his preferences?

■ What capacities has he for chewing and swallowing? Should he be assessed by a speech and language therapist? What state are his teeth and gums in?

■ Could the drugs that he is taking (for example phenytoin) interact with his food?

■ How is Raul best positioned for meals, and how much can he do for himself? Does he need a special tilted chair? What about built-up cutlery, moulded to his hand grip? Can occupational therapy help?

■ Assisting a Client to Eat and Drink

The aim of any help is to ensure, in a reasonable manner, that clients have an optimum food and fluid intake, maintaining their dignity in the process. The only food that is of any use to clients is that which they actually eat and retain. The client may need an occasional prompt or gentle reminder, constant attention or feeding. The plan of care following an assessment of needs should identify what the client requires in terms of assistance.

It helps to know when mealtimes are in order to plan the clinical workload appropriately. Food can and should be an enjoyable break, a pause or punctuation in the day, rather than just fuel. It is important to consider the environment and in non-acute settings, it is normally possible to take clients into a dining room or day room for meals, although a person who needs help with feeding may be best served in privacy to reduce embarrassment to the client. Clients should always be involved in decisions about where they should eat their food.

If a client is frightened, nauseated or in pain, appetite will be affected, therefore these factors need to be addressed before the food is served. Pain relief or antiemetic medication should be given in time for it to be working well and any other medication, such as insulin, should be given before the meal if required.

It is important to ensure that those needing help with elimination have been encouraged to perform well before mealtimes in order to reduce unpleasant noises and smells, which act as an appetite suppressant. If a client does need a commode at a mealtime, they should be wheeled out to a bathroom for privacy. Bedpans, urinals, commodes and toilet rolls should be removed from bedside tables and bedsides before presenting food. Relatives and carers may wish to assist the client to eat and drink. They may also bring in favourite foods, provided hospital policy is adhered to. Prior to serving the meal, it should be ensured that the client's mouth is clean and that their dentures are in place and fit. In a non-acute setting, sherry can be useful as an appetite stimulant for elderly clients (Simpson, 1992).

Sitting the client as upright as possible allows the client to swallow food and fluid more easily. If possible, an upright chair drawn up to a table of comfortable height should be used. The client in an armchair may find even an adjustable bedside table too high. In such a case, consider putting a firm pillow under the client to raise him to a more comfortable height. Clients in bed need to be sitting upright with their pillows arranged so that they can lean forward.

When serving food, it is important for staff and clients to wash their hands and wear an appropriate apron as per hospital policy. Presentation of the food counts. The cleanliness of the surroundings must be considered by ensuring that smells are neutral, fresh air is available, and the environment is clear of things such as rubbish bags, sputum pots and drainage bags. The food should be made to look appealing. In clinical areas where plated meals are offered, food presentation is considered in the kitchen. In areas where food is served from a trolley, the nurse should consider this carefully. When serving food to the client who is blind, the 'clock face' should be used to describe what is where on the plate. In some settings, staff can eat their meals with clients to enhance the social function. This can be a useful reminder to those with limited memory who just forget to eat without the external prompt of seeing others doing so.

The contents of the tray should be arranged so the client can reach and access everything. Hot foods should be offered hot and cold foods cold to enhance their palatability. Condiments should be available to flavour food. Appropriate cutlery should be provided and food cut up as required. A drink should be made available. Clients should be provided with protection for their clothes if they want this.

If the client requires assistance to eat, the following guidance should be observed:

● Check the client/patient's dietary needs
● Introduce yourself
● Obtain consent and explain procedure
● Ensure bed area is safe (bed brakes on!) and set up appropriately
● Position the client correctly
● Ensure mouth is clean and dentures in place
● Wash hands and put on appropriate apron
● Prepare equipment needed
● Sit at the same level
● Check the food is not too hot
● Try not to rush them or give them too much food at a time – between one half and a full teaspoonful per mouthful is plenty
● Ensure each mouthful is swallowed
● After a pause, offer the next mouthful
● Offer fluid periodically
● Foods with a smooth texture such as ice cream, yoghurt, custard, purée, baked beans (without toast) and mashed potato are easier to swallow. Food types to be avoided by the client with eating or swallowing difficulties are those which are stringy, crumbly, tough or of mixed texture, as well as items such as peas, nuts and sweetcorn. If a pureed diet is offered, component foods should be kept separate so that an unappetising greyish sludge is avoided
● Communicate to the client throughout
● Stop giving the patient food and report to a registered nurse if:
  – The client's voice sounds wet or gurgly
  – The client shows signs of choking

– Food is pocketing in the client's mouth
- When the client has finished, offer a mouthwash or check mouth for retained food – clear with drink, swab or toothbrush if necessary
- The client should stay sitting upright for about 30 minutes to reduce the chance of **reflux**
- Document how much the client has eaten and any other factors of importance.

reflux

a backward flow of food and fluid up the gastrointestinal tract

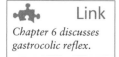   Link

Chapter 6 discusses gastrocolic reflex.

Drinking or eating may trigger the gastrocolic reflex, so patients' needs can be anticipated by offering toilet facilities. Some clients who cannot tell you what they need may go red in the face after tea, coffee or meals, which can mean that they need to defaecate.

Clients may need help with completing the menu cards. The types of food chosen should be discussed with the patient if necessary. Soup and ice cream is an option but is low in energy and micronutrients. This can be a nutritional disaster if allowed to go on for more than a couple of days. Supplementary puddings or other food choices on the menu may be a better option. Some clients may find it easier to eat little and often and a snack between meals should be encouraged to maximise nutritional intake.

Oral fluid intake

If it is suspected that a client is dehydrated or overhydrated, then this issue should be reported to a registered nurse (RN) or doctor. Fluid balance is a complex process in the body and there are many factors that can cause dehydration or overhydration. It may be that the client requires intravenous or subcutaneous fluid or a change in the types of medication they are taking. If the fluid chart identifies that the client who is able to drink is drinking insufficient amounts, then oral fluid intake should be encouraged.

■ Nutritional Support

The decision to give nutritional support is a decision that should be made by key members of the multidisciplinary team, particularly the dietitian, doctor and nurse and of course the client. The mainstay of nutritional support is to use the gastrointestinal tract if it is working (enteral feeding) and to use the intravenous (parenteral) route only if the gut is unavailable, for example as a result of complete intestinal obstruction. Parenteral support is beyond the scope of this text.

If the client is able to swallow, then oral dietary supplements may be offered in the first instance. Oral dietary supplements are usually given in the form of milk or fruit-flavoured energy- and nutrient-dense beverages. These may be termed 'sip feeds'. Nutrient-rich puddings and soups are also available and may be used by clients with dysphagia to supplement the diet. Vitamin or mineral supplements may be prescribed if there is evidence of a specific deficiency. A multivitamin supplement may be considered necessary by the health-care team if dietary intake of energy, protein, fat and carbohydrate is adequate but the diet is considered to be limited and therefore lacking in micronutrients. Oral dietary supplements are generally used to complement normal food and fluid intake.

If the client is unable to swallow adequately or is unable to eat sufficient amounts to meet their nutritional needs, enteral feeding by tube may be given. This decision is not taken lightly, as enteral feeding via tube has psychological and social implications for the client and complications may occur. Enteral feeding by tube may be used to provide all the client's requirements or simply be supplemental feeding in those who find it difficult to take enough in orally. Contraindications for enteral feeding by tube include persistent vomiting, delayed gastric emptying, an oesophago-gastric fistula, oesophageal reflux and **paralytic ileus**. The patient's medical condition will be considered carefully before the route by which enteral feeding is given is decided.

paralytic ileus

paralysis of the intestinal muscle

The most straightforward route for gut access is the nasogastric route. A fine-bore polyurethane or PVC nasogastric tube is inserted for the delivery of liquid feeds. The smallest possible tube is used to reduce the discomfort of leaving it in place and minimise the risk of nasal mucosal ulceration. Insertion is by a trained nurse or doctor. Doctors are responsible for the insertion of fine-bore tubes in clients with maxillofacial disorders or surgery, laryngectomy and disorders of the oesophagus due to the high risk of perforation.

The procedure for inserting a tube can be seen in Dougherty and Lister (2004). Local policy and guidelines should be adhered to. It is essential to check the position of the tip of the tube in the stomach before feeding begins. This should be done by aspiration of the tube for acid residual or by X-ray (see National Patient Safety Agency, 2005). The tube should be flushed with 30–50 mls of water before and after each feed and before and after drug administration. Sterile water should be used to flush tubes in acute health-care settings and all tubes that terminate in the jejunum (Skipper et al., 2003). In the community setting, cooled, freshly boiled water or sterile water from a newly opened container should be used if the individual is immunosuppressed (NICE, 2003). Fifty ml bladder tip syringes should be used and syringes should be discarded after use. Warm water should be used to dislodge blocks in the tube. Fluids or air should never be forced into the tube though, as the tube may split. The giving set tubing should be changed according to local policy and procedure. The type and rate of feed to be given should be prescribed by the dietitian or in some specialist units may be prescribed by the doctor. The client's head and shoulders should be elevated by at least 30 degrees when the feed is in progress and for one hour after it has stopped unless contraindicated.

Critically ill clients may not absorb feeding solution in the stomach so the residual volume in the stomach is aspirated and measured soon after the feed has commenced in order to determine whether the feed is being digested and absorbed. Algorithms detailing what should be done according to how much is absorbed are usually available in units where this is carried out.

Complications of nasogastric tube placement include malposition at insertion, displacement after insertion, nasopharyngeal irritation, occlusion of the tube, biochemical disturbances and infection. Malpositioning of the tube in the trachea or bronchus may cause the accidental intrapulmonary administration of feed, or pulmonary or oesophageal perforation. The response to feeds should be documented by recording the amount given against the client's prescription, noting any side-effects, for example diarrhoea, and assessing the client's nutritional status at agreed intervals. Other routes via the nose include nasoduodenal and nasojejunal tubes. These types of tube are used in specialist areas.

> **Link**
>
> *Chapter 4 covers the administration of drugs via a nasogastric tube.*

Enterostomies

For clients who need enteral feeding for a long period (usually more than four weeks), a tube is inserted directly into the gastrointestinal tract across the abdominal wall known as an **enterostomy**. Usually tubes are inserted into the stomach (gastrostomy) (Figure 5.2) but in some specialist areas they may be inserted into the jejunum (jejunostomy). This procedure can be carried out in endoscopy, radiology or the operating theatre. A local anaesthetic and sedation may be given or it may be performed as part of an operation. Clients with long-term problems with eating, such as those who have had a stroke or brain injury or have motorneurone disease, multiple sclerosis or learning disabilities with multiple physical handicaps, may have a gastrostomy. Contraindications to the insertion of gastrostomy feeding tubes include **ascites**, severe obesity, blood clotting abnormalities and gastric malignancy.

Instructions as to when feeding can be started – usually on same day the tube has been inserted – should be issued by the person who inserted the tube. As with tubes via the nose, the enterostomy tubes should be flushed with the same frequency and in the same way as nasogastric tubes. The gastrostomy site must be observed daily for signs of gastric acid leakage and infection. Before it is healed, the gastrostomy site should be cleaned aseptically with normal saline, but once it is healed, it should be cleaned daily with soap and water. A dressing is not required unless there is discharge. It may be advised that the gastrostomy tube is pushed in by 1 cm and rotated daily once the tract is healed to avoid tissue adhering to the tube. Local guidelines should be consulted on this issue, as practice does vary according to policy and the type of tube used.

enterostomy
the formation of an external opening into the small gastrointestinal tract

ascites
excess fluid in the peritoneal cavity

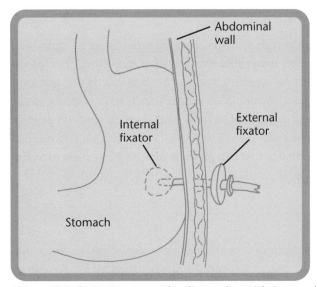

Figure 5.2 ● Gastrostomy feeding tube with internal and external retention discs

Complications of gastrostomy feeding tube insertion include peritonitis (inflammation of the peritoneal cavity), pulmonary aspiration of the feed, peristomal (around the hole) infection, ischaemic pressure necrosis (tissue death from a lack of blood supply as a result of pressure) and migration of the tube.

Clients who receive their nutritional needs via a tube may be unable to keep their mouth clean and moist without assistance. It is important therefore that the client is assisted to clean his mouth regularly and use lip salve as required. The client's mouth should be inspected daily for signs of infection and for observation of general condition.

The nurse must be aware of the psychosocial impact of enteral feeding by tube. Clients who are tube-fed miss out on the social and emotional bonds that can be part of eating together with family and friends. Some clients may eat and drink small amounts and this should be encouraged if they can. Another issue of paramount importance when considering the care of a client requiring nutritional support is the ethics of **hydration** and nutrition. Foods and fluid cannot be given to a client without their consent, unless a client is being treated under the appropriate part of the Mental Health Act. This is a complex topic and is discussed by Lennard-Jones (1999).

hydration
the state of fluid balance of the body

Drugs may be given via feeding tubes in accordance with guidelines. For further information, see the British Association of Parenteral and Enteral Nutrition website (BAPEN, 2005b).

Drug–nutrient interactions

Food intake, absorption and metabolism can be influenced by some drugs and some nutrients may influence drug absorption and metabolism. This is an important issue for nurses to be aware of because of their role in the administration of medications. A good example of a drug–nutrient interaction is the interaction of the antiepileptic drug phenytoin with enteral feed. Phenytoin needs to be administered when the client's stomach is empty to ensure optimal absorption of the drug. The pharmacist can provide advice on this issue in a clinical setting (see also Jordan et al., 2003).

■ Obesity

For many clients, obesity is more of a problem than undernutrition. The equation is deceptively simple: the energy expended must be balanced by the energy gained. The body's metabolism slows over time, so as people become less active because of age, they need to adjust their intake downwards and try to keep their activity level up. Nearly half of Britain's population is overweight (a BMI of over 25), and one in five is clinically obese (a BMI of over 30).

diabetes mellitus

diabetes mellitus is the inadequate production or utilisation of insulin, causing a chronic disorder of glucose metabolism. In type I diabetes mellitus there is a lack of insulin due to destruction of the islet cells in the pancreas. Type II diabetes mellitus is characterised by insulin resistance and changed levels of insulin secretion

Obesity can reduce a person's life expectancy, the increased weight relating to conditions such as type II **diabetes mellitus**, osteoarthritis, sleep apnoea and coronary heart disease. The client with obesity may well experience psychological and social penalties too (Thomas, 1998). The treatment of obesity should be individualised and include assessment and goal-setting. It should be based on diet, activity and behavioural change (Green and O'Kane, 2002). The initial aim of obesity management is to stabilise weight and prevent further weight gain. Following this, a moderate weight loss can be attempted followed by further weight loss and weight maintenance. If diet, activity and behavioural change are unsuccessful in isolation, surgery or drug therapy may be offered. Prevention is, however, better than cure and currently there are lots of national and local initiatives to try to address the significant public health problem of obesity in this country.

■ Chapter Summary

This chapter has reviewed the basic essentials of nutrition and hydration. Macronutrients, micronutrients and current recommendations concerning nutritional intake have been described, and the screening and assessment of clients' nutritional status, planning of nutritional interventions and the nurse's role in common nutritional interventions have been considered. Throughout this process, it must be remembered that securing the well-being and dignity of the client is paramount.

Test Yourself!

1. List the five sections that make up the plate model.

2. What should you try to eat less of, and no more than 6 g a day?

3. What foods are rich in carbohydrates?

4. If your BMI was in the range of 25.0–29.9, what would you be classed as?

5. How much water should you flush a nasogastric tube with before and after each feed and after drug administration?

■ Further reading

Barasi, M.E. (2003) Human *Nutrition. A Health Perspective.* Arnold, London.

Bowling, T. (2004) *Nutritional Support for Adults and Children.* Radcliffe Medical Press, Abingdon.

BAPEN (British Association for Parenteral and Enteral Nutrition) (2005) *Welcome to BAPEN.* BAPEN, Redditch. http://www.bapen.org.uk.

British Nutrition Foundation (2004) *Welcome to the British Nutrition Foundation.* BNF, London. http://www.nutrition.org.uk.

DoH (Department of Health) (2003) *The Essence of Care: Patient-focused Benchmarks for Clinical Governance.* HMSO, London.

Dougherty, L. and Lister, S. (eds) (2004) *The Royal Marsden Hospital Manual of Clinical Nursing Procedures,* 6th edn. Blackwell Science, Oxford.

Geissler, C. and Powers, H. (eds) (2005) *Human Nutrition,* 11th edn. Elsevier, Edinburgh.

Lennard-Jones, J. (1999) *Ethical and Legal Aspects of Fluid and Nutrients in Clinical Practice.* Nursing Times Books, London.

■ References

BDA (British Dietetic Association) (2003) Effective Practice Bulletin issue 32: Challenging the use of body mass index (BMI) to assess under-nutrition in older people. *Dietetics Today* **38**(3):15–19.

Barasi, M.E. (2003) *Human Nutrition: A Health Perspective.* Arnold, London.

BAPEN (British Association for Parenteral and Enteral Nutrition) (2005a) *Malnutrition Universal Screening Tool (the MUST).* BAPEN, Redditch. http://www.bapen.org.uk/the-must.htm.

BAPEN (British Association for Parenteral and Enteral Nutrition) (2005b) *Drug Administration via Enteral Feeding Tubes*. BAPEN, Redditch. http://www.bapen.org.uk/drugs-enteral.htm.

Dougherty, L. and Lister, S. (eds) (2004) *The Royal Marsden Hospital Manual of Clinical Nursing Procedures*, 6th edn. Blackwell Science, Oxford.

DoH (Department of Health) (1991) *Dietary Reference Values for Food Energy and Nutrients for the United Kingdom*. Report of the Panel on Dietary Reference Values of the Committee on Medical Aspects of Food Policy. HMSO, London.

DoH (Department of Health) (2003a) *5 a day, UK*. Department of Health, Leeds. http://www.doh.gov.uk/fiveaday/index.htm.

DoH (Department of Health) (2003b) *The Essence of Care: Patient-focused Benchmarks for Clinical Governance*. HMSO, London.

Elia, M. (2003) *The MUST Report*. BAPEN, Redditch.

Field, A.E., Coakley, E.H., Must, A. et al. (2001) Impact of overweight on the risk of developing chronic diseases during a 10-year period. *Archives of Internal Medicine* **161**(13): 1581–6.

Fieldhouse, P. (1995) *Food and Nutrition. Customs and Culture*, 2nd edn. Chapman & Hall, London.

FSA (Food Standards Agency) (2003) *Safe Upper Levels for Vitamins and Minerals*. FSA Publications, London.

FSA (Food Standards Agency) (2004/05) Homepage, London, FSA. http://www.food.gov.uk/.

Gibney, M.J., Elia, M., Ljungqvist, O. and Dowsett, J. (2005) *Clinical Nutrition*. Blackwell Science, Oxford.

Green, S. and O'Kane, M. (2002) Learning to support practice: management of obesity in adults. *Practice Nurse* **23**(2): 36, 38, 40, 42–6.

Green, S.M. and Watson, R. (2005) Nutritional screening and assessment tools for use by nurses: literature review. *Journal of Advanced Nursing* **50**(1): 69–83.

International Obesity Task Force (2000) *About Obesity*. International Obesity Task Force, Quebec. http://www.iotf.org.

Jordan, S., Griffiths, H. and Griffith, R. (2003) Administration of medicines part 2: pharmacology. *Nursing Standard* **18**(3): 45–54.

Lean, M.E.J. (2000) Pathophysiology of obesity. *Proceedings of the Nutrition Society* **59**: 331–6.

Lennard-Jones, J. (1999) *Ethical and Legal Aspects of Fluid and Nutrients in Clinical Practice*. Nursing Times Books, London.

McLaren, S. and Green, S. 1998 Nutritional screening and assessment. *Professional Nurse* (study supplement) **13**(6): S9–14.

National Patient Safety Agency (2005) *Advice to the NHS on reducing harm caused by the misplacement of nasogastric feeding tubes*, London, NPSA. http://www.npsa.nhs.uk/display?contentId=3525.

NICE (National Institute for Clinical Excellence) (2003) *Prevention of Healthcare-associated Infections in Primary and Community Care*. NICE, London.

Nursing and Midwifery Practice Development Unit (2002) *Best Practice Statement: Nutrition Assessment and Referral in the Care of Adults in Hospital.* Nursing and Midwifery Practice Development Unit, Edinburgh.

Rollins, H. (1997) Nutrition and wound healing. *Nursing Standard* **11**(51): 49–52.

Skipper, L., Cuffling, J. and Pratelli, N. (2003) *Enteral Feeding Infection Control Guidelines.* Infection Control Nurses Association, Bathgate.

Simpson, P.M. (1992) Alcohol consumption in the elderly. *Nutrition Research Reviews* **5**: 153–66.

Thomas, D. (1998) Managing obesity: the nutritional aspects. *Nursing Standard* **12**(18): 49–55.

UKCC (United Kingdom Central Council for Nursing, Midwifery and Health Visiting) (1997) *Feeding of Patients* (letter). UKCC, London.

▧ Useful Websites

www.nutrition.org.uk **British Nutrition Foundation**
Provides healthy eating information, resources for schools, news items and recipes

www.food.gov.uk **Food Standards Agency**

www.bapen.org.uk **British Association for Parenteral and Enteral Nutrition**

6

Elimination

Contents

Learning Outcomes

The purpose of this chapter is to explore the urinary and faecal elements of elimination, explaining the normal and abnormal processes and influences on it. At the end of the chapter, you should be able to:

- Explain the development of elimination that an individual experiences throughout the life span

- Identify specimens that may be collected and common abnormalities that may be found

- Understand the causes of constipation and diarrhoea, and the nursing care of clients experiencing these

- Outline the types of urinary and faecal incontinence and the possible treatments and interventions available

- Introduce the different types of stoma and the specific care that clients with them require.

The chapter provides an opportunity for you to undertake activities that will assist you in your understanding of some aspects of client care. It also includes case study scenarios to illustrate points made in the text.

■ Faecal Elimination

Elimination of excess water and wastes is a basic need for all forms of life.
(Lewis and Timby, 1993)

Successful elimination in humans depends on the individual having an intact and
fully functioning gastrointestinal tract, urinary tract and nervous system.

The lower gastrointestinal tract (Figure 6.1) includes the small and large
intestines. The small intestine (duodenum, jejunum and ileum) is approximately
610 cm (20 feet) long and 2.5 cm (1 inch) in diameter in an adult. The partially
digested food (chyme) leaving the stomach is moved along the small intestine by
peristalsis. The large intestine (caecum, colon, rectum and anus) is approximately 152 cm (5 feet) long and 6 cm (2.5 inches) in diameter. The faeces – the
waste material of digestion that is passed out of the body via the anus or any
other opening (stoma) designed for this purpose following surgery (see below) –
are moved along the length of the large intestine in response to food entering the
stomach. This **gastrocolic reflex**, which propels the faeces by mass peristalsis
and is associated with eating, usually occurs three or four times a day, during or
immediately after a meal.

peristalsis

the coordinated serial
contraction of smooth
muscle propelling food
through the digestive
tract

gastrocolic reflex

a mass peristaltic
movement of the large
intestine occurring
shortly after food enters
the stomach

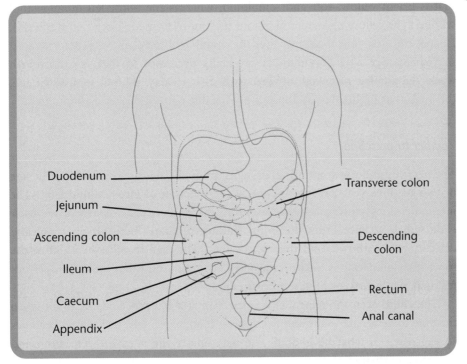

Figure 6.1 ● The main structures of the lower gastrointestinal tract

The defaecation reflex is initiated by the response to faeces entering the rectum. This reflex encourages the internal anal sphincter to relax, the need to defaecate being conveyed to the brain and interpreted by the individual as an awareness of the requirement to eliminate faeces. The 'normal' defaecation pattern varies from one individual to another, some defaecating three times a day, others only once a week.

Development of faecal elimination

Infant

At birth, the muscles of the infant's intestines are poorly developed and control by the nervous system is immature. The intestines contain some simple digestive enzymes but are unable to break down complex carbohydrates or proteins, so the infant can, therefore, digest only simple foods (Cox et al., 1993).

meconium

the thick, sticky material that accumulates in the intestines of the foetus and forms the newborn's first stools

The infant's first bowel movement usually occurs within the first 24 hours of birth and comprises **meconium**, which contains salts, amniotic fluid, mucus, bile and epithelial cells. It is greenish-black to light brown in colour, almost odourless and of a tarry consistency. With the introduction of milk feeding, the characteristics of the infant's faeces change. The infant who is breastfed will have a stool that is bright yellow, soft and semiliquid, whereas the bottle-fed infant's stool will be light yellow to brown in colour and more formed (Kozier et al., 2004). During the first four weeks of life, the infant will have up to 4–8 soft bowel movements per day. This number gradually decreases so that, by the fourth week, the number of bowel movements is 2–4 per day. By four months of age, the infant has gradually developed a predictable pattern of faecal elimination.

Toddler to preschool

The nervous and gastrointestinal systems gradually mature and are, by the age of two to three years, ready to control the function of faecal elimination. The infant develops patterns of defecation so the parents can identify when their child will have success on the potty. Eating stimulates peristaltic activity and defecation (see above), and this can be used as a sign to take the child to the toilet. As elimination is a natural process, it is important that the child does not feel that it is a dirty or unnatural procedure.

The child, even though toilet trained, can still have 'accidents', often when the urge to defaecate is allowed to progress inappropriately. If the child becomes so engrossed in what he is doing, he may ignore the need for defecation and become constipated.

School-aged child

During the school years, the gastrointestinal system attains adult functional maturity. Individuals with learning disabilities may not reach the indicated maturation milestones because of their disability or lack of perception.

Adolescent

Adolescence is important, as the developing bowel habits will take them through their adult life. Adolescents often find it difficult to talk about any elimination problem as they develop sexually.

Adult

A healthy adult usually eliminates 100–400 g of faeces per day (this varies with dietary intake), 25 per cent being solids and the remaining 75 per cent water (Kozier et al., 2004). The solids are made up of cellulose, epithelial cells shed from the lining of the gastrointestinal tract, bacteria, some salts and the brown pigment stercobilin. The brown-coloured faeces occur as a result of the breakdown of bile by the intestinal bacteria. If bile is unable to enter the intestines as a result of obstruction of the bile ducts (which transport bile from the gall-bladder to the duodenum), the faeces are white.

There may be an increasing incidence of intestinal disorders (colonic and rectal carcinoma, and other gastrointestinal conditions such as **irritable bowel syndrome** and **Crohn's disease**) in adulthood. These can be caused by a decrease in the excretion of digestive enzymes (pepsin, ptyalin and pancreatic enzymes) and gastric acid. Elimination patterns are affected by changing lifestyle, for example marriage, having children and changes in employment, which may precipitate stress and anxiety.

Ageing adult

The decrease in the excretion of digestive enzymes continues with age. The elimination process may be affected by changing dietary intake caused by a reduced production of saliva, fewer taste buds and the loss of natural teeth, which are replaced by dentures, caps, crowns and bridges. There are increasing numbers of individuals with learning disabilities living into old age, resulting in 59 per cent of them who live 50–65+ years experiencing continence and excretory health problems (Walker and Walker, 1998; Bland et al., 2003).

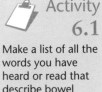

Activity 6.1

Make a list of all the words you have heard or read that describe bowel habit. You may like to discuss this list with your colleagues. This will help you to understand some of the 'language' your clients may use.

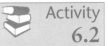

Activity 6.2

For further information on physiology and factors affecting defecation, read Kozier et al., 2004, pp. 1225–8.

irritable bowel syndrome

abnormally increased motility of the bowel, often associated with emotional stress

Crohn's disease

a chronic, often patchy, inflammatory bowel disease of unknown origin, usually affecting the ileum

Specimen collection

specimens

samples of tissue, body
fluids, secretions or
excretions

Specimens are samples of tissue, body fluids, secretions or excretions (Chart 6.1). Nurses often have responsibility for the collection, labelling and timely, safe transport of samples to the laboratory. The validity of test results therefore depends on good practice.

The most common observations the nurse will be required to make of the patient and the specimen are:

● Colour
● Frequency/time
● Amount
● Consistency
● Odour
● Foreign substances (presence or absence)
● Any pain/discomfort expressed by the client on eliminating.

Using these observations, it is important that the nurse makes a clear, accurate and concise report in the client's records.

Activity 6.3

For further infor-
mation on
specimen collection,
read Dougherty and
Lister, 2004,
pp. 663–75.

Faecal specimens

Faeces may be analysed to detect abnormal characteristics or contents, for example blood, parasites, parasite eggs and pathogens.

It is essential that the faecal specimen is not contaminated, so the client is asked to void urine separately into a toilet, bedpan or urinal; urine can interfere with the examination of the faeces, for example destroying some parasites. The client is then asked to pass the faeces into a bedpan. The nurse transfers approximately 15 g (3 teaspoons) of the faeces into the specimen collection container. Care should be taken not to contaminate the outside of the specimen container with the faeces (containers usually have a built-in spatula to assist with this).

Chart 6.1 ● Reasons we collect specimens

Specimens are collected:
● To identify the nature of any disease or for diagnosis
● To assess the effect of treatment
● To confirm or eliminate a specific site of the body as a focus of infection or colonisation
● To determine whether a client who has had an infection is still harbouring the pathogen responsible for it. Clients who have *Salmonella* food poisoning may, for example, still harbour the bacteria in their stools even though their signs and symptoms have disappeared

Altered faecal elimination

Constipation

Constipation refers to the abnormally difficult or infrequent passage of hard faeces and is caused by a decreased motility of the intestines. Some elderly individuals find it difficult to pass soft, bulky faeces. The longer the faeces remain in the intestine, the more water is absorbed from them, which makes them become harder and dryer.

Many individuals wrongly regard themselves as being constipated if they do not defaecate every day. Some individuals who are constipated have episodes of diarrhoea that can be the result of the hard faeces irritating the colon (often termed constipation with overflow). It is, therefore, essential that a note of the normal bowel habits of clients is included in the admission procedure and recorded.

constipation

the abnormally difficult, infrequent or incomplete passage of hard faeces

Causes of constipation

Causes of constipation include the following:

- *Drugs:* tranquillisers, analgesics (especially those containing codeine), opiates, diuretics, anti-Parkinsonian drugs, anticholinergics and antacids containing aluminium as these reduce the motility of the intestines
- *Laxatives:* the abuse of laxatives or frequent enemas. The normal reflexes then diminish, causing the abuser to need more laxative to provide a result and thus become dependent on laxatives
- *Pregnancy:* limits the space for the faeces to pass through the intestine. Peristalsis slows because progesterone causes an excessive absorption of water from the faeces
- *Disease:* obstruction from outside or within the intestine, for example from an abdominal or intestinal tumour, adhesions, interfering with the passage of faeces. Other causes include irritable bowel syndrome, **diverticular disease** and neurological deficiencies such as **paraplegia**, multiple sclerosis and Parkinson's disease and endocrine disorders, for example hypothyroidism.
- *Pain:* for example from an anal fissure (a longitudinal ulcer in the anal canal) or external haemorrhoids (varicose veins in the anal canal, colloquially known as piles)
- *Psychiatric reasons:* depression, leading to a lack of interest in the surroundings and diet, chronic psychoses and anorexia nervosa, which can cause an imbalanced or inappropriate dietary intake and therefore a low fibre and fluid intake
- *Diet:* food low in fibre or an inadequate food intake

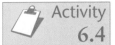

Activity
6.4

List all the factors that may predispose an individual to constipation.

diverticular disease

a condition in which pouch-like extensions develop through the muscular layer of the colon, affecting the passage of faeces

paraplegia

paralysis or sensory loss of the lower limbs, usually including the bladder and rectum

- *Lack of fluid:* either an insufficient intake of fluid or, rarely, an excessive loss of fluid through vomiting and/or sweating
- *Immobility:* any disease that predisposes to immobility or any enforced immobility from bedrest reducing the motility of the gastrointestinal tract
- *Ignoring the call to defaecate:* this allows more fluid to be absorbed from the faeces, thus making them harder and more difficult to eliminate
- *Psychological factors:* unfavourable lavatory conditions, poor hygiene or having to use commodes and bedpans, which may result in the client delaying the defecation process.

There are increasing numbers of individuals with learning disabilities who live to old age and with this comes the normal ageing factors. Added to this, individuals with Down's syndrome experience an increased risk of hypothyroidism, an Alzhiemer's type disease, which can result in an increasing risk of constipation (Holland et al., 1998; Hutchinson, 1999; Evenhuis et al., 2000).

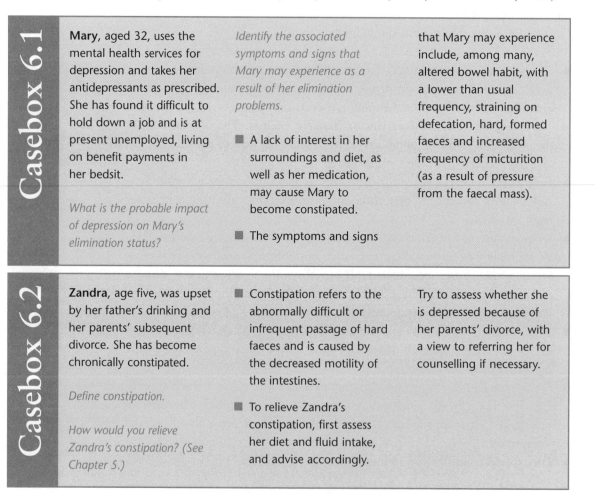

Casebox 6.1

Mary, aged 32, uses the mental health services for depression and takes her antidepressants as prescribed. She has found it difficult to hold down a job and is at present unemployed, living on benefit payments in her bedsit.

What is the probable impact of depression on Mary's elimination status?

Identify the associated symptoms and signs that Mary may experience as a result of her elimination problems.

■ A lack of interest in her surroundings and diet, as well as her medication, may cause Mary to become constipated.

■ The symptoms and signs

that Mary may experience include, among many, altered bowel habit, with a lower than usual frequency, straining on defecation, hard, formed faeces and increased frequency of micturition (as a result of pressure from the faecal mass).

Casebox 6.2

Zandra, age five, was upset by her father's drinking and her parents' subsequent divorce. She has become chronically constipated.

Define constipation.

How would you relieve Zandra's constipation? (See Chapter 5.)

■ Constipation refers to the abnormally difficult or infrequent passage of hard faeces and is caused by the decreased motility of the intestines.

■ To relieve Zandra's constipation, first assess her diet and fluid intake, and advise accordingly.

Try to assess whether she is depressed because of her parents' divorce, with a view to referring her for counselling if necessary.

Care of client with constipation

With his or her help, a history must be taken of the patient's normal elimination pattern. If a diagnosis of constipation is made, an assessment can be undertaken to aid the planning of the client's care.

It is the nurse's responsibility to promote an understanding of the measures available to overcome constipation. The client needs to be educated in the signs and symptoms that are associated with constipation, for example:

● Altered bowel habit, with a lower than usual frequency
● Straining on defecation
● Abdominal and/or back pain
● Changing shape of the faeces
● Hard, formed faeces
● A palpable abdominal mass
● Halitosis (bad breath)
● Headache (owing to possible dehydration and the build-up of toxins)
● Impaired appetite
● An increased frequency of **micturition** because of increased pressure on the bladder from an increased mass in the large intestines.

micturition
_____
the voiding of urine

Clients may require advice on:

● *Dietary intake:* increasing the proportion of fibre
● *Fluid intake:* increasing fluids and avoiding excess alcohol as this acts as a diuretic. The client should be advised to drink 30–35 ml/kg per day (unless other medical conditions restrict this)
● *Mobility:* doing more exercise, if other medical conditions allow, to help to increase the motility of the gastrointestinal tract.

Activity
6.5
Calculate your fluid intake over 24 hours and compare it with the recommendation of 30–35 ml/kg per day.

Although laxatives should be avoided, they may be used only as a short-term measure as prolonged use can lead to dependency, which may result in faecal impaction at a future date.

Other measures to treat constipation include the use of enemas and suppositories. Suppositories are bullet shaped and are designed to melt once they have been inserted into the rectum. Some suppositories soften the faeces and some lubricate the anal canal, whereas others use chemicals to stimulate peristalsis. Other types of suppository that the nurse may use do not promote elimination but are treatments for other conditions, for example infections and pain; these include antibiotic and analgesic preparations. Enemas are solutions that are instilled into the large intestine, the most common being a type of cleansing solution used to empty the lower intestinal tract of faeces.

To insert or introduce a suppository or enema, the client is asked to lie on his left side with his knees bent and drawn up gently towards his abdomen (Figure 6.2). The left side is the preferred side for lying on as the bowel will be angled downward, which will aid the retention of the suppository or enema and help to prevent trauma to the rectum. The suppository or enema is gently introduced into the rectum and the client is asked to retain it for approximately 15 minutes to allow the chemicals to stimulate defecation. Clients often feel that they wish to defaecate as soon as the suppository or enema has been introduced into the rectum because of stimulation caused by the insertion: the anus and rectum react to the stretching of the muscle by sending the information to the brain that the rectum is full.

For some clients, for example those who are paraplegic/quadriplegic or grossly constipated, the only method of faecal elimination available to them is manual evacuation. The client is required to lie on the left side, and the nurse will remove the impacted faeces by hooking them out of the rectum using a gloved finger or two fingers to break them up. This should be used only in exceptional circumstances and not as a routine alternative to other methods of aiding faecal elimination. **Do not employ the procedure without specific instruction** as there is an associated danger of perforation of the lower gastrointestinal tract.

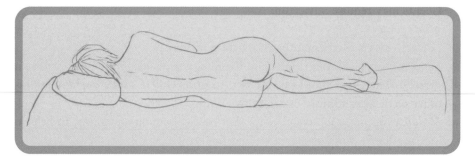

Figure 6.2 ● Left lateral position

<table>
<tr><td rowspan="10" style="writing-mode: vertical;">Casebox 6.3</td><td>

Mrs Ghosh is 89 and has been living in a residential care home for three years. She used to walk in the garden each day but now finds it difficult, requiring a helping hand for safety. Mrs Ghosh spends most of her day sitting in either the lounge or her bedroom. Her

</td><td>

gums are very sore as her dentures are not fitting properly, so she will only eat 'sloppy' food.

Why does Mrs Ghosh have a potential risk of suffering from constipation? (See Chapters 5 and 9.)

</td><td>

What drugs can treat constipation but when abused can cause it?

■ There is a risk of constipation because of immobility, ignoring the call to defaecate, possible depression, leading to a lack of interest in her

</td></tr>
</table>

Casebox 6.4

surroundings and diet, a lack of fibre and, because of her immobility, drinking only the amount of fluid on offer, which may not be sufficient.

■ Laxatives can both treat and predispose to constipation.

Adam, aged 50, has learning disabilities and multiple physical disabilities. He has just moved to a group home in the community. He suffers from chronic constipation as a result of long-term care in an institution where he had a poor diet (lacking in fruit and vegetables), restricted access to fluids and little exercise. Previous care to relieve his constipation included enemas and laxatives.

Adam's new GP has advised the discontinuation of the enemas and laxatives in order to treat his constipation.

What changes to Adam's lifestyle would you consider to improve his elimination problems? (See also Chapters 5 and 9.)

■ Adam needs to increase his mobility. His diet should be assessed and relevant advice given, emphasising an increase in the amount of fruit and vegetables. Fluid intake should also be assessed, the target being an intake of 30–35 ml/kg per day. Discourage Adam from ignoring the call to defaecate, and gradually reduce his enemas and laxatives.

Diarrhoea

Diarrhoea results when movements of the intestine occur too rapidly for water to be absorbed. Faeces are therefore produced in large amounts and may range from being 'loose' to being entirely liquid. If the diarrhoea is severe, large amounts of fluid, consisting of ingested fluids and digestive juices, together with sodium and potassium, are lost in the faeces; this can rapidly result in dehydration and electrolyte imbalance.

diarrhoea
the frequent passage of loose, watery stools

Causes of diarrhoea
The causes of diarrhoea include:

- *Lack of hygiene:* poor hygiene when preparing food after elimination, causing the contamination of ingested food
- *Laxatives:* laxative abuse
- *Infected food: Staphylococcus pyogenes, Salmonella, Escherichia coli* and *Campylobacter*
- *Stress:* excitement, stress and anxiety, causing an increased rate of peristalsis so that the faecal material moves faster through the intestines and less water is absorbed

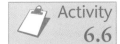
Activity
6.6
List all the factors that may predispose an individual to diarrhoea.

- *Diet:* excessive fibre-rich foods, drinks high in caffeine, which stimulate intestinal motility, and allergy to some foodstuffs, causing irritation of the intestine
- *Disease:* diseases such as chronic pancreatitis, **ulcerative colitis**, Crohn's disease, diverticular disease and irritable bowel syndrome can result in swings between diarrhoea and constipation. Malabsorption syndrome can cause fatty diarrhoea (**steatorrhoea**).

ulcerative colitis

a chronic but inflammatory disease of the large bowel

steatorrhoea

fatty diarrhoea

Care of the patient with diarrhoea

It is essential that fluid balance is maintained as the client can quickly become dehydrated. The nurse must therefore assess the client for signs of dehydration (tachycardia and decreased skin turgor), and the client's input and output of fluid must be accurately recorded. Oral fluid should be high in added potassium and sodium, for example commercially prepared drinks such as Dioralyte or flat cola with a pinch of salt. In severe cases, an intravenous infusion may be required. Some herbal teas, for example rosehip, orange and rhubarb, should be avoided as they exacerbate diarrhoea (Newell et al., 1996).

A careful and thorough history must be taken from the client to ascertain the possible cause of the diarrhoea. All clients suffering from diarrhoea must be treated as potentially infectious until proved otherwise by laboratory examination of the faeces.

Skin care of the perianal region must be maintained, as faecal matter is made up of 60 per cent bacteria that can destroy the skin's cellular defence, leading to skin breakdown and infection. This can also result in the bacteria tracking up the urethra and causing a urinary tract infection (Whitman, 1991 cited in Le Lievre, 2002). Barrier creams may be applied to the area once it has been thoroughly but gently cleaned and dried.

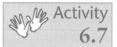 **Activity 6.7**

Try the following exercise to assess skin turgor. Pinch the supraclavicular skin (above the collar bone). If a person is dehydrated, the skin fold will remain. In normal hydration, the skin will return to its normal position almost immediately. Older skin reacts more slowly than younger.

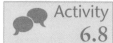 **Activity 6.8**

Identify the impact of diarrhoea on an individual's lifestyle.

Faecal incontinence

Faecal incontinence is the inability to control faecal and gaseous discharge through the anal sphincter (Kozier et al., 2004) and is distressing for the individual as it is difficult to disguise expelled faeces and/or flatus. Soffer and Hull (2000) suggest that the incidence of faecal incontinence in the total population is 1–2 per cent. However, they also suggest that the prevalence increases with age and is as high as 7 per cent in individuals over 65 years, who are otherwise healthy. It is essential that a complete history is taken from the client as it may identify possible causes of the incontinence. These include:

- Disease or injury: permanent or progressive conditions such as spinal cord damage, cerebrovascular accident (stroke) or multiple sclerosis: 50 per cent of patients with multiple sclerosis and 61 per cent of those with spinal injuries suffer from faecal incontinence (Kamm, 1998)

- Impacted faeces with overflow (spurious diarrhoea)
- Temporary loss of control caused by diarrhoea
- Laxative abuse
- Caffeine abuse – as this acts by stimulating colonic motor activity, giving a laxative effect
- Pudendal nerve damage after childbirth
- Infection
- Ulcerative colitis or Crohn's disease, which can lead to faecal urge incontinence
- Stress incontinence caused by chronic straining, trauma or a congenital defect, or arising postpartum
- Congenital malformation, for example anal atresia
- Rectal prolapse, rectal **intussusception**
- Iatrogenic injury (trauma/injury to anal sphincter)
- Megarectum (rectum grossly dilated – Horton, 2004)
- Anxiety.

intussusception
a part of the bowel slips into the lower part and causes intestinal obstruction

Management of faecal incontinence

The management will depend on the cause but will include:

- Administering suppositories or an enema every two to three days if the condition has been caused by faecal impaction, and then instigating a regimen to prevent recurrence
- Advice on changing the diet to one that is well balanced and high in fibre, with an increased fluid intake (if other medical conditions allow)
- The treatment of any diarrhoea
- Controlling and trying to eliminate laxative intake if the condition has been caused by laxative abuse
- Advising clients to attend to their elimination needs after a meal to take advantage of the body's normal gastrocolic reflex
- The use of incontinence aids, such as pads, pants and bed protection
- Pelvic floor exercises (see below). For severe cases of stress incontinence, surgery is indicated, for example post-anal repair or repair after **rectoplexy** for rectal prolapse
- Surgery – sphincter repair, neosphincter (Boyd-Carson, 2003)
- When caring for clients with learning disabilities, a behavioural programme that involves prompt sitting on the toilet and other measures such as increased fluid intake and the use of fibre supplements or bulking agents to help normal bowel function (Smith et al., 1994).

rectoplexy
the fixation of the rectum by suturing to surrounding tissue

Stoma care

The word 'stoma' is derived from Greek meaning mouth or opening. A stoma is formed following surgical intervention for a disease process, its full name being determined by its site. A stoma for elimination purposes is therefore an opening on to the surface of the abdomen through which faecal elimination from either the small or large intestine (or urinary elimination; see below) takes place.

The formation of either a temporary or permanent stoma may be the result of elective surgery or an emergency procedure.

Colostomy

colostomy

an opening of the colon on to the abdominal wall

A **colostomy** is an opening from the colon, which may be temporary or permanent and is indicated for the treatment of the following conditions:

- Malignancy of the colon or rectum, Black (2000) reporting that colorectal cancer is the second most common malignancy in the Western world
- Diverticular disease
- Inflammatory disease of the intestine (for example Crohn's disease or ulcerative colitis)
- Trauma to the large intestine
- The relief of acute intestinal obstruction or perforation

anastomosis

the joining of two hollow structures

- The protection of a distal **anastomosis**, the stoma being formed in a position higher in the gastrointestinal tract than the join between the two ends of intestine that remain after a section of bowel has been removed.

A permanent colostomy is required when the distal segment of the large intestine has been removed, for example when the rectum has been excised because of cancer. The stoma is created by bringing the proximal end of the colon out through an opening on to the anterior wall of the abdomen.

A temporary colostomy is usually necessary to divert the flow of faeces away from the distal part of the large intestine. The surgical technique permits the stoma to be closed once the condition requiring the surgery has been resolved.

The faecal material eliminated from a colostomy, especially if it is on the transverse or descending colon, will be semisolid once the initial postoperative period is complete and the client returns to a 'normal' diet.

Ileostomy

ileostomy

an opening of the ileum on to the abdominal wall

An **ileostomy** is an opening into the ileum and can be indicated for the treatment of inflammatory diseases of the intestine, for example Crohn's disease or ulcerative colitis, or as a temporary measure to rest the large intestine after major large bowel surgery. An ileostomy can be a permanent stoma when the colon has been removed (panproctocolectomy) or temporary to allow the disease process to resolve. A temporary stoma can be closed by anastomosis at a later date and the intestine returned to normal functioning.

The faecal material eliminated through an ileostomy (Chart 6.2) is liquid in consistency, containing digestive enzymes that can cause **excoriation** and erosion of the skin if it is not well protected.

excoriation

injury to the skin caused by trauma such as scratching, rubbing or chemicals, for example the combination of urine and/or faeces and air

Chart 6.2 ● Faecal consistency

- *Ileostomy:* fluid faeces (of a porridge-like consistency), normally 500–800 ml every 24 hours
- *Transverse colostomy:* unformed faeces, semiliquid
- *Descending colostomy:* more formed faeces, near to the normal output for that patient

Management of a client with a stoma

Preoperative care

The client will require a rigorous preoperative assessment, particularly if presenting with a history of chronic disease, weight loss or anorexia. Such clients may be debilitated, so malnutrition and electrolyte imbalances must be corrected to ensure optimum recovery to facilitate wound healing (Kozier et al., 2004). Clients also require psychological preparation to prepare them for the change in body image, to reduce anxiety and for reassurance that they can return to their previous place in society.

The stoma nurse should ensure that the client is offered counselling prior to surgery. She or he, or the consultant if no stoma nurse is available, should mark appropriate sites for the stoma so that the surgery does not interfere postoperatively with normal activities of living (Chart 6.3). The client should be shown and allowed to discuss the appliances available (Figure 6.3).

Chart 6.3 ● Sites to be avoided to facilitate the easy management of a stoma

- Old scars
- Bony prominences
- The umbilicus
- The pubic area
- Skin folds

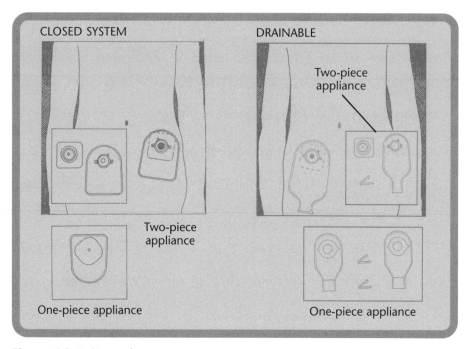

Figure 6.3 ● Stoma bags

Postoperative care

Up to 20 per cent of clients who have a stoma experience significant psycholog-ical problems postoperatively (White, 1998; Black, 2000) and will therefore require a great deal of support, especially in the initial days, weeks and months after its formation. The elimination process of the body has changed, as has body image. Clients therefore have to be helped to adapt to the changes: preop-erative counselling may help them to make a full recovery, returning home to a 'normal' life. Patients may initially demonstrate evidence of withdrawal and depression. Overcoming this is an important part of nursing care; if nurses can show that they accept the clients, this will give their clients confidence.

The formation of the stoma concerns not only clients, but also their partners; one reason being that the change in body image may cause their partners psychological difficulties because of an inability to accept it. Clients who have an ileostomy or colostomy may experience sexual dysfunction (impotence in males and **dyspareunia** in females), but even if they suffer no problems, clients may not be able to return to their normal activities, including sexual activity, for two or three months after the operation. This may be because of the trauma and oedema at the site of the surgery, or sometimes because of nerve damage.

Within our multicultural society, care must be provided that is appropriate to the health practices, values and beliefs of the client. As an example, clients who

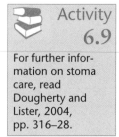

Activity 6.9

For further infor-mation on stoma care, read Dougherty and Lister, 2004, pp. 316–28.

Link

Chapter 8 mentions the impact of stoma surgery on body image.

dyspareunia

the occurrence of pain in the labial, vaginal or pelvic region during or after sexual intercourse

practise the Muslim religion of Islam are required to pray five times a day, before which they are required to perform a washing ritual called *al-wadhu* to signify the body's cleanliness inside and out. The client will need to apply a clean stoma appliance at each prayer time, so a two-piece appliance may be most suitable (Black, 2000).

Care specific to the stoma

Postoperatively, the stoma must be checked regularly – its colour and size, whether it is retracting or prolapsing (Chart 6.4) and its function – to ensure its viability. The stoma may initially discharge some **haemoserous** fluid, and this will be followed, once bowel sounds return, by the passage of some **flatus**, mucus and fluid. Once solid food has been reintroduced, the stoma will discharge faecal matter that is often very liquid at first but gradually becomes less fluid or semi-solid, depending on the stoma site, over the following few days or weeks.

haemoserous fluid

serous fluid containing small amount of blood

flatus

gas in the gastrointestinal tract, which is often expelled through a body orifice, especially the anus

Chart 6.4 ● Appearance of a normal stoma

● Pinkish red (the colour resembling that of the inside of the mouth)
● Initially postoperatively, the stoma is oedematous

The client will require dietary advice as some gas-forming foods (for example onions, cabbage, baked beans and spicy food) may produce excess flatus and pain. The client is therefore advised to try out foods gradually in order to identify which ones cause problems. Clients who have an ileostomy should be advised to increase their fluid intake as their faeces will contain a large amount of water that would previously have been absorbed by the large intestine.

It is important that clients are shown how to care for their own stoma and that, prior to discharge, they are proficient in its management, for example in changing stoma bags, cleaning the stoma and disposing of equipment and soiled stoma bags.

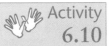

Activity 6.10

To gain some appreciation of what the stoma client experiences, stick a stoma bag full of slushy Weet-abix on to your abdomen and wear it for a few hours, engaging in as many 'normal' activities as possible.

■ Urinary Elimination

The normal anatomy of the urinary system is shown in Figure 6.4.

Development of urinary elimination

Infant

At birth, both nervous system control and renal function are immature, so there is an inability to concentrate the urine and urinary elimination is involuntary.

Urinary output is affected by fluid intake, the amount of activity and the environmental temperature. If the infant is more active or the temperature is raised, more fluid will be excreted through the skin and more water vapour via exhaled air.

Toddler to preschool

The bladder increases in size with the growth of the child and is now able to hold more urine. By two years of age, the kidneys are maturing and can conserve water and concentrate urine almost as well as those of the adult. The nervous system is mature enough for the toddler to control bladder functioning and, as Martini (2002) suggests, toilet training is not physiologically possible until this time.

Day-time bladder control is attained first, followed by night-time control. Even when toilet training has been achieved, however, there may be times of regression and 'accidents'.

School-aged child

The urinary system has now reached maturity.

Adolescent and young adult

There are no noticeable changes in urinary elimination during this time.

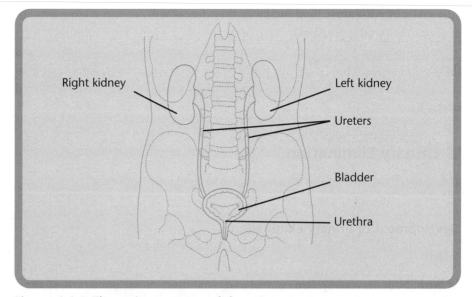

Figure 6.4 ● The main structures of the urinary system

Adult

There is a decrease in renal function with ageing as the result of a gradual decrease in the number of nephrons. Bladder tone gradually diminishes and urinary elimination is therefore more frequent, as the ability to store urine prior to voiding decreases. In a healthy adult, the decrease in renal function is so gradual that the effects are minimal until later in the ageing process (Cox et al., 1993).

Ageing adult

The nephrons continue to decrease in number so renal function gradually lessens. This, combined with vascular **sclerosis**, decreases the glomerular filtration rate, thus decreasing the concentrating ability of the kidneys. Waste products are still processed effectively by the kidneys, but this takes longer than before (Cox et al., 1993).

sclerosis
hardening or induration of an organ or tissue

The loss of smooth muscle elasticity affects the bladder and reduces its capacity. Inhibited bladder contraction can result in frequency and a premature urge to urinate. In the older male, the enlargement of the prostate gland can lead to **urethritis**, especially if there is urinary stasis, which may result in a urinary tract infection (UTI). This leads to dribbling of urine, difficulty in commencing urination, a poor stream, incomplete emptying of the bladder and increased frequency. These changes can cause nocturia (the need to urinate at night) and therefore disturbed sleep. The decrease in oestrogen level in females can predispose to stress incontinence.

urethritis
inflammation of the urethra

Specimen collection

Urine specimens commonly collected are:

- Urine test for *routine screening*, for example on admission or as an outpatient screening procedure
- *Early morning urine* (EMU): because of **diurnal** variation, the first voided urine of the day is usually the most concentrated and is the preferred specimen when testing for substances present in a low concentration, for example hormones in a pregnancy test

diurnal
occurring over a 24-hour period

- *24-hour urine collection*: used to assess the amount of a substance that is lost in the urine. Depending on the substance to be measured, a preservative may be required in the collection bottle, as in the creatinine clearance test (an increased amount of creatinine being found in the urine in the advanced stages of renal disease)
- *Midstream specimen of urine* (MSU), the object of collection being to obtain a specimen of urine uncontaminated by bacteria that may be present on the:

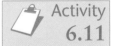
Activity
6.11
List the types of urine specimen you have been asked to collect and why.

– skin
– external genital tract
– perianal region
– distal third of the urethra.

When a UTI is suspected, macroscopic and microscopic examination of an MSU will identify changes in the urine:

1. *Macroscopic examination:* although this is by no means diagnostic, the appearance of the urine can provide evidence of infection. Urinary infection, like any other bacterial infection, is associated with an increased number of white cells at the site of the infection and an inflammatory response that results in the production of pus. Pus in the urine (pyuria) renders it cloudy, so the majority of infected urine is cloudy and some is foul-smelling.
2. *Microscopic examination:* the number of white and red cells per mm^3 of urine is routinely counted. In good health, urine often contains a small number of these cells along with the occasional epithelial cell shed from the lining of the urinary tract. Fewer than 10 white cells/mm^3 is generally considered to be normal. Counts of between 20 and 50/mm^3 are most probably caused by infection but are also a feature of renal disease, so further tests may be requested to confirm the diagnosis. A count greater than 50/mm^3 indicates acute bacterial infection. Infected urine and urinary stasis can lead to crystallisation of the urine; both this and foreign bodies can cause urinary tract stones (Chart 6.5).

Chart 6.5 ● Factors predisposing to urinary stone formation

idiopathic

of unknown or spontaneous origin

- Dehydration
- **Idiopathic (most common)**
- Urinary stasis
- Chronic urinary infection
- Foreign bodies (for example fragments of catheter tubing)
- Disease processes (for example gout and hyperparathyroidism)
- Immobility

Source: Burkitt et al. (1990).

Principles of collecting an MSU

Any bacteria present in the urethra are washed away in the first portion of urine voided, which is not collected. An avoidance of contamination by other bacteria is achieved by thorough cleansing and a good clean technique (Chart 6.6).

Chart 6.6 ● Collection of a midstream specimen of urine

Protocol for women

1. The client should thoroughly wash her hands with soap and water
2. The area around the urinary **meatus** must be cleaned from front to back with soap and water
3. With one hand, the client should spread her labia, keeping them apart until the specimen has been collected
4. The client voids approximately the first 20 ml into the toilet and then passes a portion of the remaining urine into a sterile container. The remaining urine is passed into the toilet
5. The client's fingers should be kept away from the rim and inner surface of the container
6. The specimen is then labelled and, along with the investigation request slip, is forwarded to the laboratory for testing

Protocol for men

1. The client should thoroughly wash his hands with soap and water
2. The foreskin (if present) is retracted and the urinary meatus cleansed
3. The client voids approximately the first 20 ml into the toilet and then passes a portion of the remaining urine into a sterile container. The remaining urine is passed into the toilet
4. The client's fingers should be kept away from the rim and inner surface of the container
5. The client's foreskin (if present) should be returned to its normal position
6. The specimen is then labelled and, along with the investigation request slip, is forwarded to the laboratory for testing

meatus

a passage or opening

Catheter specimen of urine

A catheter specimen of urine (CSU) is taken using an aseptic technique. The catheter bag tubing is clamped (taking care not to damage the tubing) above the specimen portal and left for approximately one hour. The specimen portal is cleaned using an injection/alcohol swab and allowed to dry. A sterile needle (21 G × 1½ inches) is inserted into the portal, and a specimen of approximately 10–20 ml of urine is withdrawn into the syringe, the needle then being removed and the catheter bag tubing unclamped. The specimen should then be transferred to a sterile container, ensuring that the container is not contaminated. It is important that specimens are taken only from the portal that has been designed for this procedure, as using any other site may cause the catheter, catheter bag or tube to leak. Urine taken from the catheter bag is too old and possibly too contaminated for an accurate test result.

Urine specimens should, if possible, be taken before antibiotics are commenced as any treatment may affect the result.

Urine testing for screening

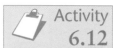

Activity 6.12

List the observations that may be made on a specimen of urine without using a test.

It is important to remember that urine is a body fluid, so all precautions (as identified in a care setting's control of infection procedure book) must be taken for the nurse's safety.

All clients being admitted to hospital should have a urine test. This is one of the few times that urine is screened, and it can highlight any previously undiagnosed medical conditions, for example diabetes mellitus. It will also give baseline information on the client and may precipitate further investigations.

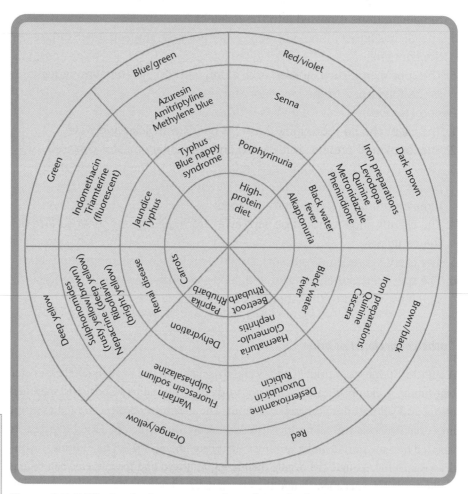

Figure 6.5 ● Effects of substances on the colour of urine (adapted from Ford, 1992)

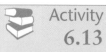

Activity 6.13

For exact details on how to test urine during routine screening, read the guidelines that are enclosed with all containers of urine test strips; these will be stocked in your clinical area.

The client is asked to void a specimen of urine into a urinal, bedpan, jug or other clean receptacle. The urine must be observed for its colour and odour before being tested with a reagent stick. Normal urine is pale and straw-coloured, but the urine may be darker because of a loss of extra fluid through perspiration during hot weather, or from a limited fluid intake. Normal urine, when fresh, has little smell, but if left it may develop an odour of ammonia. Infected urine may be foul-smelling immediately after voiding and become worse on standing. The normal 'straw' colour may alter because of substances present in the urine (Figure 6.5).

Fluids containing alcohol increase the urinary output by inhibiting the production of the antidiuretic hormone. Likewise, fluids that contain caffeine (for example tea, coffee, cola drinks) have a diuretic property so increasing urine production (Kozier et al., 2004).

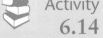

Activity 6.14

For further information on urine testing, read Dougherty and Lister, 2004, pp. 472–3.

Casebox 6.5

Mrs MacDonnell, aged 72, has visited her GP complaining that her urine has been red.

What urinary test will the GP perform, and what do you expect the result to be?

What foods could Mrs MacDonnell have been eating that would turn her urine red?

■ A routine urine test and an MSU will be taken. These findings may be positive for haematuria, or negative if the problem is diet related. Even though

Mrs MacDonnell is aged 72, vaginal bleeding (which could be disease related) should not be ruled out.

■ Beetroot or rhubarb could have this effect on her urine.

Altered urinary elimination

Incontinence

Incontinence can be either permanent or temporary. It can be defined as the involuntary loss of urine and/or faeces at an inappropriate time or in an inappropriate place. This is a 'silent problem', many individuals being thought not to seek medical help because of embarrassment. It is identified that 5–7 per cent of 15–44-year-olds, 8–15 per cent of 45–64-year-olds and 10–20 per cent of over-65-year-olds experience incontinence, 20 per cent of women aged over 40 years being affected by urinary incontinence, with 23 per cent of males aged 40–79 years experiencing dribbling and 14.5 per cent wet clothing (Thakar and Stanton, 2000; Hunskaar et al., 2004). As well as causing clients considerable distress and discomfort, urinary incontinence costs the NHS approximately £424 million per year (Continence Foundation, 2000).

Incontinence is not a disease but a symptom of an underlying disorder that can be mental, physical, social or environmental and affects both sexes at all ages. It may be primary, as in childhood **enuresis** or learning disability, or secondary to another cause such as multiple sclerosis, prostatic enlargement,

incontinence

the involuntary loss of urine and/or faeces at an inappropriate time or in an inappropriate place

enuresis

an involuntary discharge of urine after the age by which bladder control should have been established. In children, a voluntary control of urination is usually established by the age of five. Nocturnal enuresis is, however, present in about 10 per cent of otherwise healthy children at age five, and 1 per cent at age fifteen

obesity or constipation. It can also result from a combination of these, that is, the cause can be multifactorial. As Hunskaar et al. (2004) have identified, urinary incontinence affects the psychosocial, social, economic and physical well-being of individuals and their families. Urinary incontinence has an impact on feelings of sexuality, in its broadest sense, including sexual relationships, appearance, intimacy and caring (Roe, 1999). In a study of Pakistani women's perception of urinary incontinence, Wilkinson (2001) identified feelings of being unclean and sinful. For practising members of the Muslim religion, urinary incontinence has implications on religious obligations – their daily ritual of ablutions and prayer. They also felt more embarrassment when talking to males about incontinence issues.

When assessing clients, their oral fluid intake should be reviewed, as some herbal teas, for example elderberry, strawberry, rose, wild blackberry and nettle, act as diuretics (Newell et al., 1996).

There are four main types of urinary incontinence:

- Stress incontinence
- Urge incontinence
- Reflex incontinence
- Overflow incontinence.

The male and female urethras are shown in Figures 6.6 and 6.7 respectively (see also Chart 6.7).

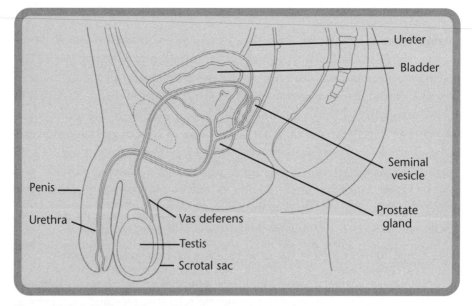

Figure 6.6 ● The position of the urethra in a male

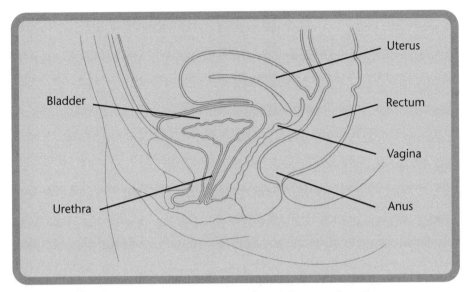

Figure 6.7 ● The position and angle of the urethra in a female

Chart 6.7 ● The female urethra
....

- The urethra is embedded in the anterior wall of the vagina
- It runs downwards and forwards behind the symphysis pubis and opens at the external urethral orifice, which lies just in front of the opening of the vagina
- Its diameter is approximately 0.7 mm
- It is approximately 4 cm long
- The urethra is 'slit-shaped' rather than cylindrical
- If there is a weakness of the pelvic floor muscles and the urethra becomes more vertical, it is easier for urine to leak out (incontinence)

....

Source: Haslam (1997).

Stress incontinence

This type of incontinence is more common in females than males and it is both a neuromuscular and anatomical condition. The main cause is sphincter deficiency – pelvic floor dysfunction, pudental/pelvic nerve damage, injury or degenerative changes as a result of hormonal deficiency, or age-related atrophy of the tissues (Bardsley, 2004). A small amount of urine is leaked on physical exertion, coughing, sneezing or laughing. This results from an incompetent urethral sphincter, which is caused by a weakness of the supporting pelvic floor muscles. Predisposing factors include childbirth, hormonal changes owing to the menopause, vaginal prolapse, obesity, inactivity and constipation; in men, stress incontinence can occur after prostatectomy.

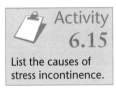

Activity
6.15
List the causes of stress incontinence.

Treatment includes pelvic floor exercises, weighted vaginal cones, electrical therapy that stimulates the nerves, causing the muscles to contract, periurethral bulking injections, pharmacological therapy, special tampons, vaginal pessary and, in the case of postmenopausal women, oestrogen hormone replacement therapy (Bardsley, 2004). Surgical intervention may include **vaginal repair** or insertion of sub-urethral tape, which is inserted between the urethra and vagina, therefore lifting the middle part of the vagina.

Urge incontinence

Urge incontinence causes the loss of a variable amount of urine and is caused by **detrusor muscle** instability (an unstable bladder), neuropathic conditions and outflow obstruction. The individual often complains that he has little or no warning of a need to micturate and is often incontinent on the way to the toilet. Causes include urinary tract infection, bladder stones, an enlarged prostate gland, a urethral stricture, faecal impaction, Alzheimer's disease, cerebrovascular accident, spinal cord lesions and Parkinson's disease. Residual volumes of urine, left in the bladder after micturition, may occur, causing urinary stasis and a subsequent UTI.

Treatment rarely involves surgery but does include bladder retraining exercises, **antimuscarinic** drug therapy and relaxation exercises.

There is a high level of mixed stress and urge incontinence, especially in the elderly.

Reflex incontinence

This type of incontinence manifests itself as the individual's failure to recognise the need to micturate and is usually caused by damage of the peripheral nerves to the bladder or of the spinal cord. The bladder fills and empties on a reflex cycle, and the condition may be combined with incomplete voiding and a high residual urinary volume.

Treatment may involve surgery, for example urinary diversion or urostomy (see below). In addition, catheterisation (indwelling urethral, suprapubic or intermittent self-catheterisation) and other techniques, such as the Valsalva or Credé manoeuvres (Chart 6.8), may be used.

Chart 6.8 ● Valsalva and Credé manoeuvres

Valsalva manoeuvre

The client is asked to inhale and then attempt to forcibly exhale, with the glottis (vocal cords), nose and mouth closed. This causes the diaphragm to flatten, thus increasing the intra-abdominal pressure. Unless the urethral

---

vaginal repair

following prolapse of the vagina and uterus, surgical repair is performed to return the structures to their normal position

detrusor muscle

the external longitudinal layer of the muscular coat of the bladder

antimuscarinic

opposing the action of muscarine or agents that mimic it, for example atropine and scopolamine

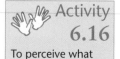 Activity 6.16

To perceive what clients experience when they are incontinent, wet a pad with water and wear it next to your skin in the perineal area. Undertake as many everyday activities as possible.

sphincter is in complete spasm, the increased pressure forces urine to be voided. Clients with cardiac problems should not attempt this

Credé manoeuvre
The client is asked to apply pressure over the symphysis pubis. The pressure may be enough to produce spasm of the bladder or cause voiding of the urine

Overflow incontinence

Overflow incontinence is caused by urinary retention with overflow, which is caused by:

● *An obstruction* from an enlarged prostate, prostatic cancer, urethral stricture or faecal impaction; treatment includes prostatectomy, urethrotomy and the clearance of any faecal impaction
● *A hypotonic bladder* (ineffective contraction of the bladder when voiding urine) caused by neuropathy (as in diabetes) or anticholinergic medication (such as imipramine); treatment includes intermittent self-catheterisation, drug therapy (for example carbachol) to enhance detrusor contractility and a review of drug regimens to ensure that other medication is not the cause of the hypotonia
● *Detrusor–sphincter dyssynergia* (uncoordinated muscle activity) caused by neuropathic conditions, for example paraplegia and multiple sclerosis; treatment includes intermittent self-catheterisation and **biofeedback** to teach coordination.

biofeedback
a training programme designed to develop one's ability to control the autonomic (involuntary) nervous system

An indwelling catheter should be used only as a last resort for clients with voiding difficulties.

Cystitis

Cystitis is inflammation of the bladder usually occurring secondary to an ascending UTI. It is more common in sexually active females because of the close proximity of the urethra and the vagina. In the acute stage, clients complain of frequent and painful micturition; in the chronic stage, it is secondary to a lesion that may have pyuria as its only symptom. Antibiotics are used to treat the infection, and the client should be encouraged to drink 2–3 litres of fluid per day (if the medical condition allows) to dilute the urine and decrease the pain on micturition.

cystitis
inflammation of the bladder, usually secondary to an ascending UTI

Pelvic floor exercises

Activity 6.17

If you do not already practise pelvic floor exercises regularly, you should start now by following the instructions in Chart 6.9.

Pelvic floor exercises (Chart 6.9) are primarily intended to increase the strength of the levator ani muscles. In women, pelvic floor exercises involve the contraction and relaxation of the muscles that surround the vagina and anus, thus improving their tone. This helps to restore the normal anatomical relationships of the surrounding structures as well as the function of the urethral sphincter.

In males, pelvic floor exercises should be taught before prostatectomy so that they can help to stop post-micturition dribbling following prostatectomy by improving urethral sphincter function.

Chart 6.9 ● Pelvic floor exercises
....

The client needs to sit, stand or lie in a comfortable position and tighten the pelvic floor for approximately 10 seconds – there should be feeling of tightening the anus but not the buttocks, abdomen or legs. This should be repeated 10 times. Clients need to imagine that they are stopping a flow of urine. For females learning this exercise, a finger can be inserted into the vagina and 'squeezed'. Clients should progress so that, when passing urine, they can stop and start mid-flow; this should be carried out once a week to check the progress of the exercise regimen. Pelvic floor exercises should be performed at least twice daily

....

Urinary catheterisation

A urinary catheter is designed to remove fluid from or instil fluid into the bladder. Urinary catheterisation is a common procedure, with 12 per cent of hospital clients (Crow et al., 1996) and 4 per cent of clients in the community (Getliffe, 1990) being catheterised at any one time.

Indications for catheterisation are:

cytotoxic

toxic to cells; the term is usually applied to drugs used in the treatment of cancer

- Pre- and postoperatively to empty the bladder before or after abdominal, rectal or pelvic surgery
- The acute or chronic retention of urine
- To introduce drugs, for example antibiotics and **cytotoxic** drugs
- To irrigate the bladder in order to remove sediment and/or blood clots
- Trauma, for example any trauma to the pelvis or lower urinary tract (as any oedema resulting from the trauma may cause obstruction), in order to monitor for blood, and following burns to monitor urinary output
- The accurate measurement of urinary output

- Diagnostic investigations of bladder function
- Incontinence, when all other methods have failed.

Catheters

The nurse should assess the client prior to catheterisation and identify the reason for undertaking the procedure, the length of time the catheter is to remain in situ and the sex of the client. This will help to determine the type of catheter required. The size of catheter will depend upon whether clear urine or haematuria is to be drained (Chart 6.10). Catheters designed for women are shorter than those designed for men because the adult urethra is approximately 4 cm long in a woman and 20–23 cm in a man.

In the majority of cases, a retaining balloon 5 ml in volume will be sufficient. The catheter will require 10 ml of sterile water for its insertion: 5 ml to fill the balloon and 5 ml the balloon's inlet tubing. A balloon size of 30 ml volume should be discouraged, its main use being for clients following urological surgery, in particular prostatic surgery.

Chart 6.10 ● Catheter size (for an adult)

- Clients with clear urine: 12–16 Fr (Ch)
- Clients with haematuria: 18–22 Fr (Ch)

1 Fr (Ch) is equivalent to 0.3 mm, catheters being measured across their external diameter

Common types of catheter

- *Teflon:* the latex is teflon coated to reduce urethral irritation; such catheters can be used for clients requiring short- or medium-term, up to one month, catheterisation
- *Silicone:* these catheters are very soft, are less irritating and cause less crystal formation than the latex variety. They should be used for clients who require catheterising for more than two weeks, the catheters having a life span of approximately three months
- *Hydrogel:* these catheters absorb water to produce a slippery surface and therefore decrease friction to the urethra. They are more resistant to encrustation and adherent bacteria, and have a life span of up to 14 weeks
- *Conformable catheter:* these are designed to conform to the shape of the female urethra (slit-shaped) and allow partial filling of the bladder. They are approximately 3 cm longer than conventional female catheters.

Types of catheterisation

Activity 6.18

For further information on urinary catheterisation, refer to Dougherty and Lister, 2004, pp. 330–47 and Kozier et al., 2004, pp. 1284–5.

There are three types of catheterisation. The most common and probably the best known is indwelling catheterisation, the other two being intermittent self-catheterisation and suprapubic catheterisation.

Indwelling catheters

The insertion of a urethral catheter requires an aseptic technique, and it is preferable for the client to have a shower or bath prior to catheterisation to ensure good hygiene. The balloon size, the type of material and the size of the catheter used will depend on the reason for catheterisation.

Once the catheter is in situ, meatal and perineal hygiene should be performed. Soap and water are sufficient to clean the meatal and perineal areas, but the nurse or client must ensure that the area is thoroughly dried afterwards (Brown, 1992).

The type of urinary drainage bag will be determined by whether the client is mobile (for example clients able to continue normal mobility activities or clients in wheelchairs) or has limited mobility (for example after surgery or with a medical condition reducing mobility). Clients who are normally mobile may benefit from wearing a leg bag during the day, changing to a full-size drainage bag at night. Clients with limited mobility will wear a full-size bag until the catheter has been removed or 'normal' mobility restored.

To empty a urinary drainage bag, the nurse must wash her hands prior to and after carrying out the procedure, as well as wear gloves during the procedure. The outlet tap of the catheter system should be opened and the urine allowed to drain into a single-use receptacle, the outlet tap being closed after emptying. The urinary drainage bag must hang below the level of the bladder to ensure that urine does not seep back into the bladder; the bag can be supported by attaching it either to the side of the bed or to a stand specially designed for this purpose. If a leg bag is worn, it must be secured to the client's leg without causing traction to the catheter and therefore trauma to the urethra and bladder neck. The tap of the urinary drainage bag must not touch the floor as this will result in contamination and a possible UTI (Figure 6.8).

It is important that meatal and perineal hygiene is maintained to reduce the risk of encrustation around the catheter and meatus. The client should be encouraged to drink 20–35 ml/kg per day (unless other medical conditions restrict this) in order to reduce the risk of UTI, constipation (as this may cause pressure on the bladder and urethra) and the irritant effect of concentrated urine on the bladder. Constipation should also be avoided as it can contribute towards leakage around the catheter.

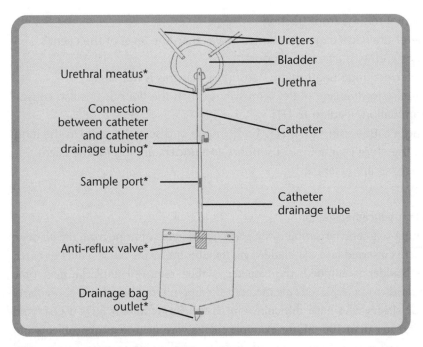

Figure 6.8 ● Points (*) at which pathogens can enter a closed urinary drainage system

Pomfret (2000) identified a number of risk factors or serious complications associated with urinary catheterisation, including urethral perforation, trauma, stricture formation, urinary tract infection, encrustation and bladder calculi and possible carcinoma of the bladder. Urinary tract infections are the most common complaint for individuals with indwelling catheters (Simpson, 2001) and the incidence increases with the longer the catheter is in situ (Curran, 2001). This is particularly increased when individuals have other infections, the catheter is being used to measure urinary output, or individuals have existing chronic conditions, for example diabetes or malnutrition. Also, females are at greater risk than males (Maki and Tambyah, 2001). The principles of care of the patient with a urinary catheter are shown in Chart 6.11.

Chart 6.11 ● Principles of care for the client with a urinary catheter in situ

● Meatal hygiene – to minimise encrustation
● Fluid intake – adequate intake to reduce the risk of concentrated urine irritating the bladder and to lessen the risk of constipation
● Catheter selection – the appropriate size of catheter and balloon, in a material appropriate to the time proposed in situ, and of a length appropriate to gender; a shorter length for women can, for example, prevent

accidental trauma from traction
- Catheter drainage bag – positioned lower than the level of the client's bladder and with effective support
- Catheter drainage bag tubing – ensuring that this is not kinked
- Catheter bag drainage outlet – must not touch the floor as this can cause contamination, leading to UTI
- Having a catheter in situ affects body image and sexual activity in the long term, therefore psychological support and understanding for the client and partner are essential

Link

Chapter 8 investigates issues of body image.

Intermittent self-catheterisation

Intermittent self-catheterisation is the periodic drainage of urine from the bladder. A catheter is inserted into the bladder via the urethra by the nurse, client or carer, and the bladder is emptied; the catheter is then removed until the next time voiding needs to take place. This method of emptying the bladder is particularly useful for clients who have difficulties in passing urine and/or have a post-void residual greater than 100 ml, for example clients with neurological problems and those who suffer from urinary incontinence, thus allowing them to gain control of their bladder. Prior to instruction, clients and/or carers should be assessed in terms of whether they are suitable to undertake this procedure (Chart 6.12).

Chart 6.12 ● Criteria for clients undertaking intermittent self-catheterisation

Clients should:
- Be incontinent of urine (overflow incontinence)
- Have good manual dexterity and mobility
- Have the mental ability to learn and understand
- Show good motivation
- Possess an intact urethra
- Have a bladder capacity of 100 ml or more

The catheter's length will be determined by the client's gender. For a man, the catheter should be 38 cm long, and for a woman 20 cm as the female urethra is shorter than the male.

The actual principles and procedure of intermittent self-catheterisation are the same as for the insertion of an indwelling catheter, but this is a 'clean' procedure rather than an aseptic one. Catheters may be used more than once and may be self-lubricating. Urinary tract infections are lower in incidence in this group than in clients with indwelling catheters.

Suprapubic bladder drainage

A self-retaining catheter is inserted through a suprapubic incision or puncture into the bladder (Figure 6.9). This is a temporary measure to divert the flow of urine from the urethra when the urethral route is impassable or impossible because of, for example:

- Trauma
- Stricture
- Prostatic obstruction
- Pelvic fractures
- Gynaecological operations: vaginal hysterectomy and vaginal repair.

Drainage can be maintained for several months.

Bond and Harris (2005) suggest that, for suprapubic catheterisation, the catheter used should be no smaller than 16 Ch with a 10 ml balloon as this ensures that the tract between the bladder and skin is maintained.

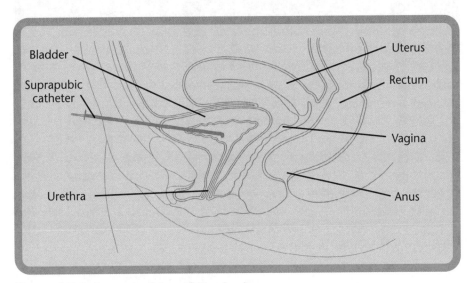

Figure 6.9 ● A suprapubic catheter in situ

Urostomy

A **urostomy** is performed when the bladder is being removed or is diseased (Chart 6.13). It is an opening from the ureters into a resected section of (usually) ileum, approximately 15 cm in length, which then channels the urine through a stoma that has been formed on the abdominal wall (known as an ileal conduit) and is fashioned into a spout to aid drainage.

urostomy

an opening in the abdominal wall to allow the diversion of urine

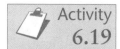
Activity
6.19

For further infor-
mation on
urostomy, read
Dougherty and
Lister, 2004, p. 317
and Kozier et al.,
2004, pp. 1283–4.

Urine that is eliminated through a urostomy can excoriate the surrounding skin if it is not well protected. The urine will constantly 'dribble' from the stoma into a urostomy drainage bag (Figure 6.10). The management of a urostomy is the same as for stoma care.

Chart 6.13 ● Indications for urostomy formation

- Malignant disease of the bladder
- Malignant disease of the pelvis
- Trauma
- Neurological damage
- Congenital disorders
- Intractable incontinence

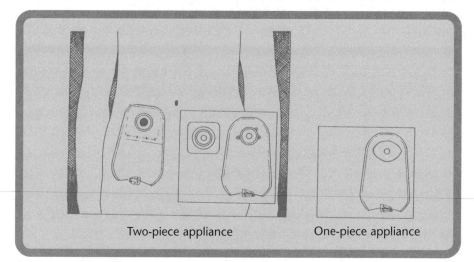

Two-piece appliance   One-piece appliance

Figure 6.10 ● Urostomy bags

■ Chapter Summary

This chapter has explored both the urinary and faecal elements of elimination. It explains the normal anatomy and physiology and then identifies the abnormal processes of and influences on elimination. It explores possible treatments, the advice available and nursing care for the conditions identified.

Test Yourself!

1. What information do you need to obtain when making an assessment of your clients' elimination needs?

2. List and explain the factors that may cause a client to become constipated.

3. Identify four types of incontinence.

4. What is the difference between an ileostomy, a colostomy and a urostomy?

5. Identify the psychological factors that affect both urinary and faecal elimination.

6. How much fluid should a healthy individual weighing 65 kg drink in a day?

■ Further Reading

Benson, D. (2003) The importance of a thorough continence assessment. *Nursing Times* **99**(29): 53.

Fultz, N.H. and Herzog, A. (2001) Self-reported social and emotional impact of urinary incontinence. *Journal of the American Geriatrics Society* **49**: 892–9.

Getliffe, K. (2003) How to manage encrustation and blockage of Foley catheters. *Nursing Times* **99**(29): 59.

Marieb, E. (2004) *Human Anatomy and Physiology*, 6th edn. Benjamin Pearson Cummings, Redwood City, CA.

Marklew, A. (2004) Urinary catheter care in the intensive care unit. *Nursing in Critical Care* **9**(1): 21–7.

Peate, I. (2003) Nursing role in the management of constipation: use of laxatives. *British Journal of Nursing* **12**(19): 1130–6.

■ References

Bardsley, A. (2004) Key trends in the management and treatment of stress urinary incontinence. *Professional Nurse* **19**(10): 30–2.

Black, P. (2000) Practical stoma care. *Nursing Standard* **14**(41): 47–53.

Bland, R., Hutchinson, N., Oakes, P. and Yates, C. (2003) Double jeopardy? Needs and services for older people who have learning disabilities. *Journal of Learning Disabilities* **7**(4): 323–44.

Bond, P. and Harris, C. (2005) Best practice in urinary catheterisation and catheter care. *Nursing Times* **101**(8): 54–8.

Boyd-Carson, W. (2003) Faecal incontinence in adults. *Nursing Standard* **18**(8): 45–51.

Britton, P.M. and Wright, E.S. (1990) Nursing care of catheterized patients. *Professional Nurse* **5**(5): 231–4.

Brown, M. (1992) Urinary catheters: patient management. *Nursing Standard* **6**(19): 29–31.

Burkitt, H., Quick, C. and Gatt, D. (1990) *Essential Surgery: Problems, Diagnosis and Management*. Churchill Livingstone, Edinburgh.

Continence Foundation (2000) Making the case for investment in an integral continence service: a source book for continence services. In Thakar, R. and Stanton, S. Management of urinary incontinence in women. *British Medical Journal* **321**: 1326–31.

Cox, H., Hinz, M., Lubno, M. et al. (1993) *Clinical Applications of Nursing Diagnosis: Adult, Child, Mental Health, Gerontic and Home Health Considerations*, 2nd edn. F.A. Davis, Philadelphia.

Crow, R., Chapman, R., Roe, B. and Wilson, J. (1996) *A Study of Patients with an Indwelling Urethral Catheter and Related Nursing Practice*. Nursing Practice Research Unit, University of Surrey, Guildford.

Curran, E. (2001) Reducing the risk of health-acquired infections. *Nursing Standard* **16**: 45–52.

Dougherty, L. and Lister, S. (2004) *The Royal Marsden Hospital Manual of Clinical Nursing Procedures*, 6th edn. Blackwell Publishing, Oxford.

Evenhuis, H., Henderson, C.M., Beange, H., Lennox, N. and Chicione, B. (2000) *Healthy Aging: Adults with Intellectual Disabilities: Physical Health Issues*. World Health Organization, Geneva.

Ford, A. (1992) Feeling off-colour. *Nursing Times* **88**(5): 64–8.

Getliffe, K. (1990) Catheter blockage in community patients. *Nursing Standard* **5**(9): 33–6.

Haslam, J. (1997) Floor plan. *Nursing Times* **93**(15): 67–70.

Holland, A.J., Hon, J., Huppert, F.A., Stevens, F. and Watson, P. (1998) Population based study of the prevalence and presentation of dementia in adults with Down's syndrome. *British Journal of Psychiatry* **172**: 493–8.

Horton, N. (2004) Behavioural and biofeedback therapy for evacuation disorders. In Norton, C. and Chelvanayagam, S. (eds) *Bowel Continence Nursing*. Beaconsfield Publishers, Beaconsfield.

Hutchinson, N.J. (1999) Association between Down's syndrome and Alzheimer's disease: review of the literature. *Journal of Learning Disabilities for Nursing, Health and Developmental Disabilities* **15**: 329–36.

Hunskaar, S., Lose, G., Sykes, D. and Voss, S. (2004) The prevalence of urinary incontinence in woman in four European countries. *British Journal of Urology International* **93**(3): 324–30.

Kamm, M.A. (1998) Faecal incontinence. *British Medical Journal* **316**: 528–32.

Kozier, B., Erb, G., Berman, A. and Snyder, S. (2004) *Fundamentals of Nursing: Concepts, Process and Practice*, 7th edn. Pearson Education, Upper Saddle River, NJ.

Lewis, L.W. and Timby, B.K. (1993) *Fundamental Skills and Concepts in Patient Care.* Chapman & Hall, London.

Maki, D.G. and Tambyah, P.A. (2001) Engineering out the risk of infection with urinary catheters. *Emerging Infectious Disease* **7**: 342–7.

Martini, F.H. (2002) *Fundamentals of Anatomy and Physiology*, Prentice Hall, Englewood Cliffs, NJ.

Newell, C.A. Anderson, L.A. and Phillipson J.D. (1996) *Herbal Medicines. A Guide for Healthcare Professions.* Pharmaceutical Press, London.

Pomfret, I.J. (2000) Multidisciplinary continence care. *Nursing Times* **99**(19): 59.

Roe, B. (1999) Incontinence and sexuality: findings from a qualitative perspective. *Journal of Advanced Nursing* **30**(3): 573–9.

Simpson, L. (2001) Indwelling urethral catheters. *Nursing Standard* **15**(46): 47–53.

Smith, L.J., Franchetti, B., McCoull, K., Pattison, D. and Pickstock, J. (1994) A behavioural approach to retraining bowel function after long-standing constipation and faecal impact in people with learning disabilities. *Developmental Medicine and Child Psychology* **34**: 41–9.

Soffer, E. and Hull, T. (2000) Fecal incontinence: a practical approach to evaluation and treatment. *American Journal of Gastroenterology* **95**(8): 1873–9.

Thakar, R. and Stanton, S. (2000) Management of urinary incontinence in women. *British Medical Journal* **321**: 1326–31.

Walker, C. and Walker, A. (1998) *Uncertain Futures: People with Learning Difficulties and their Aging Family Carers.* Pavilion/Joseph Rowntree Foundation, London.

White, C. (1998) Psychological management of stoma related concerns. *Nursing Standard* **12**(36): 35–8.

Whitman, D. (1991) Intra-abdominal infections: pathophysiology and treatment. Hoechst, Frankfurt. In Le Lievre, S. (2002) An overview of skin care and faecal incontinence *Nursing Times* **98**(41): 58–9.

Wilkinson, K. (2001) Pakistani women's perceptions and experiences of incontinence. *Nursing Standard* **16**(5): 30–2.

■ Useful Websites

www.aca.uk.com Association for Continence Advice
A membership organisation for health and social care professionals concerned with the progression of care for continence

www.continence-foundation.org.uk Continence Foundation
Provides advice for people with bladder or bowel problems

www.wocn.org Wound Ostomy and Continence Nurses' Society

www.dh.gov.uk Department of Health

www.health.gov.au/internet/wcms/publishing.nsf/content/continence-2 Australian government Department of Health and Ageing
Provides information about continence

Chapter

7

RUTH SADIK, CHRIS WALKER AND DEBRA ELLIOTT

Respiration and Circulation

Contents

- Respiration
- Circulation
- Chapter Summary

- Test Yourself!
- Further Reading
- References

Learning Outcomes

The purpose of this chapter is to examine factors associated with respiratory and cardiac function. It will explore the nurse's role in relation to assessing and implementing care with clients who experience difficulties with maintaining breathing and circulation. At the end of the chapter, you should be able to:

- Monitor and interpret a client's respiratory and cardiac vital signs

- Rationalise common deviations from normal values

- Identify techniques for maintaining cardiorespiratory function

- Assist clients in maintaining effective cardiorespiratory function

- Recognise the signs of cardiorespiratory arrest

- Describe the appropriate response and initial management of a collapsed client.

Respiration

Respiration and circulation before birth

During fetal life, the function of the heart and lungs is minimal, as the maternal placenta is employed in supplying the oxygen, nutrition and waste removal required to sustain growth and development in the uterus for 37–40 weeks (term) (Tucker Blackburn, 2003). By this time the lungs are anatomically and physiologically fully functional; however, the maturation process will continue until the end of the eighth year of life, with a marked increase in lung dimensions and number of alveoli.

Lung development commences approximately 22 days after fertilisation, with the appearance of buds on the wall of the rudimentary alimentary tract that will form the trachea and major bronchi. One week later the bud is seen to have bifurcated and, in the following week, two secondary buds form on the left branch and three on the right, which correspond to the lobes of the fully formed lung. This process constitutes the embryonic phase of development; however, there are three further stages prior to birth:

- *Pseudoglandular* (weeks 6–17) – further branching occurs and primitive cartilage, smooth muscle and epithelial cells can be found, and fetal breathing movements can be detected
- *Canalicular* (weeks 16–20) – vascular beds are laid down and primitive air sacs are present by the latter week; also lung fluid starts to be secreted, which appears to dictate the normal structure and size of the internal air space (Tucker Blackburn, 2003)
- *Sacular/alveolar* – further growth and development of the respiratory tree; pneumocytes types I and II can be found in the alveolar walls that are responsible for surfactant secretion; and by 26 weeks, bronchioles with their surrounding capilliaries are evident, increasing the chances of independent survival if born at this time.

The prenatal lungs are filled with fluid, secreted by the alveolar cells, that contains a complex lipoprotein substance, known as surfactant, which is also needed for normal lung function. An immature form of it is found as early as 24 weeks gestation, but the mature form is not secreted until 32–34 weeks gestation (Coad, 2002). In the postnatal period, surfactant prevents the alveoli collapsing during inspiration. In readiness for the transition to breathing air, the fetal breathing movements increase to approximately 70 per minute in the weeks leading up to birth.

If born before 34 weeks gestation, many infants will experience breathing difficulties, either because the alveoli or the capilliaries surrounding the alveoli have not yet matured, meaning that an effective mechanism for gaseous exchange is not available.

The heart and blood vessels develop during the fourth week of pregnancy and are complete by the end of the eighth week. The speed of development corresponds to the embryo's increasing need for nutrients that cannot be met by the yolk sac. Until around day 21, the primitive heart is merely two tubes lying parallel to each other, known as endocardial tubes. These fuse to become the single cardiac tube. Over the next few days, this tube elongates and coils back on itself, to the right (dextra or D-looping), creating a single chambered vessel. If you have difficulty envisioning this, there are some fantastic websites, such as www.visembryo.com, that allow you to see heart development in three dimensions. By 28 days, the heart has started to beat, and by week five it has taken on the characteristic conical shape with identifiable structures (Tucker Blackburn, 2003).

Inside the heart, the single chamber is divided into four chambers by the formation of septa. One, dividing the heart horizontally into atria and ventricles, is composed of two sections that overlap approximately at the level of the atria, creating the foramen ovale. The other septum divides the heart vertically into right and left sides, and gives rise to the valves of the heart. This process is complete by week eight, and if any disruption occurs, congenital abnormalities such as ventricular or atrial septal defects may result.

The heart is also adapted to intrauterine life, and not yet prepared for the work of sending deoxygenated blood to the lungs (pulmonary circulation) or oxygenated blood around the body (systemic circulation), as the fetal circulation only has to manage oxygen and waste exchange with the placenta. This is achieved by an ingenious series of diversions that do not persist beyond the neonatal period, aimed at providing the developing brain and vital structures with appropriate nutrients while avoiding flooding the immature lungs with blood. You will need to refer to Figure 7.1 while reading this next section.

Maternal blood enters the placenta through the intervillous spaces, while the fetal blood flows through chorionic villi capilliaries, which project into the intervillous spaces. Although the maternal and fetal bloods do not mix, water, oxygen, nutrients and waste products such as carbon dioxide cross the placental barrier, selectively in both directions.

Blood on the fetal side of the placenta is approximately 80–90 per cent saturated with oxygen, and flows into the inferior vena cava, via the umbilical vein, to mix with deoxygenated blood returning from the lower part of the fetus, thus decreasing oxygenation even further (70–75 per cent saturated). The blood continues towards the underside of the liver, where it separates; a small amount of blood enters the portal and hepatic circulation of the liver, and the remainder travels directly to the inferior vena cava via the ductus venosus. It enters the right atrium at 55–60 per cent oxygenation and, due to the higher pressure from the placenta, its path is directed in an almost straight line across the atrium, through the foramen ovale, and into the left atrium. It is by this mechanism that the highest possible concentration of oxygen passes to the left ventricle to be pumped, via the aorta, to the brain (Tucker Blackburn, 2003).

Deoxygenated blood from the head and upper extremities enters the right atrium and, because it is only subject to the fetus's systemic circulation, is directed downwards through the tricuspid valve into the right ventricle. From here it is pumped through the pulmonary artery, where the majority is shunted through the ductus arteriosus to the descending aorta. The remainder is pumped to the non-functional lungs, where small amounts return to the left atrium via the pulmonary veins. Blood then returns to the placenta, from the descending aorta, via the hypogastric arteries and two umbilical arteries.

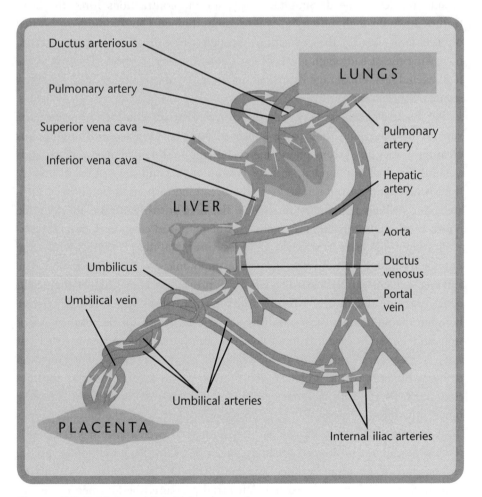

Figure 7.1 ● Maternal/fetal blood supply

Prior to birth, the high pulmonary vascular resistance created by the collapsed fetal lungs creates greater pressures in the right side of the heart and pulmonary artery. At the same time the free-flowing placental circulation and ductus arteriosus produce a lower systemic vascular resistance in the rest of the fetus's vascular system. The onset of labour brings about many profound changes in both systemic and pulmonary circulations.

The onset of birth involves a complex set of processes orchestrated between the fetus and mother, although the precise mechanism remains a mystery. In the final weeks prior to, and during birth, the fetal blood system is flooded with chemicals whose function is to prepare the cardiac and respiratory systems for extrauterine adaptation. As the majority of births involve the fetus lying head down in the uterus, the transition to the outside world is all part of this adaptation.

The fetal head, in contact with the maternal cervix, causes the cervix to open around the fetus's head. Simultaneously, uterine contractions force the head further down through the cervix, as it becomes thinner. The compression exerted on the fetus during the transition through the birth canal creates stress, increasing the already high levels of catecholamine and cortisol. These increase fetal excitability, encourage breathing, increase the absorption of lung fluid and stimulate surfactant release.

As the fetal head is delivered, the thorax remains compressed within the vagina, allowing lung fluid to be squeezed out via the nose and mouth, thus creating a vacuum. Atmospheric air rushes into the fetal lungs and expands them. If this does not happen, perhaps because the second stage of birth is rapid, fluid is not cleared from the lungs or the breathing response has not been initiated, due to high pulmonary resistance, the first breath can take considerable effort, resulting in the diaphragm and ribs being pulled concave (Coad, 2002).

Systemic vascular resistance doubles after the first breath, while the pulmonary vasculature dilates, decreasing pulmonary vascular resistance. The foramen ovale is pushed closed as left atrial pressure becomes higher than right atrial pressure and the flow reverses in the ductus arteriosis, preventing flow between the pulmonary artery and the aorta. The reason for this closure is not fully understood. As the infant is fully delivered, the umbilical cord is either left until it has ceased pulsating to be clamped, or is clamped immediately on delivery. Either way, the umbilical vein flow ceases at birth. Muscular contraction shuts off the ductus venosus and portal venous pressure rises, directing blood flow through the liver.

A postnatal condition known as 'persistent fetal circulation' may develop if the infant requires prolonged resuscitation at birth. In this condition, hypoxia, carbon dioxide retention and acidosis can precipitate pulmonary vasoconstriction. If right atrial pressure exceeds left atrial pressure, the foramen ovale can open and lead to deoxygenated blood pouring into the left atria, via the shunt.

Conversely, if the ductus arteriosus fails to close, a right-to-left shunt may continue. In both these cases, the result is deoxygenated blood being circulated around the body, exacerbating hypoxia and hypercarbia. Surgical intervention is usually required.

While fetal heart structures may never fully close, they are usually functionally closed eight days after birth. Changes in systemic or pulmonary blood flow, due to congenital defects or disease, may result in these structures either remaining open or functionally opening, days or weeks later. In relation to breathing, the majority of infants will breathe within six seconds of birth and have normal respiratory patterns within 15 minutes (Coad, 2002).

Mature respiration

The purpose of respiration is to ensure that the cells of the body are provided with oxygen and that the waste products of their metabolism, carbon dioxide and water, are excreted. Effective respiration is achieved through the exchange of these two gases within the lungs, which in turn depends on the competence of the related structures of respiration. The regulation of respiration is, however, controlled by the brain in response to both neural and chemical factors.

Although brief overviews will be provided within this chapter, you should consult specialist texts on the subject in order fully to understand the anatomical and physiological principles of respiration, including the organs of respiration, pulmonary ventilation, lung volumes and capacities, gaseous exchange, the transport of gases and the control of respiration. Your lecturers may recommend alternative texts, but Marieb (2006) has a valuable chapter entitled 'The Respiratory System', which will give you the background to the relevant structures and their function in facilitating effective respiration. Whichever text you choose, it should be available for reference while working through this chapter.

Respiratory overview

In order to make a comprehensive assessment, one first needs to understand the way in which air is taken into and expelled from the lungs, carried around the body and utilised by the cells.

Spontaneous respiration depends on regular neural impulses from groups of neurones in the medulla oblongata and pons Varolli. The medulla contains two areas of specialised nerves, known as the 'inspiratory and expiratory centres', whereas the pons contains nuclei referred to as the 'pneumotaxic and apneustic centres', which influence and modify the medullary neurones. These areas are required to work together to bring about effective respiration, both voluntary (under our conscious control) and involuntary (unconsciously). The voluntary mechanisms include actions that are non-gaseous in nature, for example coughing, swallowing, vomiting and speech. Involuntary or subconscious respiration, which is needed to sustain life, consists of inspiration, expiration and the fine-tuning of the system relating to increased need, such as when exercising, and decreased need during sleep.

During inspiration, nerve impulses pass from the medulla to the diaphragm and intercostal muscles (Figure 7.2), causing them to contract and thus enlarge the thoracic cage, therefore lowering the intrapleural pressure. As the outside air pressure is greater than the air pressure inside the lungs, air flows into the alveoli until the intrapleural pressure is equal to atmospheric pressure.

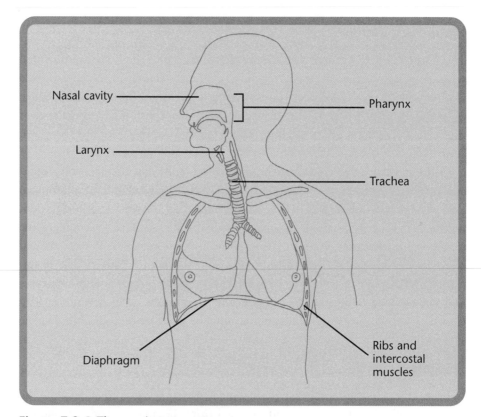

Figure 7.2 ● The respiratory system

As the lungs expand, stretch receptors within the lung tissue convey nerve impulses to the pneumotaxic centre, which further inhibits inspiration. When muscle contraction ceases and relaxation commences, the stretched muscles recoil to their original length. The thoracic cage and lungs return to their normal sizes, and intrapleural air pressure exceeds atmospheric pressure, forcing air out of the airways and into the atmosphere. Expiration is a passive process, dependent only on the inhibition of inspiration.

The chemical control of respiration is attained by groups of specialised cells in the walls of the aorta and carotid arteries known as **chemoreceptors**. Their function is to monitor and respond to changes in the **partial pressure** (denoted by the letter P, see below) of either carbon dioxide (CO_2) or oxygen (O_2) in the blood. Any increase in PCO_2 is transmitted to the respiratory centre, where inspiration is initiated. A small drop in PO_2 acts as a similar trigger, although a substantial decrease in level can have the effect of depressing respiration. The body can normally maintain the balance between blood PCO_2 and PO_2 through quiet respiration.

chemoreceptors
nerve endings or groups of cells that are stimulated by chemicals

partial pressure
the pressure of a gas in a mixture of gases, related to its concentration

The notion of partial pressure is explained by the fact that all gases in a mixture exert their own pressure as if the other gases did not exist. If we take air as an example, this is a mixture primarily of oxygen (two molecules of oxygen), carbon dioxide (one molecule of carbon and two oxygen), nitrogen (two molecules of nitrogen) and water vapour (two molecules of hydrogen and one of oxygen). The pressure that these gases exert allows them to move across membranes from an area of high concentration to one of a lower concentration. So, when the PO_2 is high, as in the arterial beds of the lungs, oxygen combines with haemoglobin, and when the PO_2 is low, as in the peripheral tissues, oxygen is released from the haemoglobin. For carbon dioxide, the process is the same, and forms the basis of normal gaseous transport.

Increases in respiratory rate occur in relation to the demands of body tissues for oxygen. Factors that increase the demand for oxygen in healthy individuals are exercise, increased body temperature and emotional responses such as laughing or crying. Ineffective breathing patterns occur when the oxygen demands of the individual are not met by the amount of oxygen available (Marieb, 2006).

The health worker's role as part of the multidisciplinary team approach lies in the accurate assessment and diagnosis of factors affecting clients' breathing, in planning and carrying out effective interventions and in evaluating the degree of success.

Physical assessment

Nursing assessment can be made by collecting data from:

- The client, significant others and previous notes
- Observation of the client
- Physical examination
- Laboratory investigations.

The following sections will cover assessment in terms of the quality, rate, pattern and depth of breathing, the colour of the mucous membranes and skin,

accessory muscles of respiration

muscle groups in the neck, back and abdomen that aid respiration by moving the rib cage

the presence of any cough, the shape of the chest, the equality of movement on both sides of the chest and the use of any **accessory muscles of respiration.**

Respiratory rate

Respiratory rate is the number of inspirations and expirations recorded in one minute without the client's knowledge while he is at rest (Chart 7.1). The normal respiratory rates for children and adults are shown in Table 7.1, and the effects of exercise on respiration are described in Chart 7.2.

Chart 7.1 ● Hints for assessing the respiration rate

Sitting at the client's right side, reach across and take the pulse in his left wrist while laying his hand on his upper abdominal area. When you have completed this observation, keep hold of the wrist as if you were still counting the pulse; you can then feel the chest or abdomen moving against your hand. Count the frequency of movement for one minute and then make the other necessary observations

Chart 7.2 ● Effects of exercise on respiration

During exercise, the muscles of the body utilise oxygen and provide carbon dioxide in higher concentrations than when resting. This reduction in PO_2 is identified by the aortic and carotid bodies, and stimulates the respiratory centre to increase the rate of inspiration. This consequently increases oxygen intake and carbon dioxide output

Table 7.1 Resting respiratory rates by age

Age	Rate (breaths/minute)
Under 1 year	30–40
1–2 years	25–35
2–5 years	25–30
5–12 years	20–25
12 years and older	15–20

Source: Weiteska et al. (2005).

In certain conditions, abnormalities of the rate of breathing may occur:

bradypnoea

slow but regular breathing as a result of depression of the respiratory centre

● **Bradypnoea:** slow but regular breathing as a result of depression of the respiratory centre. It is a normal phenomenon during sleep but in ill-health may indicate oversedation, opiate poisoning or the presence of a cerebral lesion

- Tachypnoea: an increased respiratory rate caused by the body's demands for extra oxygen or by a decreased amount of oxygen being available when the circulation is diminished or respiration impeded. Tachypnoea may be present in **anaemia**, **shock**, **cardiac failure** or **alkalosis**. It may also indicate infections such as meningitis or pneumonia.

- Apnoea: cessation of breathing, which is usually abnormal and constitutes a medical emergency. Short periods of apnoea that can last beyond 20 seconds may, however, be deemed normal in infants and children (Poets et al. 1993).

Respiratory rhythm

Normal breathing is effortless, regular and quiet. Each breath takes approximately as long as four or five heart beats, so for a child with a pulse rate of 120 beats per minute, one would expect a respiratory rate of 24–30 breaths per minute, while for an adult with a pulse rate of 80 beats per minute, one would anticipate a respiratory rate of 16–20 breaths per minute.

As the regulatory centres in their brains are immature, the respiratory pattern of newborn babies is more erratic, periods of bradypnoea and tachypnoea being interspersed with periods of apnoea of up to 20 seconds in duration. A typical pattern is represented in Figure 7.3.

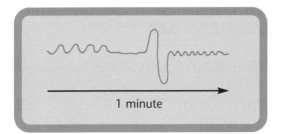

Figure 7.3 ● Normal respiratory pattern of the newborn

Changes from the normal pattern of respiration are known as:

- Dyspnoea: difficult, laboured breathing, present when the airways are obstructed, as in asthma, chronic obstructive airways disease or **pulmonary oedema**. It is frequently accompanied by sweating and pallor

- Orthopnoea: the ability to breathe without difficulty only when sitting upright. It may be a result of heart failure with pulmonary oedema, or occur in an infant or small child when abdominal pressure is exerted on the diaphragm

- Cheyne–Stokes respiration: breathing cycles of gradually decreasing rate and depth, followed by cycles of increasing rate and depth. This alternating

---

tachypnoea
an increased respiratory rate caused by a lack of oxygen or a need for extra oxygen

anaemia
a deficiency of haemoglobin in the blood

shock
shock results from an acute failure of circulatory function (Advanced Life Support Group, 2005)

cardiac failure
occurs when the heart muscle is unable to pump blood effectively around the body

alkalosis
an increase in the amount of alkali in the blood

apnoea
cessation of breathing

dyspnoea
difficult, laboured breathing

pulmonary oedema
fluid in the alveoli and lung tissue

orthopnoea
the ability to breathe without difficulty only when sitting upright

Cheyne–Stokes respiration
breathing cycles of gradually decreasing rate and depth, followed by cycles of increasing rate and depth

pattern is repeated at intervals of between 45 seconds and 3 minutes, and there may be periods of apnoea during the cycles. Cheyne–Stokes respiration frequently indicates impending death

- *Biot's respiration:* periods of rapid, deep breathing interspersed with periods of apnoea, which may indicate fear or metabolic **acidosis**
- *Kussmaul's respiration:* an increased rate and depth of breathing associated with metabolic acidosis
- *Asthmatic breathing:* prolonged expiration (greater than two seconds) accompanied by a wheeze.

Respiratory depth and effort

Respiratory depth is assessed by observing the degree of movement in the abdominal wall in children under the age of seven years and in the chest wall in older children and adults (Hazinski, 1999). The total amount of air inspired and expired in one normal breath is known as the **tidal volume** and can be assessed using a spirometer. Its value differs depending on the gender, age, height and weight of the client, but an approximate figure of 6–7 cm^3/kg can be used, if required.

Hyperpnoea is shallow, rapid breathing, usually in an attempt to avoid pain of either a thoracic or an abdominal nature.

Accessory muscles are not usually used when at rest; however, as effort increases, various groups of muscles become involved:

- *Nasal flaring:* the alae nasi in the nostrils flare in order to decrease resistance to air entry
- *Recession:* may be supraclavicular, suprasternal (known as 'tracheal tug'), intercostal, subcostal or substernal. In clients of all ages, any of these signs represent severe respiratory distress.

Respiratory sounds

Whereas normal respiration is soundless, there are a variety of sounds associated with respiratory assessment that indicate respiratory disease:

- *Stridor:* a harsh sound heard on inspiration, indicating obstruction of the larynx
- *Snoring:* a noise that occurs on inspiration through the nose, usually during sleep. It is indicative of partial obstruction of the upper airway. Causes include inflammation of the nasal mucosa, deviation of the nasal septum, the tongue relaxing into the airway, or enlarged tonsils or adenoids. In severe cases, short stoppages in respiration, known as sleep apnoea, may occur

---

acidosis

a loss of alkali from or an increase in acid in the blood

tidal volume

the total amount of air inspired and expired in one normal breath

hyperpnoea

shallow, rapid breathing

- *Wheeze:* a melodic whistling or rasping noise heard during respiration. While most common at the end of expiration, it may also be heard during the whole of respiration; it is indicative of an obstruction to the airflow in the respiratory tract
- *Grunting:* the noise heard on expiration in infants with severe respiratory difficulty; it is a compensatory mechanism to keep the alveoli from collapsing
- *Rattle:* audible to the ear on inspiration or expiration and associated with excessive mucus secretion or retention. If a hand is placed on the mid-sternum, rattles can be felt as a 'fluttering' on forced expiration
- *Râles and crepitations:* audible with a stethoscope, these are associated with excess fluid in the lungs
- *Head bobbing:* the involuntary movement of the head observed in infants with severe respiratory distress. It is caused by the use of the sternomastoid muscle in respiration.

Colour

In healthy individuals, the skin is warm and well perfused, with pink mucous membranes and nail beds. If, however, tissue oxygenation is low (**hypoxia**) or unusually high, there may be noticeable changes in the client's colour. The palms of the hands and feet, the nail beds and the mucous membranes of the mouth and eyes are good places to look for possible changes in clients of all nationalities:

- *Cyanosis:* blue tinging of the skin with or without involvement of the mucous membranes indicates that there is an abnormally high level of carbon dioxide in the blood. This may be observed in overdoses of drugs that depress the respiratory centre, for example opiates, or in cases where there is a mixing of oxygenated and deoxygenated blood, as in right-to-left intracardiac shunts. There are two kinds:
  - peripheral cyanosis: a blue tinge to the hands and feet
  - central cyanosis: blueness of the mucous membranes of the mouth, lips and conjunctivae
- *Cyanosis with dyspnoea:* laboured breathing and blue extremities may be indicative of damage to the chest wall or lung tissue.

Cough

This is part of a response group that defends the bronchi, trachea and lungs against irritation from a foreign body or excessive secretions. A cough is a sudden, violent expulsion of air from the lungs, which may contain a mix of mucus, cell debris, pus and microorganisms.

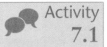

Activity 7.1

Observe a colleague laughing, excited or upset and assess their respiratory rate, depth and rhythm without their knowledge. Describe the event and behaviour, for example was the laugh a giggle or a 'belly' laugh? Did you notice that there were changes in all three aspects of the respiratory pattern? In what ways were the rate, depth and rhythm affected?

hypoxia

a low oxygen concentration at the cellular level

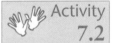

Activity 7.2

To help you to identify some respiratory sounds, use a stethoscope to listen to the chest of a colleague or client, preferably one with a smoker's cough or respiratory infection. Is there any difficulty differentiating between the noises made on inspiration and those on expiration? Can you hear the heart beat as well?

There are numerous types of sputum, amounts varying from 100 to 500 ml (Law, 2000), which are indicative of differing disease processes:

- *Mucoid:* has the appearance of raw egg white and occurs in chronic bronchitis
- *Tenacious mucoid:* as above but is sticky and difficult to expel; this occurs in asthma
- *Mucopurulent:* thick, sticky and green/yellow in colour, indicating the presence of infection in the lungs; also occurs in smokers and asthmatics
- *Purulent:* slimy and green or yellow in colour, produced during bronchopneumonial infection
- *Frothy:* a bubbly, white secretion that may appear pink if tinged with blood, which is produced when the client has pulmonary oedema
- **Haemoptysis:** indicates that the client is bleeding into the lungs. The expectorate, that is, the secretions coughed up from the lungs, is bright red and frothy. Haemoptysis may indicate that the client is suffering from tuberculosis, carcinoma of the lung or **pulmonary embolism**.

To enable an accurate diagnosis to be made, the nurse may be asked to collect a sputum specimen to be sent to the laboratory. It may be easier to collect the specimen in the morning when the client awakens, prior to breakfast (Middleton and Middleton, 1998). This is because, while the client is recumbent overnight and respiration is shallow, a high volume of secretions may have accumulated, which will be expectorated as the respiratory depth increases. If the client has eaten, food particles may be present in the specimen, making analysis difficult. The principles of collection are outlined below:

1. If appropriate, ensure that the client has drunk sufficient fluid the night prior to sputum collection.
2. Ensure that the client's mouth is clean and free from foreign material such as food. This may necessitate cleaning the mouth with clean water. Do not allow the client to use toothpaste or mouthwash as they may have an antiseptic effect.
3. Explain to the client, using methods appropriate to her understanding, that the substance you want to collect is mucus from the lungs rather than saliva from the mouth.
4. If the client is able to comply with self-collection, give her a covered, wide-necked sterile collecting pot to expectorate into the next time she coughs.
5. Explain to the client that accidental contamination of the inside of the container by her fingers should be avoided, as the laboratory staff need to be certain that any organisms found in the specimen have come from the client's lungs.

haemoptysis

coughing up blood from the respiratory tract

pulmonary embolism

blockage of the pulmonary artery or one of its branches by foreign matter, usually a thrombus originating somewhere in the venous system

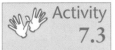 Activity 7.3

Ask a physiotherapist to show you how he or she intervenes with clients who experience difficulty expectorating. Interventions may include **postural drainage**, **percussion** and vibration.

postural drainage

positioning the patient in a way that allows gravity to move fluid from one part of the body to another

percussion

tapping with the fingers on parts of the body

6. If coughing is difficult or the client is exhausted, there are a variety of techniques that the nurse can utilise to ease expectoration. A warm drink or a eucalyptus inhalation may be beneficial. You can also involve the physiotherapist who may either physically help the client to expectorate or provide a variety of breathing exercises.

Once the client has provided a specimen, and you are happy that it is sputum, the pot should be labelled with the client's name, the ward and the date and time of collection, and be dispatched to the laboratory within the hour along with the doctor's request form.

The client needs the opportunity to clean her teeth or rinse her mouth after providing the sputum specimen as it may taste unpleasant.

Chest shape

The thoracic cage is circular in infants, whereas in the older child and adult, the chest becomes wider from side to side than it is from front to back. Deviations from these shapes are indicative of chronic disease processes. The classical 'barrel' chest that occurs in asthma or chronic bronchitis is probably the most common abnormality.

When examining the thorax, the nurse should ensure that the chest moves equally from anterior (front) to posterior (back), and laterally (side to side) (Dougherty and Lister, 2004).

Nursing interventions

Airway maintenance

'Airway' is the generic term for those parts of the respiratory system through which atmospheric air containing oxygen is inspired to reach the lungs, and expired. If a loss of **patency** occurs in any part of the airway, the flow to the lungs of oxygen-containing air is impeded and a state of hypoxia results. Blockages to airflow may result from a disease process or from mechanical reasons – either a foreign body being inhaled or the tongue relaxing into the airway during periods of unconsciousness. The causes of airway obstruction are listed in Chart 7.3.

In either event, it is essential that the student nurse is able to assist the client in maintaining an effective airway and thus sustaining oxygen delivery to the tissues. Airway maintenance can be achieved by the following methods.

Activity 7.4

Find a client or colleague with a known respiratory infection or cough. Ask him or her to describe the type of cough and sputum produced. What could be the cause of the cough? Did you review the text to help you to determine a cause? Did you perform a respiratory assessment to provide more clues?

patency

being freely open

Chart 7.3 ● Causes of airway obstruction

- Anaphylaxis
- Foreign body
- Coma
- Trauma
- Chemical irritants
- Infection
- Near-drowning
- Neurogenic or cardiac causes of pulmonary oedema

Head tilt/chin lift

This is performed when the client experiences a loss of consciousness; it forces the tongue forward into the mouth and away from the airway. The head tilt can be accomplished in adults, children and infants by placing one hand on the client's forehead and applying a firm backward pressure. The fingers of the other hand are placed underneath the chin to support and lift the chin forward. The preferred degree of tilt is neutral in infants (defined as under one year old), sniffing in the child (defined as between one year and puberty) and hyperextension in the adult (Wietska et al., 2005; www.resus.org.uk) as shown in Figure 7.4.

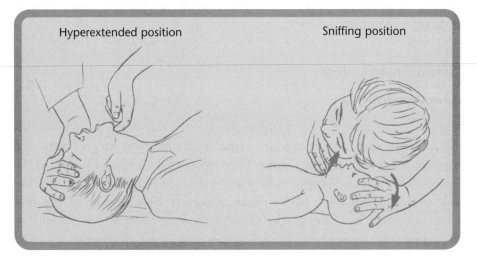

Figure 7.4 ● Airway opening manoeuvres

Insertion of a Guedel's (oropharyngeal) airway

oropharynx

the area behind the mouth from the soft palate to the hyoid bone

An artificial airway (Figure 7.5) is used when the client is unconscious, or the airway is occluded and she is unable to support respiration unaided. The Guedel's airway extends from the teeth to the **oropharynx**, keeping the tongue in its normal anatomical position. The airway is a concave structure that fits over the tongue, although the insertion technique differs depending on the age of the client. If a gag reflex is present, an oropharyngeal airway is not used as it may cause vomiting, choking or **laryngospasm**.

Although you need to be aware of the technique, you are unlikely to participate in this procedure during your common foundation experience.

laryngospasm

the prolonged contraction of the muscles controlling the vocal chords, which results in the airway being blocked off

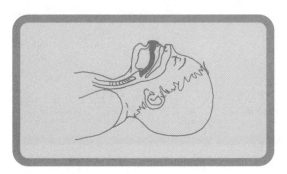

Figure 7.5 ● Guedel's (oropharngeal) airway

Heimlich manoeuvre

The Heimlich manoeuvre (Figure 7.6) may be applied if a foreign body has been aspirated into the airway and is obstructing the flow of air entry to the lungs. It is an alternating series of mouth-to-mouth ventilations, abdominal or chest thrusts and interscapular back blows. The full manoeuvre is performed only on clients who have stopped breathing as it can prove hazardous if executed while they are still breathing.

If used, up to five back blows should be administered as a series of sharp blows with the heel of the hand between the shoulder blades. If possible, the client should be head down and prone, to facilitate removal of the foreign body. In infancy and childhood, this can be achieved by holding the child prone across your forearm or thigh. If back blows fail to dislodge the foreign body, abdominal thrusts should be used in the child and adult, and chest thrusts in the infant.

Abdominal thrusts can be achieved by standing behind the client with your hands situated between his breastbone (sternum) and navel. With one fist under the bottom of the breastbone, in the region of the xiphoid process, clench the other fist and pull your arms sharply upwards. This action increases the intrathoracic pressure, forcing the foreign body out of the airway.

Chest thrusts resemble chest compressions but are much sharper and performed at a speed of about 10 per minute in the adult (www.resus.org.uk).

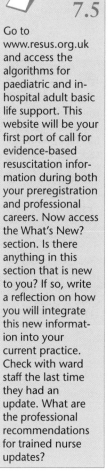

Activity
7.5

Go to www.resus.org.uk and access the algorithms for paediatric and in-hospital adult basic life support. This website will be your first port of call for evidence-based resuscitation information during both your preregistration and professional careers. Now access the What's New? section. Is there anything in this section that is new to you? If so, write a reflection on how you will integrate this new information into your current practice. Check with ward staff the last time they had an update. What are the professional recommendations for trained nurse updates?

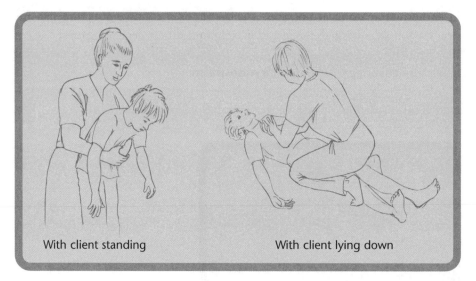

With client standing   With client lying down

Figure 7.6 ● Heimlich manoeuvre

Cardiac/respiratory arrest

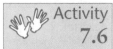 Activity
7.6

Find out the policy
in your clinical area
for clients who
suddenly collapse
or are expected to
die. Does the policy
include boundaries
related to age or
mental or physical
competence? If
there is no policy,
do all staff share a
common under-
standing of what to
do in such an
event?

Clinical death is characterised by respiratory and cardiac arrest. In some cases, this is reversible by the prompt application of resuscitative measures, the aim of resuscitation being to 'prevent or reverse premature death in patients with severely compromised or arrested respiration and circulation' (Baskett and Chamberlain, 1997). There are, however, also times when the order to attempt resuscitation is withheld. This is frequently applied on moral grounds, if resuscitation will deny the client the right to a dignified death, each case being considered individually. In most instances, the client who is not for attempted resuscitation is known to be going to die or might potentially die from their injuries or disease, and as there can be no generic rules applied to the 'Do not attempt resuscitation' (DNAR) order, each establishment should have published guidelines relating to this policy. In all cases where a DNAR order is not in place, full resuscitation measures should be employed. The Resuscitation Council website (www.resus.org.uk) has guidelines for medical and nursing staff about initiating DNAR orders.

The arrest will, in many instances, be unwitnessed, and the rescuer will have no idea of either the cause or any underlying disease. Assessment should therefore follow a methodical process to establish whether the client has airway obstruction, respiratory arrest or cardiopulmonary arrest. This process of assessment is known as 'ABC', which denotes the sequence of checking the airway, breathing and circulation. Only a preliminary assessment of the environment and client is required before resuscitator action is commenced. First aid principles should be followed at all times, including the principle that the rescuer will come to no harm by undertaking resuscitation.

In an attempt to simplify the resuscitation procedure, the Resuscitation Council (2005a) has brought the process for children over the age of one year and adults into line; however, infants continue to have some differences.

Principles of resuscitation

Once an initial assessment has been made, and there is no evidence of cervical injury, stimulate the client by shaking his shoulder gently and asking him whether he is OK. If the client responds, maintain an open airway, provide supplemental oxygen and call the resuscitation team if required.

Open the client's airway using the chin lift or head tilt and look, listen and feel for signs of breathing. In the event that opening the client's airway fails to restore ventilation, he requires someone to do it for him. In an emergency situation, this is achieved artificially through mouth-to-mouth or mouth-to-nose resuscitation:

1. With the client lying supine (on his back), open the airway using the chin lift, or the jaw thrust shown in Figure 7.7.
2. If using the mouth-to-mouth technique, close off the client's nostrils with the hand that is holding the head up, while supporting the chin with the other (Figure 7.8). In the infant, if using mouth-to-nose-and-mouth, this is not required.
3. The rescuer takes a normal breath, seals his lips over the client's mouth, or in the case of an infant the nose and mouth, and exhales over the next 1–1.5 seconds until the chest rises by one-third, as with a normal breath. This is said to be an 'effective breath'.
4. Once the client's chest has risen, the rescuer removes his own mouth and observes the chest fall during exhalation. This should be repeated up to five times.
5. The client should then be assessed for signs of circulation. In the infant, this is achieved by feeling the brachial pulse, and in all other age groups by palpating the carotid pulse for 10 seconds. If you are confident that you have identified signs of circulation and adequate oxygenation, including an appropriate pulse rate, place the client in a recovery position (Figure 7.9). If signs of adequate circulation appear to be absent, commence chest compressions.

If the client has a pulse but is not breathing, continue to ventilate until help arrives.

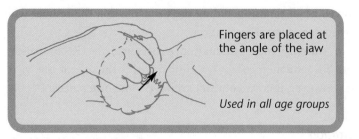

Figure 7.7 ● Jaw thrust

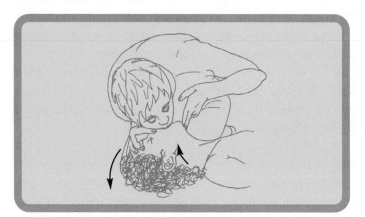

Figure 7.8 ● Mouth-to-mouth seal

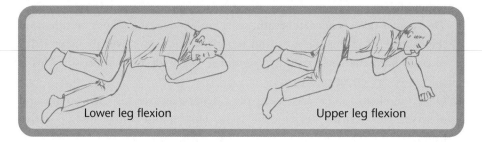

Figure 7.9 ● Recovery positions

Compression of the heart is needed when the client's heart abruptly stops circulating blood, and therefore oxygen, around the body. To reinstate the cardiac output, the rescuer must perform these compressions at the same rate per minute as the client's normal pulse rate. To perform this on an older child and adult:

1. Ensure that the client is lying on his back and that his chest area is resting on a firm surface.
2. Kneel at the side of the client and locate the site for compression by

following the rib margin up to the xiphoid process and place one finger on this notch. Place the heel of the other hand immediately above it on the sternum (Figure 7.10).

3. Remove your finger from the xiphisternum and place this hand over the other one, either grasping the wrist with the thumb or intertwining the fingers. Raise your fingers away from the chest wall, leaving just the heels of the hands in contact (Figure 7.11). This manoeuvre decreases the risk of fracturing the ribs.

4. Position yourself vertically above the client's chest and use sufficient force to depress the sternum by one-third of its depth (www.resus.org.uk). **Note:** This may vary from using one or two hands depending on the size and strength of the rescuer and size and age of the victim.

5. Release the pressure and repeat at a rate of approximately 100 beats per minute.

For infants, the rescuer should use the same anatomical landmarks but use only two fingers to depress the sternum.

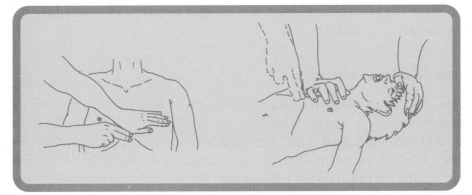

Figure 7.10 ● Location of the cardiac compression site in an older child and adult

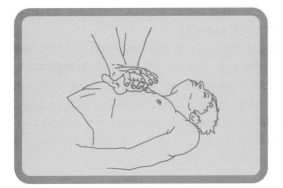

Figure 7.11 ● Finger position during cardiac compression

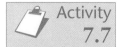

The above procedures of artificial respiration and cardiac compression are frequently carried out in combination to maintain effective oxygen delivery to the major organs. The ratio for a one-person resuscitation with infants and children is 15 cardiac compressions to 2 respiratory insufflations (15:2), while for an adult, it is 30 cardiac compressions to 2 respiratory insufflations (30:2). **Remember that it is your responsibility to regularly check the Resuscitation Council website to ensure that you are carrying out up-to-date practices.**

Now do Activity 7.7. Did you ascertain that acute hospital wards tend to have a 'crash' trolley where all the equipment and drugs are kept together? On less acute wards and in community areas, minimal resuscitation equipment, such as a back board, oxygen, ventilatory equipment and suction, is available. If the ward has its own trolley, a nurse will usually be first on the scene to fetch it. If, however, a group of wards or areas share equipment, a porter may be delegated. Equipment and drugs should be checked, and replaced if necessary, immediately following use. If emergencies occur regularly, a first-level nurse usually checks the 'crash' trolley every day, whereas in less acute settings, this may be done once a week or even monthly.

Have you asked your assessor or a senior colleague to show you how the equipment works and connects?

Volume measurements

functional residual capacity
the amount of air remaining in the lung on completion of normal expiration

expiratory reserve volume
the maximum volume of air that can be expired from the resting level

residual volume
the amount of air remaining in the lungs after a maximum expiration

total lung capacity
the total amount of air in the lungs following maximal inspiration

inspiratory capacity
the maximal amount of air inspired

peak expiratory flow rate
the maximum flow during forced expiration from full capacity

The common units for recording measurements of lung function are volumes and capacities, one capacity comprising two or more volumes (Figure 7.12). In healthy individuals, these values are reliant upon age, height, gender and nationality (Kendrick and Smith, 1992). During one normal respiration, the amount of air inhaled and exhaled is the tidal volume. The amount of air remaining in the lung on completion of normal expiration is the **functional residual capacity** (FRC), which in turn is made up of the **expiratory reserve volume** (ERV) and the **residual volume** (RV). The total amount of air in the lungs following maximal inspiration is called the **total lung capacity** (TLC), and the maximal amount of air inspired is the **inspiratory capacity** (IC).

As airflow obstruction is the main symptom of respiratory disease, the two most important measurements are the TLC and the RV. The **peak expiratory flow rate** (PEFR) is the maximum flow during forced expiration from TLC and is usually measured by a Wright's meter or mini-Wright's meter (Figure 7.13), the latter device being available in low and standard versions. The former is used for clients with severe dyspnoea, elderly clients and young children, whereas the latter is for adults and older children (Booker, 2003).

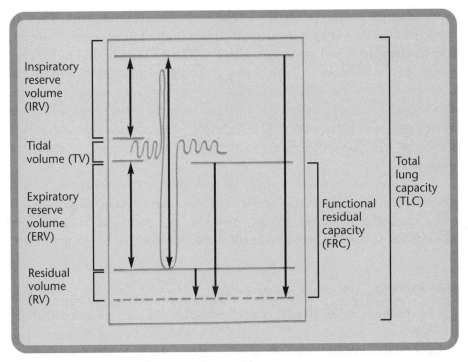

Figure 7.12 ● Lung volumes and capacities

Serial measurements of PEFR can help to identify the variable airflow obstruction of asthma and chronic obstructive pulmonary disease. In nursing it is becoming more common to have to record pre and post bronchodilator medication PEFRs, although there remain challenges to accurate recording (Booker, 2003).

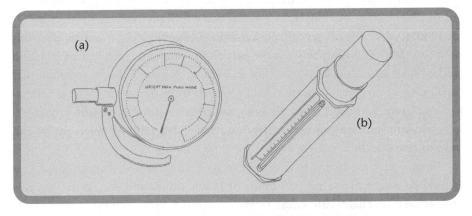

Figure 7.13 ● (a) Wright's meter   (b) Mini-Wright's meter

When recording a PEFR, any drugs that the client is taking should be known.

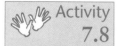

Activity 7.8

Ask the physiotherapist or respiratory nurse specialist whether you can arrange to observe spirometry testing. What instructions do clients need to adhere to in preparation for spirometry? What five aspects does the nurse need to consider in order to ensure an effective spirometry result? If in doubt, refer to Booker, 2003.

Ensure that the pointer or marker on the flow meter is set at zero. When all restrictive clothing has been loosened, the client is asked to stand or sit upright, with head and neck looking straight ahead and take a deep breath in. With the mouthpiece between the teeth and lips sealed tightly around the outside of the mouthpiece, she is then asked to breathe out as hard and for as long as she can. Three sequential readings should be made, allowing the client to rest for at least 30 seconds between attempts. The highest reading is then recorded. There should be less than 30 litres/minute difference between them in normality (Booker, 2003).

The second test that is increasingly being performed by nurses is spirometry, which is used for the more chronic phase of obstructive airways disease, as it is exhausting and exacting for ill clients. You may see it performed in ambulatory care settings where nurses have undertaken special training to carry out this test.

Pulse oximetry

Pulse oximetry is a non-invasive way of providing constant information about the client's cardiovascular and respiratory systems by measuring the percentage of haemoglobin available to carry oxygen around the body. Oxygen is mainly transported by binding to haemoglobin as oxyhaemoglobin, although a small amount may be dissolved in plasma. Each molecule of haemoglobin can combine with up to four molecules of oxygen, and when it is, this state is known as '100 per cent saturated'. However, not all molecules of heamoglobin are fully saturated, and some may carry only one or two molecules of oxygen, leading to a state of hypoxia. This may explain why normal values for oxygenation are 97–99 per cent (Chandler, 2001).

kPa

kilo Pascal unit of pressure

Oxygen saturation is a difficult, but important concept for practitioners to grasp (Popovich et al., 2004), as a saturation of 97 per cent may reflect a PO_2 of 13 **kPa**, while a reading of 90 per cent may indicate a PO_2 of only 9 kPa. This is due to the relationship between the partial pressure of oxygen in arterial blood and oxygen saturation not being linear, but forming an S-shape, meaning that small drops in oxygen saturation lead to much more dramatic drops in arterial oxygen levels. Although relatively high, an oxygen saturation reading of 85–90 per cent can indicate significant hypoxia, and if left without intervention can lead to brain death.

When caring for clients having their oxygen saturation levels monitored, you should be aware of the normal limits of blood values and the limitations this may impose on clients' lifestyles.

Pulse oximetry is now considered to be a component of routine vital signs (Popovitch et al., 2004), in conjunction with understanding normal limits, so it is important to recognise how it works.

Pulse oximetry combines a light-emitting diode (sensor) that transmits red and infrared light waves through the peripheral vascular bed to be received by a light-sensitive photodiode (detector). As arterial blood is red, it filters out infrared light but allows red light to pass through, whereas venous blood is blue, which filters out red and allows infrared light to pass. The photodiode records the intensity of both infrared and red light transmitted through the haemoglobin. To work accurately, the sensor and detector must lie opposite each other. The pulse oximeter has various types of sensor depending on the site of use, usually a finger or toe, an ear lobe or the bridge of the nose. Research carried out by Sun et al. (2003) demonstrated that forehead monitoring can result in the overestimation of tissue oxygenation status and recommend that it is not used in critically ill clients.

When a sensor is in place, the skin underneath it should be checked regularly for signs of abrasion or circulatory impairment. Chandler (2001) has also noted that sites should be changed at least two hourly to safeguard against skin burns. The nurse is expected to record the date, time and site of sensor in the client's notes.

Pulse oximetry may prove inaccurate in cases in which the client has severe anaemia, is in shock, is experiencing **vasoconstriction** or has dark skin colouring. Cautious use should also be made of oximetry if the client smokes heavily or is suffering from carbon monoxide poisoning, as these factors can compromise the accuracy of the reading. One of the main problems with accuracy of recordings is the mobility of the client, with reliability of the reading decreasing with movement. New generation devices are replacing the older 'motion intolerant' ones with good results; however, research carried out by Giuliano and Higgins (2005) illustrates the need for further studies to ascertain how much more reliable they really are.

vasoconstriction
contraction of the blood vessel wall, causing the lumen to narrow

Oxygen delivery

Most cells in the body need oxygen to survive and carry out their functions. As cells work, they use oxygen and produce carbon dioxide as a waste product, which must be excreted. It is the ultimate function of the cardiovascular and respiratory systems, alongside red cells in the blood, to deliver oxygenated blood to the tissues. If either of these systems becomes diseased or compromised, the level of oxygen in the tissues falls. Hypoxia (a low oxygen level) occurs and the continuance of this state leads to cellular death, as oxygen is essential to life. Many of the body's cells are able to regenerate and/or compensate, but brain cells lack this capacity and their function may be lost for ever. In severe hypoxia, brain cell death may be so widespread as to bring about the death of the individual. Extra (supplemental) oxygen can be administered to support cellular function.

Activity 7.9

When on your clinical placement, find out whether there is a policy governing the use of oxygen, and if so, what it recommends. What type of oxygen delivery system is available in your clinical area?

Atmospheric air, containing 21 per cent oxygen, is breathed in through the nose or mouth. This figure can also be expressed as the partial pressure of the constituent gases (see above). The oxygen exerts 21 per cent of the total atmospheric pressure, so the proportion of the pressure caused by the oxygen can also be stated as 21 kPa. Some of the oxygen, however, is lost during the journey to the alveolar air sacs, which at this point contain just 13.2 per cent or kPa of oxygen. Whereas the blood in the capillaries surrounding the air sacs already contains some oxygen (5.3 kPa), this value is less than that encountered in the alveolus. Gases diffuse from an area of high to one of low concentration, so oxygen moves from the alveoli into the blood until equilibrium has been reached. Carbon dioxide leaves the blood in the same way, diffusing from a high concentration in the blood (6 kPa) to a lower concentration in the alveoli (5.3 kPa). Once in the blood, a small amount of the oxygen dissolves directly, but the majority combines with haemoglobin in the red cells to become oxyhaemoglobin and be conveyed around the body to the cells. The situation with carbon dioxide is more complex, the gas being carried in several forms – carbonic acid, hydrogen carbonate ions and bound to protein elements, where it becomes known as a carbamino compound.

Tissues differ in their requirement for oxygen, three main areas accounting for 60 per cent of oxygen consumption:

● The brain
● The liver
● Skeletal muscle.

Once in the tissues, oxygen is used to produce adenosine triphosphate (ATP), the fuel for cell maintenance and survival.

Hypoxia can arise when the control mechanisms that ensure an adequate oxygen delivery to the cells fail. This may be due to:

ventricular septal defect

an abnormal opening in the septum between the right and left ventricles of the heart

persistent patent ductus arteriosus

a developmental defect leading to an abnormal connection between the pulmonary artery and the aorta

● Deficient oxygenation of the blood through being in a low oxygen environment, for example during strangulation, suffocation, drowning, inadequate ventilation of the lungs following major abdominal surgery, chest injury, prematurity or paralysis of the respiratory muscles, shunts between the right and left heart (as in infant **ventricular septal defect** and **persistent patent ductus arteriosus**) and inflammatory lung diseases such as asthma and bronchitis
● Inadequate transport of oxygen by haemoglobin as a result of anaemia, a sudden loss of blood or carbon monoxide poisoning
● Circulatory inadequacy due to low blood pressure or heart failure
● Inability of the cells to use oxygen, which is usually an indication of cyanide poisoning.

The consequences to the client may be that the cells' ability to produce ATP is lost, so, depending on which tissues are affected, the signs and symptoms observed by the nurse will vary:

- Disorientation and drowsiness if the brain is affected
- Decreased urine output if there is kidney damage
- Muscle weakness
- The skin appearing blue (peripheral cyanosis) or, in central cyanosis, the whites of the eyes, the lips, the tongue and the nails taking on a blue tinge
- Tachycardia (a rapid pulse rate)
- Changes in respiratory rate and depth
- The infant's skin becoming grey and mottled
- The hands and feet becoming cool or cold.

This list is not comprehensive and you may like to add any other observations you make.

Oxygen therapy is, according to Thomson et al. (2002), the provision of increased oxygenation with or without the use of specialised equipment. It is used when the adult's blood oxygen saturation is less than 90 per cent (Thiagamoorthy et al., 2000) and the infant or young child's is 94 per cent or less (Hazinski, 1999). This difference in level is related to the young child's larger consumption of oxygen for cellular growth and function.

As a result of potential dangers, oxygen is treated in the same way as drugs and as such should be prescribed by a doctor. The prescription should include:

- The percentage of oxygen to be administered
- The flow rate in litres per minute and mode of delivery
- Whether it is to be continuous or intermittent, or to be given immediately.

As oxygen may need to be administered in an emergency without a doctor present, the ward, hospital or unit should have an agreed written policy to cover this eventuality.

Each oxygen delivery system comprises five basic components:

1. *An oxygen supply:* which may be piped to the ward or come from a portable cylinder that is universally coloured black with a white top and is marked 'Oxygen'. These come in a variety of sizes and are often confused with cylinders containing medical air; a careful check thus needs to be made for accuracy. A portable cylinder for home use holds 300 litres, whereas cylinders for use with adults in an acute setting hold 3,400 litres.
2. *A flow meter:* a device that measures the flow of oxygen in litres per minute.

3. *Tubing:* usually green in colour, albeit found in different lengths and diameters, which connects the source to the patient or client.
4. *A delivery mechanism:* mask, cannula, hood, incubator and mechanical ventilator.
5. *A humidifier:* which may be used to warm and moisten the oxygen during delivery.

The choice of method of administration depends upon:

- The concentration of oxygen required
- The client's compliance.

For infants, oxygen is provided via a head hood or box that can provide up to 100 per cent oxygen, the flow rate being set at 7 litres per minute to prevent carbon dioxide accumulation inside the hood. The hood or box allows both good visibility of the patient's face and access to the infant or child's body without disrupting the flow of oxygen. If, however, humidification is used, visibility may be decreased and the child may become cold and wet, which can in turn lead to cold stress and skin irritation. There should be no impedance to the outflow of carbon dioxide, and an oxygen analyser must be used (Frey and Shann, 2003).

Oxygen delivery to newborn babies may be carried out inside an incubator, which allows for the control of environmental temperature and high visibility. The disadvantages are that the oxygen concentration is poorly controlled and that, in the humid environment, microorganisms such as *Pseudomonas* may grow. The oxygen flow should normally be between 4 and 5 litres per minute; a concentration of up to 40 per cent can be consistently delivered if a head box is used.

A Derbyshire chair can be used optimally for infants and young children as the oxygen can be consistently administered while the child is sitting in an upright position, allowing for downward displacement of the diaphragm.

Several kinds of disposable face mask, similar to that illustrated in Figure 7.14, are available for both adults and children, these being capable of delivering a concentration of oxygen ranging from 24 per cent to 60 per cent. The nurse should ensure that the client's nose and mouth are just covered. Masks provide a rapid and accurate delivery to the client, with high visibility. The client may also move around within the confines of the length of oxygen tubing. Disadvantages are that clients cannot eat or speak with the mask on, and if they vomit, this may not be easily noticed.

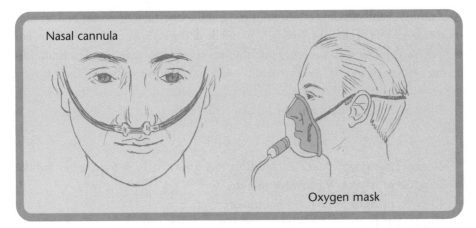

Figure 7.14 ● Oxygen delivery devices

If oxygen is being administered via a face mask, the nurse should ensure that the mask fits snugly around the client's nose, otherwise oxygen may blow into the eyes, causing discomfort and possible damage. As oxygen can cause mucous membranes to become dry, leading to inflammation and trauma, both eye and mouth care are required for clients wearing oxygen masks. When used for infants and children, it can help to position the mask upside down if the oxygen flow causes problems with the eyes.

Nasal cannulae are reserved for flows of less than 1 litre per minute or if an infant or child requires less than 24 per cent oxygen. Nasal prongs are usually more comfortable for children and infants, who can eat and vocalise while they are in situ. They are not advocated if the client is mouth-breathing.

Nasal catheters are not usually used for infants, who rely predominantly on nose breathing, because irritation to the airways on insertion and removal may cause further respiratory distress. They are advocated for adults and are positioned at the level of the uvula.

Thus, adults can be given nasal cannulae, catheters or face masks. The advantages and disadvantages are the same in adults and children for all three types of system, although an oxygen flow of more than 1 litre per minute is administered to adults, up to a maximum of 3 litres per minute. Fluid intake should also be closely monitored to ensure adequate hydration.

Oxygen may need to be humidified because:

● Oxygen from piped or cylinder sources is dry
● Dry gases lead to drying out of the mucous membrane lining the respiratory system
● Dry mucous membranes may become inflamed, causing excessive mucus production.

Activity
7.10

Find out whether your area's policy is routinely to humidify oxygen. If so, how long should a client be prescribed oxygen before it is humidified? Is there any recent research linking respiratory infection and humidification? If there is, have you shared it with the staff in your clinical area?

As a result, clients needing continuous oxygen therapy may be prescribed humidification. In this technique, oxygen is bubbled through sterile water at room temperature, picking up moisture and thus increasing its humidity. The humidification of oxygen has, however, recently been linked to waterborne infections of the respiratory tract, so it appears to be losing favour as a routine procedure.

Oxygen concentration should be assessed at the point of delivery, but as a guide:

- 28 per cent oxygen can be achieved from a flow rate of 5–6 litres per minute
- 35 per cent from 6–9 litres per minute
- 40 per cent from 8–12 litres per minute
- 60 per cent from 10–14 litres per minute.

Dangers associated with oxygen administration are linked to the fact that it is a colourless, tasteless, odourless, transparent gas that is heavier than air and supports combustion. As such, there are various precautions that must be taken when caring for clients receiving oxygen therapy:

1. Avoid the use of grease or oil on any part of the system delivering oxygen to the client, as it may support combustion.
2. No electrical devices should be operated when the client is receiving oxygen. This includes battery-operated shaving equipment and battery-operated toys for children.
3. Volatile solutions should be used cautiously. Petroleum-based products, which may be inflammable, should not be used to moisten patients' lips.
4. Explain that the client or visitors should not smoke near oxygen supplies.
5. Make sure that you know where the fire extinguishers are positioned or accessed.

Complications of oxygen therapy arise because the prolonged breathing of a high level of inspired oxygen can cause changes in the brain and lung tissue, resulting in fibrosis and decreased efficiency of the relevant organ. In infants, it can also cause a type of blindness known as 'retrolental fibroplasia'.

Clients of all ages with certain types of chronic respiratory disorder need to have a relatively low oxygen level to maintain their breathing. This is known as the 'hypoxic drive'. If oxygen is delivered without due consideration to the underlying disease, it can lead to the cessation of respiration.

Some clients complain of pain behind their breastbone, which is thought to be related to tracheitis (inflammation of the trachea) and may be an indication for humidification. Humidification during oxygen therapy has itself been linked to an increased risk of chest infection.

When caring for a client receiving oxygen therapy, the nurse should make regular checks (the patient care plan detailing the exact frequency and the observations to be made) on:

- Vital signs, such as respiratory rate, pulse rate, temperature and blood pressure
- The colour of the client's skin and mucous membranes
- The oxygen saturation level if a pulse oximeter is in use.

Now do Activity 7.11. Did you remember to prepare an upright position for the client, with a backrest and four pillows for an adult and a chair for an infant? The client should be easily observable from the nurses' station. You also need the appropriately sized oxygen equipment with humidity, suction and pulse oximetry. As the client is probably mouth-breathing, equipment for oral hygiene, a drink and, in the event of the client having a productive cough, a sputum pot and tissues will be needed. If breathlessness is severe, the older client may appreciate being close to a window or fan to give the impression of an airy environment.

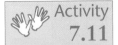

Activity 7.11

You are informed by the accident and emergency department that a client (of the age group appropriate to your area) with severe dyspnoea is to be admitted to your ward within the hour. The client has bilateral chest movement, an obvious use of accessory muscles and an oxygen saturation value of 87 per cent. You are asked by the staff nurse to prepare a bed space for the new arrival. What do you need to do?

Airway suctioning

Although it is unlikely that you will be asked to undertake this procedure, it is frequently performed on medical and surgical wards, and clients with severe physical disabilities often require airway clearance. As such, it is necessary to have some background knowledge on the rationale for airway suctioning. Suctioning is an essential skill for the nurse caring for the patient who has respiratory compromise. It is used to help to maintain a patent airway in cases where the patient is unable to do this herself.

Ineffective airway clearance is the state in which the client experiences a real or potential threat to respiratory status related to an inability to cough effectively. Clients at risk of accumulating secretions in the airway may be diagnosed as demonstrating:

- An ineffective cough reflex
- The inability to remove secretions
- Abnormal breath sounds
- An abnormal respiratory rate, depth or rhythm
- An increased pulse rate
- Pallor or cyanosis of the skin.

This may be as the result of:

chronic obstructive
airways disease

a disease process that
causes irreversibly
decreased lung function

- An acute or chronic inflammatory response, such as pneumonia or **chronic obstructive airways disease**
- Burns or trauma to the face, chest or abdomen
- Having an endotracheal or tracheostomy tube in place, which may cause narrowing of the airway or increase the amount of secretion present
- Paralysis of the muscles of respiration because of medication or disease.

In episodes of unconsciousness or paralysis involving the muscles of respiration and the stomach, the patient may be at risk of vomiting and subsequently inhaling vomitus into the respiratory system. This is most acutely possible during, or immediately following, the reversal of anaesthetic agents within the operating department. An impaired level of consciousness through the ingestion of noxious substances, for example alcohol, or through head injury is a cause likely to be seen in the accident and emergency department.

Although the art of airway suctioning may appear somewhat barbaric and distressing because of the visual, auditory and aesthetic images it conveys, it is the most effective way of maintaining a clear airway and sustaining life. The nurse is placed in the position of observing a patient who is ineffectively ventilating and showing all the signs of respiratory distress, but knowing that the procedure she is about to perform could potentially either save the patient's life or cause untold damage. Both prior to and following the procedure, the patient's respiratory rate, rhythm, depth, effort and sounds should be reassessed.

Inhaled drug delivery methods

Drugs administered directly into the lungs are rapidly absorbed through the alveolar–capillary network into the bloodstream, therefore avoiding many of the side-effects associated with oral forms of the drug. This method is known as 'inhalation' therapy and consists of drugs in either powder or liquid form being breathed into the lungs, thus penetrating the cells directly.

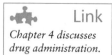

Link

Chapter 4 discusses drug administration.

Metered-dose inhalers, which deliver a high dosage of drug locally to the lung tissues, rely on pressurised air passing over powder to force the drug deep into the lungs. This is the method frequently used to administer bronchodilators or steroids to clients with asthma or chronic obstructive airways disease, but the effectiveness of this method is determined by the client's ability to combine activation of the inhaler with inhalation of the drug. Elderly clients, the very young and those with learning disabilities may be unable to achieve this degree of coordination.

The nebulisation of drugs involves compressed gas (either oxygen or air) passing through a quantity of liquid drug within a nebuliser attached to a face mask; this then forms an aerosol spray that is inhaled into the lungs. Little coordination is needed so there is a greater compliance of clients who may experience difficulty with a metered-dose inhaler. A number of machines are available that deliver nebulised drugs to the lungs through a process known as 'intermittent positive-pressure ventilation'. The nurse should familiarise herself with the equipment in order to understand the nature of the therapy being given.

Teaching a client to use a metered-dose inhaler

Although there are a variety of devices on the market, the principles of action remain the same:

1. Remove the cover of the inhaler.
2. Load the inhaler as instructed by the manufacturer.
3. Ask the client to breathe out gently but not fully.
4. With the client's head tilted slightly backwards, place the mouthpiece between his lips and ask him to breathe in as deeply as possible.
5. Remove the inhaler from between his lips.
6. Tell the client to hold his breath for 10 seconds and then breathe out slowly.
7. Repeat the procedure if necessary.

■ Circulation

The purpose of the circulatory system is to provide an adequate blood flow to vital organs such as the heart and brain. An adequate circulation ensures the delivery of oxygen and nutrients to the body tissues; the removal of carbon dioxide and waste products; and the dissipation of heat from active organs to ensure temperature regulation. Effective circulation is achieved via two separate circuits, the systemic and pulmonary circulations, both of which originate and terminate within the heart.

In order to understand the physiological and anatomical principles of circulation, including the cardiovascular system and its components, coronary and peripheral blood flow, the cardiac conduction system and the cardiac cycle, your lecturers may recommend specialist texts on the subject, such as Marieb (2004).

Circulatory assessment

As described above, an adequate circulation of blood is necessary to deliver oxygen and other nutrients to the tissues. Indeed, significant cardiovascular dysfunction can result in circulatory shock, whereby tissue perfusion with oxygen and nutrients is inadequate for the body's metabolic requirements. Some of the more common causes of shock are listed in Chart 7.4. Another common reason for hospital admission is coronary heart disease (CHD), which leads to conditions such as angina and myocardial infarction. At present CHD remains the biggest killer in the UK (DoH, 2005). Due to the prevalence of conditions such as these, it is essential that a thorough physical assessment of cardiovascular function should be undertaken as an integral part of the nursing process. This assessment should include an examination of heart rate, blood pressure, peripheral perfusion and fluid balance. In the context of chest pain, an electrocardiogram (ECG) and pain assessment should also be undertaken.

> **Link**
>
> *Chapter 1 has more information related to assessment.*

Chart 7.4 ● Common causes of shock

● Hypovolaemic	for example	Haemorrhage
		Gastroenteritis
		Burns
● Cardiogenic	for example	Heart failure
		Arrhythmias
● Distributive	for example	Sepsis
		Anaphylaxis
● Obstructive	for example	Tension pneumothorax
		Cardiac tamponade
		Pulmonary embolus
● Dissociative	for example	Anaemia
		Carbon monoxide poisoning

Source: Advanced Life Support Group (2005).

Physical examination

As discussed in Chapter 1, a physical examination will frequently commence with an initial rapid observation of the client. Consider the client in Casebox 7.1 and determine what general information could be obtained from a rapid initial assessment prior to a detailed cardiovascular assessment.

Casebox 7.1

Davol Singh is a 62-year-old gentleman who has presented to the nurse at his general practice. He reports that he has had several episodes of central chest pain and shortness of breath while undertaking his daily walk over the past few weeks. His last episode of chest pain was one hour ago, and he remains slightly short of breath on arrival at the GP surgery. He is accompanied by his wife, who is extremely anxious and worried about his condition. Mr Singh is known to be a heavy smoker (30 a day) and suffers from raised cholesterol.

What is the nurse's first task?

■ Prior to undertaking a full cardiovascular assessment, the nurse could observe the texture, temperature and colour of Mr Singh's skin. This may reveal signs of physiological and emotional stress, such as clamminess and pallor, as well as the presence of any cyanosis, which would indicate decreased oxygenation of the tissues.

■ A simple question such as 'How are you feeling?' will also help to establish mental alertness and the degree of respiratory difficulty: can the client complete sentences or only gasp individual words? Also, it will be important to note whether the patient continues to have any degree of chest pain.

Heart rate

The heart rate is most commonly assessed by calculating the pulse rate. As the left ventricle of the heart contracts, blood is forced from the left ventricle into the aorta. This creates an arterial pressure change, which in turn leads to a wave of distension that can be felt in the arterial wall. This is known as the **pulse** (Chart 7.5).

pulse
the wave of distension felt in an artery as the heart contracts

Chart 7.5 ● Hints for pulse measurement

The pulse is detected by placing two fingers over an artery close to a bony or firm surface. The most common site used for pulse rate detection in adults and children over the age of two years is the radial pulse because it is one of the most easily detected and accessible sites. This can be felt on the anterior aspect of the wrist (Figure 7.15). The arm should be supported and relaxed, and the palm rotated uppermost. The pulse should be felt with the index and middle fingers over the groove along the thumb side of the inner wrist. Toddlers may need distracting to ensure accurate counting of the pulse. Further sites available for pulse rate palpation are shown in Figure 7.16. In infants and children under two years, the most reliable method used for calculating the heart rate is to measure the apical rate by placing a stethoscope over the chest at the apex of the heart (Wong et al., 2003). When assessing a person's pulse, three factors should be observed: its rate, rhythm and strength

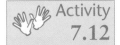 Activity 7.12

Count your resting pulse and respiratory rate. Run up a flight of about 10 stairs five times. Count your pulse and respiratory rate now and again after two minutes. Chart these readings and note the correlation between the respiratory and pulse rates. Consider what physiological changes have occurred. There is usually a 1:4 or 1:5 differential between the respiratory and pulse rates.

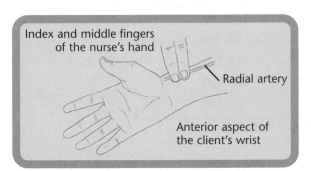

Index and middle fingers of the nurse's hand

Radial artery

Anterior aspect of the client's wrist

Figure 7.15 ● Locating the radial pulse

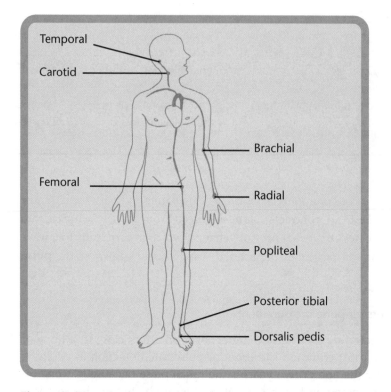

Figure 7.16 ● Common sites in the body for pulse rate palpation

The pulse rate is the number of beats in a 60-second period. It is calculated most accurately by counting the number of beats felt within a full period of 60 seconds or, at a minimum, over a 30-second period, then doubling the result. Accuracy is particularly important and is most difficult in patients who have a fast or irregular heart rate. Normal heart rates for children and adults are shown in Table 7.2.

Table 7.2 Normal heart rates for children and adults

Age (years)	Heart rate (beats per minute)
<1	110–160
1–2	100–150
2–5	95–140
5–12	80–120
12–Adult	60–100

Source: Advanced Life Support Group (2005).

A heart rate faster than the normal values shown in Table 7.2 is known as a tachycardia. In adults this is considered to occur when the heart rate is over 100 beats per minute. Causes of an increased heart rate include exercise, stress, fear, excitement, pyrexia (fever), blood or fluid loss, certain drugs and heart conditions (for example **atrial fibrillation** and cardiac failure).

A heart rate slower than the normal values shown in Table 7.2 is known as a **bradycardia**. In adults this is considered to occur when the heart rate is less than 60 beats per minute. Causes of a slow heart rate include hypothermia, certain drugs (for example **digoxin** and **beta-blockers**), activation of the parasympathetic nervous system (for example during sleep or rest), certain heart conditions (such as heart block, which results from a disorder of the conduction system) and raised intracranial pressure following a brain haemorrhage. A slow heart rate may also be a normal finding in fit athletic individuals.

Now carry out Activity 7.13. Did you consider:

● *Atropine*: increases the heart rate by inhibiting the parasympathetic nervous system. It can be used in asystolic cardiac arrests, with patients who are unwell with bradycardias, and pre-operatively to limit the effects of the vagal nerve

● *Thyroxine*: replacement therapy for clients with an underactive thyroid gland. When taken in excess, this drug will increase the metabolic rate and heart rate

● *Adrenaline* (epinephrine): its actions resemble those of the sympathetic nervous system, thereby increasing heart rate and strength of contraction. It also causes peripheral vasoconstriction, which allows more blood to be diverted to the central organs, such as the heart and brain (Resuscitation Council (UK), 2005a). It is for this reason that adrenaline is one of the key drugs used in cardiac arrest.

The accurate recording and reporting of an abnormally fast or slow heart rate is essential. It will often indicate a sudden change in a person's condition that needs to be further assessed and possibly treated. Furthermore, extreme bradycardia and tachycardia result in inadequate filling of the coronary arteries, which can lead to myocardial **ischaemia** and **infarction**. In addition, a lack of oxygenated blood to the brain (hypoxia) initially leads to confusion and disorientation, and can ultimately lead to brain damage.

The strength or volume of the pulse is important because it can provide an indication of the person's cardiac function, cardiac output and probable blood pressure. Table 7.3 outlines the relationship between palpable pulse sites and systolic blood pressure. A pulse that is weak and difficult to feel is often described as 'thready'. A thready pulse will usually be rapid and may be obliterated by pressure on the artery, suggesting that the patient is dehydrated, bleeding

tachycardia
a heart rate faster than 100 beats per minute in an adult

atrial fibrillation
an irregular and ineffective heart rhythm

bradycardia
a heart rate slower than 60 beats per minute in an adult

digoxin
a drug that slows, steadies and strengthens the heart beat, and is used for arrhythmias such as atrial fibrillation

beta-blockers
drugs that slow the heart rate and reduce the blood pressure

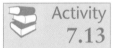
Activity 7.13

Identify three drugs that can alter the heart rate. Look up how they do this in a pharmacology reference book.

ischaemia
insufficient blood supply to the tissues. May result in infarction

infarction
the death of tissues (necrosis) due to the lack of an oxygenated blood supply

or exhausted. In such cases, it may be necessary to feel the carotid or femoral pulse. A very strong and bounding pulse may be the result of infection, stress, anaemia or exercise. A pulse which quickly disappears or 'collapses' may indicate a Corrigan's or waterhammer pulse, which is a feature of aortic valve regurgitation (Swanton, 2003). The first half of the pulse is normal or full but after reaching its peak, the wave suddenly recedes under the finger.

The rhythm of the pulse is the pattern in which the beats occur. In a healthy person, the pattern or rhythm is regular because the chambers of the heart are contracting in a coordinated manner, producing a regular pulse beat. In children and young adults, the pulse is regular but there is a slight acceleration during inspiration and a slight deceleration during expiration, known as **sinus arrhythmia**. This is uncommon over the age of 40 years (Houghton and Gray, 1997).

sinus arrhythmia

an irregular heart rhythm following the pattern of respiration

Table 7.3 The correlation between palpable pulses and systolic blood pressure

Palpable pulse site	Systolic blood pressure
Radial	>80 mmHg
Femoral	>70 mmHg
Carotid	>60 mmHg

Source: Greaves et al. (2001).

Irregularity of pulse rhythm can be divided into three types: occasional irregularity, regular irregularity and irregular irregularity. An occasional irregularity may be perceived as a missed pulse or 'dropped beat' and is often the result of an occasional ventricular ectopic (an extra beat, followed by a compensatory pause). This should be reported but might not be treated. A regularly occurring irregularity may be detected as a cyclical event and may be the result of a heart block. Again, this should be reported as it may well compromise the circulation, sometimes with catastrophic effects. An irregularly irregular rhythm is often a result of atrial fibrillation, which is one of the most common irregular cardiac rhythms. Its prevalence increases with age: 0.5 per cent of the population aged 50–59 have this condition, compared with 8.8 per cent of the 80–89 age group (Swanton, 2003).

Apical pulse rate measurements (heard through a stethoscope placed over the apex of the patient's heart; Figure 7.17) are advocated in children from birth to 24 months of age, and should be counted for one minute (Wong et al., 2003). The apical pulse rate is also incorporated into the assessment of adults who have an irregular heart rate and/or when a measurement of **pulse deficit** (the difference between the apical and peripheral pulse rates) is required.

pulse deficit

the difference between the apical and peripheral pulse rates

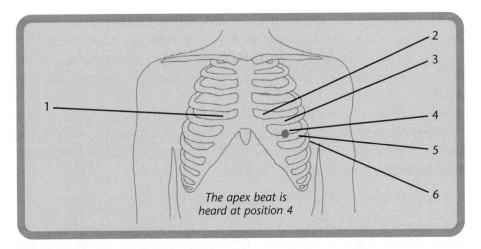

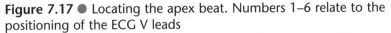

The apex beat is heard at position 4

Figure 7.17 ● Locating the apex beat. Numbers 1–6 relate to the positioning of the ECG V leads

Blood pressure

Blood pressure is the pressure exerted by the blood on the walls of a blood vessel. Each blood vessel has its own pressure, the pressure in the vessels falling continuously from the aorta to the end of systemic circulation. This pressure gradient or fall needs to exist for blood to flow. During contraction of the ventricles of the heart, blood is ejected into the systemic and pulmonary circulations, causing a distension of the arteries and an increase in arterial pressure. When contraction ends, the arterial walls recoil passively and blood is driven further through the arterial circulation. Arterial pressure therefore rises and falls during the contraction and relaxation of the heart. The maximum pressure is known as the **systolic pressure** and the minimum pressure that occurs during relaxation of the heart is known as the **diastolic pressure**.

A number of factors determine blood pressure, including peripheral resistance, intravascular blood volume and the **stroke volume**.

Peripheral resistance is the opposition to the blood flow and is determined by:

- *Blood viscosity ('stickiness')*: the greater the viscosity, the greater the resistance
- *Blood vessel length*: the longer the vessel, the greater the resistance
- *Blood vessel diameter*: the smaller the tube, the greater the resistance
- *Elasticity of the vessels*: the greater the stretch, the less the resistance.

Reductions in intravascular blood volume can directly and dramatically decrease blood pressure, especially if the blood loss (such as haemorrhage) or

systolic pressure
the blood pressure relating to the contraction of the heart

diastolic pressure
the blood pressure relating to the resting phase of the heart

stroke volume
the amount of blood ejected from the ventricle during each heart beat

fluid loss (as in burns or dehydration) is rapid. In these circumstances, the body attempts to rectify the problem via the sympathetic nervous system. For example, vasoconstriction of the peripheral circulation redirects blood to the major arteries and vital organs such as the brain, heart and kidneys. Treatment for blood volume loss involves the replacement of blood, plasma or fluid at a rate determined to be appropriate to the patient's condition.

The stroke volume plays an integral part in the cardiac function. Indeed, the cardiac output (ml per minute) is equal to the stroke volume (ml per beat) multiplied by the heart rate (beats per minute).

$$\text{Cardiac output} = \text{Stroke volume} \times \text{Heart rate}$$

Normal cardiac output is approximately 5 litres per minute (Marieb, 2004). The stroke volume is in turn affected by factors such as the venous return to the heart, the resistance against which the heart is pumping, and the contractility of the heart. Thus, patients who develop cardiogenic shock following myocardial infarction have a decreased stroke volume due to the decreased strength of the heart beat, and the blood pressure falls.

For a more detailed explanation of the physiology of blood pressure, see Hinchliff et al. (1996) or Marieb (2004).

A routine component of the cardiovascular assessment is the measurement and recording of blood pressure. The most frequent, non-invasive method of measuring arterial blood pressure employs a sphygmomanometer. The frequency of recording will depend on the patient's condition, the reason for admission and the results of the reading. It is therefore essential that the technique is performed accurately, on the same arm each time, and that the patient is prepared prior to the procedure. Other factors that should be considered when undertaking an accurate blood pressure measurement are detailed in Chart 7.6 and Figure 7.18.

Chart 7.6 ● Technique for accurately measuring blood pressure

- Use a properly maintained and calibrated device
- The patient should be comfortably seated, tight clothing around the arm removed and the arm supported at heart level
- An appropriately sized cuff should be used
- If a mercury manometer is used, the observer needs to be at eye level with the device, and the column of mercury needs to be lowered slowly. The blood pressure should be read to the nearest 2 mmHg
- The diastolic value should be measured at the disappearance of sounds (Korotkoff phase V – see Table 7.4)
- Document findings

Source: Williams et al. (2004).

The effects of anxiety should also be considered, and ideally patients should be as relaxed as possible prior to a blood pressure recording. However, it is notable that in some groups of patients, a phenomena known as 'white coat hypertension' or the 'white coat effect' can occur (Williams et al., 2004). In these circumstances, anxiety relating to an anticipated recording results is a stress effect that artificially raises the blood pressure. This effect needs to be considered, and can be overcome via repeated measurements, especially with the use of ambulatory blood pressure monitors in a community setting.

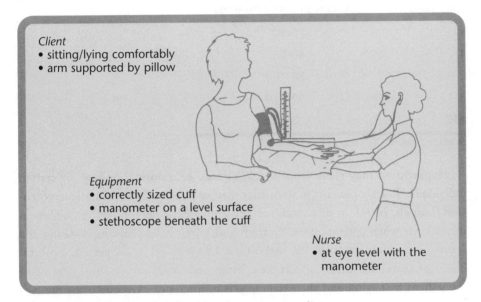

Client
• sitting/lying comfortably
• arm supported by pillow

Equipment
• correctly sized cuff
• manometer on a level surface
• stethoscope beneath the cuff

Nurse
• at eye level with the manometer

Figure 7.18 ● Preparation for blood pressure reading

Table 7.4 Korotkoff sounds with examples of pressure values

Phase	Sound	mmHg	Pressure
1	Tapping that is sharp and clear	120	Systolic
2	Blowing or swishing	110	
3	Sharp but softer than phase 1	100	
4	Muffled and fading	90	
5	No sound	80	Diastolic

Source: Dougherty and Lister (2004).

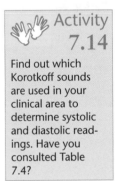

Activity
7.14

Find out which Korotkoff sounds are used in your clinical area to determine systolic and diastolic readings. Have you consulted Table 7.4?

Normal values for blood pressure readings are shown in Table 7.5. A persistently high blood pressure reading is known as **hypertension**. Williams et al. (2004) identify that hypertension exists when the systolic value is greater than

hypertension
_____
high blood pressure

139 mmHg, and/or the diastolic value is greater than 89 mmHg. Clinicians are concerned with blood pressure readings because a significantly increased mortality exists for individuals who are hypertensive, especially in relation to CHD and stroke (Williams et al., 2004; Royal College of Physicians, 2004). A low blood pressure reading is known as **hypotension**, and exists in adults when the systolic blood pressure is lower then 100 mmHg (Marieb, 2004).

hypotension

low blood pressure

Table 7.5 Average systolic blood pressure values

Age (years)	Systolic pressure (mmHg)
<1	70–90
1–2	80–95
2–5	80–100
5–12	90–110
>12	100–120

Source: Advanced Life Support Group (2005).

Hypotension may result from shock, or may be a normal finding for certain individuals. Elderly patients in particular may be affected by orthostatic hypotension (Marieb, 2004). In this condition, the sympathetic nervous system is slow in its response when patients stand up from a sitting or lying position, resulting in a syncopal (fainting) episode. If orthostatic hypotension is suspected, postural blood pressures should be undertaken, being performed on the same arm, with the patient first lying and then standing. If a difference exists between the two systolic pressures, the patient is said to have a postural fall in blood pressure, which is especially significant if the difference is 20 mmHg or more. Care is necessary when undertaking this procedure, as it may provoke a syncopal episode.

On occasions, it may be necessary to compare blood pressures between left and right arms. In cases of suspected aortic dissection, a difference in blood pressure readings of more than 20 mmHg can indicate a tear in the ascending aorta, which in turn affects the circulation of blood into the arteries supplying the arms (Manning, 2005).

Activity 7.15

Measure a colleague's resting blood pressure. Ask them to complete 20 sit-ups. Take the blood pressure again. Note the difference and consider the physiological changes that have occurred.

Peripheral perfusion

Peripheral perfusion is assessed by considering the colour, texture and temperature of the skin, the presence of peripheral pulses or **oedema** and the capillary refill time.

When assessing the colour of the skin, any pallor and/or cyanosis should be

oedema

an excessive accumulation of fluid in the tissue spaces

noted. Pallor may indicate shock, haemorrhage or poor perfusion and is easier to detect in Caucasian skin. Darker skin may become grey or ashen if severe haemorrhage has occurred. The conjunctiva of the eyes can also be inspected as a lack of their usual reddish colour indicates anaemia. Central cyanosis, such as blue lips, is an indicator of poor gaseous exchange and reflects decreased oxygen levels in the blood (Jarvis, 2003). Peripheral cyanosis is an indicator of decreased blood flow and perfusion, reflecting decreased oxygen delivery to the tissues (Jarvis, 2003). This can be noted in the extremities and the nail beds.

The texture and temperature of the skin will reveal any localised or generalised warmth or coolness and any signs of sweating. A localised heat reaction may occur following a bite or sting, whereas generalised heat may be present with an underlying pyrexia or sepsis. Sweating (diaphoresis) may indicate that the patient is pyrexial; and the skin may become cold and clammy in situations such as circulatory shock and pain, reflecting peripheral vasoconstriction secondary to the action of the sympathetic nervous system (Marieb, 2004).

Palpation of the peripheral pulses (see Figure 7.16) will indicate the presence of arterial blood flow to the extremities, and both limbs should always be checked for pulses or blood flow as this may vary considerably from limb to limb. If an area of tissue is not adequately perfused, it becomes ischaemic, the metabolic function of the tissue deteriorates and the damage eventually becomes irreversible (necrosis). Arterial insufficiency may lead to the following signs: ulceration of skin; thickening and slow growth of the nails; and skin which is shiny, scaly and hairless. Oedema and pain may also be present in the limb. Characteristically, the patient will awake in pain at night and hang the limb over the edge of the bed to increase the blood supply, thus alleviating the pain. Clinical investigations can include Doppler testing, which utilises non-invasive, continuous-wave ultrasound.

A capillary refill test (CRT) can be utilised when assessing the adequacy of tissue perfusion. This can be assessed peripherally by applying firm pressure for five seconds on a fingertip held at heart level (Resuscitation Council (UK), 2005b); or centrally by pressing for five seconds on the centre of the sternum (Advanced Life Support Group, 2005). This cutaneous pressure squeezes the blood out of the capillaries, and the length of time taken for the skin to turn pink again indicates the speed of capillary refill. A CRT greater than two seconds may be an indicator of decreased tissue perfusion, but a prolonged CRT may also occur if the patient is cold. This finding should thus be used in conjunction with other clinical signs, and a central CRT is considered to be more reliable than a peripheral CRT when assessing for circulatory shock (Advanced Life Support Group, 2005).

Peripheral oedema may result from changes in osmotic pressure (for example decreased protein levels in the blood, which might occur in liver failure), conges-

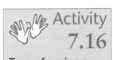

Activity 7.16

Try performing a capillary refill test on yourself and then on a colleague. Read the text to ascertain the normal values.

tion (for example in congestive heart failure), or if there is poor lymphatic drainage. Oedema is usually gravitational and may be observed in the feet or legs, or even in the genital area or sacral region if it is excessive. Patients may be taking diuretic therapy, so fluid balance and/or daily weights should be accurately ascertained to determine fluid loss.

Pulmonary oedema is characterised by acute breathlessness, often with frothy sputum, and is caused by acute left-sided heart failure. These patients are often seriously ill and are frequently unable to talk, feeling as if they are 'drowning'. Urgent medical assistance is necessary, and the patients will usually be prescribed oxygen and diuretics.

Casebox 7.2

Frances Riteur is an 80-year-old lady with known congestive heart failure. Her diuretic therapy has been altered, and the practice nurse is monitoring the effects of her new treatment.

What will the nurse be monitoring?

■ Frances will probably be weighed weekly. A weight loss of 1 kg per day represents a loss of 1 litre of fluid per day.

■ Any reduction in peripheral oedema will be noted.

■ Any reduction in breathlessness will be noted.

■ Any improvement in exercise tolerance, appetite and bowel function will also be noted, as it may indicate a lessening of her cardiac failure.

Fluid balance

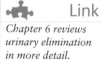

Link

Chapter 6 reviews urinary elimination in more detail.

A fluid balance record may be requested for clients who have circulatory compromise. An accurate recording of all forms of input and output is essential, as it will compare total input and output and show whether these are optimal. Urinary output for an adult normally ranges from 1.5 to 2 litres per day (1 ml/kg per hour), but this depends on normally functioning kidneys, the kidneys receiving an adequate blood supply and a lack of obstruction to urinary flow (Smith, 2000). Problems with any of these three mechanisms can therefore affect urinary output. If, for example, a patient becomes hypovolaemic post surgery, the decreased cardiac output will result in decreased renal perfusion, and hence the urinary output will drop. A reduced urinary output may thus be an early indicator that a patient's condition is deteriorating, and **oliguria** should be reported. Oliguria is said to exist when the urine output is less than 0.5 ml/kg/hour in adults (Smith, 2000), 1 ml/kg/hour in children and 2 ml/kg/hour in infants (Advanced Life Support Group, 2005).

oliguria

inadequate production of urine

Fluid charts can also reveal the effects of diuretic therapy, which is used to improve urinary output. Additionally, patients may be weighed daily or twice weekly as a method of assessing the weight/fluid balance, as 1 kg of weight is equivalent to 1 litre of water. Total fluid balance figures are often transferred onto a cumulative fluid balance chart, which allows several days or weeks of recording to be easily viewed. Continuous fluid balance over a longer period of time is vital in some groups of patients, for example those with renal or cardiac failure.

Pain

The ability to assess and effectively manage a patient's pain is an essential nursing skill. Pain was discussed in Chapter 1, and this section specifically details the assessment, recording and monitoring of pain arising from circulatory problems. As part of the pain assessment, the nurse should identify the location, severity and description of a patient's pain and consider whether there are any precipitating or alleviating factors.

An individual may be able to state the location of their pain (for example central chest pain) or point to it, but a site may be difficult to establish in individuals if there is a language barrier, for example young children and those who do not have English as their first language. Anatomical diagrams and multilanguage tools may be helpful with such patients. Some departments use graphical tools to chart a patient's pain, and these can be referred to again in subsequent reviews and evaluations.

It is important to establish the severity of the pain, and three types of scale exist to assist with this process. The first main tool to assess pain severity is the verbal descriptor scale (Chart 7.7), in which an individual is asked to select a word that describes their pain. These scales are quick and easy to use, but do require an understanding of English or translation into other languages. A second tool is the visual analogue scale (Figure 7.19), which is usually a straight line with either numbers or describers along it. These are quick to use, but they require abstract conceptualising by the patient, which may be difficult in young children or those with learning disabilities. The third type of scale is the pain behaviour tool. This relies on the principle that patients who are in pain exhibit certain types of behaviour (Chart 7.8), which can be objectively assessed.

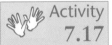

Link

Chapter 1 gives further examples of pain assessment methods.

Activity 7.17

Identify the pain assessment tools used in your clinical area. Ascertain whether pain scores are linked to an analgesic protocol, for example a pain score of 8 out of 10 equates to the need for opiate analgesia. Do nurses make their own judgements of what pain clients are experiencing? Do particular clients express more pain than others?

Chart 7.7 ● Verbal descriptor pain scale

- None
- Slight
- Moderate
- Severe
- Agony

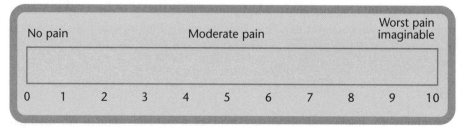

Figure 7.19 ● Visual analogue pain scale

Chart 7.8 ● Pain behaviour scale

- Verbal response
- Body language
- Facial expression
- Behavioural change
- Conscious level
- Physiological change

An ideal pain assessment tool should allow for a quick but comprehensive pain assessment, which combines the patient's subjective interpretation of their pain with an objective assessment by the nurse of the effects of this pain on the patient's behaviour. Such a tool should also facilitate the ongoing assessment and evaluation of pain and pain control. Figure 7.20 shows a pain ruler that meets these criteria, while the Manchester Triage Group has also designed a pain ruler aimed at emergency departments, but with obvious value to other clinical environments (Mackway-Jones, 1997). The Manchester tool combines the verbal descriptor, visual analogue and pain behaviour tools, which provides for both patient and practitioner assessment.

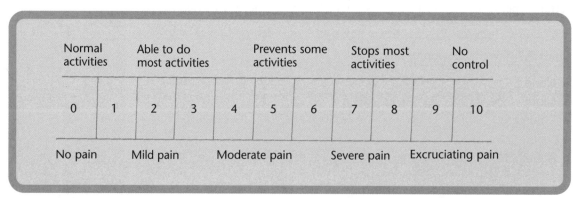

Figure 7.20 ● A pain ruler

It is important to remember that patients frequently understate the amount of pain they are in. This may be especially true with older clients, specifically those who have lived with chronic pain and have found ways of adapting to and coping with pain. Children may also understate pain, possibly because of fear of the consequences, such as having to go to hospital.

A description of the pain is necessary to clarify and confirm its location and severity, and may also indicate its probable cause. For example, a client who describes leg pain that is cramping and excruciating, being worse on walking, may have intermittent **claudication** secondary to arterial insufficiency. Investigations obviously need to be performed to confirm the initial suspicion, but the description helps the practitioner to prioritise the management of these patients.

claudication
_____
pain in the lower limbs due to insufficient arterial blood supply

Precipitating factors such as exercise, stress, movement, respiration, position, time and duration are helpful in determining the probable cause and possible effects of the pain. Chest pain on respiration, particularly inspiration, may, for example, arise from the pleura or pericardium.

Alleviating factors such as heat, cold, rest, analgesics, position and distraction may again indicate the cause of pain but may also help with pain management strategies. A patient with angina, for example, who complains of chest pain when walking in the cold can be advised to alter her walking habits or try prophylactic vasodilators such as glyceryl trinitrate prior to exercise.

The physiological effects of pain may be minimal, but on occasion marked tachycardia and hypertension might develop in response to the stress effect; while vagal stimulation might result in bradycardia, hypotension and syncope. Chronic pain can certainly curtail a patient's activities or lifestyle, and health education advice may be appropriate. For further information, see Macintyre and Ready (2001) or Park et al. (2000).

Nursing interventions

Cardiac monitoring

A cardiac monitor displays a graphical representation of the electrical activity occurring within the heart. It is a useful tool to assess a client's heart rhythm and also provides information about their condition and progress. Whereas cardiac monitors were once the domain of specialist units, now they are increasingly used in a variety of clinical settings. Chart 7.9 outlines hints on using cardiac monitors.

Chart 7.9 ● Hints on using a cardiac monitor

● Ensure that the cardiac monitor is situated in a safe, observable position
● Switch it on at the wall and on the monitor (if appropriate)
● Set the monitor to lead 2 unless told otherwise
● Attach the electrodes to the client's skin surface as shown in Figure 7.21
● The electrodes need to be firmly attached to the patient's skin. This may be difficult if the patient is shocked and sweating. If the leads do not adhere, the following may be useful: shave the chest if necessary (in the area where the electrodes need placing); abrade the skin lightly (most electrodes have a rough edge to achieve this); and dry the skin.
● Ensure that the rhythm tracing is visible and observe it regularly

It is important to always match what is seen on the cardiac monitor to the patient's condition. For example, leads dislodged from a patient may mimic asystole. Likewise, it is also important to note that during some cardiac arrests, patients can have a near normal ECG rhythm. This is known as 'pulseless electrical activity' (PEA) and occurs when the electrical activity is compatible with a cardiac output, and yet there is no mechanical activity to propel blood around the body. There are various causes of PEA (and indeed cardiac arrest in general) including **hypovolaemia**, hypothermia, hypoxia, hypo/hyperkalaemia and other metabolic disorders, tension pneumothorax, cardiac tamponade, toxic/therapeutic disorders and thromboembolic and mechanical obstruction (otherwise known as the '4 Hs and 4 Ts'; Resuscitation Council (UK), 2005a). The guiding principle is to look at the patient first and the monitor second.

The normal cardiac rhythm, or **sinus rhythm**, has characteristic waveforms (Figure 7.22), and an understanding of these, in addition to the physiology of normal cardiac conduction, will enable you to identify any deviations from the normal ECG. What follows is a basic introduction to ECG interpretation; for a more detailed approach, see books such as *The ECG Made Easy* (Hampton, 1998).

hypovolaemia
an abnormally low circulating blood volume

sinus rhythm
the normal rhythm of the heart

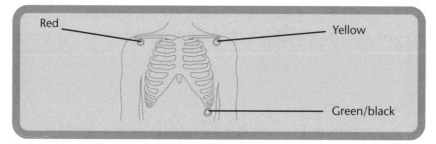

Figure 7.21 ● ECG chest lead placement

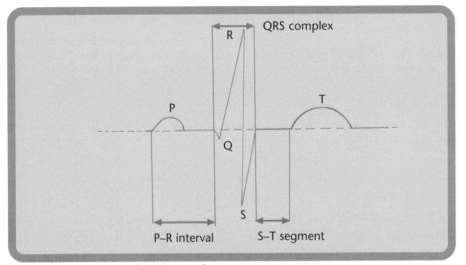

Figure 7.22 ● Normal ECG waveform

The isoelectric line, or baseline, is seen as a straight line. The first wave of the ECG is the P wave, representing the **depolarisation** of the atrial myocardium. Atrial depolarisation leads to atrial contraction (systole), during which blood is expelled from the atria into the ventricles. The P wave is followed by the QRS complex, which represents ventricular depolarisation. The Q wave is the first downward (or negative) deflection after the P wave, but is not always present in normal conduction. The R wave is the first upward (or positive) deflection after the P wave, and the S wave is the downward deflection that follows an R wave. Following ventricular depolarisation, ventricular systole occurs, resulting in blood being expelled into the systemic and pulmonary circulations. The next deflection on the ECG is the T wave, representing ventricular muscle repolarisation, which corresponds with ventricular diastole. It is in this period that the ventricles fill with blood prior to the next systolic contraction. Atrial repolarisation occurs during ventricular depolarisation, but the waveform is masked by the greater electrical activity occurring in the ventricles. A normal or sinus beat therefore has a P wave, a QRS complex, a T wave, and an S–T segment that is on the isoelectric line. Alterations to these waveforms indicate cardiac arrhythmia, disease or damage.

When analysing the ECG rhythm, various pieces of information are required to ascertain whether the rhythm is sinus in origin or whether there is an arrhythmia. What follows is a six-stage process that can be used for the basic analysis of an ECG rhythm:

1. Heart rate.
2. Regularity of heart rhythm.

depolarisation

loss of the polarised state of the plasma membrane, involving a loss or reduction of the negative membrane potential

3. Presence/absence of P waves.
4. P–R interval.
5. QRS complex duration/width.
6. Rhythm interpretation.

Heart rate

The heart rate can be obtained in several ways. If the rhythm is regular, count the number of large squares between two consecutive R waves and divide the number into 300 to determine the heart rate. For example, 5 large squares between two R waves divided into 300 gives a heart rate of 60. However, if the heart rate is irregular, such as with atrial fibrillation, this method is clearly unreliable. In such situations, an alternative method is necessary, which involves counting the number of QRS complexes that occur in a 6-second period on an ECG strip (that is, 30 large squares). The resultant number of QRS complexes is then multiplied by 10, which indicates the number of complexes that occur in a 60-second period.

Regularity

The regularity of the rhythm should be noted. If this is not obvious, it can be ascertained using a ruler or ECG rule, or merely by marking a piece of paper at the top of two complexes and moving it along the rhythm strip to see whether the other complexes fall regularly. Irregular rhythms are unlikely to be sinus in origin except for sinus arrhythmia, in which acceleration and deceleration occur with respiration.

P waves

The presence of a P wave should be noted, as it is an essential component of sinus rhythm.

P–R interval

The P–R interval is measured from the beginning of the P wave to the beginning of the QRS complex. It can be measured in either time (0.12–0.20 seconds) or squares (3–5 small squares on the ECG paper). For the rhythm to be sinus rhythm, the P–R interval must fall within this duration. If the P–R interval is greater, it may indicate atrioventricular heart block.

QRS complex

The QRS duration is measured from the beginning to the end of the QRS complex. Again, it can be measured in time (less than 0.12 seconds) or squares (less than 3 small squares on the ECG paper). Beats that are sinus in origin and are conducted normally through the conduction system will fall within these parameters.

Rhythm interpretation

Having followed the processes outlined above, it should be possible to decide whether or not the rhythm is sinus in origin. Further skills are then necessary to determine which other rhythm it might be, but these are beyond the scope of this section.

Anti-embolic precautionary measures

The British Thoracic Society (2003) identifies that the classification of venous thromboembolism (VTE) includes both deep vein thrombosis (DVT) and pulmonary embolus (PE). Major risk factors for the development of a VTE include major abdominal/pelvic surgery, the later stages of pregnancy, lower limb fractures, malignancy, reduced mobility and a history of previous VTE (British Thoracic Society, 2003). A PE results when thrombi, especially from the pelvic veins and the deep veins of the leg, dislodge and follow the venous system through to the pulmonary arterial system (Goldhaber, 1997). These emboli can then lead to a range of clinical signs and symptoms, ranging from dyspnoea, chest pain, circulatory collapse and sudden death. It is for this reason that the prevention of VTE is vitally important.

Anti-embolic stockings and heparin

Ball and Phillips (2001) identify that thigh-length graduated compression stockings should be used in situations where patients have a risk of developing VTE, such as those patients undergoing major surgery and those who have poor mobility while in hospital. Meta-analysis has revealed that when these stockings are worn until discharge, they significantly reduce both DVT and PE (Ball and Phillips, 2001). It is also recognised that the addition of low molecular weight heparin to these patients further reduces the incidence of VTE (Agnelli et al., 1998).

Exercises

Passive/active exercises are an important measure to promote venous return and decrease venous stasis in order to prevent a DVT. Preoperative and bed-bound patients can be taught and encouraged to combine deep breathing techniques and active leg exercises to achieve this. Exercises can be performed passively for unconscious or immobile individuals. Further measures to encourage blood flow are regular changes of position, the use of bed cradles to relieve pressure on the limbs and ensuring that the top sheets are not tightly tucked in. In some units, intermittent pneumatic compression devices are applied to the calves to assist venous return.

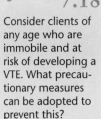

Activity 7.18

Consider clients of any age who are immobile and at risk of developing a VTE. What precautionary measures can be adopted to prevent this?

Joan Hammett is a 52-year-old lady who is recovering from minor surgery that was carried out two days ago. She suddenly complains of crushing central chest pain, which is making her feel dizzy, sick and short of breath. She is known to suffer from CHD but says that this is a lot worse than her usual angina pain.

What could you ask her about the description of pain to help you in your management?

- The site of the pain and any radiation, for example to the neck, arms or back.

- The intensity of the pain and whether anything relieves it.

- The onset and duration of the pain, for example sudden or gradual.

- The consequences of the pain. For example, when she says that she feels dizzy and nauseated, can she concentrate or is the pain too distracting for her to think normally.

- Anyone presenting with chest pain potentially has a serious condition such as a myocardial infarction and you should always seek help.

- The questions above will help the assessor to determine whether the pain is likely to be cardiac in origin.

Blood transfusion

A blood transfusion involves the administration of either whole blood or one of its components from one person to another. The types of blood or blood product commonly used are whole blood, concentrated (packed) red cells, washed red cells, platelets, plasma and plasma substitutes. In this process, however, it must be remembered that problems can arise.

Safety precautions prior to transfusion are as follows. Blood should be stored in a specific fridge (not a domestic fridge) whose temperature is constantly maintained between 2°C and 6°C to prevent bacterial contamination and be removed from the fridge no longer than 15 minutes prior to its use. Each hospital will have a local procedure for checking blood that usually involves two nurses, one of whom is a trained nurse, and includes confirming the patient's name, date of birth and hospital number, the expiry date of the blood, the blood groups of the donor and recipient, and the serial number of the unit of blood. Once checked, this information is recorded either in the patient's notes or on a prescription sheet or checklist. The unit should also be checked for signs of deterioration or damage. If there is any doubt, the blood should not be given but returned to the laboratory and advice requested. The transfusion should be prepared aseptically, and a specific blood administration set with an integral in-line filter should be used. In addition, some units use additional filters, and local policies must be checked. The giving set may be primed with saline prior to the administration of blood, as this can prevent the adherence of the blood to the set.

Observations during transfusion are an integral and essential part of the client's care and should commence with a set of baseline observations prior to commencement of the transfusion (pulse, blood pressure, temperature and respiratory rate). Local policies vary, but the patient should be constantly observed and regularly monitored for any signs of a transfusion reaction. Reactions can occur very rapidly and are most likely to occur during the initial administration of each unit. Most hospital policies include 15-minute observations during the first hour, followed by either half-hourly or hourly observations of pulse, temperature, blood pressure and respiration for the remainder of the unit, and at the completion of the unit's transfusion (Dougherty and Lister, 2004). This pattern is repeated for all new units of blood.

Transfusion complications

Circulatory overload occurs from an excessive intravascular volume that usually results in pulmonary oedema. This is most likely to occur in chronically anaemic patients who require the additional oxygen-carrying capacity of red blood cells but not the volume. The problem is prevented by using packed cells and giving diuretics. If circulatory overload occurs, the patient should be seated upright and reassured, the transfusion should be discontinued immediately and medical advice should be sought.

Haemolytic mismatch is one of the most serious complications of a blood transfusion, and clinical problems can arise rapidly following as little as a 10–15 ml infusion of incompatible blood. Problems are caused by antigen–antibody reactions, leading to acute intravascular **agglutination** and **haemolysis**. Early symptoms include fever, shivering, tachycardia, wheeze, rash and hypotension. Further complications are chest tightness, loin pain, shock and disseminated intravascular coagulation (DIC). DIC results in inappropriate clumping of platelets in the microcirculation, which results in tissue ischaemia secondary to these thrombi, as well as bleeding due to the overconsumption of coagulation factors (Barkin and Rosen, 2003). The degree of the haemolytic reaction therefore ranges from mild to severe, with shock and death in some instances. The transfusion should be stopped immediately and any remaining blood sent for analysis. Contact medical help immediately, as aggressive treatment may be necessary.

Allergic reactions are fairly common, ranging from mild irritation to anaphylactic shock. Symptoms include flushing, **urticarial hives**, wheezing, chest tightness, laryngeal oedema and peri-orbital oedema. **Anaphylaxis** is potentially fatal and requires urgent treatment. This may include intramuscular adrenaline, intravenous chlorpheniramine (an antihistamine), intravenous hydrocortisone (acting as an anti-inflammatory agent), and nebulised salbutamol (acting as as a bronchodilator).

Disease transmission is theoretically possible following transfusion and has occurred in the past, but today all blood in the UK is routinely screened for HIV

agglutination

the clumping of foreign cells due to an antigen–antibody reaction

haemolysis

the disintegration of red blood cells, causing severe anaemia and possibly jaundice

urticarial hives

a skin condition that manifests as red weals causing intense irritation; it is usually a result of hypersensitivity

anaphylaxis

a form of allergic or hypersensitivity reaction to a foreign protein and can lead to anaphylactic shock, which is potentially fatal

and hepatitis. It is also extremely rare for blood to be contaminated with other microorganisms, although Gram-negative bacteria can reproduce at 4°C. Reactions include pyrexia, rigor, chest and abdominal pain and the development of septic shock.

Cold blood can cause hypothermia when given in large quantities, and this can provoke further coagulopathies (disorders of coagulation; Greaves et al., 2001). In most instances, active blood warming is not indicated, especially as a temperature greater than 38°C can cause haemolysis of red cells (Dougherty and Lister, 2004). However, if large amounts of blood are to be transfused in an emergency, then blood should be warmed to 37°C.

Intravenous fluid therapy

A patient may receive intravenous fluid therapy if they are unable to maintain their fluid balance orally. Causes include dehydration because of a lack of oral intake, severe vomiting or diarrhoea, excess urine output or perspiration, severe burns, surgical procedures and unconsciousness. Intravenous fluid therapy is common in acute hospital settings, but it must be remembered that it is an invasive procedure with many potential complications. These include:

- Infection
- Inflammation
- Thrombophlebitis
- Extravasation (infiltration of fluid into the surrounding tissues)
- Septicaemia
- Air or particle embolism
- Circulatory overload
- Anaphylactic reaction.

The nurse's role is described in Chart 7.10.

Chart 7.10 ● Hints for intravenous therapy

- Ensure that whoever sites the cannula selects an appropriate position and uses an aseptic procedure
- When sited, the cannula should be firmly secured
- The cannula should be regularly inspected (at least twice a day) for signs of infection and inflammation
- If fluids are being delivered via the cannula, it is essential to ensure that the right fluid is given to the right patient via the right route at the right time at the correct rate (the five Rs)

Link

Chapter 4 discusses the five Rs in greater depth.

● Most hospitals operate a policy whereby intravenous fluids need to be checked prior to delivery by two nurses, one of whom is a qualified nurse. To ensure that fluids are delivered at the correct rate, electronic pump devices are frequently used in many clinical settings. If these are not available, a formula for calculating the number of drips per minute is required. One such formula is described in Figure 7.23

● The system that is used for delivering the fluid must be inspected for damage and sterility

● It is essential to ensure that the system is free of air bubbles when primed with fluids and during the process of fluid delivery

● All contact with the intravenous system should be aseptic to reduce the risk of infection

● You may also see drugs added to the fluid system. The additives may be prepacked or require adding. In most hospitals, this is a procedure for a trained nurse

$$\frac{\text{(Number of ml x drops per ml)}}{\text{(Number of hours x 60}} = \text{drops/minute}$$

The following example represents a client who is prescribed 1000 ml (1 litre) of fluid over four hours. The giving set in use delivers 10 drops per ml. The figure 60 is a given constant representing 60 minutes in one hour.

Therefore:

$$\frac{(1000 \times 10)}{(4 \times 60)} = 41.7 \text{ or } 42 \text{ drops/minute}$$

Note: The giving set package must be carefully inspected for the number of drops per ml, as this may vary.

Figure 7.23 ● Formula for drip rate calculation

■ Chapter Summary

This chapter has examined the key factors related to a client's respiratory and cardiac function. You have learnt how to monitor and interpret respiratory and cardiac vital signs and how to differentiate deviations from normal values. You have considered how to assist and maintain respiratory function with supplemental oxygenation, physiotherapy and drugs delivered via inhaler devices. In addition, you will have examined techniques to optimise cardiac function, for example pain assessment, cardiac monitoring, anti-embolic therapy, blood transfusion and intravenous therapy. Finally, you have learnt how to recognise and initially manage a cardiorespiratory arrest.

Test Yourself!

1. What is the normal respiratory rate for a two-year-old child?

2. What are Cheyne–Stokes respirations?

3. List six sounds associated with respiratory disease.

4. Describe four types of sputum.

5. List five common causes of shock.

6. Describe the types of pain assessment tool available.

7. Describe five complications of a blood transfusion.

■ Further Reading

Chandler, T. (2000) Oxygen saturation monitoring. *Paediatric Nursing* **12**(8): 37–43.

Peate, I. and Lancaster, J. (2000) Safe use of medical gases. *British Journal of Nursing* **9**(4): 231–6.

Resuscitation Council (UK) (2000) *Advanced Life Support Course Provider Manual*, 4th edn. Resuscitation Council, London.

Woodrow, P. (1999) Pulse oximetry. *Nursing Standard* **13**(42): 42–6.

■ References

Advanced Life Support Group (2005) *Advanced Paediatric Life Support*. Blackwell, Oxford.

Agnelli, G., Piovella, F., Buoncristiani, P. et al. (1998) Enoxaparin plus compression stockings compared with compression stockings alone in the prevention of venous thromboembolism after elective neurosurgery. *New England Journal of Medicine* **339**: 80–5.

Ball, C.M. and Phillips, R.S. (2001) *Evidence Based on Call: Acute Medicine*. Churchill Livingstone, Edinburgh.

Barkin, R.M. and Rosen, P. (2003) *Emergency Pediatrics*. Mosby, Philadelphia.

Baskett, P.J.F. and Chamberlain, D. (eds) (1977) The ILCOR Advisory Statement. *Resuscitation* **34**: 97–8.

Booker, R. (2003) Lung function testing. *Practice Nursing* **14**(5): 215–20.

British Thoracic Society (2003) British Thoracic Society guidelines for the management of suspected pulmonary embolism. *Thorax* **58**: 470–84.

Chandler, T. (2001) Oxygen administration. *Paediatric Nursing* **13**(8): 37–43.

Coad, J. (2002) *Anatomy and Physiology for Midwives*. Mosby, London.

DoH (Department of Health) (2005) *Coronary Heart Disease National Service Framework: Leading the Way,* Progress Report 2005. HMSO, London.

Dougherty, L. and Lister, S. (2004) *The Royal Marsden Hospital Manual of Clinical Nursing Procedures*, 6th edn. Blackwell, Oxford.

Frey, B. and Shann, F. (2003) Oxygen administration in infants. *Archives of Diseases in Childhood* **88**(2): 84–8.

Giuliano, K.K and Higgins, T. (2005) New-generation pulse oximetry in the care of critically ill patients. *American Journal of Nursing* **14**(1): 26–39.

Goldhaber, S.Z. (1997) Pulmonary embolism. In E. Braunwald (ed.) *Heart Disease: A Textbook of Cardiovascular Medicine*, 5th edn. W.B. Saunders, Philadelphia.

Greaves, I., Porter, K. and Ryan, J. (2001) *Trauma Care Manual*. Arnold, London.

Hampton, J.R. (1998) *The ECG Made Easy*, 5th edn. Churchill Livingstone, Edinburgh.

Hazinski, M.F. (1999) *Manual of Nursing Care of the Critically Ill Child*. C.V. Mosby, St Louis.

Hinchliff, S.M., Montague, S.E. and Watson, R. (1996) *Physiology for Nursing Practice*, 2nd edn. Baillière Tindall, London.

Houghton, A.R. and Gray, D. (1997) *Making Sense of the ECG*. Arnold, London.

Jarvis, C. (2003) *Physical Examination and Health Assessment*, 4th edn. W.B. Saunders, Philadelphia.

Kendrick, A.H. and Smith, E.C. (1992) Simple measurements of lung function. *Professional Nurse* **7**(6): 395–402.

Law, C. (2000) A guide to assessing sputum. *Nursing Times* **96**(24): 7–10.

Macintyre, P.E. and Ready, L.B. (2001) *Acute Pain Management: A Practical Guide*, 2nd edn. W.B. Saunders, London.

Mackway-Jones, K. (ed.) (1997) *Emergency Triage*. BMJ Publishing, London.

Manning, W.J. (2005) Clinical manifestations and diagnosis of aortic dissection. http://uptodateonline.com/application/topic.asp?file=valve_hd/5587&type=A&selected Title=1–35.

Marieb, E. (2004) *Human Anatomy and Physiology*, 6th edn. Benjamin Pearson Cummings, San Francisco.

Marieb, E. (2006) *Essentials of Human Anatomy and Physiology*, 8th edn. Benjamin Cummings, San Francisco.

Middleton, S. and Middleton, P.G. (1998) Assessment. In Pryor, J.A. and Webber, B.A. (eds) *Physiotherapy for Respiratory and Cardiac Problems*. Churchill Livingstone, Edinburgh.

Park, G., Fulton, B. and Senthuran, S. (2000) *The Management of Acute Pain*, 2nd edn. Oxford University Press, Oxford.

Poets, C.F., Stebbens, V.A., Samuels, M.P., Southall, D.P. (1993) Oxygen saturations and breathing patterns in children. *Pediatrics* **92**(5): 686–90.

Popovich, D.M., Richiuso, N. and Danck, G. (2004) Pediatric health care providers' knowledge of pulse oximetry. *Pediatric Nursing* **30**(1): 14–20.

Ramsey, J. (1989) *Nursing the Child with Respiratory Problems*. Chapman & Hall, London.

Resuscitation Council (UK) (2005a) *The Resuscitation Guidelines 2005*. Resuscitation Council (UK), London.

Resuscitation Council (UK) (2005b) *A Systematic Approach to the Acutely Ill Patient*. Resuscitation Council (UK), London.

Royal College of Physicians (2004) *Primary Care Concise Guidelines for Stroke 2004*. Royal College of Physicians, London.

Smith, G. (2000) *Alert: a Multiprofessional Course in Care of the Acutely Ill Patient*. University of Portsmouth.

Sun, S.W., Patel, B., Gangoo, W. and Carrey, Z. (2003) Reliability of forehead pulse oximetry in critically ill patients. *Chest* **124**(4): 179(s).

Swanton, R.H. (2003) *Cardiology*, 5th edn. Blackwell Science, Oxford.

Thiagamoorthy, S., Merchant, S., Carter, M., Jarvis, D. and Bateman, N. (2000) An audit of oxygen therapy: is oxygen prescribed, administered, monitored and withdrawn according to guidelines? *Journal of Clinical Excellence* **2**(2): 127–9.

Thomson, A.J., Webb, D.J. and Maxwell, S.R. (2002) Oxygen therapy in acute medical care. *British Medical Journal* **324**: 1407–8.

Tucker Blackburn, S. (2003) *Maternal, Fetal, and Neonatal Physiology*. Saunders, Washington.

Williams, B., Poulter, N.R., Brown, M.J., Davis, M., McInnes, G.T., Potter, J.F., Sever, P.S. and Thom, S. (2004) Guidelines for management of hypertension: report of the fourth working party of the British Hypertension Society. *Journal of Human Hypertension* **18**: 139–85.

Wieteska, S., Mackaway-Jones, K. and Phillips, B. (2005) *Advanced Paediatric Life Support: the Practical Approach*, 4th edn. BMJ Publishing, London.

Wong, D.L., Hockenberry, M.J., Wilson, D., Winkelstein, M.L., and Kline, N.E. (2003) *Wong's Nursing Care of Infants and Children*, 7th edn. Mosby, St Loius, MO.

Useful Websites

www.resus.org.uk Resuscitation Council UK
Provides education and reference materials to health-care professionals and the general public on the most effective methods of resuscitation

www.nelh.nhs.uk National Electronic Library for Health Programme
Works with NHS Libraries to develop a digital library for NHS staff, patients and the public

www.visembryo.com A comprehensive resource of information on human development from conception to birth, designed for both practitioners and interested laypeople

SID CARTER AND ANITA GREEN

Chapter

Body Image and Sexuality

8

Contents

Learning Outcomes

The expression of sexuality and body image appear to be interrelated, particularly when associated with physical or mental illness, disease or physical trauma. Sexuality, sexual health and body image when negatively affected can decrease a person's self-image and self-esteem. When a person has contact with a health-care setting, their illness or disability will probably impact on their sexuality (RCN, 2000) and body image. There can be many adjustments to sexuality and body image, and with these can come changes to self-care (Salter, 1997). It is important that nurses understand the interrelationship between sexuality and body image and their responsibility in understanding these two important aspects of a person. Nurses need to recognise the part they play in helping patients and clients when body image and sexuality need to be addressed as part of patient care. Nurses must also recognise their own feelings around these areas and the importance of their own self-awareness when communicating with patients and clients who want support and guidance with their sexuality and altered body image needs. The nurse has a vital role to play here in the physical and psychological care, support and treatment that she or he offers.

At the end of this chapter, you should be able to:

- Understand the interrelationship between sexuality and body image and your responsibility in understanding these two important aspects of a person

- Recognise the part you will play in helping patients and clients when body image and sexuality need to be addressed as an aspect of patient care

- Recognise your own feelings with respect to these areas

- Realise the importance of your own self-awareness when communicating with patients and clients who want support and guidance with their sexuality and altered body image needs.

■ What Are Self-image and Normal Body Image?

Link

Chapter 10 briefly discusses spirituality and nursing care.

self-image

our own assessment of our social worth

body image

the mental picture we have of our body and feelings towards it

Over the past two or three decades, nursing has integrated holistic perspectives and approaches into the care and treatment of patients and clients. We now consider the psychosocial, cultural and spiritual wants and needs of the patient and client when the nurse tends to their physical requirements. To perceive the patient and client as a 'whole' and not as a set of components that need separate attention is an important ideal and can help the nurse be more receptive to the patient's self-image and self-esteem. According to Price (1990, p. 12), **self-image** is 'our own assessment of our social worth'. Positive self-image gives us confidence and can increase our self-esteem.

An important element of self-image is **body image**, the mental picture each person has of his or her body. At birth, infants do not have a body image. As babies develop, their awareness expands and they begin to explore parts of their body. As they receive sensory stimulation through physical contact with others, they become aware of their own separateness (Sundeen et al., 1994, p. 65). Children have a relatively simple view of their own bodies. When children are asked to draw pictures of themselves and the different parts of their bodies, their view of the body and the way it functions will be drawn using elementary shapes to represent organs. Once at school, these concepts are developed and become more sophisticated as the child starts to view body image within the context of gender identification (Price, 1998, p. 50). Towards the end of primary education, children's concept of themselves, their body and its functions are influenced by the attitude of their parental figures through what they say and do and the things that are discussed or not discussed within the family context (Sundeen et al., 1994, p. 65). Adolescence, a time of rapid physical development, can bring with it feelings of awkwardness. Secondary sexual characteristics have to be incorporated into the individual's developing body image. With this go society's expectations of conforming to the social roles of being a man or woman, for example the different ways we groom and adorn ourselves when in the social arena.

Inevitably, if body image is affected either positively or negatively, this will influence the person's self-image. McCrea et al. (1982, p. 226) state that body image as a term: 'Refers to the body as a psychological experience and focuses on the individual's feelings and attitudes towards his own body.' Chilton (1984, p. 158, cited in Salter, 1997, p. 2) demonstrates the links between self-esteem and body image when stating:

> Body image also plays an important part in self-understanding. How a person feels about himself is basically related to how he feels about his body. The body is a most visible and material part of one's self and occupies the central part in a person's perceptions. Body image is the sum of the conscious and unconscious attitudes that the individual has towards his body. Present and past perceptions and feelings about size, function, appearance and potential are included. A person with a high level of self-esteem will tend to have a much clearer understanding of himself.

Added to this complex concept of body image is the element of change. How the individual perceives him or herself can alter depending on external and/or internal influences. These could be psychosocial, cultural or physiological or any combination of these. An example of this is when a woman menstruates. There are hormonal changes occurring in the body associated with the menstrual cycle. These hormonal changes cause physiological changes, for example when the level of progesterone is at its lowest, menstruation occurs. This may affect the woman's mood, and also influence how she perceives herself when menstruating. Added to this could be the woman's view of whether or not she wanted to be pregnant and how she associates menstruation with being womanly and feminine. There are cultural differences towards the menstruating woman: historically, the West has used terms like 'the curse' to describe the process of menstruating; this can affect the way women view their menstrual blood and their bodies when menstruating (Kitzinger, 1985, p. 38).

Ageing will also influence body image. As well as physiological changes, which could affect mobility and independent living, society's views on ageing are also an influence on the older person's body image (Price, 1990, p. 31). Changes in body function and appearance are a feature of health as well as illness and can be usefully viewed along an age continuum. To understand how the body is affected by normal physiological change, illness, ageing and hospitalisation and how this influences self-image is important for nurses to understand. Nurses' self-awareness in relation to how they perceive their own bodies and the bodies of others is an important contribution to this process of understanding. Even admission to hospital, before any procedures are commenced, will affect a person's body image and self-image. Removing one's day clothes and getting into bed

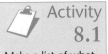

Activity 8.1

Make a list of what you like and dislike about your body.

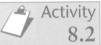

Activity 8.2

How do you perceive yourself in your later years? List the changes you envisage occurring as you age. Your list could be influenced by how you view your body now and how it functions, your older family members and how they have changed and learned to adapt. Your list could be affected by someone you know who has taken on new challenges as they have aged.

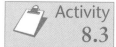

Activity 8.3

Think about how you present your body to others. Write down what you do, for example through the use of make-up, clothes and hairstyle, in order to 'face the world' when you go out to meet others. Does this change depending on who you are meeting or what you are doing?

could bring about feelings of dependency, loss and passivity. Changes to or loss of self-image due to hospitalisation have been well documented and can be linked with the changes or loss of self-identity observed in people who spend more than a few days in hospital (Goffman 1961; Sanderson, 1985, cited in Savage, 1987).

Trying to understand an individual's feelings about their body image should also include how they value the different parts of their body. This is very individual. However, the nurse can explore this with the patient when completing the initial assessment. For example, a jockey putting on weight would seriously affect his or her career, and an orchestral conductor with a damaged shoulder would be unable to work without suffering pain.

Body reality, body presentation and body ideal

Price (1990, p. 4) defines body image using three fundamental and interrelated concepts: body reality, body presentation and body ideal. This is a helpful starting point for understanding and exploring issues relating to body image.

Body reality

body reality

the body as it actually is in terms of its objective physical characteristics

Body reality refers to the body as it is, an objective representation, for example stating the height of someone, the colour of their hair and the colour of their eyes. Body reality is dynamic; our bodies undergo constant physiological change. Some of these changes we may be more aware of than others, for example the physiological changes that occur during puberty such as developing pubic hair and breasts or facial hair. These will have a dramatic effect on body reality and inevitably affect body image, self-image and self-esteem. From birth to older age, there are clear examples of how the body reality changes.

Body ideal

body ideal

how we believe our body should look and perform, this being influenced by our beliefs and attitudes and by changes in fashion

Body ideal represents how we believe our body should look like and perform. Our body ideal is influenced by the beliefs, norms and attitudes that we develop from early childhood as part of primary socialisation. During adolescence, the body ideal appears to require constant updating in the light of new trends, with the media offering examples of the most recent 'role models', for example popular music bands and the accompanying style of dress. The adolescent age group more than any other has to adjust body reality in light of new changes in fashion and social behaviour. Both conventional and non-conventional body piercing and tattooing have increased (Langford, 1996; Larkin, 2004), are attractive to young people and may be considered as permanent body reality change. These body changes may be viewed as a rite of passage and may also have cultural value. There may, however, be implications for the person when body piercing and tattooing are no longer part of their body ideal following changes in fashion or a change of view of these types of body decoration as the person ages. Body ideal also includes how we think we should smell and age, what we should weigh, and how our body should be proportioned, for example the size of our breasts and penis. Body ideal is also influenced by cultural standards, for example over the past two decades, exercise and fitness leading to a slim, toned body has led to a 'body-conscious' society (Sundeen et al., 1994, p. 67). Body ideal may also be influenced by how plastic surgery is portrayed in the media. More information is now available, with 'live' surgery on television and adverts for plastic surgery clinics in magazines, which may persuade women to seek surgical interventions to enhance their bodies.

Body presentation

Body presentation is linked with body ideal and represents how we present our body to others in a social context and in intimate situations. Body presentation includes the way we dress, adorn our body, groom, and use posture and gesture (Price, 1990, p. 10, 1998, p. 50). Body image can include how we smell. Whether or not we chose to wear deodorant and/or perfumes and, if we do, the type of perfumes we want others to smell on us can play an important part in how we want to be perceived and the association society places on particular smells and perfumes. We have a level of control over how we present our body to others. We are also influenced by what is expected of us, for example policies regarding the wearing of uniform and how it should be worn, and policies for those who are not required to wear a uniform to work but have guidelines for what is acceptable as 'non-uniform'. We are also aware of the limits and boundaries of how we can present our body to others, for example when working in the community as a community psychiatric nurse or district nurse.

Being unhappy with our body image affects the way we behave and inevitably affects those around us, even if this unhappiness is temporary. When we feel good about our body image and others notice this and offer positive comments to support us, usually this will positively affect our self-image so that we feel good about ourselves, and it is seen as approval.

■ What is Altered Body Image?

Early developments, particularly from childhood to adolescence, pregnancy and ageing, are evident through visual physiological changes to body reality and are perceived as part of normal human functioning. **Altered body image** may not be evident through obvious physiological change to the normal body; however, it

body presentation

how we present our bodies to others in a social context, including our clothes, make-up and hairstyle

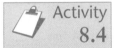

Activity 8.4

Breast and testicular self-examination should be a routine part of every woman's/man's personal health care. Do you examine yourself? List the reasons why you do/do not regularly practise this self-examination. Ask your close friends the same question. What reasons do they give for regularly self-examining. What reasons are given by those who do not? What is altered body image?

altered body image

the state of distress and lowered self-esteem that occurs when coping strategies to deal with changes in body reality, ideal or present, are overwhelmed may still have a devastating effect on the person even though there may be no external evidence to the observer. Price (1995, p. 2) defines altered body image as:

> A state of personal distress, defined by the patient, which indicates that the body no longer supports self-esteem, and which is dysfunctional to individuals, limiting their social engagement with others. Altered body image exists when coping strategies (individual and social) to deal with changes in body reality, ideal or presentation, are overwhelmed by injury, disease, disability, or social stigma.

This definition appears to recognise the importance of the person in their social and cultural environment and their spiritual awareness and its significance to how they perceive their altered body image.

Loss of self model

loss of self model

a model that aims to understand altered body image by considering loss of psychological self, loss of sociocultural self and loss of physical self

Blackmore (1989, p. 36) applies Watson's (1980) description of 'loss of self' using the **loss of self model** to explain altered body image: loss of psychological self, loss of sociocultural self and loss of physical self.

Loss of psychological self is when a person's self-concept and self-esteem is diminished. Loss of sociocultural self is when a person experiences loss of social identity, social role, family groupings or linkages with cultural background. Loss of physical self refers to the loss of bodily function or functions, a body part or parts or quality of physiological functioning. Loss of self will affect the person in different ways, depending on the disease, illness or trauma and the treatment involved, how the person perceives these and their significance to the person's life. An example using this model could be a man who has experienced ostomy surgery. The mutilation and relocation of a body orifice could have a serious effect on body image.

Link

Chapter 6 explains ostomy surgery.

Loss of psychological self

Loss of psychological self would include the patient feeling as though they have returned to an infantile stage of development, unable to control their excretory functions. This could affect how the man views his masculinity and his sexuality. He may question his sexual role and functioning. He may ask questions such as 'Do I smell?', 'Am I still attractive?', 'Will my partner still find me attractive?', 'Will people be able to see my ostomy bag?', 'Will I still be able to have sex?' and 'Will my partner still want to have sex with me?' A man involved with sporting activities may question how other men perceive him: is he seen as disabled?

Loss of sociocultural self

Loss of sociocultural self arises because society has particular attitudes towards excretion. For adults, urination and defaecation usually occur in private and are not usually discussed with others. There is also the stigma attached to having a disease of the bowel. Postoperatively, there may be a degree of unpredictability as the body adjusts to the physiological change and the person adapts to using an appliance. During this time, the person may choose to socially isolate himself. Family relationships can also be affected. Apart from the change in role within the partnership or family to that of patient, which may or may not be temporary, the man has to decide how to include his partner and other family members in the knowledge of his illness and its effects on his day-to-day life. Added to this is any cultural and religious attitude towards excretion. This can be a problem when caring for a stoma site, for example keeping the right hand clean for preparing and eating food (Bell, 1989).

Loss of physical self

Loss of physical self can occur in different ways after surgery. The loss of the normal way of defaecating can be difficult and having to adapt to having a bag on your stomach can affect how you view your body. Physical changes could include the effects of other treatments after surgery for a stoma formation, such as radiotherapy, which could cause fatigue, sore skin, and nausea and vomiting. Chemotherapy can lead to hair loss, skin discolouration and infertility. Sexual problems and a decreased libido can be suffered by a high percentage of patients (de Marquiegui and Huish, 1999). The general quality of body functioning can be affected (Blackmore, 1989).

Examples of altered body image

There are many different types of altered body image. Some of the examples given in Table 8.1 can be placed in either an **open** or **concealed altered body image** category. A woman who has recently developed anorexia nervosa may not be seen as experiencing anorexia nervosa by others; however, if the illness progresses and her eating patterns change along with weight loss and other physiological changes associated with anorexia nervosa, then her illness will become 'open' and evident to others.

Along with the idea of altered body image being open or concealed within the categories identified is the consideration of whether or not an injury, illness or disease is permanent or temporary. The person may not know this in the early stages of their condition as a prognosis may not have been given. Once the

open altered body image

an alteration in body image that can be clearly seen by others

concealed altered body image

an alteration in body image that is hidden from others

Table 8.1 Examples of altered body image

Congenital	Hereditary	Degenerative	Trauma
		OPEN	
Muscular dystrophy Cleft palate/lip Spina bifida Facial birthmarks	Huntington's chorea Retinitis pigmentosa Hair loss Acne Psoriasis, eczema	Parkinson's disease Multiple sclerosis Arthritis	Facial burns Amputation
		CONCEALED	
Hypospadias	Diabetes mellitus	Conduction deafness	Burns to main body Body scarring (abuse) and bruising

Psychological	Surgical	Medical	Miscellaneous
		OPEN	
Anorexia nervosa Schizophrenia Obsessive disorders	Mastectomy Reconstruction Amputation of limb Miscarriage Disfigurative surgery, for example for cancer of the neck Breast reduction/ enhancement Liposuction	Medication – Chemotherapy – Psychotropic – HRT Alopecia Halitosis	Tattoos Body piercing (non-exotic) – ears, eyebrows, nose Limb prosthesis Pregnancy Obesity Use of wheelchair Birthmarks Intravenous infusion Body scarring (cultural)
		CONCEALED	
Nasogastric tube Body dysmorphic disorder Body scarring (cutting) Bulimia nervosa	Circumcision Hysterectomy Orchidectomy Lumpectomy Stoma Termination Male and female genital enhancement Blepharoplasty	Sexually transmitted diseases Medication Perianal abscess Caesarean section Impotence Sterility Premature ejaculation	Crohn's disease Body piercing (exotic) – tongue, nipples, clitoris, penis

Source: Adapted from Salter (1997) and Price (1990).

person is aware of both a diagnosis and prognosis, they will have an idea of whether or not there is any permanence. Being given this information will influence how the person adapts and manages any alteration to body image. Another consideration is that those who have sustained extensive or severe disfigurement will not necessarily have more problems and greater psychological distress than people with minor body image changes (Robinson, 1997).

The role of the nurse

Assessment

It is important to assess how a person perceives their body and how this influences their self-image and self-esteem. Observing the way someone presents, for example their posture, hair, dress and make-up, can give important information. Conversations about the patient's cultural background, age and occupation can further help the nurse to make sense of the patient's body image and self-image. The nurse may ask the patient specific questions about their body image and body ideal, for example the importance the patient places on their appearance and physical functioning. The nurse will then start to understand the significance of health and illness for the patient. If a body image change has occurred from being ill or is to occur, for example from surgery, what effect could this have on the patient's body image, self-image and self-esteem in the future? The loss of self model (Watson, 1980) could be used as a framework to assess the significance and context of the altered body image for the patient.

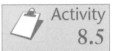

Activity 8.5

Think of a patient you have cared for who was experiencing altered body image. Write down what you observed and found out about this patient.

During the assessment process, the nurse could have contact with relatives, partners, carers and friends of the patient. Assessing their perception and expectations of the patient is important and the nurse needs to be aware of how the relative/partner/carer/friend is managing the situation. How well informed are they? What strategies are they able to use to manage their own feelings about the patient's altered body image? Are they able to continue supporting the patient (Price, 1990, p. 75)? If the altered body image is permanent, how will this affect the relationship on a psychological, sociocultural and physical level? It is important to recognise the needs of the relative/partner/carer/friend and be proactive with the support and information they require. It is also important to be aware of issues of confidentiality for the patient; ideally, communication with relatives, partners, carers and friends should only be done with the patient's permission. Some of the areas considered above could be discussed with both the patient and relatives, carers, partner and friends together.

Nurses must be aware of, particularly in relation to open or visible disfigurement leading to unfavourable views of the self (Rumsey, 2002; Koo and Young, 2002), negative effects such as lowered self-esteem, depression and anxiety (Kent and Thomson, 2002) and unfavourable reactions from others.

Engaging in social activities with those close to the patient is less of a threat than being exposed to those unknown (Rumsey et al., 2004), and encourages the patient to develop strategies in a safer environment to be used when in unfamiliar situations.

Nursing skills

Any change in body image, particularly when the change is viewed as negative, requires time for adjustment. For some patients, this adjustment may be too difficult to contemplate or totally accept. The patient can feel vulnerable and not in control of their situation. The nurse should be available for the patient to articulate their concerns and fears when the patient feels ready. It may be that the patient is only able to manage hearing small amounts of information about their illness at one time.

As discussed previously, an alteration in body image is a loss and can affect the patient in different ways, depending on what the altered body image signifies to the person. The manifestation of this loss is to experience a grief reaction. The patient may experience anger or denial as part of this reaction to their altered body image.

Once the patient has experienced the altered body image, there should be a period of rehabilitation. This time could include access to specialist practitioners, for example the stoma care nurse and breast care nurse. Provision of information about support organisations and self-help groups can also be helpful. The adaptation to any change in body image will be influenced by a number of factors, including gender, age, altered body image severity, pre- and postoperative preparation, including patient/client education, beliefs and values, coping mechanisms and sexual functioning. Anyone in a position of caring will be observed by the patient for their reactions and acceptance to the change in body image (Salter, 1997). The qualities and skills of the nurse will help the patient to adjust and find their own way of coming to terms with the alteration to their body image. The nurse must not underestimate the challenge this brings to the patient. The nurse must value and respect this process of adjustment. In turn, the nurse has a responsibility to ensure that she or he is able to work with the patient in a meaningful way on both a physical and psychological level. Insight into his or her own emotions about his or her body may help when trying to understand the distress the patient may be experiencing when they have to face a radical alteration to their appearance and body function (Price, 1998). To ensure this, he or she should access regular clinical supervision with someone who is able to help him or her to make sense of the caring relationship he or she has formed.

Link
Chapter 10 provides further information on bereavement.

Link
Chapter 14 looks at therapeutic communication and working in groups.

Casebox 8.1

Sally is a 24-year-old married mother of two young children, who was admitted to an acute mental health unit for treatment of her depression. She has been resident on the unit for three weeks, and has been treated with antidepressants and attended counselling sessions with her care coordinator. Sally is being prepared for discharge home to her supportive family and will receive regular visits from a community psychiatric nurse. Sally has stated to her care coordinator that she is worried about sleeping with her husband in case he wants to be intimate with her. She also stated that she does not feel very attractive and thinks that she is 'right off sex'.

What could be the main reasons for Sally feeling this way?

- Any long stay in hospital can influence how someone feels about themselves.

- Not being able to attend to our 'body presentation' in our normal way could mean that we become dissatisfied with the way we look as the gap between body presentation and body ideal widens.

- The antidepressants that Sally has been prescribed could affect her sexual functioning and libido. She may have become more aware of this as the depressants start to work and she begins to focus her attention on being back at home.

- Sally's body weight and appearance may have changed during the period of time she has felt depressed. This could affect how she perceives and feels about her body.

Casebox 8.2

Janice is a 38-year-old woman who has been living with her partner Lisa for 11 years. Janice has been diagnosed with Crohn's disease after suffering with chronic diarrhoea, abdominal pain and weight loss for nearly a year and a number of admissions to hospital. She has been taking medication to treat the diarrhoea and analgesics to reduce the pain. Her physician has informed her that she has a partial obstruction of her small bowel. He has referred her to a surgeon who has informed her that surgery may be necessary to remove the obstruction. Janice was also told that she will require a temporary stoma. Janice is devastated and has asked if she can discuss this with Lisa before she agrees to surgery.

List some of the concerns that Janice may have concerning the formation of a stoma.

- How the stoma will look.

- How it will function.

- How she will manage the appliance.

- How it will affect her everyday life.

- How to broach the subject with Lisa and the effect this will have on their relationship.

- One of Janice's worries could be whether she may require a permanent stoma in the future.

- Janice will also be working out how to cope with social situations and any other activities that could involve others becoming aware of her stoma.

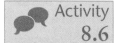

Activity 8.6

If you had to choose just one sexual behaviour that you would want entirely forbidden, what would it be? Ask a few other people what they would forbid, then ask yourselves, why? What is so bad about these examples of sexual behaviour? The reasons are usually complicated!

Activity 8.7

Think about how important sexuality is to you – your gender, your sexual orientation, fancying people, being fancied, being a parent, dreading being a parent, your body and how it feels, your wardrobe, your haircut … the list is endless. Now think about services you have participated in, and service users you have worked with. Is any of this richness expressed in what is written or said about them, the buildings the services are provided in, the materials promoting the service? Do the services have specific policies or guidelines to help workers deal with sexuality issues?

■ Human Sexuality

Sexuality is an issue that health professionals are often uncomfortable with, although it is part of everyday life. For various reasons, individuals who cope reasonably well with the uncertainties of sexuality in their own lives find this more difficult when in a professional role. In this section, we will be looking at why sexuality can create difficulties generally, and can be even more complex in the context of health care. The most common responses to the challenges of understanding human sexuality are either to ignore it and hope it goes away, or to make some hard-and-fast rules in an attempt to make it easier for everyone. Neither of these approaches has proved to work particularly well in the past, and so we will be advocating a different way. This is to accept the intricacies and paradoxes of human sexuality, try to understand them and work with them.

Dos and don'ts

Sex and sexuality are fundamental to what humans are, so if nurses ignore this part of people's lives, they are missing a large chunk of the whole person. It is also potentially harmful to the person not to have their sexuality acknowledged. Michel Foucault, a French philosopher, has written extensively about sexuality, and talks about the 'triple edict of taboo, non-existence and silence' surrounding sexuality (Foucault, 1978, p. 5). What does he mean by this? By using the word 'taboo', he is referring to the largely unwritten rules on sexual behaviour, the beliefs and myths that have developed over time. These appear to be real, but a closer examination reveals that humans have created these systems to guide their behaviour. We will be exploring the derivation of some 'common-sense truths' later on in this chapter. Now try Activity 8.6.

'Non-existence' is Foucault's way of expressing one of the ways that sexuality is dealt with, that is, by totally denying its existence, by repressing any mention of sex and sexuality. Many health-care practices appear to be attempting to do this, and it was only relatively recently in Western societies that this approach has reduced. Foucault's mention of silence is linked to the idea of non-existence, but conveys subtle differences. Silence conveys a notion that sex and sexuality exist, but are not to be talked about, just accepted as given, suffered in silence. To get a better idea of these concepts, try Activity 8.7.

The skill of the nurse in dealing with sexuality is to balance the biomedical realities of sexual function, sexual health and the reproductive process with what sexuality means to the individual person. This personal meaning is to do with the sorts of issues we looked at in Activity 8.2. It has to do with the way a person was brought up, current thinking in society in general, their race, culture or religion. The Nursing and Midwifery Council (NMC) makes it plain in the

Code of Professional Conduct (NMC, 2004), and the competences required to register as a nurse (NMC, 2001), that nurses must respect each individual's point of view. It is also a requirement that the individual's views be actively included in care planning.

The nurse's role

The ways in which nurses will encounter sexuality could be divided into two. The first is where a patient's condition is likely to have a direct and obvious effect on their sexual functioning and sexuality. Examples might be a young woman having a hysterectomy, a man having prostate surgery that may lead to impotence, and a girl with extensive burns to body and face. More positive examples could be orthodontic treatment, cosmetic plastic surgery and IVF. To take this thinking further, spend a little time considering Activity 8.8. (It is interesting to note that many of the examples of health interventions that 'obviously' relate to sexuality are also linked to the person's body image.)

A second way that nurses encounter sexuality is in the sense that everyone has one. Many writers believe that sexuality is a fundamental component of the person – you are not you without it. Nurses routinely have access to people's most intimate details, but are open to criticism for often ignoring this crucial component of any individual's life. This is an appropriate moment to make it clear that we are not advocating prying unnecessarily into an individual's private life. It is rarely necessary for a nurse to know any details of a patient's sexual functioning and relationships. However, we are advocating that nurses should be sensitive to this crucial aspect of their patients' lives, and that they should be confident and competent in discussing sexual issues if they arise.

Sexuality and self-awareness

Self-awareness is an important attribute for nurses generally, but is perhaps especially so in the case of sexuality, given its possible sensitivity. It is perfectly acceptable for nurses to have strong views on issues to do with sexuality, but potentially harmful to blindly impose them on patients/clients. Being a nurse does not mean having to subscribe to a particular set of beliefs about sex and sexuality. However, it does mean appreciating that there are many viewpoints, yours being simply another version. It is an essential skill to know what your standpoint is, and how that relates to other people. Whatever our views are, they did not come out of nowhere. It can be helpful to our understanding to know where our beliefs originated from, giving us a chance to look at them a bit more closely. Two important issues within sexuality are gender and sexual orientation, which will be explored next. Gender and sexual orientation have both been

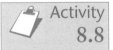

Activity 8.8

Divide a piece of paper into two columns, labelling one column 'Health interventions with a negative impact on sex and sexuality' and the other 'Health interventions with a positive impact on sex and sexuality'. Carrying on from the examples given in the text, write as many examples as you can think of under each heading. Having done this relatively quickly, reconsider the interventions you've chosen. Are they as clearly good or bad as you first thought? For example, IVF is a positive intervention to help couples achieve their need to have children. However, the difficulties that couples having infertility treatment can experience are well known, to the extent that they appear regularly in television documentaries, popular novels and dramas.

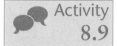

Activity 8.9

Consider the following ideas, where do you think they originate from? We are not suggesting that any of them are either right or wrong, but you may find yourself agreeing or disagreeing. Asking yourself 'why?' is working towards self-awareness:

- Gay and lesbian individuals should have freedom of sexual expression
- Anal sex is unnatural
- Women are passive receivers of male sexual advances.

gender

a social group's interpretation of being a man or a woman. It concerns the status and role of the sexes rather than their physical characteristics

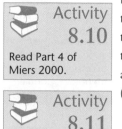

Activity 8.10

Read Part 4 of Miers 2000.

Activity 8.11

Read selected sections of Nye 1999 that particularly interest you.

hugely influenced by ancient cultural, historical, political and religious viewpoints. As a result, views vary widely and can be hotly contested. Before reading the following sections, spend some time on Activity 8.9, as it should make the material more relevant.

■ Gender

Gender is a crucial issue in health care and nursing, going way beyond the physical characteristics of being male or female. The study of gender is the study of how being a man or a woman has an impact on how much money you have, how well educated you are, what diseases you are most likely to have, your life expectancy, your mental health, diet and weight. The literature on gender needs to be studied in its own right (see Activity 8.10, for example) to do it justice. However, nurses can learn from the major finding of the social science of gender. This finding is that gender operates through members of a society learning to make assumptions about the roles and capabilities of the sexes. Most societies are heavily biased to the advantage of men, so the widely held assumptions about women tend to discriminate against them, for example men are physically and mentally stronger than women, women gossip and men think deep thoughts and so on.

Nurses can contribute towards reducing health inequalities based on gender by challenging the unsupported (and often false) assumptions about the differences between men and women. Study of the historical development of sexuality reveals that women have been regarded as inferior to men since prehistoric times. Records from the ancient civilisations of Egypt, Greece and Rome make it clear that what we now regard as sexism or patriarchy have been considered the norm for many thousands of years (Nye, 1999). As a result, the principle that men and women are equal is a relatively new one, and still has some way to go before being universally accepted. Nurses can also help by acknowledging that men and women are equal, but often have different attitudes and approaches to health, this acknowledgement being called 'gender sensitivity' (Miers, 2000).

Casebox 8.3

You are working with a school nurse in a secondary school, and have become involved in the sexual health component of the curriculum. This involves planning and running a series of sessions about sexual behaviour to a group of 12-year-old boys and girls.

The following questions will help you to understand the kinds of issues involved.

Should boys and girls be taught separately?

Do boys and girls need to be taught different things?

Could stereotyped gender differences be avoided?

■ Sexual Orientation

There is now an enormous amount of material available to explore what is known about sexual orientation, in academic literature, books, films, television, newspapers, magazines and so on. Despite this, gay and lesbian individuals can still experience discrimination in society in general, and health services in particular (Wilton, 2000). In recognition of this, the Royal College of Nursing (2005) issued a statement guiding nurses in how to combat discriminatory practice and make positive health contributions to lesbians and gay men. Recent changes in the law have made the legal position of gay and lesbian couples clearer. Couples registering under the Civil Partnership Act 2004 will have a legal status that has parity with married couples, including inheriting property after death. The main difficulties experienced by individuals with alternative sexual lifestyles seem to come from a combination of factors, but you may find it useful to ask yourself these questions:

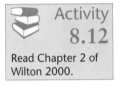

Activity
8.12

Read Chapter 2 of Wilton 2000.

1. Do I know much about gay, lesbian, transvestite, transsexual and other alternative lifestyles?
2. Do I really know how I feel about people who have different sexualities to mine?

Your personal answers to these questions really indicate the way to competent and effective nursing practice with people who have alternative sexualities. Make it your business to find out more about the richness and diversity of our sexual lives, and find out if you have some unsupported prejudices that influence your behaviour without you really being aware of it.

It is worth noting that attitudes towards homosexual behaviour are very different depending on the culture and the period of history being considered. Ancient Jewish law prohibited sexual contact between men absolutely, whereas ancient Greek civilisations considered love between men as on a higher spiritual plane than heterosexual love (Nye, 1999). Within the Christian tradition, it was only really in the Middle Ages that the Catholic Church firmly established homosexuality as wrong, while the Eastern Orthodox Churches remained more flexible. The wide range of approaches to being gay or lesbian is further demonstrated by the fact that homosexuality is actually punishable by death in some parts of the world, and yet is totally ignored in others, demonstrating how widely opinion differs. Before becoming too complacent, remember that within the past 200 years, Britain also had the death penalty for homosexuality.

This may be starting to feel a bit deep and difficult, so an example of nursing practice told to one of the authors and given in Casebox 8.5 may make the point clearer.

Casebox 8.4

Dawn has been admitted to a medical ward for some straightforward treatment. Many of the staff were cold and remote towards her because she was a lesbian. Dawn herself did not say much, and was quite bad-tempered in her interactions with all health-care staff. Lucy, one of the nurses, noticed this and found it upsetting, although she could not think of a specific intervention that would help. On one occasion, Lucy saw Dawn's partner Julie walking across the hospital car park. Lucy turned to Dawn, smiled, and said 'Hey, Dawn, that's great, your partner Julie is coming to visit you!' Dawn's demeanour immediately softened, and she started to chat about her and Julie's home life together. From then on, Dawn would talk freely to Lucy and was more relaxed. The nursing care that Dawn received was more effective and her treatment was successful.

Why do you think Lucy's simple intervention made such a difference?

Have you had, or heard of, similar experiences?

Desire

Casebox 8.4 demonstrates that being aware of sexuality in your practice does not require superhuman interpersonal skills or encyclopedic knowledge. It is mainly about listening, observing, and showing some sensitivity to different views. One way of viewing alternative sexualities is to think of all sexuality in terms of desire. Some men like tall women with brown hair who want a family. Some women like men who are reliable and have steady jobs. As far as we know, there are no specific labels for these desires, and the people who practise them are left to do so without interference. However, a man who likes men with brown hair who want a family, and a woman who likes reliable women with steady jobs may well experience interference. We all have preferences in terms of what kinds of people and activities arouse us sexually. Use Activity 8.13 to think about your own desires.

It is difficult to avoid the conclusion that society chooses what is acceptable sexual behaviour, but often not clearly and often based on outdated and unacceptable prejudices. Some of the restrictions are clearly to our benefit, for example laws against rape and sex with children. Others are more difficult to justify outside artificial and misguided belief systems.

Working with vulnerable adults

One area where the sorts of restrictions on sexual behaviour talked about above are justifiable is in the care of vulnerable adults. Just as awareness of the abuse of children grew over a period of time, so it is becoming known that some adults are at greater risk of being abused. This abuse can be sexual, but can take other forms: physical, financial, psychological, neglect or discriminatory abuse (DoH, 2000). Defining who is a vulnerable adult is not precise, but generally a vulnerable adult can be regarded as a person over the age of 18 who uses community care services and finds it more difficult than most to protect themselves from harm. This may include some older people, people with learning disabilities, disabled people and people with mental health problems.

Sant Angelo (2000) suggests some likely features of the lives of people with learning difficulties:

- High incidence of sexually abusive experiences
- Multiple experiences of bereavement and loss
- Difficulties in talking about emotions
- Limited sex education
- Limited expectations and low self-esteem
- A lack of assertiveness about sex and relationships
- A lack of privacy.

Activity 8.13

Describe your ideal partner(s), preferably by writing it down, although imagining will work too. What do they look like, what are they wearing, what are they interested in, how do they treat you? How would the relationship run: a quick fling, living together, big white wedding, eloping to an exotic destination? Would there be children? Now think about this ideal scenario you have created. Does it have a specific label that conjures up your desire in complete detail?

Casebox 8.5

Rob is 33 years old and has a learning disability. Until recently, he lived in his family home, but chose to move to a housing association flat to live on his own. He visits his local health centre regularly for a minor health problem, and the nurses have got to know him quite well. Rob has started talking to the health centre nurses about how he would like to have a girlfriend, but is starting to feel down because he is still on his own.

What simple interventions could be made with Rob to empower him to achieve his desired lifestyle?

■ Rob could be encouraged to talk about his feelings. If Rob's needs were simple advice and education, the health centre nurses could perhaps provide this intervention.

■ If Rob's needs went beyond this, he could be offered access to other services, for example self-help groups run by people with learning disabilities, learning disability community nursing, a range of independent and voluntary services to do with increasing his social network, counselling or other services as appropriate.

■ Most importantly, Rob needs to be listened to with respect and sensitivity, so that he can find the best way to achieve his goals.

In practice, nurses need to be aware of the potential sexual harm that could befall vulnerable adults. The document *No Secrets* (DoH, 2000) gives guidance on awareness, preventing and dealing with the abuse of vulnerable adults. Some findings from learning disability research give an idea of the nature of the problem. McCormack et al. (2005) surveyed 15 years of allegations of sexual abuse of people with learning disabilities, finding that just under half were confirmed. Of these, the most common location was the family home, where almost a quarter of the perpetrators of sexual abuse were family members. Most of the abuse was sexual touch, although nearly a third was penetration or attempted penetration. Joyce (2003) conducted a similar survey in a different locality, finding that people with learning disabilities were most at risk from the people they lived with, the people who cared for them or their family members. Not being taken seriously when reporting sexual abuse was also a feature. To compound the problem, Murphy (2003) found that the sexual knowledge of adults with learning disabilities was significantly lower than non-disabled adolescents, leaving them open to harm through lack of knowledge of acceptable sexual behaviour.

This small selection of the available evidence indicates why nurses have to be vigilant when working with vulnerable adults. Clearly such abuse occurs in a minority of cases, but often enough for nurses to at least be aware of the possibility.

Sexuality and skilled nursing care

Even a cursory exploration quickly reveals the complexity, richness and change-ability of human sexuality. Further examination demonstrates that if nursing is to take a holistic approach, it can no longer routinely ignore this aspect of human life. But the depth and diversity of human sexuality can make it seem unmanageable at times. A well-known framework that attempts to make sexu-ality issues more manageable for nurses is the PLISSIT model (Fogel and Lauver, 1990). The **PLISSIT model** categorises a nurse's potential interventions into four levels, each level becoming increasingly intimate and needing more specialist knowledge. The idea behind the model is that all nurses can include sexuality in

PLISSIT model
a model comprising four levels of nursing intervention to take sexuality and body image into account

their practice, but should operate at a level where they feel safe and well informed. The four levels are:

1. *Permission:* it is suggested that sexual history should be a routine part of assessment. This will raise sexuality as a legitimate concern, and gives patients permission to ask questions about it in their own care. Although this is the most basic level, success is dependent on a non-judgemental, accepting approach by nurses.
2. *Limited Information:* misconceptions and myths are clarified. Many of the difficulties experienced by people in dealing with their sexuality can be solved quickly by good quality, evidence-based information. To be told that many people have similar difficulties and to be given a few simple solutions can be liberating and takes very little time. All the nurse needs is a sound (but not necessarily encyclopedic) knowledge base and a straightforward, adult communication style.
3. *Specific Suggestions:* can relieve anxiety, promote creativity and help individuals to solve their own problems in partnerships, rather than being the passive receivers of advice.
4. *Intensive Therapy:* the person is referred to a specialist sex therapist, who may also be a nurse. It is important if nurses are to make competent interventions that they be clear about the limitations of their knowledge and skill. In some cases, solutions may not be simple and so expert intervention is needed.

Modernisation of services and sexuality in nursing

The PLISSIT model is a useful tool, and goes a long way to guide nurses to give sexuality much needed importance in nursing practice. The model can potentially relieve anxiety among nurses who are so concerned about not being 'experts' that they ignore sexuality issues altogether. However, it is important to build on the helpful principles established in the PLISSIT model, and take them further by putting them in the context of current and future health-care trends.

At the same time, at a national, more structural level, government policy for health-care services is relevant to our discussion. It is clearly the intention that health services in the future are driven by the people who use them. The version of *The NHS Plan* directed at nurses emphasises **holistic** care, listening to patients, respecting their dignity and including them in their own health care (DoH, 2001). *The NHS Plan* as a whole aims to reduce health inequalities, prevent discrimination and help individuals to know more about, and take responsibility for, their own health. All these aims are partly fulfilled by nurses

holistic

the view that individuals function as complete units and cannot be reduced to the sum of their parts

taking account of body image and sexuality, which can have impacts far beyond more obvious biomedical concerns.

As we have seen, sexuality can be about people in different groups having different amounts of power: adults and children, men and women, heterosexual and homosexual. Sometimes these differences in power can lead to abuse, perhaps linked to a powerful person or group not being willing to accept views other than their own. So nurses do need to be sensitive to each individual's notion of body image and sexuality in their face-to-face interactions, as demonstrated in the PLISSIT model, but the broader picture needs to be taken into account if our care is to be truly holistic.

■ Chapter Summary

To conclude the chapter, we need to bring body image and sexuality back together again. We looked at them separately to make the material easier to absorb, but in our daily lives they are inextricably linked. If we consider our bodies and health, either to celebrate our good fortune or bemoan an unkind fate, some part of that consideration is to do with sexuality. This could encompass our gender, our orientation, whether we think others will find us attractive or the physical ways in which we express our sexual selves. This process accelerates considerably when perceptions of our bodies change, as is nearly always the case when we access health services. So, to practise holistic care, nurses need to be aware of body image and sexuality and how they are linked. These links take many forms, but we propose a four-factor analysis that takes account of the complexity of human life and provides a framework for nurses to work in:

1. *Intimacy*: nursing can be extraordinarily intimate at times, so it is safer to be aware of the range of potential impacts that intimacy might have, for example breaking a cultural taboo.

antidiscriminatory practice

practice that aims to acknowledge the sources of oppression in people's lives and actively works to reduce them

2. **Antidiscriminatory practice** (ADP): without discrimination, body image and sexuality would cease to be difficulties in individual's lives. It is only because humans choose to make judgements about each other, based on particular characteristics, that we might be concerned about how we look, or how we express ourselves sexually. ADP appears regularly in the competences required for nurses (NMC, 2004), and is an especially important way of working in terms of body image and sexuality. Practising in an antidiscriminatory way means acknowledging the sources of oppression in people's lives, but also actively working towards reducing them (Thompson, 1998). So, you may be accepting of a person who is gay, but you may also have to work to make sure that your colleagues are as accepting as you are.

3. **Empowerment**: this can be an elusive concept (see Thompson, 1998, pp. 210–14) for a readable overview) but, put simply, means focusing your work on enabling the individuals you work with to find their own solutions and progress independently. Health-care professionals have traditionally had tremendous power over individuals, with a great unwillingness to share it. There is no place for this approach in modern health services; individuals need to regard themselves as having a large say in their own destiny. The issues surrounding body image and sexuality are often related to personal power, so nurses can make a positive contribution by understanding how much power they themselves hold through often being perceived as 'experts'. Patients undoubtedly need us to have expertise, but can do without experts. Also, by practising in an empowering way, nurses can actively demonstrate how power can be shared successfully.

empowerment
working with individuals to enable them to find their own solutions and progress independently

4. **Partnership**: empowerment does not imply that nurses should not actively help individuals. Rather, it means that the care given is within a particular type of relationship – a partnership. Working in partnership with clients prevents them from relying too much on professionals and services, in other words, from becoming dependent.

partnership
the situation that occurs when separate individuals or groups contribute as equals to devising a useful solution to a problem

This framework applies strongly in nursing practice to do with body image and sexuality. Dealing with these issues may well leave people feeling vulnerable and distressed, for example when facing mastectomy, use of a stoma, disfigurement and many more. Running the nurse–patient relationship as a partnership in these high emotion circumstances has several benefits for both parties. Partnership means that a nurse can retain qualities such as warmth and genuineness that are so important, but because they are not 'leading' the process, dependence is avoided. This makes practice safer professionally for the nurse and also for patients, who need to be able to deal with the world in their own right. You will not always be around, so it is much better for patients to learn to use their existing support networks (family, friends and so on) or be helped to find new ones (specialist support groups, voluntary services and so on).

It would be misleading to suggest that dealing with body image and sexuality issues is always easy. However, a little knowledge and a lot of openness, acceptance and willingness to talk will form a strong foundation for competent practice.

Test Yourself!

1. Using your own words, describe what is meant by the term 'body image'.

2. What are the three fundamental interrelated concepts used by Price (1990) to define body image?

3. Give five examples of surgical procedures not evident to others (concealed) that could affect body image.

4. Name some factors that may affect the sexual experiences of people with learning disabilities.

5. What does PLISSIT stand for?

6. What are the four principles suggested as a framework for practice in body image and sexuality issues?

Further Reading

Carlowe, J. (1997) Face values. *Nursing Times* **93**(42): 34–5.

Grogan, S. (1999) *Body Image: Understanding Body Dissatisfaction in Men, Women and Children.* Routledge, London.

Harrison, T. (ed.) (1998) *Children and Sexuality: Perspectives in Health Care.* Baillière Tindall, London.

References

Bell, N. (1989) Sexuality and the ostomist. *Nursing Times* **85**(5): 28–30.

Blackmore, C. (1989) Altered images. *Nursing Times* **85**(12): 36–9.

Chilton, S. (1984) Identity crisis. *Nursing Mirror* **158**(13 Jun): ii–iii.

De Marquiegui, A. and Huish, M. (1999) A woman's sexual life after an operation. *British Medical Journal* **318**: 178–81.

DoH (Department of Health) (2000) *No Secrets.* Department of Health, London.

DoH (Department of Health) (2001) *The NHS Plan – An Action Guide for Nurses, Midwives and Health Visitors.* Department of Health, London.

Foucault, M. (1978) *The History of Sexuality:* Volume 1, *An Introduction.* Penguin, Harmondsworth.

Fogel, C. and Lauver, D. (1990) *Sexual Health Promotion.* WB Saunders, Philadelphia.

Goffman, E. (1961) *Asylums: Essays on the Social Situation of Mental Patients and Other Inmates.* Anchor, New York.

Joyce, T.A. (2003) An audit of investigations into allegations of abuse involving adults with intellectual disability. *Journal of Intellectual Disability Research* **47**(8): 606–16.

Kent, G. and Thompson, A. (2002) The development and maintenance of shame in disfigurement: implications for treatment. In Gilbert, P. and Miles, J. (eds) *Body Shame.* Brunner-Routledge, Hove.

Kitzinger, S. (1985) *Woman's Experience of Sex*. Penguin, London.

Koo, J. and Young, J. (2002) Body image issues in dermatology. In Cash, T.F. and Pruzinsky, T. (eds) *Body Image: A Handbook of Theory, Research and Clinical Practice*. Guildford Press, New York.

Langford, R. (1996) The hole truth. *Nursing Times* **92**(40): 46–7.

Larkin, B.G. (2004) The ins and outs of body piercing. *The Association of Perioperative Registered Nurses* **79**(2): 3330–46. http://gateway.uk.ovid/gw1/ovidweb.cgi.

McCormack, B., Kavanagh, D., Caffrey, S. and Power, A. (2005) Investigating sexual abuse: Findings of a 15-year longitudinal study. *Journal of Applied Research in Intellectual Disability* **18**: 217–27.

McCrea, C.W., Summerfield, A.B. and Rosen, B. (1982) Body image: A selective review of existing measurement techniques. *British Journal of Medical Psychology* **55**(3): 225–33.

Miers, M. (2000) *Gender Issues and Nursing Practice*. Macmillan – now Palgrave Macmillan, Basingstoke.

Murphy, G.H. (2003) Capacity to consent to sexual relationships in adults with learning disabilities. *Journal of Family Planning and Reproductive Health Care* **29**(3): 148–9.

NMC (Nursing and Midwifery Council) (2001) *Requirements for Pre-registration Nursing Programmes*. NMC, London.

NMC (Nursing and Midwifery Council) (2004) *The NMC Code of Professional Conduct: Standards for Conduct, Performance and Ethics*. NMC, London.

Nye, R.A. (ed.) (1999) *Sexuality*. Oxford University Press, Oxford.

Price, B. (1990) *Body Image: Nursing Concepts and Care*. Prentice Hall, London.

Price, B. (1995) Assessing altered body image. *Journal of Psychiatric and Mental Health Nursing* **2**(3): 169–75.

Price, B. (1998) Cancer: Altered body Image. *Nursing Standard* **12**(21): 49–55.

Robinson, E. (1997) Psychological research on visible difference disfigurement. In Lansdown, R., Rumsey, N., Bradbury, E., Carr, A. and Partridge, J. (eds) *Visibly Different: Coping with Disfigurement*. Butterworth-Heinemann, London.

RCN (Royal College of Nursing) (2000) *Sexuality and Sexual Health in Nursing Practice*. Royal College of Nursing, London.

RCN (Royal College of Nursing) (2005) Not 'just' a friend: Best practice guidance on health care for lesbian, gay and bisexual service users and their families. www.rn.org.uk/london/downloads/notjustafriend.pdf.

Rumsey, N. (2002) Body image and congenital conditions with viable differences. In Cash, T.F. and Pruzinsky, T. (eds) *Body Image: A Handbook of Theory, Research and Clinical Practice*. Guildford Press, New York.

Rumsey, N., Clarke, A., White, P., Wyn-Williams, M. and Garlick, W. (2004) Altered body image: appearance-related concerns of people with visible disfigurement. *Journal of Advanced Nursing* **48**(5): 443–53.

Salter, M. (1997) *Altered Body Image: The Nurse's Role*. Baillière Tindall, London.

Sanderson, E. (1985) Nursing patience. *Lampada* **4**: 36–7.

Sant Angelo, D. (2000) Learning disability community nursing: Addressing emotional and sexual needs. In Astor, R. and Jeffereys, K. (eds) *Positive Initiatives for People with*

Learning Difficulties: Promoting Healthy Lifestyles. Macmillan – now Palgrave Macmillan, Basingstoke.

Savage, J. (1987) *Nurses, Gender and Sexuality*. Heinemann, London.

Sundeen, J., Stuart, G.W., Rankin, E.A.D. and Cohen, S.A. (1994) *Nurse–Client Interaction*. Mosby, St Louis.

Thompson, N. (1998) *Promoting Equality: Challenging Discrimination and Oppression in the Human Services*. Macmillan – now Palgrave Macmillan, Basingstoke.

Watson, J. (1980) Altered body image and the self. In Brown, M.S. (ed.) *Nursing and the Concept of Loss*. Wiley, New York.

Wilton, T. (2000) *Sexualities in Health and Social Care: A Textbook*. Open University Press, Buckingham.

■ Useful Websites

www.mentalhealth.org.uk Mental Health Foundation
Features information about anorexia nervosa

www.thesite.org/sexandrelationships Website aimed at young people, containing information about sexual health

www.netdoctor.co.uk Online medical guide. Information about body image and/or sexuality can be accessed via the search function

www.changingfaces.co.uk Changing Faces
A national charity based in the UK that supports and represents people who have disfigurements of the face or body from any cause

www.mariestopes.org.uk Marie Stopes International
A charity that provides sexual and reproductive health information and services

WAYNE ARNETT AND IAN DOUGLAS

Chapter

9

Movement and Mobility

Contents

Learning Outcomes

At the end of this chapter, you should be able to:

- Relate the importance of mobility to systemic homeostasis

- In relation to the activities of living, determine the influence of mobility and potential consequences

- Demonstrate enhanced awareness of the complications of immobility

- Relate further understanding of the nursing diagnoses associated with mobility and immobility

- Propose nursing strategies to prevent or meet immobility complications or impaired mobility

- Describe and explain the principles of moving and handling

- Describe a range of strategies for the optimum safety for staff and patients/clients when moving and handling, including a risk assessment.

■ Mobility and Immobility

This section will explore how nurses can assist their client groups in identifying the importance of physical movement, not only for everyday health, but, more importantly, in assuring uncomplicated recovery from ill-health.

Our species, *Homo sapiens*, would at first seem to be singularly ill-equipped to have attained its place at the top of the food chain: too slow to outrun any but the slowest predator; physically weak compared to larger mammals; and comparatively hairless so unsuited to all but the mildest climate. Yet, despite these serious handicaps, we have not only survived, but prospered enormously in comparison to our closest primate relatives. Arguably, coupled with superior cognitive abilities, this supreme survival story could simply be attributed to a couple of incredibly simple feats of musculoskeletal function:

1. Initially, as *Homo erectus*, to simply have achieved the ability to stand erect and reach, thus outstripping rival species in now being able to reach higher food sources, throw a weapon or climb to a place of shelter.
2. By achieving opposition of fingers and thumb, the species was given a tool capable of such incredibly meticulous manual dexterity, initially capable of crafting tools, but ultimately to make vehicles capable of space travel. Simple and unique musculoskeletal functions they may be, yet without them, man would probably have been consigned to the obscurity of extinction eons ago (Lewin, 1999).

Thus two simple, yet unique acts of movement have forged man's superior position among the species, and illustrate the importance of mobility in our everyday lives.

Mobility and healthy living

homeostatic

state of equilibrium of the internal environment of the body

More than any other species, the physiological (or **homeostatic**) characteristics of our bodies demand that we must remain active in order to remain healthy. In a Western society obsessed with image, exercise is constantly being held up as an essential attribute to healthy living, although it remains a fact that while only a minority are actively doing it, the majority are probably talking about it or at least their intention to imminently do more of it. Despite this, it has been estimated that around 40 per cent of adults and, more worryingly, around 15 per cent of under-16s take little or no regular exercise (Egger et al., 2004). Coupled with rising levels of obesity, especially among children, this bodes a terrible legacy for the future unless the trend can be arrested and reversed (DoH, 2004).

Back in our primeval history, exercise, or the lack of it, was hardly a problem. As a nomadic species, the need to travel with herds, hunt and gather, search for shelter or fight to ward off predators, even intertribal rivals, ensured one certainty – we either remained physically fit and able to keep up, or we died. It is unlikely that obesity was a public health concern for our prehistoric ancestors. In contemporary health and health care, it is frequently forgotten that apart from being considerably taller, heavier and perhaps a little less hirsute, modern man and woman has changed remarkably little in the 200,000 years or so of our existence as a species. Yet now, certainly within Western culture, the physical demands (and indulgences) of daily life are clearly far less arduous than when the species first evolved. We no longer have to hunt or gather, or even walk much to be assured of a range of food sources beyond the imaginings of our grandparents, let alone our prehistoric forebears. Social outlets, work, play, home and sustenance are all merely a bus or car ride away. A sedentary convenience culture has taken over from the perilous, physically demanding, evolving world of prehistory.

As stated, anatomically and physiologically, we are still fundamentally the same organism of a quarter of a million years, only without the physical demands. We can assume that the structure we have inherited had reached its evolutionary peak then. It is therefore likely that with the reduced stress on our bodies associated with modern Western living, we have, as a natural organism, become far less physically efficient than when our species first evolved.

Today, we survive illnesses and injuries that would have immediately ended the life of early *Homo sapiens*. Most 'modern' illnesses are unlikely to have existed or been encountered in primeval times, and have only emerged in recent history as man's life span has increased. Early man simply did not live long enough to develop conditions such as diabetes, schizophrenia or end stage liver disease. A simple condition such as appendicitis, easily resolved today, would, until a few centuries ago, have ended life with certainty.

Now we have an expectation of a much longer life span, despite our softer lifestyle (with its frequent abuses). Appropriate physical stress is a desirable part of this, as exercise strengthens and enhances the efficiency of homeostasis, strengthens bodily structures and enhances physical activity (Tortora and Grabowski, 2003). Exercise is therefore a substitute for the physical stresses our forebears once endured just to survive. However, the concept is not new. The benefits of fitness and exercise were being advocated by Hippocrates and Galen 2,500 and 1,900 years ago respectively (cited in Refshauge and Gass, 1995).

With a population gradually becoming less fit and more obese (DoH, 2004), health professionals have to recognise their broader responsibilities in working towards reversing these trends. The nurse plays a key role in advocating the benefits of regular exercise through his or her role as a health educator and health promoter. Certainly this was always a part of nursing in the acute hospital setting but, increasingly, nurses as primary care practitioners or practice nurses are in a pivotal position to bring the message home. Fitness and exercise, no matter at what age, have a beneficial effect in allaying the degeneration of ageing and off-setting many of the more serious illnesses associated with an oversedentary lifestyle. Malik et al. (1998, p. 426) list the potential benefits that regular exercise can bring;

osteoporosis

any disease process that results in the reduction in the bone mass

- Increased metabolic rate thus preventing obesity
- Improved strength to muscles and ligaments
- Prevention of disuse – **osteoporosis**
- Improved cardiovascular function
- Maintenance of normal blood glucose levels
- Reduced stress and anxiety
- Increased sense of well-being.

It should be remembered that it is not only the nurse's client groups who can benefit from regular exercise. Nursing is regularly a physically exhausting occupation, and nurses must remain physically fit to ensure they remain effective in meeting the demands of the job. Many health and fitness centres and clubs offer discount rates for health professionals and most large hospitals have staff fitness facilities. All nurses should give serious consideration to availing themselves of such facilities while they are working. Additionally, a fit nurse projects a positive role model, adding credibility to his or her health promotional and educational activities.

Systemic effects of immobility

It has been stated that immobility, either induced or voluntary, has a potentially damaging effect on health and well-being. When we are young, this may simply result in a loss or absence of muscular definition and obesity, but as we get older, the effects of immobility become more systemic, affecting most systems of the body. However, in illness or old age, these changes, and how they affect each of the systems of the body, can be the difference between recovery and death, seen as we consider each system in turn.

Link

Chapter 7 has more information related to respiratory and cardiovascular systems.

Respiratory system

Respiration functions at its best when we are upright and active. Even sitting down can restrict full respiratory function, as the abdominal organs are forced up under the diaphragm, thus partially limiting inspiration and gaseous exchange. Lying recumbent adds gravity bearing down on the outer chest to the equation and breathing becomes shallower. Malik et al. (1998) state that oxygen intake can drop by as much as 26 per cent after only three weeks of bedrest. Impairment of the accessory muscles of respiration will reduce the effectiveness of coughing in order to expectorate and mucous in the airways will be retained and become more tenacious. The longer the secretions remain, providing a rich cocktail ripe for bacterial contamination, the greater the likelihood of a chest infection.

Cardiovascular system

In recent years, we have become all too aware of the dangers of long-haul air travel and their association with an enhanced risk of deep vein thrombosis (DVT). It will therefore be clear that extended inactivity or bedrest can result in venous stasis and a greater likelihood of clotting due to fibrin breakdown. Venous return is almost entirely dependant on the muscle pump provided by the muscles of the lower limb, mainly the gastrocnemius muscle of the calf (Tortora and Grabowski, 2003). The patient is left prone to pooling of blood in the lower limbs, resulting in **thrombophlebitis** which could precipitate ulceration, or **thrombosis**, carrying life-threatening consequences such as pulmonary or cerebral **embolus**. Moreover, immobility will result in increased cardiac workload, which could also have serious consequences if there is a pre-existing cardiac illness (de Wit, 2001). Poor circulation may also result in reduced cerebral perfusion, resulting in problems with cognition, communication and compliance with care regimes.

thrombophlebitis
inflammation of the wall of a vein with a secondary thrombosis within the involved segment

thrombosis
a blood clot within a vein/artery

embolus
a mass of undissolved matter in a blood vessel

Gastrointestinal system

Inactivity such as that imposed by prolonged bedrest will naturally result in far less expenditure of energy as the basal metabolic rate drops. As less fluid and nutrient replacement occurs, anorexia and dehydration can result (de Wit, 2001), although, paradoxically, this usually leads to an increased laying down of body fat (Malik et al., 1998). Peristalsis will reduce and this, combined with dehydration, will result in the cardinal complication associated with immobility, constipation.

Healthy mobilisation, walking, stooping, climbing stairs and so on, assists gastrointestinal motility by applying intermittent compression forces and fluctuating intra-abdominal pressure on the small and large intestine, which greatly assists peristalsis and thus regular defaecation (Walsh, 2002). When this aid to peristalsis is absent such as in prolonged immobility, the transit of waste matter through the distal gastrointestinal tract slows. As this is also the site for reabsorption of water from the faecal matter, the faeces becomes dry, hard and ultimately impacted.

Link
Chapter 6 has more information related to the urinary and gastrointestinal systems.

Urinary system

Normal activity and movement also has a beneficial effect on normal urinary function. Regular hydration and mobility will ensure the urine remains highly diluted and micturition occurs regularly, thus eliminating waste products on a regular basis. The urinary bladder, which functions best when we are in a vertical position, is constantly cleansed of waste products as the dilute urine constantly 'washes' the bladder walls between micturition. Conversely, reduced hydration, a consequence of prolonged immobility, can lead to increased viscosity of urine as it becomes more concentrated. Within the urinary bladder itself, especially when the patient is lying recumbent, there can be precipitation of salts, byproducts and dead cells, normally eliminated when we micturate. This concentration can form a sediment in the ridges (rugae) in the bladder wall and fails to be effectively eliminated. It is highly favourable to bacterial growth and leaves the immobile patient at serious risk of urinary tract infection.

Malik et al. (1998) warn that after as little as four days immobilisation, **hypercalcaemia** can occur, as immobility (disuse) osteoporosis follows calcium reabsorption from the skeleton. Coupled with increased dehydration, this can overload the renal tubules' capacity to eliminate the increased calcium levels and this in time can build to form renal calculi.

Urinary tract infections are also commonly associated with patients with restricted mobility, simply because of physical restrictions impeding adequate cleansing, especially of the perineum after toileting.

hypercalcaemia

excess amount of calcium in the blood

Musculoskeletal system

Earlier we mentioned the fact that the stress of physical activity is essential to ensure normal replenishment of bone tissue. Conversely, inactivity and immobility lead to a reduction in bone mass through immobility osteoporosis (Walsh, 2002). In the same way, the soft tissues of the musculoskeletal system can also suffer a reduction in quality and efficacy. Underused muscle will waste and lose density. This in turn can lead to contractures and stiff joints, seriously impeding rehabilitation if left unaddressed, and even increasing the risk of falls, especially in the elderly (DoH, 2003).

Integumentary system

Although the skin in relation to wound care will be thoroughly discussed in Chapter 11, no discussion of immobility could proceed without exploration of the pressure issue. Every generation of nurses will have been made aware that a major consequence of prolonged bedrest is the risk of pressure ulcers (decubitus ulcers, pressure sores). Such was the association that these lesions were actually referred to as 'bedsores'. Pressure ulcers are the result of a combination of factors, for example age, nutritional status, mobility, skin quality and general state of health of the patient. However, pressure, friction and shearing are the leading factors to their formation and the need for early and accurate assessment of risk cannot be overemphasised (Alexander et al., 1996).

Where bony prominences pass relatively close to the skin, such as at the sacrum, shoulders, heels, elbows and hips, the dermal layer containing the blood vessels is compressed. Burman (1993) states that normal mean capillary pressure is between 12–32 mm/Hg, so if pressure at these points exceeds these values for a prolonged period of time, **ischaemia** and **tissue necrosis** will result. Livesley (1992) cautions that ischaemia can occur in as little as 20 minutes, therefore early assessment of mobility and pressure risk is essential.

ischaemia

local and temporary
reduction/loss of blood
supply due to
obstruction

tissue necrosis

death of areas of tissue
or bone that are
surrounded by healthy
parts

Reproductive system

Although often difficult to discuss, and thus frequently avoided, problems of sexual function or expression may often accompany conditions that restrict mobility. From simply being prevented from moving to a place of privacy in order to satisfy a sexual need, to the far more serious permanent impairment of sexual function, perhaps following spinal injury, immobility can present real challenges to health care at a number of levels. It is vital that nurses, who work in any discipline that involves sexually active clients with restricted mobility, and regardless of the complexity or even discomfiture that it may impose, do not shirk from supporting the patient in meeting these needs with sensitivity and objectivity.

Psychological issues

Sadly, many nurses, although undoubtedly as hard working and committed as any of their colleagues, still only tend to nurse what they can see. Yet it is likely that the factors causing patients the most concern – fear, ignorance about their condition, anxiety, depression, stress and boredom – lie invisible, and thus unaddressed (de Wit, 2001). It is these invisible factors that can impinge most significantly on patient morale, and be pivotal in the success or failure of care regimes, even the most sophisticated. If the patient has lost the will to comply, then all care can be doomed to failure. Immobility gives patients time to ruminate alone on the possible changes in their lives that may present after discharge, for example loss of employment, loss of social network, altered body image, effects on relationships and so on. Immobility restricts opportunities to seek help or pursue diversions, to talk to staff or other patients, to simply find a quiet spot in order to think, to pursue a hobby, access a telephone or just walk.

Nursing strategies in immobility

Link

Chapter 1 has further information related to the activities of living model (Roper et al., 2000).

Although frequently a source for derision by many nursing purists, theorists and scholars (Mitchell, 1984; Walsh, 1991; Fraser, 1996), this section will be guided by the Roper-Logan-Tierney model of nursing (Roper et al., 2000). The rationale for using this model is that it is easy to use and understand, comprehensive and familiar to the overwhelming majority of nurses and, despite its detractors, still the most accessible nursing model in use today (Newton, 1991; Holland et al., 2003).

Regardless of the severity of the illness, injury or prognosis, it is frequently not the primary diagnosed condition that accounts for the patient's deterioration or death. All too often it can be attributed to complications of immobility impinging on the function of one or more of the systems discussed above. For the very ill or elderly, even in the absence of a terminal prognosis, these complications can still seriously challenge recovery and survival. It is the long-held (although, sadly, largely anecdotal) view of the authors that the nurse's failure to recognise the potential for these complications, act effectively on that recognition and/or educate the patient to adopt a self-help approach from an informed knowledge base is a fundamental, yet persistent flaw in contemporary nursing.

Focusing on the activities of living (Roper et al., 2000), this section will briefly discuss the risks and possible nursing strategies in relation to a patient with impaired mobility. It will further seek to demonstrate how the actions of the nurse, in unison with the multidisciplinary team of health professionals, can address all the potential complications associated with immobility.

Maintaining a safe environment

In keeping with previous adaptations of the model for living and for reasons of clarity, consideration of maintaining a safe environment can best be interpreted by applying this in a broader sense to potential needs within either the internal or external environment.

Internal environment

Related to immobility, consideration of the patient's internal environment can be applied to the risk of venous stasis and the potential for developing DVT. DVT is notoriously common in immobilised adults, although rarely seen in children or adolescents. In the large veins of the lower leg, most commonly the soleal and gastrocnemius veins, activation of the clotting factor Factor XII occurs when the innermost endothelial layer is damaged or compressed. Such damage or trauma frequently occurs in surgery, or following prolonged periods of inactivity (Coleridge-Smith et al., 1991). The resulting platelet aggregation, thrombin formation and fibrin generation forms a thrombus or clot. The major threat lies in the propensity for a fragment (embolus) to break away from the thrombus to eventually occlude a pulmonary vessel in the lungs (pulmonary embolus – PE), which, if large enough, could be instantly fatal.

When DVT has occurred, the problem can be minimised by monitoring closely and giving anticoagulants. However, by far the best course of action should lie with prevention, which is the essence of good nursing care. This starts with careful consideration of risk factors, as shown in Chart 9.1.

Chart 9.1 ● Risk factors for deep vein thrombosis

- History of varicose veins
- Dehydration
- Age of 40 years
- Past or family history of DVT or PE
- Prolonged immobility/degree of mobility
- Prolonged surgical procedures (over 30 minutes)
- Pregnancy
- Serious illness, for example myocardial infarction, heart failure, sepsis
- History of clotting disorders
- Obesity
- Underlying malignancy
- (Possibly) recent long-haul air travel

Source: Adapted from Walsh (2002).

External environment

Related to mobility, risk to the external environment can manifest from two sources. First, if bed-bound, the patient may be restricted or physically incapable of mobilising around the bed, and so unable to self-help, eat or drink, thus raising the risk of dehydration and DVT. Second, the newly mobilising (or elderly) patient may at first have stiff joints or wasted muscles, leaving them more prone to the risk of falls (DoH, 2003). Time spent in building up muscle groups, advising the patient on walking aids and educating them to walk – **only within the limitations of their returning mobility** – prior to discharge is time well spent. Early lifestyle assessment and adaptation of the home environment to limitations in mobility is as vital as any other aspect of treatment and care.

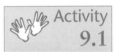
Activity 9.1
Take time to talk or work with occupational therapy colleagues. Ascertain what aids and adaptations may be appropriate to a newly discharged patient, from your client focus, with mobility problems.

Communicating

Related to mobility, communication between nurse and patient is essential. It is central to what nurses do, and without effective communication – verbal, non-verbal and paralinguistic – nursing could not take place. Too often, nurses fail to

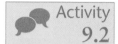

Activity 9.2

When you next engage with a patient or client, and the patient shares a concern or anxiety with you, identify and reflect on the verbal, non-verbal and paralinguistic components of the interaction.

Activity 9.3

Where language is a barrier to compliance due to ethnic or cultural isolation, reflect on ways that the importance of compliance might be communicated.

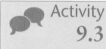

Activity 9.4

Go back to your textbooks or lecture notes and remind yourself of alterations in fluid requirements and fluid loss: (a) in the elderly, (b) when ill and bed-bound and (c) when fit and active.

engage with their patients for fear of it getting in the way of nursing care. The reality is that nursing care and patient satisfaction is maximised when clients are fully involved and kept fully informed (Newton, 1996). How can we expect them to comply with a particular nursing regime or strategy if its importance has not been fully explained to them, especially if what is being recommended seems to be at odds with what is comfortable, or conflicts with a personal belief of what constitutes recovery, for example early mobilisation following surgery?

Breathing

Naturally breathing is an involuntary activity of living essential to life and largely taken for granted. However, when mobility is restricted, even this may become impaired. Your life science studies will have told you that respiration occurs as an interaction between diaphragm, ribs and intercostals and the accessory muscles of respiration. It functions at its optimum efficiency when we stand upright, with gravity not restricting maximal vital capacity. Walking briskly or exercising increase respiratory rate and thus optimise ventilation. Movement will also facilitate expectoration of mucous secretions from the airways, thus allowing removal of contaminants that might otherwise cause congestion and possible infection. Immobility, through illness or ageing, may render patients chair- or bed-bound, losing the respiratory benefits of active movement, restricting vital capacity as abdominal organs limit movement of the diaphragm, and reducing ciliary action, thus increasing secretions and the risk of pulmonary infections (Tortora and Grabowski, 2003).

Eating and drinking

Nutrition and hydration are also essentials of life. Yet we take for granted water, as literally on tap, and the widest selection of food perennially available in our local supermarket, or even delivered to our door. Takeaway outlets have even relieved us of the need to prepare and cook our meals, and are (dubiously for health) an increasingly popular, if expensive, option for meeting our food needs. However, restricted mobility through age, infirmity or illness will severely restrict choice and access. Financial constraints, perhaps after retirement or loss of a spouse, or reliance on public transport may make shopping difficult as local amenities close down in favour of out-of-town shopping centres. When in hospital, little choice is available regarding what and when we eat and drink. Cultural and ethnic factors may demand food preparation in a specific way, not possible in the hospital setting, and thus not available to the inpatient who requires it. When nursing the patient with restricted mobility, mealtimes become major events, and carers must ensure that meals are presented in the most attractive and edible way possible. It must be remembered that many of the complications of immobility are in some way associated with dehydration (see Chart 9.2). If nothing else, immobile patients must be encouraged to drink adequately and frequently.

Chart 9.2 ● Complications of immobility associated with inadequate hydration

- **Constipation** – reduced motility following dehydration slows transit of faecal matter through the intestine, leading to increased reabsorption and possible impaction. May result in toxic effects as intestinal waste toxins are taken up into the circulation and may manifest as confusion, delirium and so on
- **Urinary tract infection** – reduced hydration and movement may cause concentration of urine and sedimentation of urinary solutes in the bladder, which may provide a site for increased bacterial growth, resulting in infection
- **Respiratory infections** – restricted chest movement due to reduced mobility combined with dehydration can result in increased viscosity of respiratory secretions, increasing their tenacity and hampering expectoration or removal. Retained secretions may provide a site for increased bacterial growth, resulting in infection
- **Deep vein thrombosis** – reduced hydration and mobility may alter blood viscosity so increasing the risk of clotting
- **Renal calculi** – long-term immobilisation may result in immobility osteoporosis. Less hydration and renal filtration may concentrate calcium and other solutes in the renal tubules, increasing the risk of kidney stone formation

Eliminating

As we mobilise – walking, running, climbing, turning, stooping, reaching and so on – we actively assist peristalsis and the transit of the products of digestion through the digestive tract. When mobility is restricted, through ageing, infirmity or illness, this support to motility is lost and constipation may result. Mobility also has implications for urinary elimination.

Simply by encouraging mobilisation within the patient's limitations can go far in avoiding complications; however, avoidance might well lie simply with ensuring that patients hydrate adequately. But reduced mobility leading to restricted access or reliance on others to meet toileting needs might, conversely, lead to a cognitive decision not to drink. If nurses and carers cannot be trusted to immediately respond to the patient's request to go to the toilet, then the patient

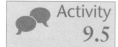

**Activity
9.5**

As uncomfortable
as this may be, next
time you go to the
toilet, consciously
reflect on all
aspects of mobility
that it involved.

will not risk incontinence, regardless of how important hydration may be. We only need to let the patient down once in this way and that trust cannot be regained (Sander, 1999). It may falsely be believed that time spent not assisting the patient in meeting their toileting needs is time saved. However, when this leads to incontinence, constipation, infection and confusion, that time 'saved' is rapidly lost. Neglect is a poor substitute for quality care and timely intervention and is thus a false economy, with no place in contemporary nursing care.

Personal cleansing and dressing

When attending to your personal cleansing needs today, consider the physical activity involved. First, we physically needed the upper body strength to turn off the alarm, switch on the lamp and get out of bed and into a standing posture. Lower limb strength enabled us to walk to the bathroom. Grip and upper arm strength opened all doors en route and, coupled with vision and dexterity, enabled the men to shave and all to clean their teeth. Similar feats of locomotion and mobility, but now coupled with balance, got us in and out of the shower. Think about the physical agility necessary to thoroughly wash all parts of our bodies. After drying our hair and the women applying make-up (highly dexterous and requiring meticulous hand-to-eye coordination), we dress, and again wildly contort our bodies to put on and adjust our clothing to our satisfaction.

Now consider how illness, infirmity or ageing will seriously impinge on this activity. Inevitably, cleansing and dressing will be far less efficient or adequate when dependent on others, despite the patient's desire to look as clean and well turned out as you do. Yet think how much time we spend on our own personal hygiene and grooming, and contrast this with how much time we can allow to each of our higher dependency patients. Reflection on this point will fully illustrate the primacy of mobility.

Controlling body temperature

The controlling body temperature activity of living is frequently applied to monitoring the patient for the development of infections, some of which have been already discussed earlier (respiratory and urinary tract infection). Related to mobility and immobility, a low grade rise in temperature may be the first indicator of a DVT (Marieb, 2004).

When fit and well, we give little thought to the ways we control our body temperature, and yet again, mobility is central to doing so. Conversely, lack of mobility can impinge upon it. We need to be mobile to select and buy appropriate clothing, according to the climate. Yet, mobility may influence socioeconomic status, which may restrict choice and quality, especially when elderly or chronically ill. The simple acts of getting dressed or undressed, putting on extra or discarding clothing, switching on heating or opening and closing windows all depend on degrees of mobility. At its most extreme, perhaps when severely ill or incapacitated, we may have a total absence of control or awareness of our thermoregulatory needs. An example here might relate to patients with high spinal injuries resulting in **tetraplegia**. In this permanent condition, many thermoregulatory functions, such as shivering and even the sensation of cold, may be lost to the patient. In extreme cases, the patient may be totally unaware that their temperature is rising or dropping to that of the surrounding environment (poikilothermia). In the latter, a patient could be blissfully aware that they are dying of **hypothermia**.

tetraplegia

paralysis of both arms and legs

hypothermia

having a body temperature below normal ranges

Mobilising

As we have seen so far, mobilising is an essential activity of living in order to maintain maximum independence. Conversely, as we have shown, immobility can lead to a whole array of potentially life-threatening complications. One serious complication of prolonged bedrest is the risk of developing pressure ulcers, discussed earlier. In some areas of care, these can be present in almost endemic numbers. Although intrinsically linked to immobility, the care of this condition will on this occasion be discussed in Chapter 11, where wound care is considered in greater detail than allowed here. There can be little doubt now that the longer we remain physically mobile, preferably beyond just sedentary activity, life, in terms of both quality and quantity, is considerably enhanced (Uglow and Dewing, 2004).

Link

Chapter 11 discusses wound healing.

Working and playing

We are an active and social organism, working or physically occupied, either for employment or pleasure, for the majority of our lives. Mobility in employment increases options and choice and thus the potential for prosperity and success. Immobility restricts and confines choice and thus is linked to less opportunities and lower income. When not at work, or even after retirement, we still retain the desire to remain active and stimulated. It is a factor which prolongs life, self-esteem and independence (Uglow and Dewing, 2004).

Expressing sexuality

Right to the end of our lives, most of us like to present ourselves at our best. This is largely linked to self-esteem, dignity and personality, and a central component of our personality is our sexuality (Bancroft, 1983). Many nurses find this the most awkward activity of living to enquire about because of its difficult association with sexual orientation and practices. Sexuality is far greater than that. It is essentially that factor which determines us as the man or woman we wish the world to regard us as. It is the need for the 90-year-old man to shave every day, long after anyone notices that he is always clean shaven. It is the 85-year-old woman who still has her hair styled every fortnight, decades after she became comfortable with the absence of a sexual partner. It is the clothes we wear or don't wear, the way we smell and the way we interact, and mobility is central to it. When ill or infirm, patients cannot get up to change their nightdress, stained with soup for several days, and cannot get up to wash thoroughly the food stains from the corners of their mouth that their carers' 'topping and tailing' perpetually miss. Yet have no doubt that if our patients were aware of how their failing eyesight and mobility had frequently allowed them to become unkempt, to the degree that they could not see it or get up to rectify it, potentially it could be of greater concern than any other aspect of their care, more important even than pain, a poor prognosis, the advance of age or even impending death.

Death can be dealt with, but a loss of dignity can often be perceived as worse even than death. Our sexuality and how we are allowed to express it to the world is central to all this, and mobility plays a major part. It enables us to shop and browse, experiment and get it wrong, dress and groom, wash and cleanse, and generally present to the world the image of ourselves we wish to project. And when we start to fail, through ageing, illness or infirmity, we look to our carers, acting at the peak of their professional practice and perceptiveness, to make up the deficits.

Sleeping

The environment where care takes place is also, for some, a place of work. The business of professional nursing is a 24/7 activity, sadly not always conducive to the sleep and rest patterns of our patients and client groups. In its broadest sense, in relation to mobility, a person would not choose to sleep in a hospital. A key attraction of private health care is that one is at least assured of a private room, sadly not yet an option for the majority of patients in this country. Sleep is an important activity of living. It is the recuperative and restorative phase of the circadian cycle (Chokroverty, 1999; Lower and Bonsack, 2002; Tortora and Grabowski, 2003). Illness and infirmity impinge on the quality of sleep (Redeker and Hedges, 2002), while insomnia is a frequent feature of ageing. Lack of mobility associated with each of these states can encroach on the quality and quantity of sleep. Pain may be alleviated by a simple change of position, but prevented by a mobility deficit. The shedding or acquiring of blankets or clothing, required if one is too hot or too cold, is prevented by immobility. Day-time sleeping, which might otherwise be allayed by walking or socialising, will, for the bed-bound patient, inevitably disrupt night-time sleep patterns – by far the most desirable in terms of sleep quality.

Dying

Death is perhaps the final but, nonetheless for the nurse, important activity of living. Related to mobility, we have already read that immobility alone can hasten the deterioration and death of patients through its exacerbation of potentially fatal complications. Equally, though, immobility can impinge on the process and, for many, the rites of death. For many dying patients, there is an imperative to revisit or enhance their spiritual ties. Immobility may prevent their access to temple, mosque, synagogue or church at this important end stage of life. Access and mobility issues, especially among minority faiths, may prevent death rites being fully completed or their importance fully understood. Finally, social isolation and the obscure location of hospitals, hospices and care facilities may make the attendance of significant others and relatives during the final hours of a person's life difficult to share due to access issues. As longer life expectation increasingly takes life into advanced old age, higher pressure workloads and fluid workforces can make the pressures on carers so great that the niceties of an 'ideal' death become ever more a luxury rather than the norm. Ironically for many, nursing is the main care discipline that has primacy at this all-important end stage of life, and it is timely nursing interventions and interactions, coupled with socio-cultural insight and knowledge, which make the difference between care that is barely adequate or exceptional at this most crucial time in a person's life.

■ Moving and Handling

According to the Health and Safety Executive (HSE, 2005), the health services is one of Britain's biggest employers, with approximately 1.2 million employed by the NHS and approximately 0.7 million in the private sector. This high volume of employment and the associated work-related injuries are reflected within the figures for the period 1996/7–2000/1. The HSE has stated that over 61,100 health-care workers suffered an injury reportable to the HSE under the Reporting of Injuries, Diseases and Dangerous Occurrences Regulations (RIDDOR) 1995 (HSE, 2003a), which equates to an average of 12,233 injuries per year.

Many health and social care professionals see musculoskeletal injuries as an occupational hazard. By reflecting upon current statistics, we must not accept the so-called 'consequences of the profession', but each person must strive to amend the clinical culture they work within, their own personal and professional thinking and attitudes towards moving and handling and by these actions influence colleagues and clients alike. Within the health service, moving and handling is the commonest form of over-3-day injuries (injuries that incur an absence of work for three or more days) in nurses (51 per cent), care assistants (51 per cent) and assistant nurses (54 per cent) (HSC, 2004).

The Health and Safety Commission (2004) has also stated that the number and rate of over-3-day injuries in the health services have been declining over recent years, and the number of injuries has fallen by 16 per cent since 1997/98 and the rate of injury by 27 per cent since 1998/99. However, over the past five years, moving and handling injuries have still accounted for approximately 53 per cent of all over-3-day injuries in the health services and moving and handling accidents made up 12 per cent of all reported major injuries in 2002/03. These kinds of accidents have risen by 13 per cent since 1999/2000. This remains an unnecessary and worrying statistic within the health service.

These over-3-day injuries equate to 9,551 reported incidents in 2002/03 (8 per cent of all over-3-day employee injuries in industry), the same proportion as that for 2001/02 (10,077). The Labour Force Survey for 1998/99 identified that health and social work (a wider definition than just health care) had an above-average rate of injury. Ambulance workers and nurses were 2.8 times more at risk than clerical workers (HSC, 2004).

In 1995, the HSE produced a Self-reported Work-related Illness Survey, which clearly identified that moving and handling was a major contributing factor in musculoskeletal, work-related illness. These included back-related injuries, upper limb and neck injuries and lower limb injuries. Over half the respondents reporting a musculoskeletal disorder said it affected their back, with 79 per cent reporting that their condition *only* affected their back. The survey also identified that nurses have one of the highest rates of musculoskeletal disorders (an estimated rate of 5.8 per cent compared to the average of 2.5 per cent), which is often associated with moving and handling incidents (HSE, 1998, 2000).

When one considers the working culture, we often work towards nonsensical time schedules that force the majority of 'heavy' work to be allocated in the morning, almost immediately after handover. From an HSC (2004) study, nurses, assistant nurses and care assistants all incur more over-3-day handling injuries between 8 am and 12 noon than at any other time of the day. The number of over-3-day handling injuries sharply decline throughout the rest of the working day from noon onwards.

It is clear that being injured while moving and handling or supporting a person within a health service continues to be the most common reason for over-3-day injuries, with 2,005 reported incidents/accidents in 2002/03, which should alone be a reason to reflect upon your moving and handling practices and the practices of others.

Chart 9.3 ● Main causes of work-related absences

The main causes of injury (resulting in over-3-day absences) continue to be:

● Moving and handling/musculoskeletal injury
● Slips and trips
● Assault/violence
● Struck by something (for example sharp knives or falling objects)

The main causes of occupational ill-health continue to be:

● Musculoskeletal injury
● Dermatitis
● Work-related stress

Source: HSE (2005).

Worldwide, health-care professions have been identified as having a higher incidence of back-related injury from manual handling technique injuries (Norton, 1970; Kidd, 1995; Love, 1996; Retsas and Pinikahana, 2000). Incidences of associated absence from work have been estimated at over 764,000 days per year (Bannister, 1996, p. 25). It is estimated that the true cost of workplace accidents to the British economy could be as much as £16 billion per annum (Zindani, 1998).

A survey by the HSE estimated that, in 2001/02, 1.1 million people in Great Britain suffered from musculoskeletal disorders (MSDs) caused or made worse by their current or past work. An estimated 12.3 million working days were lost due to these work-related MSDs, and on average each sufferer took about 20 days off in that 12-month period (HSE, 2004).

Compensation claims can routinely cost employers in excess of a million pounds in awards and legal costs where workers are retired through ill-health. Nursing compensation claims in 1996 cost the NHS approximately £8.5 million for back injuries alone, as a result of patient moving and handling, which roughly translates to 5 per cent of the total running expense of an average hospital (Zindani, 1998).

Media reports are still prevalent and identify large awards such as:

● Back pain nurse awarded £420,000 (BBC News, 16 October, 2002)
● Nurse wins £800,000 for back injury (BBC News, 15 February, 2000)

However, one can also find articles about the high sickness rate in nursing that relate to 'severe back strain' (BBC News, 26 June, 2005).

These headlines can lead to confusion among staff and students. Many believe that the compensation culture allows us to obtain a successful claim against an employer. It is recognised that a 'no lifting policy' has now been seen as impractical. It may at times, when assessed as safe to do so, be necessary to assist the patient or lift an inanimate load; however, it is only acceptable if the physical effort required to do so is as low as is reasonably practicable, taking into consideration alternative methods and equipment. Nurses must also reflect upon what is seen as an emergency. Some may consider an emergency a reason for 'unsafe practices' and 'controversial techniques' to be employed. Any emergency task within the health service should, where possible, have a procedure/ policy in place to safeguard all staff and clients' well-being. It is the responsibility of the organisation and the workplace to ensure that appropriate equipment and staffing numbers are available.

Researchers have found that the possible reason for back injuries are all linked to 'non-compliance'. Many researchers, such as Norton (1970), Bell (1987, p. 24), Venning (1988, p. 327) and McGuire and Dewar (1995, p. 35), showed that aiding devices such as hoists and sliding sheets are not being used when required, and many pieces of equipment were being left to 'gather cobwebs'.

It is clear through discussions with students and qualified members of staff that they are well aware of the policies and procedures available for drug administration and the subsequent consequences of drug errors. However, ask the same question in relationship to moving and handling and a very different awareness is apparent. Many would not even consider administering an injection without fully following the stated policy/procedure, but ask the same health-care professional to assist in standing a patient using a 'drag lift' and many would oblige without reflecting upon the consequences to themselves, colleagues, patients and relatives.

Health and social care professionals can relate to and accept the potential harm and even death following a drug error, but when asked the worst complication of carrying out 'controversial' (unsafe) moving and handling techniques, many respond with 'back pain', 'musculoskeletal injury' and laugh openly when informed that death is the worst event that can occur.

Moving and handling is so inbred within our culture that in many cases the rationale for the use of controversial techniques is seen as 'this is what is always done', or 'it is necessary for nursing care'. I have heard staff refer to the adages: 'I have done it this way for 20 years and not injured myself' or 'If I injure myself, I will get sick pay and then sue for compensation.' One aspect that is recurrent within the statements above is that staff members have referred to themselves and not the consequences of their actions on patients and colleagues or the accumulative damage that is being done.

Awareness of the relevant current regulations, governing bodies and recommended risk/generic assessments is imperative, because, without it, adaptations to outdated techniques and the continuation of controversial manoeuvres will continue (see Chart 9.4). Many NHS Trusts now support disciplinary action when staff members continue to use these outdated and controversial techniques. One must consider that current law and legislation applies to all health and social care professionals. If you travel at 35 mph in a 30 mph limit, you will expect to be caught and accept the consequences of your actions – the same should apply to moving and handling.

Student and staff members must be aware of current regulations, governing bodies and risk assessment. This not only highlights the 'boundaries' in which we need to work to promote a safe working environment for ourselves, colleagues, patients and relatives, it also clearly demonstrates the scope and complexities that are inherent in today's moving and handling culture. Zindani (1998, p. 10) believes that 'the regulations are a radical departure from the old statutory framework, going well beyond simple 'lifting' accidents and covering a multitude of moving and handling tasks'.

Chart 9.4 ● Governing bodies, regulations and Acts relevant to health and safety

- Nursing and Midwifery Council (2005)
- Royal College of Nursing (2003)
- Manual Handling Operations Regulations 1992 (HSE, 2003a)
- Reporting of Injuries, Diseases and Dangerous Occurrences Regulations (RIDDOR) 1995 (HSC, 2002)
- Provision and Use of Work Equipment Regulations (PUWER) 1998 (HSE, 1999)
- Lifting Operations and Lifting Equipment Regulations (LOLER) 1998 (HSE, 2002)
- Management of Health and Safety at Work Regulations 1999
- Health and Safety at Work Act 1974
- Human Rights Act 1998
- Disability Discrimination Act 2000

The law as it relates to manual handling is regulated by statute principally in the form of the Health and Safety at Work Act 1974 and the Manual Handling Operations Regulations 1992, the latter introduced under the provisions of the Health and Safety at Work Act to enable the UK to implement the requirements of European Directives on the manual handling of loads. Manual handling operations have been defined within HSE directives (HSE, 2003a) as:

Transporting or supporting a load, including lifting, putting down, pushing, pulling, carrying or moving by hand or bodily force. This also includes the intentional dropping or throwing of a load.

Within these regulations, employers have a general duty 'To ensure, so far as is reasonably practicable, the health, safety and welfare at work of all employees' (Health and Safety at Work Act 1974) and must avoid the need for hazardous manual handling operations. An example of employers' responsibilities are listed in Table 9.1. There may be occasions when this is not reasonably practicable, and for these the HSE recommends that employers make a suitable and sufficient assessment and take appropriate steps to reduce the risk of injury to the lowest level reasonably possible.

Employees have a duty under the Act to take reasonable care of their own health and safety and that of other people who may be affected by their actions, and it is essential that all health-care workers adhere to these regulations. As a student nurse, preparing to take on a professional role, faced with moving and handling operations throughout your career, you will need to continue to review any relevant new legislation. All employers are required by law to update their employees annually on the principles and practice of moving and handling operations.

As the safety of the nurse and patient is paramount, nurse education will include instruction on moving and handling operations, and guidance on local practice and the use of moving and handling equipment. Teaching staff have a responsibility to provide the correct information, as indicated by law, and students contracted within a school must, also by law, undergo regular updating. Failure to do so may affect their ability to practice.

Table 9.1 Example of the comparison between employer and employee responsibilities under relevant regulations

Employers' responsibilities	Employees' responsibilities
Paragraph 167 of the Manual Handling Operation Regulations 1999, Section 2 of the Health and Safety at Work Act and Regulations 10 and 13 of the Management of Health and Safety at Work Regulations 1999	Paragraph 182 of the Manual Handling Operation Regulations 1999, as well as the Management of Health and Safety at Work Regulations 1999
Require employers to provide their employees with health and safety information and training	Require employees to make use of appropriate equipment provided for them, in accordance with their training and the instructions their employer has given them

When considering the abundance of regulations and guidance from regulatory and governing bodies, it is surprising that injuries, incidence and accidents occur. It is often due to ignorance that many avoid the implementation of training, make incorrect judgements and not use the relevant equipment such as hoists and slide sheets. They are often surprised when disciplined for carrying out controversial techniques such as the drag lift. One must consider that for every regulation that conveys a duty to an employer, there is often a duty ensuring that the employee works within the safe systems provided (see Table 9.1).

Assessment of safe principles of moving and handling

Many clinical/back care advisers and trainers within moving and handling have moved away from the teaching/facilitation of 'techniques' and instead work within the boundaries of teaching and facilitating 'principles' of safe moving and handling. This method of teaching and facilitation of moving and handling give the practitioners a 'toolkit' of safe principles that can be adapted when completing a 'generic' and/or a 'patient risk assessment'.

A generic assessment is an assessment that can provide solutions and/or possible solutions to ALL moving and handling scenarios possible within an area. This may lead to the purchase of new equipment, as current practice is unsatisfactory. (BackCare, 1999)

Protocols, generic assessments and the use of standard procedures can help the nurse/healthcare worker choose the strategy for a particular situation but in many cases an individual plan is required [that is, a] risk assessment. (BackCare et al., 2005, p. 105).

Risk assessments

Risk assessments (or 'individual patient handling profile') and generic assessments must be completed to comply with current laws and legislation: Manual Handling Operations Regulations 1992 (HSE, 2003a); *The Guide to the Handling of Patients* (BackCare et al., 2005); and the Health and Safety at Work Act 1974.

It is strongly recommended that you assess and be aware of your own and client limitations when assessing a client's needs. Seek relevant supervision and support, and ensure that you have sufficient staff to assess the patient safely, that is, one nurse is not enough to assess a patient's standing or sitting ability for the first time.

The following five categories (using the acronym ELIOT) are an example of a simple risk assessment and must be remembered and acted upon before actually becoming involved in the facilitation of patient or inanimate load moving and handling (BackCare et al., 2005, p. 91):

- *Environment*
  Space constraints within the working area, or the area moving to? Ventilation? Poor lighting? Where is the task to be carried out – indoors or outside? Flooring type and level of surface? Trailing wires? Pets? And so on
- *Load*
  As an inanimate load:
  Unwieldy, that is, size, shape, weight and complexity of the object? Difficult to grasp? Unstable? Sharp? Hot or cold? And so on
  As a patient:
  How much can the patient participate? What are their expectations/wishes? Are they in pain? Are they prone to falls? Have you considered cultural issues? Does their underlying condition prevent or complicate compliance? Are they likely to become agitated and aggressive? And so on
- *Individual capacity* (the handler and the patient)
  Does it require unusual strength? Create a hazard? Require special information, education, training and demonstrations? Are all the individual members fit and able for the task ahead? And so on.
- *Other factors and the interaction between these components*
  Does clothing affect the task? Have the views of the person being assisted been considered? Could a generic assessment save time and still meet the needs? Does the handler undertake regular manual handling? Does everyone involved fully understand the task ahead? And so on.
- *Task*
  What is the task – is it clearly defined? What does it involve – twisting, stooping, carrying over distances and so on? Does it need to be done – are there alternative measures? Does additional time need to be allocated? And so on.

As with any assessment, such as a care plan or care pathway, it requires regular and ongoing evaluation as within the nursing process:

1. Assessment
2. Diagnosis
3. Planning
4. Intervention
5. Evaluation.

The risk assessment or individual patient handling profile should reflect the patient's individual requirements (Table 9.2) and incorporate the clients ever changing needs and abilities, for example can the patient participate more after breakfast than before? Does the patient require temporary moving and handling equipment following clinical intervention or treatment? For example, while a

> **Link**
> Chapter 1 has more information related to the nursing process.

profiling bed is being delivered, you may decide that to lower the risk as far as reasonably practicable, you will use a mattress variator (V-shaped frame that is positioned under the head end of the mattress. The inflation of a cushion opens the frame to bend the mattress to aid sitting) to ensure that the client is able to sit forward in bed with minimal assistance.

Table 9.2 Example of an individual patient handling profile, identifying varying options according to health needs

Task	Date	Additional information
Floor to bed/chair	30 October 2006	1. Mrs Jones, who has a past history of falls, is generally able to get herself up from the floor with verbal guidance and demonstration and the use of two chairs and two nurses
	5 November 2006	2. Following treatment, Mrs Jones's condition deteriorates and requires mobilisation with a wheelchair and three nurses
	10 November 2006	3. If a fall occurs following her treatment, a hoist must be used to assist Mrs Jones. Minimum of three nurses

As with any care plan or care pathway, it is also vital that actual and potential needs, both nurse and patient perceived, are incorporated to ensure that all potential avenues are assessed. The risk assessment, once completed, should include safe moving and handling principles and procedures, and the correct number of staff, manoeuvres and/or recommended equipment.

The risk assessment is a legal document and should therefore incorporate exactly what the patient requires. It should include appropriate and current principles that are approved and not shown on the list of controversial techniques (see BackCare et al., 2005, pp. 273–89) or involve the use of unsafe principles that place you, your colleagues or patients in danger. Following your assessment, recommended equipment should be included and where necessary purchased, highlighted or requested from various sources. If unfamiliar with the clinical setting, it maybe wise to seek support and advice from colleagues who may recommend alternative and readily available alternatives, for example you recommend a profiling bed to sit a patient forward in bed; however, there are mattress variators available within the stores.

Within the health-care setting, the patient is referred to as the 'load'. Therefore, size, weight, shape, fragility, stability, the individual's ability to function

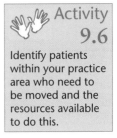

Activity
9.6

Identify patients within your practice area who need to be moved and the resources available to do this.

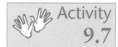

Activity 9.7

Identify one patient and undertake a risk assessment, related to moving and handling, with them.

both physically and mentally, and any attachments that may adversely affect movement, such as infusion pumps, should be considered. Human beings can display individual characteristics that may help or hinder moving and handling operations: elderly clients, for example, may suffer from arthritis.

The Manual Handling Operations Regulations 1992 (HSE, 2003a) do not contain any weight limits below which moving and handling can be considered safe; rather they suggest the avoidance of hazardous moving and handling so far as is reasonably practicable, making suitable and sufficient assessments that cannot be avoided, and reducing the risk of injury from moving and handling tasks. You should ensure that all patient handling is assessed by considering all the risk factors rather than weight alone.

The numerical guidelines (Figure 9.1) can be used to determine when an assessment is needed. As you will identify from this, the 'lifting' ability of males and females is different and must be taken into consideration when undertaking a risk assessment. The RCN (2003) believes that even here manual handling should be avoided or made less demanding wherever reasonably practicable.

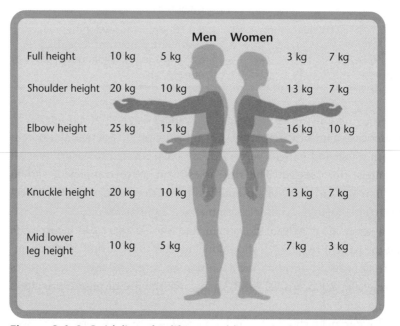

Figure 9.1 ● Guidelines for lifting and lowering for men and women (adapted from HSE, 2003a)

It is assumed that the load can easily be grasped with both hands and that the procedure is being undertaken in a safe working environment. The aim is to eliminate hazardous manual handling in all but exceptional or life-threatening situations; however, many 'life-threatening situations' will have been generically assessed and a safe action plan and procedure produced. Patients should be encouraged to assist in their own transfers and handling aids must be used whenever they can reduce the risk of injury.

Handling patients manually may continue only if it does not involve lifting most or all of a patient's weight and is not done to replace equipment or carried out frequently throughout the day, leading to accumulative injuries to nurse/client. Care must also be taken when supporting a patient, and pushing and pulling should be kept to a minimum. Staff should assess the capabilities and rehabilitation needs of a patient to decide on which, if any, handling aids are suitable.

Ergonomics

Ergonomics can be defined as the study of the relationship between the working environment and the people within it. It adapts the task to the person – rather the adapting the person to the task; it is important in the prevention of injury resulting from moving and handling activities, ensuring the optimum 'fit' between the people and the work.

Ergonomics puts people first, and by taking account of their capabilities and limitations, it aims to make sure that the tasks, equipment, information and the environment suit each worker (HSE, 2003b).

Ergonomic processes include risk assessment as well as the identification and implementation of measures to reduce the risk. Posture, the types of furnishing used, their height, position and manoeuvrability, the tasks undertaken and the environment are all assessed in order to ensure that the job is designed to fit the worker and thus reduce the incidence of manual handling injuries.

The HSE booklet *Understanding Ergonomics at Work* (2003b) discusses what type of workplace problems ergonomics can solve (Chart 9.5). By reducing and even eliminating these problems, one can reduce musculoskeletal injuries and the associated complications that may be attributed to these injuries, such as slips, trips and falls.

Chart 9.5 ● Work-based problems for moving and handling

- The load is too heavy and/or bulky, placing unreasonable demands on the person
- The load has to be lifted from the floor and/or above the shoulders
- The task involves frequent repetitive lifting
- The task requires awkward postures, such as bending or twisting
- The load cannot be gripped properly
- The task is performed on uneven, wet or sloping floor surfaces
- The task is performed under time pressures and incorporates too few rest breaks

Source: HSE (2003b) © Crown copyright (2006).

Normal body movement and associated terminology

To fully comprehend the complexities and rationale of safe moving and handling, one must first grasp a basic understanding of normal body movement, basic principles that should be applied whenever possible.

Anatomical positioning

Standing upright with arms out to the side, palms of the hands should be facing forwards, feet parallel, pointing forwards and shoulder-width apart.

Stability: stance, base of support, centre of gravity

If the line of gravity (which runs through the centre of gravity) falls within an object's base, that object is stable, that is, balanced. Once an object's line of gravity falls outside its base, the object will begin to topple and fall under gravitational forces (BackCare et al., 2005, p. 58).

Stability is a one of the key principles of safe moving and handling. One must ensure that the patient, your colleagues and you are correctly positioned when carrying out any aspect of safe moving and handling and/or mobility. To maintain a stable base, you must ensure that your feet are shoulder-width apart, with one foot slightly in front of the other (adjustment of the back foot may automatically occur). This position provides a wide base of support and ensures that you are stable in all directions (Figure 9.2).

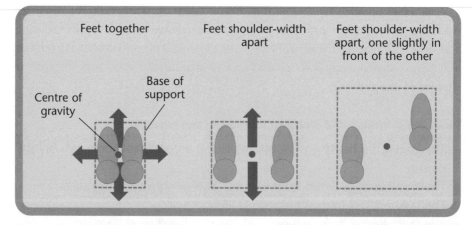

Figure 9.2 ● Positioning of feet to provide a stable base: identifying base of support and centre of gravity

It also provides a sound base and positioning to enhance weight transfer, when 'pushing or pulling', in a safe, assessed manner within a manoeuvre. This weight transfer from one foot to the other allows you to use your body weight to produce movement, rather than the strength in your arms (Figure 9.3).

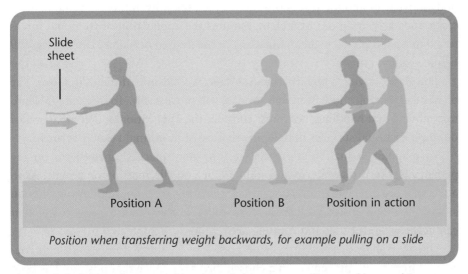

Slide sheet

Position A   Position B   Position in action

Position when transferring weight backwards, for example pulling on a slide

Figure 9.3 ● Transference of body weight when pulling and/or pushing

Leverage: muscles, joints, group actions and lever systems

Muscles, along with an insertion (generally distally located) and origin (generally proximally located) in bones, are used to create the required action that will produce a range of movement (ROM) that can be created from that joint.

Joints allow a ROM that is specific for their design. The elbow, a hinge joint, allows flexion and extension by the use of muscle group action. No one muscle can function alone, it must be accompanied by another to recreate the initial position of the joint. Flexion of the elbow is created by the contraction of the biceps (prime mover or agonist) and relaxation of the triceps (antagonist), and extension by reversal of these forces and roles. The movement must also be 'fixed' and stabilised to prevent undesirable movement, these muscles are called 'fixators'. This working relationship between muscle and bone most often produces actions and movement that involve leverage and lever systems (see Marieb, 2004, p. 325).

In your body, a 'fulcrum' is produced within the joint, your bones act as levers and muscle contraction provides the effort at the insertion point on the bone. The load is the bone, along with overlying tissue and any other load you are trying to move (Marieb, 2004, pp. 326–7). When carrying a coffee cup, this becomes a load along with the bones of the hand, wrist, forearm and surrounding tissue. The elbow joint becomes the fulcrum, and the effort is provided by the biceps (see Marieb, 2004, pp. 326–30).

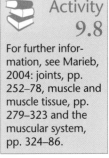

Activity
9.8

For further information, see Marieb, 2004: joints, pp. 252–78, muscle and muscle tissue, pp. 279–323 and the muscular system, pp. 324–86.

Friction: types and use

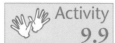

Activity 9.9

Place an eraser on your desk or work surface, next to it place an opened carrier bag. It is obvious which one will move easier, but why? How can the principles of frictional forces be applied to aid safe moving and handling?

Types and use of friction must be considered to aid the effectiveness of normal body movement and the forces produced by muscles. Even the most mundane of tasks, such as getting out of a chair, requires the application of frictional forces to aid normal body movement and assist in the desired outcome. Do Activity 9.9 before reading on.

The eraser, having a high frictional surface, will be more difficult to move. The plastic bag, having a low frictional surface, will move easily. To integrate this into safe moving and handling, one must consider the application and comparison of differing frictional surfaces in daily life that assist in normal body movement.

To maintain a high friction surface, one may place slippers/shoes on the patient's feet to promote grip and stability, or non-slip matting on a mattress to aid foot purchase when adjusting their position. To encourage a low friction surface, one may insert a 'slide sheet' to decrease frictional/shearing forces that can occur when turning and rotating are required.

One-way slide sheets will provide both low frictional forces and high frictional forces to aid movement in a chosen direction. Once that position has been reached, the material used to provide the low friction surface (now moved in the opposite direction) produces a high frictional surface. The material used is similar to corduroy. If you run your hands across the length of the corduroy strands, they appear smooth to the touch, but run your hands in the opposite direction and the material's make-up alters and the feel is different. When the material's surfaces are placed together, this alteration in make-up allows the surfaces to run smoothly in one direction and lock in the other.

Terminology of movement

As discussed previously, movement at joints can be wide and varied. It is imperative that you are aware of the potential ROM and positioning of each of the available joints. This terminology is vital to enhance interprofessional communication, both verbal (that is, handovers) and written (that is, medical notes) (see Marieb, 2004, pp. 259–63), and also shows an awareness of effective client communication and understanding, when used correctly and appropriately.

Communication

An enhanced awareness and understanding of normal body movement and its integration into safe moving and handling will provide you with a sound base to build upon when communicating instructions to your client and/or colleagues. To assess what the client is able to do for themselves, you will be required to 'talk clients through a manoeuvre' using verbalisation and demonstration. But without a holistic awareness and analysis of how you would normally carry out a manoeuvre and safe alternatives, nurses often run out of ideas and unsuccessfully assist/lift the client into position.

You should use clear and appropriate communication techniques and terminology. Demonstrate what is required of patients if they are unclear about what they are required to do. Ensure that what you require the client to do is explained fully and broken down into achievable goals. Praise them and ensure that at every stage they are well and willing to continue.

Conclusion to moving and handling

When assessing the patient's ability or assisting in any manoeuvre, the priority is to encourage and promote independent, normal body movement whenever possible, however insignificant it may at first appear. Every time the patient is distracted from participating in an independent task, or a task is carried out for them when not necessary, the patient's rehabilitation is being affected. Without the patient's involvement, muscle groups, joints and so on will ultimately weaken and reduce potential mobility, compounding underlying conditions, such as diabetes, and affect the delicate balance of the body systems – cardiac, respiratory, integumentory, gastrointestinal and so on.

Safe and appropriate moving and handling strategies should be taken into consideration when formulating the patient's risk assessment. These recommended strategies are designed to promotion the achievable level of independence and discourage the promotion of dependence.

In essence, the assessment should be graduated and build upon acquired knowledge and be conducted in a safe and conducive environment. Whenever possible, education, demonstration and training would take place prior to the manoeuvre; however, this is not always achievable. Ensure that the task in its entirety has been explained to the patient and then break it down into achievable goals/task. Throughout the task, and at the end of each stage, ensure that the patient is well and is not suffering from any ill effects of the manoeuvre. Also encourage and praise the patient's contribution and obvious effort.

To ensure that this moving and handling task is assessed correctly and graduated, a list of moving and handling questions (MHQs) (Chart 9.6) have been designed to:

- Promote the safety of you, your colleagues, your patient and their relatives
- Promote the application of safe moving and handling techniques
- Demonstrate and apply normal body movement to encourage independence
- Advocate the continual risk assessment of the task

- Prevent controversial techniques occurring
- Guide a logical and sequential process.

Chart 9.6 ● Moving and handling questions (MHQs)

1. What is normal body movement for the task?
2. Can I teach the patient to do this unaided?
   - If yes, how would this be achieved: verbal/non-verbal, demonstration, written?
   - If no, move to Q3.
3. If not completely unaided, is there equipment available that would mean the patient could do this for him or herself, for example Jacobs ladder, bed lever, bed blocks, slide sheets, profiling bed and so on?
   - If yes, how would this be achieved?
   - If no, move to Q4.
4. If unable to perform the task themselves, what is the minimum of assistance one and then two people can give (a) without equipment and (b) with equipment?
5. Are there unsafe ways of doing this I must avoid? If so, what are they?

Note: It is strongly recommended that you practise these processes under strict supervision until you are deemed safe and/or competent.
Source: Questions designed by April Brooks (School of Health Professions and Rehabilitation Sciences, Southampton University).

The introduction of equipment to enhance the patient's independence and reduce the risk of injury is governed by the Manual Handling Operations Regulations (HSE, 2003a), which state that employees should 'make full use of appropriate equipment and apply good handling techniques' – this equipment may range from hand blocks (bed blocks) to ceiling track hoists.

Casebox 9.1

Mr Patel, a 72-year-old man, has been admitted to your ward with right-sided paralysis and is unable to move his right arm and leg. He is conscious and aware of his admission but is unable to undertake any activities for himself. He weighs 80 kg (13 stone) and has also been suffering from urinary incontinence. He has been placed in a side room that has its own toilet facilities but reduced working space. Undertake a risk assessment of the above scenario and discuss your findings with your manual handling coordinator.

What would you do if the nurse you were working with asked you to lift this patient manually rather than use the appropriate equipment?

■ Assessment should ascertain whether there is likely to be any risk of injury. A more detailed assessment will consider the task involved, the load, the environment and individual capability.

■ In this case, you should politely refuse to lift Mr Patel, referring to the Manual Handling Operations Regulations

(HSE, 1998b). An alternative method of moving the patient should be employed.

■ Chapter Summary

This chapter has discussed the effects of immobility on patients/clients and demonstrated the holistic aspect of care required when assessing the patient/client. It has also identified the need for safe moving and handling and discussed the need for a good risk assessment prior to any application of this aspect of care.

Test Yourself!

1. What are the effects of immobility on each of the body's systems?

2. Describe the link between immobility and the pathophysiology of deep vein thrombosis.

3. If prolonged, unrelieved pressure is applied to any of the following – sacrum, shoulders, heels, elbows and hips – what could happen to the surrounding tissues?

4. Who has legal responsibility for moving and handling?

5. What does ELIOT stand for?

6. What is the status of a risk assessment (or individual patient handling profile)?

■ Further Reading

Disability Rights Commission (2005) *Disability Discrimination Act 1995.* http://www.drc-gb.org/thelaw/thedda.asp.

Health and Safety Commission (2000) *Key Fact Sheet on Injuries within Residential Care Homes Reported to Local Authorities 1994/95 to 1998/99.* http://www.hse.gov.uk/statistics/industry/rescar.pdf.

Health and Safety Commission (2004) *Management of Health and Safety at Work Regulations 1999: Approved Code of Practice and Guidance.* HSE, Norwich. HMSO Crown copyright.

Health and Safety Executive (2003) *Five Steps to Risk Assessment.* HSE, Norwich. HMSO Crown copyright. http://www.hse.gov.uk/pubns/indg163.pdf.

Health and Safety Executive (2004) *A Guide to Risk Assessment Requirements: Common Provisions in Health and Safety Law.* HSE, Norwich. HMSO Crown copyright. http://www.hse.gov.uk/pubns/indg218.pdf.

Royal College of Nursing (2002) *Working Well Initiative: RCN Code of Practice for Patient Handling.* RCN Publications, London. http://www.rcn.org.uk/publications/pdf/code-practice-patient-handling.pdf.

Tyldesley, B. and Grieve, J.I. (1996) *Muscle, Nerves and Movement: Kinesiology in Daily Living*, 2nd edn. Blackwell Science, London.

References

Alexander, M.F., Fawcett, J.N. and Runciman, P.J. (2006) *Nursing Practice Hospital and Home.* Churchill Livingstone, London.

BackCare (1999) *Safer Handling of People in the Community.* National Back Pain Association, Teddington.

BackCare/Royal College of Nursing/National Back Exchange (2005) *The Guide to the Handling of Patients: Introducing a Safer Handling Policy*, 5th edn. National Back Pain Association, Teddington.

Bancroft, J. (1983) *Human Sexuality and its Problems.* Churchill Livingstone, Edinburgh.

Bannister, C. (1996) Learning not to lift. *Nursing Standard* **10**(46): 34–5.

Bell, F. (1987) Ergonomics aspects of equipment. *International Journal of Nursing Studies* **24**(4): 331–7. Cited in Moody, J. and Tigar, F. (1996) A study of nurses' attitudes towards mechanical aids. *Nursing Standard* **11**(4): 37–42.

Burman, P. (1993) Using pressure measurements to evaluate different technologies. *Decubitus* **6**(3); 38–42.

Chokroverty, S. (1999) *Sleep Disorders Medicine: Basic Science, Technical Considerations and Clinical Aspects*, 2nd edn. Butterworth-Heinemann, Boston, MA.

Coleridge-Smith, P.D., Hasty, J.H. and Scurr, J.H. (1991) Deep vein thrombosis: effect of graduated compression stockings on the deep veins of the calf. *British Journal of Surgery* **78**: 724–6.

Department for Constitutional Affairs: Justice, Rights and Democracy (2002) *Human Rights Come to Life: Study Guide – Human Rights Act 1998*, 2nd edn. Crown Copyright. http://www.dca.gov.uk/hract/studyguide/.

De Wit, S.C. (2001) *Fundamental Concepts and Skills for Nursing.* WB Saunders, Philadelphia.

DoH (Department of Health) (2003) *Implementing the NSF for Older People Falls Standard – Support for Commissioning Good Services.* Stationery Office, London.

DoH (Department of Health) (2004) *Choosing Health: Making Healthier Choices Easier.* Stationery Office, London.

Egger, G., Champion, N. and Bolton, A. (2004) *The Fitness Leader's Handbook*, 4th edn. A&C Black, London.

Fraser, M. (1996) *Using Conceptual Nursing in Practice: a Research-based Approach*, 2nd edn. Harper & Row, London.

Health and Safety at Work Act (1974) *Health and Safety Homepages. Professional Health and Safety Consultants Ltd.* http://www.healthandsafety.co.uk/haswa.htm.

HSC (Health and Safety Commission) (2002) *A Guide to the Reporting of Injuries, Diseases and Dangerous Occurrences Regulations (RIDDOR) (1995).* HSE, Norwich. HMSO Crown copyright.

HSC (Health and Safety Commission) (2004) *Comprehensive Injury Statistics in Support of the Revitalising Health and Safety Programmes: Health Service.* HSE, Norwich. HMSO Crown copyright. http://www.hse.gov.uk/statistics/pdf/rhshlth.pdf.

HSE (Health and Safety Executive) (1998) *Self-reported Work-related Illness in 1995: Results from a Household Survey.* HSE, Norwich. HMSO Crown copyright. http://www.hse.gov.uk/statistics/2002/swi95.pdf.

HSE (Health and Safety Executive) (1999) *Provision and Use of Work Equipment Regulations 1998 (PUWER): Open Learning Guidance.* HSE, Norwich. HMSO Crown copyright.

HSE (Health and Safety Executive) (2000) *Information Sheet: 4/00/EMSU Secondary Analysis of the 1995 Self-reported Work-related Illness Survey* (SW195). HSE, Norwich. HMSO Crown copyright. http://www.hse.gov.uk/statistics/2002/secan95.pdf.

HSE (Health and Safety Executive) (2002) *Lifting Operations and Lifting Equipment Regulations 1998 (LOLER): Safe Use of Lifting Equipment. Approved Code of Practice and Guidance.* HSE, Norwich. HMSO Crown copyright.

HSE (Health and Safety Executive) (2003a) *Manual Handling: Manual Handling Operations Regulations (1992) Guidance on Regulations.* HSE, Norwich. HMSO Crown copyright.

HSE (Health and Safety Executive) (2003b) *Understanding Ergonomics at Work: Reduce Accidents and Ill Health and Increase Productivity by Fitting the Task to the Worker.* HSE, Norwich. HMSO Crown copyright. http://www.hse.gov.uk/pubns/indg90.pdf.

HSE (Health and Safety Executive) (2004) *Getting to Grips with Manual Handling: A Short Guide.* HSE, Norwich. HMSO Crown copyright. http://www.hse.gov.uk/pubns/indg143.pdf.

HSE (Health and Safety Executive) (2005) *Health Services.* http://www.hse.gov.uk/healthservices/index.htm.

Holland, K., Jenkins, J., Soloman, J. and Whittam, S. (eds) (2003) *Applying the Roper-Logan-Tierney Model in Practice.* Churchill Livingstone, London.

Kidd, R. (1995) Raising awareness. *Nursing Times* **91**(31): 20–1.

Lewin, R. (1999) *Human Evolution: An Illustrated Introduction.* Blackwell Scientific, London.

Livesley, B. (1992) Aetiology of pressure sores – pressure. Proceedings of the tissue viability conference in Bath. Cited in Walsh, M. (ed.) (2002) *Watson's Clinical Nursing and Related Sciences*. Baillière Tindall, London.

Love, C. (1996) Injury caused by lifting: A study of the nurses' viewpoint. *Nursing Standard* **10**(46): 34–9.

Lower, J. and Bonsack, C. (2002) High-tech, high-touch: mission possible? Creating an environment for healing. *Dimensions of Critical Care Nursing* **21**(5): 201–5.

Malik, M., Hall, C. and Howard, D. (1998) *Nursing Knowledge and Practice: A Decision-making Approach*. Ballière Tindall/RCN, London.

Marieb, H. (2004) *Human Anatomy and Physiology,* 6th edn. Benjamin Cummings Pearson, London.

McGuire, T. and Dewar, B. J. (1995) An assessment of moving and handling practices amongst Scottish nurses. *Nursing Standard* **9**(40); 35–9.

Mitchell, J.R.A. (1984) Is nursing any business of doctors? A simple guide to the nursing process. *British Medical Journal* **288**: 216–19.

Newton, C. (1991) *The Roper-Logan-Tierney Model in Action*. Macmillan – now Palgrave Macmillan, Basingstoke.

Newton, V. (1996) Care in pre-admission clinics. *Nursing Times* **92**(1): 27–8.

Norton, D. (1970) *By Accident or Design: A Study of Equipment Development in Relation to Basic Nursing Problems*. E & S Livingston, Edinburgh.

NMC (Nursing and Midwifery Council) (2005) Protecting the public through professional standards. http://www.nmc-uk.org/(e3wrbrbndj4e1f450e0h1j45)/aDefault.aspx.

Redeker, N. and Hedges, C. (2002) Sleep during hospitalisation and recovery after cardiac surgery. *Journal of Cardiovascular Nursing* **17**(1): 56–8.

Refshauge, K. and Gass, E. (eds) (1995) *Musculoskeletal Physiotherapy: Clinical Science and Practice*. Butterworth-Heinemann, Oxford.

Retsas, A. and Pinikahana, J. (2000) Manual handling activities and injuries among nurses: an Australian hospital study. *Journal of Advanced Nursing* **31**(4): 875–83.

Roper, N., Logan, W. and Tierney, A. (2000) *The Roper-Logan-Tierney Model of Nursing Based on Activities of Living*. Churchill Livingstone, Edinburgh.

RCN (Royal College of Nursing) (2003) *Working Well Initiative: RCN Guide for Manual Handling Assessments in Hospital and the Community*. RCN Publications, London. http://www.rcn.org.uk/publications/pdf/Manual_Handling_Assessment.pdf.

Sander, R. (1999) Promoting urinary continence in residential care. *Nursing Standard* **14**(13): 49–53.

Tortora, G. and Grabowski, S. (2003) *Principles of Anatomy and Physiology*, 10th edn. John Wiley & Sons, New York.

Uglow, J. and Dewing, J. (2004) Introducing a physical activity group on an intermediate care ward. *Nursing Older People* **16**(6): 19–22.

Venning, P.L. (1988) Back pain prevention amongst nursing personnel. *AAOHN Journal* **36**(8): 327–32.

Walsh, M. (1991) *Models in Clinical Nursing: The Way Forward*. Baillière Tindall, London.

Walsh, M. (ed.) (2002) *Watson's Clinical Nursing and Related Sciences*. Baillière Tindall, London.

Zindani, J.H. (1998) *Personal Injury in Practice – Manual Handling: Law and Legislation*. CLT Professional Publishing, Birmingham.

■ Useful Websites

www.nelh.nhs.uk National Electronic Library for Health Programme
Works with NHS Libraries to develop a digital library for NHS staff, patients and the public

www.hse.gov.uk Health and Safety Executive
An enforcing authority working in support of the Healthcare Commission

www.drc-gb.org Disability Rights Commission

www.rcn.org.uk The Royal College of Nursing
Represents nurses and nursing, promotes excellence in practice and shapes health policies

PHIL RUSSELL

10 Dying, Death and Spirituality

Contents

- Awareness of Death
- Health Promotion and Dying
- The Concept of Pain and Symptom Control
- Last Offices
- Bereavement

- Spirituality
- Chapter Summary
- Test Yourself!
- Further Reading
- References

Learning Outcomes

This chapter is concerned with dying, death and loss. It will introduce you to the concept of death and begin to examine some of the principal aspects of palliative care. At the end of the chapter, you should be able to:

- Reflect on the nature of death in today's society
- Discuss the concept of death
- Explore how and when people die
- Identify the key principles of palliative care
- Discuss the principles of pain and symptom control
- Reflect on the nature of communication with patients who are dying and their relatives
- Identify the measures required in caring for a body after death
- Consider your role in bereavement
- Reflect on the spiritual nature of human beings and its importance in health care.

For most of us, death seems a long way off. We hopefully enjoy our lives and are more interested in living life to the full than worrying about dying. Wilson (1975) suggests that man cannot live to the full until he has confronted death, and although this may be true, it might also be argued that with today's healthy lifestyles and an expectation of life until well into our eighties, there is no reason to concern ourselves with death. Whatever the truth of these arguments, as a nurse you have chosen to enter a profession in which you will inevitably be confronted by death. You therefore need to be able to care not only for people who are dying, but also for their relatives through this process and beyond as they are confronted by grief and bereavement and perhaps having to learn to live alone. In addition, there is a need to care for yourself and your colleagues. After all, we are dealing with one of the most powerful and emotional periods of life – the transition from the living, known world to the unknown world of death.

A word of caution here: some of the discussions and exercises in this chapter may be distressing if you have recently been bereaved or have someone close to you who is dying. Feel free to miss out this chapter and revisit it when you feel the time is right for you.

■ Awareness of Death

> Surely our attitudes to death and to life would be less riddled with fears and anxiety, if we recognised death and talked and taught about it as part of normal human experience. (Collick, 1986)

Perhaps you have not given death very much thought, or perhaps you have experienced death in your life and it has loomed large in your thoughts. Whichever is true, you are encouraged here to think about how death is viewed by society today.

It is suggested that we live in a death-denying society. In other words, even in the face of the obvious, we find it difficult to accept that we will one day die. We rarely discuss the subject and, for many, death takes place hidden away in institutions such as hospitals, hospices and nursing homes. It might be argued that this blind spot occurs partly because very often we have no need to think about death. For most of us, longevity has become the norm and we can be optimistic about achieving our three-score years and ten. Modern science and better health care could, it is suggested, leave us with a life span of up to 120 years. So, if this is the case, why should we concern ourselves with a far-off event? Nevertheless, the knowledge that we will one day die always lurks in the background. Death may face us at any time of life, sometimes suddenly and unexpectedly, sometimes creeping slowly upon us:

This existence of ours is as transient as autumn clouds.
To watch the birth and death of beings is like looking at
    the movements of a dance.
A lifetime is like a flash of lightening in the sky,
Rushing by, like a torrent down a steep mountain.

                                        (The Buddha, in Rinpoche, 1992)

Although most people recognise the inevitability of death, to a large extent it is kept in the shadows. Death rattles away at the edge of our awareness (Yalom, 1980), and in modern Western society we have fewer and fewer reminders that we will one day be faced by the reality of death. The emergence of a life-limiting disease can, however, awaken hidden fears that have lain only in the shadow of our awareness. Society's death-denying approach, in which dying is hidden away in institutions, death is rarely talked about and funeral rituals and mourning have become minimised, has little power over keeping death at bay (Aries, 1981). As Morgan (1995) comments, 'death refuses to die' – death can strike at any moment and we may be very unprepared for it:

When you are strong and healthy,
You never think of sickness coming,
But it descends with sudden force
Like a stroke of lightning.
When involved in worldly things,
You never think of death's approach;
Quick it comes like thunder
Crashing round your head. (Milarepa, in Rinpoche, 1992)

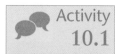

Activity 10.1

Think of some of the losses in your life. Don't think just of deaths but of all sorts of loss, such as the loss of security the first time you went to school, or when a brother or sister first left home. What effect did these losses have on you? What did you do to cope?

Sogyal Rinpoche (1992) suggests that, deep down, we know we cannot avoid facing death forever and that the more we can accept the impermanence of life, the greater freedom we can find in living. It is up to you to decide how far you will explore your own personal living and dying, but you might wish to consider this advice by La Rochefoucauld (in Walter, 1990): 'Death and the sun are not to be looked at steadily', but 'As with the sun, so with death: without staring at it, the wise person lives in its light'. Whatever your personal explorations involve, you have chosen a profession in which you will inevitably be faced with people who are dying and people who are bereaved. Although many people in society never have to face death until middle age or beyond, you will inevitably have to confront it. As Collick (1986) suggests, 'death is a crisis for the dying and for the living for which both are usually wholly unprepared'. A large part of understanding death and dying is achieved by learning through experience rather than being taught, and you might like to start this process by reflecting on some of the losses in your life.

Where and how people die

There is evidence to suggest that most people would prefer to die in their own home (Townsend et al., 1990; NICE, 2004), yet most people still die in an institutional setting. Table 10.1 shows that a significant number of people, whether or not their condition is cancer related, die in NHS hospitals. It is also evident that a considerable number of people with non-cancer-related conditions die in nursing and residential homes. Despite this, many people do spend much of their last year of life in their own home but are admitted when their condition worsens and their families feel that they are no longer able to cope (Barclay, 2001). This clearly has implications for how care is provided and where resources are needed.

Table 10.1 Place of death for cancer and non-cancer patients

	Cancer (%)	Non-cancer (%)
NHS hospitals	48.3	55.0
Voluntary hospices	13.3	0.2
Psychiatric hospitals	0.3	1.0
Own home	25.8	19.9
Nursing home	7.3	10.9
Residential home	3.6	9.6
Other home/places	1.6	3.4

Source: ONS (1997) England and Wales.

A framework has been developed to better enable people to die at home if that is their place of choice. This is known as The Gold Standard Framework and was developed by Dr Keri Thomas, adopted by Macmillan Cancer Relief and endorsed by the NHS. The framework was successfully piloted in over 76 GP practices and is now being adopted by many practices across the country. The seven key Gold Standards that underpin the framework are:

1. Communication.
2. Coordination.
3. Control of symptoms.
4. Continuity – out of hours.
5. Continued learning.
6. Carer support
7. Care in the dying phase.

The object is to set up an easy-to-use and cost-effective system that clearly identifies those in the community with palliative care needs. Where this is done, a coordinated multidisciplinary care package can be put in place to care for the patient and the family. In particular, this enables the needs of the patient and family to be met out of hours. In the last days of life, when it can be particularly difficult for the family, measures such as the the Liverpool Integrated Care Pathway for the Dying Patient can be initiated (Ellershaw and Wilkinson, 2003). This is discussed later in this chapter under the section 'In the last days of life'.

People, of course, do die at all ages and from a variety of causes, including suddenly from illness and accidents. In addition, although much of the literature on caring for the dying focuses on people dying from cancer, the main causes of death in England and Wales continue to be diseases of the circulatory systems such as heart attacks and stroke.

It is also useful to reflect on the age at which people die. Mortality tends to be high during the first year of life, decreasing during childhood and then gradually rising with age from 15 years onwards (Victor, 2000). However, unless you are a midwife or a children's nurse, the majority of people you care for will be 65 years or older and dying from a wide range of conditions, of which the cancers comprise just one specific collection of conditions. Table 10.2 shows the mean age of death from selected causes.

Table 10.2 Mean age at death from selected causes, by sex

Cause	Mean age at death	
	Male	Female
All	71.9	78.2
Stomach cancer	71.9	76.6
Colon cancer	71.5	75.7
Lung cancer	71.1	71.5
Skin cancer	62.0	66.4
Female breast cancer	–	68.9
Cervix cancer	–	62.5
Prostate cancer	77.6	–
Leukaemia	67.0	69.9
Diabetes	72.9	77.8
Ischaemic heart disease	73.2	80.1
Stroke	76.9	82.0
Bronchitis, emphysema and asthma	73.1	74.6
Liver disease	56.9	60.9
Injury and poisoning	46.5	63.9
Car accidents	38.8	49.1
Suicide/self-inflicted	43.9	50.1

Source: ONS (1997) England and Wales.

Activity
10.2

Look at Table 10.2. What are the main causes of death for people under the age of 65? Work out the average age for men and for women for all causes of death. What does the table tell you about life expectancy for men and women?

Having considered how and where people die, it is useful to consider what we mean by dying and how we define someone as being dead.

When am I dead?

If nurses are to care for people who are dying in a way that is positive, it is important to recognise that we are alive until we are dead, and that we should have the opportunity, should we choose, to live to our full potential. Life exists on a continuum from conception to death. During this time, our health varies and is affected by many factors in our internal body environment and by external influences. Despite efforts to deny death and preserve life, death continues to be the inevitable earthly end and the last stage of life.

This end point of life that we call being dead is not as easily defined as one imagines. The common understanding of death is the absence of vital signs, that is, a cessation of breathing, a lack of a palpable heart beat and fixed, dilated pupils. In most cases of expected death, these remain the usual criteria, but the situation has been complicated by modern technology, which allows people to be kept alive on life-support machines. Establishing the exact moment of death in such circumstances requires different criteria, such as brain death tests, to cope with this technologically supported extension to life (Veatch, 1995). Furthermore, although most Western societies try to make a clear distinction between being alive and being dead, some societies have a much wider differentiation. Some such societies consider the person to be alive for a considerable period after most Western cultures would regard them as dead, while other cultures grieve for people as if they were dead in a way that most Western societies would hold to be inappropriate, because the person would still be considered to be alive (Rosenblatt, 1997). But have you ever heard anyone in our own society say, 'For me she died a long time ago; now there is just an empty shell?' Perhaps in some circumstances we too have different definitions of death.

Whichever way we look at death, dying has no easily definable point. When does light become dark, and when does day become night? These are arbitrary and man-made divisions. We are all dying until we reach that ill-defined point we call death, or, to put in a more positive way, life continues until a decision is made that we have reached that end point we call death.

When am I dying?

Understanding the point at which someone is defined as dying is itself a grey area. Davis et al. (1996) emphasise that a diagnosis alone is not enough. Someone, whether it is the patient, a carer or the medical staff, needs to reach a position at which they accept the condition as being terminal. Nevertheless, dying and being in a terminal condition are not necessarily the same thing. A prognosis suggesting that there is no obvious curative treatment does not mean that the person does not have much active living to do, and even the terminal phase will differ from person to person. The whole process of dying may take various directions and shapes. Death may be sudden or lingering, expected or unexpected; it may progress slowly and then take a sudden downturn, or the process may move up and down before finally declining to death (Glaser and Strauss, 1968). For some, there may be little opportunity to reflect on the process, but many others have the opportunity for living fully right up until the moment of death. Although dying is a time of crisis, it can also be a time of opportunity for change and positive growth (Yalom, 1980).

The point of this discussion is that if we are to care for people who are dying, we first need to acknowledge that there are many grey areas: just as the person who is dying is facing uncertainty, nurses too sometimes have to face ambiguity and uncertainty. It is important, however, to focus on the fact that people are living until they are dead and that they deserve the highest quality of life that is attainable. One positive way at looking at this is to view care of the dying from a health promotion perspective.

■ Health Promotion and Dying

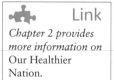

Link

Chapter 2 provides more information on Our Healthier Nation.

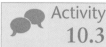

Activity 10.3

Imagine you are asked to look after a 67-year-old woman who is in the terminal stages of an illness. What would be your main concerns over how to care for her?

The concepts of health and death rarely fit comfortably together, yet if life exists until death, 'health for all' must include all people from birth up to the end of life. The White Paper *Our Healthier Nation* (DoH, 1999) is targeted at helping people to achieve healthier, more fulfilling lives. Although it makes no reference to care of the dying, it might be hoped that some aspects of the White Paper would be interpreted and acted upon within the scope of those who are defined as dying. Good health is described by the White Paper as requiring a confident and positive outlook and being able to cope with the ups and downs of life. Health is not just about how long people live but about quality of life, ensuring that they are not robbed of dignity and independence; it is equally important to all people, whatever their clinical health status.

Seedhouse (1997) emphasises the importance of allowing people to achieve their maximum potential for health whatever their starting point. This health-promoting perspective thus allows a more positive view of the dying process. It is also a view that gives patients a choice. How they choose to do their dying may be very different from how we might choose to do ours, but their decision should always be respected. This perspective on death and dying fits well with the philosophy of caring for the dying usually referred to as 'palliative care'.

Definitions of palliative care

Palliative care is the term used to refer to the care of patients whose condition is not amenable to curative treatment. Such conditions invariably lead to the person's death, but the length of time involved is extremely variable. The World Health Organization (2005a) defines palliative care as:

palliative care
care provided to people whose condition is no longer amenable to curative treatment

> an approach that improves the quality of life of patients and their families facing the problem associated with life-threatening illness, through the prevention and relief of suffering by means of early identification and impeccable assessment and treatment of pain and other problems, physical, psychosocial and spiritual. Palliative care:

- provides relief from pain and other distressing symptoms
- affirms life and regards dying as a normal process
- intends neither to hasten nor postpone death
- integrates the psychological and spiritual aspects of patient care
- offers a support system to help patients live as actively as possible until death
- offers a support system to help the family cope during the patient's illness and in their own bereavement
- uses a team approach to address the needs of patients and their families, including bereavement counselling, if indicated
- will enhance quality of life, and may also positively influence the course of illness
- is applicable early in the course of illness, in conjunction with other therapies that are intended to prolong life, such as chemotherapy or radiation therapy, and includes those investigations needed to better understand and manage distressing clinical complications.

The term **terminal illness** tends to hold highly negative connotations and can lead to patients receiving appropriate care far too late in their condition, whereas palliative care can and should start at the time of diagnosis, in some cases several years before the person reaches the terminal stages of the illness.

terminal illness
refers to a prognosis suggesting that there is no obvious curative treatment. 'Terminal care' is the term reserved for the care provided to patients in the last days, weeks or sometimes months of their life

The growth of modern palliative care grew out of the work of Dame Cicely Saunders who opened St Christopher's Hospice in Sydenham in 1967. A former nurse, she moved into the world of medical social work before finally training as a doctor. Through her work, she became very conscious of the poor care and distress of patients who were dying. Her vision was for people to die free of pain and that they should be enabled to live until they died, supported by skilled carers and with their physical, psychological, spiritual and social needs addressed. Dame Cicely Saunders caught the imagination of the country and the world and, by the year 2001, over 93 countries throughout the world had initiated hospice and palliative care interventions (Hospice Information Service, 2001).

Palliative care has now become a speciality in its own right, initially emerging through the work of the **hospice** movement, but now provided in a variety of settings, including hospices. These may be independent voluntary or fall within the NHS. Many hospices also have a day unit, providing a range of facilities from symptom control to counselling and complementary therapies.

Palliative care may also be offered in the home, supported by the primary care team, and may involve a Macmillan nurse. Macmillan nurses are invariably clinical nurse specialists funded by the organisation Macmillan Cancer Relief, and although they predominantly work in the community, some may be employed as part of the hospital palliative care team. In addition, Marie Curie nurses offer hands-on care to patients at home, usually spending their whole shift caring for one individual. These nurses are usually part-charity and part-NHS funded, and range from care assistants who have specialised in this area to highly trained palliative care nurses.

Hospital palliative care teams offer support and symptom control to patients in general hospital wards. This is often where palliative care begins, early intervention usually meaning better managed palliative care.

Whatever the setting, palliative care involves a number of specialised professionals including:

- Clinical nurse specialists in palliative care (often Macmillan nurses)
- Consultants in palliative medicine
- Social workers
- Clinical psychologists
- Other supporting professionals, such as physiotherapists, occupational therapists and in some cases complementary therapists.

One of the criticisms of palliative care has been its predominant focus on people with cancer, but although much has been learnt from the experience gained while caring for those with cancer, there is now a desire to make such expertise available in the care of people with other chronic diseases. There is also a considerable need to extend this expertise into nursing homes, where more and more people will end their lives (Komaromy et al., 2000). To this end, a **palliative care approach** is advocated in addition to specialist palliative care.

The aim is for the palliative care approach to become an integral part of all clinical practice whatever the illness or its stage (NHSE, 1996). So, for example, this would include not only patients with cancer, but also those with dementia, chronic heart disease, stoke and respiratory disorders, and those at the end of life in nursing homes. It is this notion of a palliative care approach that can be

---

hospice

voluntary or NHS-funded establishments where palliative care is provided. Hospices attempt to provide the best possible quality of life for the final stages of an illness. This includes family support and bereavement services

palliative care approach

a philosophy of care suggesting that all people with life-threatening illness should receive quality care and that this should be provided by all health-care professionals rather than just by specialist palliative care services

practised by all health-care professionals and supported by specialist palliative care teams. Like the definition of palliative care above, it is underpinned by key principles advocated by the NHSE (1996). These are:

- A focus on quality of life, including good symptom control
- A whole-person approach, taking into account the person's past life experience and current situation
- Care that encompasses both the person with the life-threatening disease and those who matter to that individual
- A respect for patient autonomy and choice, for example over place of care, treatment options and access to specialist palliative care
- An emphasis on open and sensitive communication, extending this to patients, informal carers and professional colleagues.

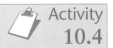

Activity 10.4

Think of each of the NHSE's key principles and make some notes about what they mean for nursing practice in caring for the dying.

This palliative care approach is very significant to the nurse because it acknowledges the importance of all nurses providing palliative care rather than this just being something left to specialists in the field.

One of the most important documents to influence the face of palliative care in recent years has been the National Institute for Clinical Excellence (NICE) document *Improving Supportive and Palliative Care for Adults with Cancer* (2004). This recognises that for some people their supportive and palliative care needs have not been met as adequately as might be hoped for. The importance of the patient and family being heard and being treated with respect is identified. It recognises that patients want to be involved in the decision-making process about their care and that face-to-face communication is important. It further notes that patients want well-coordinated services and expect quality symptom control and psychological, social and spiritual support. They want to be able to die in a place of their choosing – often their own home – and they want reassurance that their families will be supported through the illness and into bereavement (NICE, 2004, p. 5). The NICE guidance identifies 13 topic areas to tackle these issues and makes key recommendations for each area. The complete document or an executive summary can be viewed online at www.nice.org.uk.

The above discussion emphasises that palliative care is a team activity. It is not just about different team members doing their job but about working together jointly in the best interests of the patient and the family. For the moment, however, we will reflect on the role of the nurse within the team.

The nurse's role

The nurse's role in palliative care is about caring for the living, so it is primarily about providing high-quality nursing care. We will focus here on some of the important elements required to provide quality care to people facing death as a result of their illness, but first try to think about the sort of person you would like to care for you or a member of your family: what sort of person would they be and what sort of skills would you want them to have?

It is always difficult to pin down the specific skills required to be a good nurse, but Saunders (1978) offers some help in this when she talks of 'being with' people when they are suffering. It is as if we walk alongside them offering support as and when it is needed. Saunders identifies the characteristics required for this role:

non-judgemental

accepting the values of others

- Respect the identity and integrity of other human beings
- Be sensitive and **non-judgemental**
- Know when to listen and when to speak
- Have the knowledge and skills to intervene in a way that promotes the best quality of life as perceived by the patient.

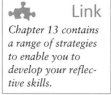

Link

Chapter 13 contains a range of strategies to enable you to develop your reflective skills.

The list may appear straightforward, but each item requires considerable skill and expertise. It is perhaps a skill that can be learnt only through experience, coupled with hard work on ourselves, through reflection, and a developing sense of self-awareness.

Davies and O'Berle (1990) also provide a useful framework that encapsulates those elements expressed by Saunders. The dimensions they describe in Figure 10.1 emerged from work interviewing patients and their families, and although the research reflects care delivered by specialist palliative care nurses, these dimensions are relevant to any nurse who subscribes to the palliative care approach.

Dimensions of care

The nurse–patient relationship

- Finding meaning
- Preserving integrity
- Connecting
- Doing for
- Empowering
- Valuing

Figure 10.1 ● Dimensions of care (adapted from Davies and O'Berle, 1990)

- *Valuing* – Valuing is very much a core element, and relates to respecting the person and being non-judgemental. These terms are part of the core conditions that Rogers felt were necessary for a therapeutic relationship

- *Connecting* – This relational aspect of caring becomes increasingly important in the care of the dying. It is through this that we connect with patients and their relatives. It is hard to describe what this actually means but it bears similarities to empathy. It is about listening, having a caring attitude that says 'You are important.' It means giving quality time to the person, even if this is only a couple of minutes.

- *Empowering* – One of the great anxieties facing people who are dying is losing control, which easily happens when vulnerable people are faced with powerful professionals and sometimes find themselves in a strange institutional environment. It is therefore important not to disempower people but to allow the person to care for themselves and make decisions for themselves as much as is possible. This can be difficult, particularly when you are faced with what might appear to you an irrational decision, such as refusing some form of treatment. It is at such times that the need to be non-judgemental, coupled with being supportive, becomes increasingly important

- *Finding meaning* – Facing death may be a daunting prospect and a time when people question why and what life has been about. They seek to sort out their life and the meaning it has for them and others around them. This is part of the spiritual aspect of our lives and will be dealt with more thoroughly later in the chapter

- *Doing for* – People who are dying often need a lot of physical care and emotional support; families too may feel inadequate and frightened. At such times, nurses may need to provide much of the care, including pain and symptom control. This may be carried out by an individual nurse but is supported by a team approach. There is an inherent danger here of taking over from the patient and relatives, so it is important in 'doing for' that this is carried out, whenever possible, in negotiation with the person and family to avoid disempowering them

- *Preserving integrity* – Caring for the dying can be a challenging experience, and it is important for nurses not to lose sight of their own self, their ability to maintain a positive view of themselves and their capacity to feel valued by themselves and others. This may mean reflecting on the care given and exploring the meaning of life and death. In maintaining integrity, it is important that the nurse has good support within and outside her professional arena. Becoming emotionally involved with and upset for someone who is dying is not a loss of integrity: it is quite normal sometimes to feel emotional turmoil, just as it is quite normal sometimes not to feel any emotional attachment. Loss of integrity comes about when these emotions incapacitate the nurse and there is a loss of self-esteem and self-worth, perhaps associated with guilt and inadequacy. At such times, it is important to seek help and support.

Link

Chapter 14 explores therapeutic relationships in more detail.

◼ The Concept of Pain and Symptom Control

🧩 **Link**

Pain assessment is described in Chapters 1 and 7.

Pain and symptom control is an important and specialist area when caring for the dying; a detailed, technical discussion will therefore be left to other texts to explore. Nevertheless, it is important to have an introduction to some of the concepts related to pain and pain management and the diversity of potentially unpleasant symptoms that need careful management in those who are dying.

Although not all patients with a life-limiting disease will experience pain, it remains one of the most feared symptoms (Clark, 1993). According to Faull et al. (1998), pain occurs in 75 per cent of patients with advanced cancer and 65 per cent of those dying from all other causes. Pain is not, however, a straightforward sensory experience but an inclusive one that is moderated by emotional, social and spiritual elements as well as physical influences. This is known as the 'concept of total pain'. We can usually tolerate quite intense pain if we know that it will go away and that it is not ultimately associated with our impending death. For individuals with a life-limiting disease, the pain is not only often chronic, but also a constant reminder that it is part of a disease process that will result in their death.

analgesics

pain-relieving drugs. An absence of pain is termed 'analgesia'

Pain is a highly personal and individual experience and as such requires detailed assessment and management that goes far beyond simply prescribing **analgesics**. As such, good pain management requires a considerable input from the nurse in terms of assessing the non-physical aspects of pain. But the physical aspects are important too. The WHO (2005b) advocates the use of a three-step analgesic ladder (Figure 10.2) when managing pain. This concept is basically simple and for most patients is effective in minimising their pain. It advises that medication should be:

Step 1: *by mouth* whenever possible
Step 2: *by the clock* (in other words, analgesia should be given at regular intervals, not just waiting until the pain is manifest)
Step 3: *by the ladder.*

non-opioid analgesics

analgesics such as paracetamol and non-steroidal anti-inflammatory drugs, for example aspirin

opioids

drugs such as morphine derived from the opium poppy; these are controlled drugs

Non-opioid analgesics for mild pain may include paracetamol; **opioids** for mild-to-moderate pain may include drugs such as dihydrocodeine; and opioids for severe pain may include morphine. You may wish to look these drugs up in your drugs handbook.

This method of pain control has been accepted worldwide as a valuable model. You are not expected to have a full grasp of its prescribing implications but instead to recognise that effective analgesia is available to patients. If the patient is to remain relatively pain-free, pain management should be started early and analgesics given regularly and reviewed regularly. With early intervention, most patients start at step 1, but it is perfectly acceptable to start at step 2. What is essential is to get the patient as pain-free as possible as quickly as possible, if that is what the patient wants.

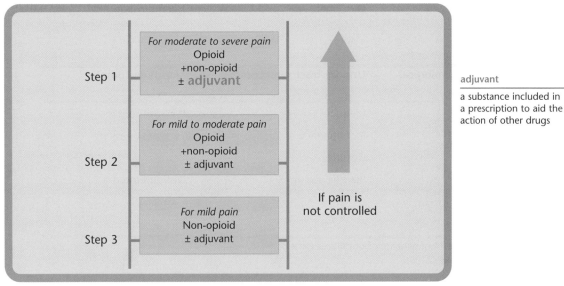

adjuvant

a substance included in a prescription to aid the action of other drugs

Figure 10.2 ● Three-step analgesic ladder (adapted from WHO, 2005b)

Other symptoms

Other distressing symptoms experienced by the patient are many and varied; some of these are shown in Table 10.3. According to Finlay (1995), the five most common symptoms are pain, weakness, constipation, nausea and vomiting, and dyspnoea. As with pain, a careful and comprehensive assessment of all symptoms is very important. What might be a minor irritation for a healthy individual can be a huge burden to a person approaching the end of their life, draining their energy, self-esteem and enjoyment of life, and leading to insomnia, fatigue and depression. Each additional symptom adds to the patient's total discomfort, yet with good nursing care many of the symptoms are treatable and/or avoidable. It is thus essential to assess thoroughly and regularly, and never dismiss any symptom of which the patient complains. Although some of the symptoms involved require specialist intervention, many can be managed by good quality nursing care, including caring therapeutic communication.

Table 10.3 Common distressing symptoms

Gastrointestinal symptoms	Respiratory symptoms	Cardiovascular symptoms
Dry mouth	Choking	Dehydration
Nausea and vomiting	Cough	Oedema
Constipation	Dyspnoea	Haemorrhage
Diarrhoea		
Anorexia		
Neurological and psychological symptoms	Urinary tract symptoms	Skin symptoms
Loss of concentration	Frequency	Pressure sore
Insomnia	Incontinence	Fungating lesions
Weakness and fatigue	Dysuria	Pruritis
Anxiety and fear	Bladder spasm	Disfigurement
Depression/sadness		
Confusion		

Note: This is not a definitive list of symptoms but outlines some of those commonly encountered.
Source: Adapted from Cooke (2000).

Communication

What is special about communication when caring for the dying? Maybe nothing. However, NICE (2004) identifies face-to-face communication as one of the key topic areas and suggests it is fundamental to good quality palliative care, yet is is often reported by patients and carers as being poor. What do you say to someone who is facing death? How do you respond to the relatives and friends? Perhaps part of the difficulty lies in our deep-rooted fears of death, referred to earlier in the chapter. Because these fears lie essentially in our subconscious, we may not even be aware of their existence. There are, however, other, more overt fears that may get in the way of open communication. Buckman (1998) identifies the following fears commonly encountered in health-care professionals:

● There is a fear of the pain we feel because of patients' and relatives' distress. Sometimes we almost hurt for them
● We fear being blamed by patients for their condition and ultimate death, as if it were our fault. This blaming does sometimes happen as patients and relatives struggle to understand why nothing can be done to cure them. Nursing and medical staff also struggle with how to manage a condition that is not amenable to treatment

- We fear not knowing what to say because we have never been taught what to say. Indeed, talking about dying is not like other clinical procedures: although you can have guidelines, there is no script for the right thing to say. But if we always wait for the right thing to say, we may end up with nothing being said, a common scenario. With the right intent and a little courage, we will gain experience and become more confident in effective therapeutic communication

- In a similar way, our desire always to have the right answer can make it difficult for us to say, 'I don't know.' Yet we may have many unanswered questions, and trying to flannel with patients and relatives will only lead to mistrust. An honest 'I don't know' can lead to a more open communication and a developing trust between the patient and the health professional

- Talking to patients and relatives can sometimes result in their giving an emotional reaction. This can lead to fears of how to manage this reaction and how to manage other staff members who may feel that you have 'upset' the patient. Nevertheless, discussing life and death issues is upsetting and we need to be prepared for a whole variety of possible reactions and learn how best to manage them

- Many people have fears about their own death. Some of these lie in the person's awareness and some may be subconsciously held. Health-care professionals are regularly confronted by death, however, so it is more difficult for them push such fears aside and out of their thoughts

- Some nurses wonder how much they should express their feelings, and fear that to do so would be unprofessional. Although it is important to remain in control of the situation, it is rare for patients or relatives to see emotion as unprofessional, and indeed a lack of any emotion can be seen as insensitive

- Finally, there is a fear of the hierarchy. What am I allowed to say? How should I respond when asked questions? Will the hierarchy blame me, especially if they have differing views about talking to patients?

These fears can lead to nurses using blocking or distancing tactics to avoid talking to patients. They may avoid patients altogether, use small talk, give false reassurances, ignore or not pick up on cues, use jargon, deal only with the positive or pass the buck (Faull et al., 1998; Jarrett and Maslin-Prothero, 2004). This may result in patients and relatives being left stranded in an uncertain world; the barriers erected may encourage them to withdraw into themselves and become even more anxious and depressed. In addition, without clear communication, patients and families are void of essential information necessary for them to be involved in the decision-making process.

Learning to cope with these fears comes easier to some than others. We all have a unique background that affects how we manage such situations, and it is important that you are gentle with yourself and develop your abilities gradually.

Just reading this chapter will certainly not be the answer, and perhaps a good place to start is reflecting on your own thoughts and experiences of death. Some guidelines, however, can help in providing at least a little scaffolding to support you through your learning:

Link

Chapter 14 discusses some of the core skills in good communication, including an intro- duction to breaking bad news. You might wish to review this now in the light of the discussion on communication in death and loss.

- Listen to patients and their relatives. Don't feel you have to have the answers; just listen and care
- Remember that not everyone wants to talk about their illness or about dying, so don't force it on people, but do be sure it is not just you who is avoiding the issue
- Don't deny people their feelings by telling them not to worry or not to be silly. Acknowledge their feelings by saying something like 'It must be worrying' or 'It seems you are very frightened'
- Offer openings such as 'Is there anything you would like to talk about?'
- Don't distance yourself. Sit with the person and, when appropriate, use touch as a way of connecting with them
- Be prepared for a variety of emotions, including anger. This is rarely personal but may be an expression of the person's fear, uncertainty and loneliness
- Don't be offended if they choose someone else to talk to. We can't always be the right person, but this does not mean that you are not a good nurse or not good at communication.

In the last days of life

The final days of a person's life can be difficult for health-care professionals to manage, especially if they do not have specific training in the care of the dying. The Liverpool Integrated Care Pathway for the Dying Patient is an evidence-based pathway developed in a hospice but able to be adapted and used in the commu- nity, acute hospital setting or nursing home. It sets out 11 initial assessment and care goals and 7 goals for after life care, which are listed below (Charts 10.1 and 10.2). Great emphasis is made of regular assessment, which is recommended to be 4 hourly for physical aspects of care and 12 hourly for psychological and spiritual aspects of care that should include the family as well as the patient.

Chart 10.1 ● Initial assessment and care goals

Comfort measures
- Goal 1: Current medication assessed and non-essentials discontinued
- Goal 2: PRN subcutaneous medication written up according to agreed guidelines
- Goal 3: Discontinue inappropriate interventions

Psychological insight
- Goal 4: Ability to communicate in English is assessed as adequate
- Goal 5: Insight into condition assessed

Religious/spiritual support
- Goal 6: Religious/spiritual needs assessed with patient/carer

Communication
- Goal 7: Identify how family/others are to be informed of patient's impending death
- Goal 8: Family/others given hospital/hospice facilities leaflet
- Goal 9: GP practice is aware of patient's condition

Summary
- Goal 10: Plan of care explained and discussed with patient/family/others
- Goal 11: Family/others express understanding of plan of care

Source: 'How to use the Liverpool Care Pathway for the Dying Patient', by Kinder, C. and Ellershaw, J. (2003) in *Care of the Dying: A Pathway to Excellence* edited by Ellershaw, J. and Wilkinson, S. (2003). By permission of Oxford University Press.

Chart 10.2 ● Care after death goals

- Goal 12: GP practice contacted regarding patient's death
- Goal 13: Procedure for laying out followed according to agreed policy
- Goal 14: Procedures following death discussed or carried out
- Goal 15: Family/others given information on hospital/hospice procedures
- Goal 16: Hospital/hospice policy followed for patient's valuables and belongings
- Goal: 17 Necessary documentation and advice given to the appropriate person
- Goal 18: Bereavement leaflet given

Source: 'How to use the Liverpool Care Pathway for the Dying Patient', by Kinder, C. and Ellershaw, J. (2003) in *Care of the Dying: A Pathway to Excellence* edited by Ellershaw, J. and Wilkinson, S. (2003). By permission of Oxford University Press.

■ Last Offices

Last offices is the term used to describe the last elements of care carried out after a person has died. For many nurses, this is their first contact with death and, handled sensitively, it can be a positive experience. Much of the procedure is not founded on research, but is based on myth and ritual. Nevertheless, ritual can itself be an important part of caring and should not be dismissed lightly. Much of the laying out of the dead provides an avenue for the nursing staff to offer their last opportunities for care and may for some act as a final closure. Procedures for last offices will vary and also depend on whether the person has

last offices

final procedures carried out after a patient has died

died in hospital, at home, in a nursing home or in a hospice. There are, however, some broad, very practical aspects to the procedure and the following principles outlined by Cooke (2000) need to be followed. Examine your local policy on last offices and reflect on each of these aspects of care:

- Appropriate care should be given to the bereaved relatives. If possible, give them the opportunity to be with the deceased before the body is removed from the ward. Prepare the area by removing as much clutter and as many clinical items as you can. Ensure that there are chairs next to the bed for the relatives to sit on
- You will need to be guided by local procedures for preparing the body, but in essence, individuals can be left in their nightwear; leaving a hand exposed allows the relatives to touch and hold the person. Covering the face with a sheet can make death frightening and unnecessarily mysterious for the relatives (Henley, 1986). Relatives should not be discouraged from talking to, hugging and kissing the person; after all, this may be the last time they are close together
- It is not a necessary routine to wash the patient, but a judgement should be made on whether, for example, a man should be shaved. If nurses choose to wash the patient as a way of saying goodbye, this will often be acceptable as long as it does not infringe any religious or cultural norms for the patient
- Be careful not to do anything that would have been out of the ordinary for the person when alive, for example do not put lipstick on a woman who would normally never have worn it
- Offer to stay with the relatives, but be equally prepared to leave them alone in privacy. Relatives will need to be given advice and help with what to do next. They may wish to talk to the doctor or nurse to ask about the circumstances of the death. It is important for them not to be left with many unanswered questions, and it is helpful for them to have a contact person should questions arise at a later date
- Ensure that there is appropriate support for the staff. Death will not always be an upsetting experience, which is perfectly acceptable. On some occasions and for some staff, however, it may be an upsetting experience, so be alert to your own feelings and the feelings of the staff around you. Be supportive and if necessary take 'time out' to reflect on what has happened. It is always useful to identify someone in your life who you can talk to at such a time, even if this is only at the other end of the telephone
- Provide appropriate support for other patients as they are invariably aware when someone has died. Do not try to hide the facts from them – they have a right to know – particularly in long-stay wards or nursing homes, and they may need an opportunity to talk

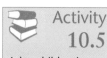

Activity 10.5

Ask a children's nurse and a community nurse how they manage last offices. Identify the differences and try to work out a rationale for these. Look at the *Royal Marsden Hospital Manual of Clinical Nursing Procedures* (Dougherty and Lister, 2004) for details of last offices and the requirements for different faiths. Look at the Age Concern website (www.ageconcern. org.uk) and search for the information contained in 'What happens when someone dies.'

- Provide dignity and privacy for deceased patients, treating them with the respect you would have given when they were alive
- Protect staff, other patients and relatives from infection and hazards. You should consult local procedures for infection control measures, but essentially those who have died are no more or less infectious then when they were alive. Universal precautions should still, however, be used. Body bags may need to be used for infectious patients
- Ensure a respect for the religious and cultural beliefs of the patient and family. If possible, find out from the family before the patient dies what specific procedures are required afterwards. Then ensure that these are adhered to
- Comply with the relevant legal requirements. Always check whether the coroner needs to be informed of the death; if so, drains, catheters, tubes and so on should normally be left in situ
- Ensure the care and safe custody of the patient's property
- Provide prompt and effective communication with other wards and departments. Remember that many people are involved – relatives, porters, mortuary staff, doctors, chaplains, infection control nurses and patient administration staff.

■ Bereavement

Death can release a whole variety of emotions. Some people may hardly be affected: perhaps the relationship was not very strong, or the death may have been a relief as it marked the end of suffering. For others, death can be difficult to come to terms with. C.S. Lewis (1961), tormented by the death of his wife, opens his book with the comment:

> No one ever told me that grief was so like fear. I am not afraid but the sensation is like being afraid. The same fluttering in the stomach, the same restlessness, the same yawning. I kept on swallowing.

What these emotions and feelings relate to and what purpose they serve have been the subject of great debate for many years. Do we have to work through **grief** in a series of stages, and do we eventually have to let go of the lost person before we can get on with life? The debate remains in a state of flux, so only a brief outline of some of the models proposed will be described here.

Many recent models of **bereavement** stem from the work of Freud and his contemporaries. Freud (1917) saw grief as a process to be worked through, something he called 'griefwork'. He hypothesised that, to recover from grief, the person needed to let go of all the energy invested in their loved one before they

grief
a natural human expression and reaction to a loss

bereavement
the state of having lost someone significant

could invest that energy in another. Although most of the bereavement models have since changed and developed, this concept is still central to many of them. One of the models emerging from this tradition is that of Worden (1983), who describes a 'tasks of grief' model in which the bereaved work through a series of tasks. These tasks are:

- To accept the reality of the loss
- To experience the pain of grief
- To adjust to an environment no longer containing the loved one
- To relocate the deceased and move on.

Parkes (1996) describes grief as a psychosocial transition in which the bereaved individual has to readjust to a new world without the deceased person. Every aspect of life becomes changed and they have to adapt to this new and altered world. Parkes also identifies a number of stages involved in the grieving process: shock and alarm; searching; anger and guilt; and finally gaining a new identity. Central to this theory is letting go of the old world and adapting to the new.

A widely published model is that of Kubler-Ross (1969), who also describes a staged model consisting of denial, anger, bargaining and acceptance. Her initial work was in fact based on people who were dying. She talked to many terminally ill patients and observed the way in which they were attempting to adapt to their illness and impending death. The work of Kubler-Ross opened up a whole new way of caring for those who were dying. The stages she observed and described were similar to those which people appeared to pass through when bereaved.

Although the theories described here all add something to the understanding of grief, they are also open to criticism in that people rarely follow such a neat pattern of bereavement and are just as likely to want to maintain a connection with the deceased as to let them go completely (Klass et al., 1996; Walter, 1999). In a study of bereaved parents, Rubin (1993) found that they still maintained a firm attachment to their child up to 13 years after the death, and there is reason to believe that such an attachment may continue for as long as the parent lives.

More recent studies have placed a greater emphasis on people's individual experience of grief, which is in turn considerably influenced by culture and social norms. It is not unusual in our current society for people to expect the bereaved to get over their grief quickly, yet for many it is a long and sometimes painful struggle. So much depends upon the relationship with the deceased, the person's usual coping strategies and the support available. In addition, factors such as the mode of death, for example a prolonged illness, suicide or an accident, can have a profound impact on how the bereaved person copes. The death of a child may be especially difficult to cope with and requires careful and sensitive management.

An alternative approach to the bereavement process has been proposed by Stroebe and Schut (1999). They have suggested a dual process model in which bereaved people oscillate between working at their grief and expressing their feelings, on the one hand, and allowing themselves to deal with everyday tasks and take on new roles, on the other (Figure 10.3). This model allows a more individualised approach to bereavement, taking into account gender and to some extent cultural differences. It acknowledges that people sometimes need to be fully immersed in the emotional aspects of their loss, whereas on other occasions, they need time to adjust to life without the deceased, manage day-to-day life and be distracted from their grief. People oscillate between these two, sometimes confronting their grief and at other times avoiding it.

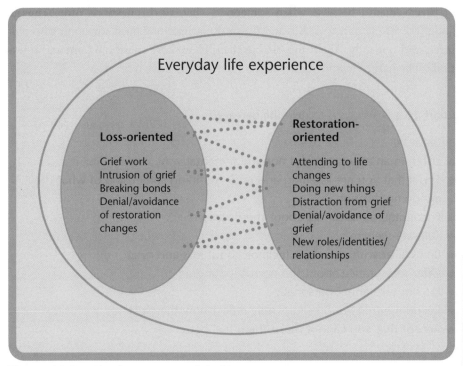

Figure 10.3 ● Dual process model of bereavement (adapted from Stroebe and Schut, 1999)

Nurses are for the most part involved with people during the acute stage of grief when someone significant has recently died. It is worth remembering, however, that many people who enter the health-care system, whether in hospital or at home, will have experienced losses during their life. In particular, older people are frequently faced with the death of family and friends, and those who move into nursing home care face many additional losses. Bereavement

Activity 10.6

List the types of loss experienced by someone who has to leave their own home and move into a nursing home. What sort of positive and negative thoughts and feelings might they experience? Think of all the types of loss that people might experience through ill-health – psychological, physical and social losses.

responses will also be manifest in people who are confronted by a social loss, such as the loss of a job or a relationship, and the associated loss of self-esteem and self-worth. Illness too brings with it many losses, including the physical loss of body parts or body function.

Whatever the cause of the loss, it is important to focus on individuals rather than a theoretical perspective. Listen to their story rather than trying to fit them into any model or stage. Accept them and their way of grieving. Helping people through grief and bereavement relies heavily on your ability to communicate effectively through listening, touch, the use of silence and sensitive responding. You might find the '10 ways to help the bereaved' (Chart 10.3) a useful starting point for deciding what you can do to help.

Perhaps you could add to the above list 'By recognising the spiritual nature of bereavement', because when someone is bereaved, questions often emerge about the whole nature of life and death. Relatives may need someone who will listen and not judge them but enable them to explore these fundamental questions. The nature of spirituality is the focus of the next section.

Chart 10.3 ● Ten ways to help the bereaved

- Be there
- Listen in an accepting and non-judgemental way
- Show that you are listening and understanding something of what they are going through
- Encourage them to talk about the deceased
- Tolerate silence
- Be familiar with your own feelings about loss and grief
- Offer reassurance about the normality of grief
- Do not take anger personally
- Recognise that your feelings may reflect how they feel
- Accept that you cannot make them feel better

Source: Adapted from Goodhall et al. (1994).

■ Spirituality

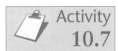

Activity 10.7

Think about the word 'spirituality', making notes about what you feel the term means to you.

Spirituality is not something that belongs only to the dying and those suffering, but is potentially an aspect of our everyday lives that is with us throughout our life. It is, therefore, an important element in all aspects of nursing, and it is discussed here partly out of convenience and partly because it is in times of crisis that many people become more acutely aware of the spiritual nature of life. Rinpoche (1992) comments:

Spiritual care is not a luxury for the few; it is *the* essential right of every human being, as essential as political liberty, medical assistance, and equality of opportunity. A real democratic ideal would include knowledgeable spiritual care for everyone as one of its essential truths.

So what is spirituality and spiritual care? It is clearly not easy to define, and the danger of defining it is that in so doing you lose its very essence. Walter (1997) argues that when you begin to examine the various definitions, you are left with the question of how some aspects are any different from 'psychological care', 'social care' and religion. However true this might be, spirituality is perhaps more than the sum of its parts: the diverse elements when enmeshed become something new and individual. Stoll (1989) captures this sentiment by expressing the relational aspect of spirituality and the religious dimension when she writes:

> Spirituality is my being; my inner person. It is who I am – unique and alive. It is me expressed through my body, my thinking, my feelings, my judgements and my creativity. My spirituality motivates me to choose meaningful relationships and pursuits. Through my spirituality I give and receive love; I respond to and appreciate God, other people, a sunset, a symphony and spring. I am driven forward, sometimes because of pain. Spirituality allows me to reflect on myself. I am a person because of my spirituality – motivated and enabled to value, to worship and to communicate with the holy, the transcendent.

Kellehear (2000) argues that, although spirituality is difficult to define, some level of definition is not only possible, but also important. Definitions provide a platform for debate and practice, and are useful, providing we recognise that they are dynamic and changing and open to dissent and challenge.

It is suggested that human beings seek to understand and transcend suffering, desiring to understand and make sense of their situation; this is no more so than when people are faced with death (Kellehear, 2000). Kellehear describes a multi-dimensional model that incorporates the situational, religious, and moral and biographical aspects of spirituality (Figure 10.4). Although not everyone will access all three areas or all the elements within the areas, they do assume the types of need that coexist in spirituality. What the areas have in common is that each reflects an attempt at transcendence, in other words, an attempt to find meaning from a given life crisis.

I will not attempt to explain all these aspects of spirituality in the model but will try to give a flavour of what Kellehear is suggesting.

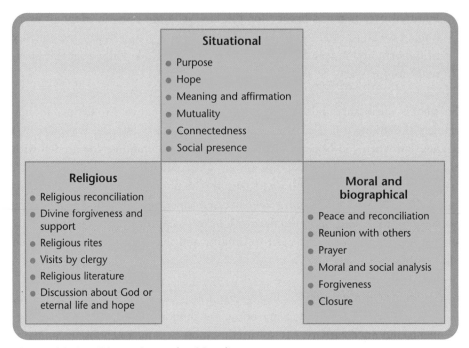

Figure 10.4 ● Dimensions of spirituality (adapted from Kellehear, 2000)

Religious

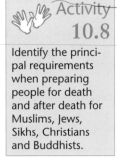

Activity

10.8

Identify the principal requirements when preparing people for death and after death for Muslims, Jews, Sikhs, Christians and Buddhists.

Religion is for many an important aspect of spiritual life. Through this vehicle many seek to find answers and guidance through prayer, meditation and ritual. It is an almost impossible task to describe the particular practices of the many religions, and even within the same religion people will have different interpretations and depths of devotion. Indeed, there is a danger of trivialising people's beliefs if we simply focus on the ritual aspect of their belief system. This makes it even more important to take care in the assessment process.

Rather than simply 'ticking the box', it is important to ask what patients' religion means to them and what they need while they are in our care. For example, do they wish their spiritual leader to visit them? What dietary needs do they have? If it is not possible to ask the patient, consult the relatives. If the patient is terminally ill, find out what the potential requirements might be in the terminal stages of the illness and after death. Sikhs, for example, may desire to have prayers said to them during the last stages of their life. Muslims may require that only Muslims touch or prepare the body after death.

In summary, be respectful of religious needs; seek advice and guidance early; keep contact numbers for local spiritual leaders and trusted local interpreters; listen to the needs of patients and relatives; and provide support to allow people to practise and meet their religious needs.

Situational

The situational aspect relates closely to trying to understand and make sense of the situations in which people find themselves. It emerges from the immediate situation, with its attendant medical problems, treatment and environment, be this hospital, hospice or their own home. People seek to discover hope and purpose in the place and situation they are in, to seek hope where there sometimes appears to be none. There can be nothing worse than to tell someone that there is nothing more we can do for them. But if we are to 'die living', there is always hope, hope to see a grandchild born, to paint a final picture, to see the sun rise, to be held by those you love, to be angry and express your emotions, to cry and seek solace, to fight and struggle. There is a need for help in this potentially frightening journey and people may want the closeness, presence and affirmation of others as they seek to find meaning from their situation.

Moral and biographical

The moral and biographical aspect also involves finding meaning in life but more from a biographical perspective: 'What has my life been about?' It is so easy just living life from day to day that we forget to ask more fundamental questions, but people faced with a life crisis frequently reflect on their life and try to make sense of it. It is also a time to seek forgiveness from loved ones, to say the things often left unsaid and to make amends. This may be done through prayer, which may have no specific religious significance. The nurse can help by using the skills already discussed, giving time, however little, listening, caring, touching, giving a smile, listening to the anger and providing privacy for visits. For those who are dying, there is a need to bring about some degree of closure on life, to make this a time to sort out and put into perspective their life history.

This section has reflected on the complex nature of spirituality and has suggested that it is concerned with more than religion, being instead something within all of us – even though some may be more aware of this than others. At a time of crisis, however, spirituality may become more central to our thinking. Narayanasamy (2001) suggests that, to develop these skills, nurses need to develop their own self-awareness of spirituality, becoming aware of their own attitudes, values and prejudices and recognising what skills they have and which they are deficient in. Some of the skills needed are listening, trust-building and giving hope, as well as a knowledge of spirituality.

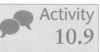

Activity 10.9

Consider the following questions in relation to the branch and client group you will be working with:

- How would you tell your client of the death of a significant person?
- How would you start to talk to someone about their illness and prognosis? (In the case of a neonate, this will be with the parents. With a child, this may, depending on age, involve the child and his or her parents or guardians.)
- How will last offices and disposal of the dead person be managed?

Be content with not knowing all the answers at this stage, but think about the difficulties these questions pose and carry them around in your head so that you can read, observe and practise as a continuous journey to knowing.

■ Chapter Summary

Death is the inevitable end to life for all of us. As a nurse, you are in a position to help many people with this transition and to help and care for the bereaved who are left behind. This chapter is only a brief introduction to this fascinating aspect of nursing; it does not pretend to be comprehensive, and in places you have perhaps been left with more questions than answers. You are encouraged to read widely around the subject and to do so critically, but just as important is your ability to learn from experience through active reflection. You may find it useful to explore a range of sources of information on death and loss, including novels, poetry and the arts; some suggestions are offered in the further reading below.

This chapter has tried to emphasise the individual nature of caring for people who are dying or bereaved. It has not been possible to include every scenario, but whether you are dealing with a dying neonate or a child, an adult or older person, someone with mental health problems or a learning disability, each requires their individual circumstances to be taken into account.

Test Yourself!

1. List the common cardinal signs of death.

2. What are the dimensions of palliative care described by Davies and O'Berle (1990)?

3. What does the term 'total pain' mean?

4. What does the term 'analgesic ladder' mean?

5. What, according to Finlay (1995), are the five most common symptoms seen in the dying patient?

6. What does the term 'last offices' mean?

7. What are the elements of loss-oriented grief and restoration-oriented grief, as described by Strobe and Schut (1999)?

8. Identify at least four ways in which you can help bereaved relatives.

9. What are the three elements of spirituality, as defined by Kellehear (2000)?

10. Make notes on your feelings about caring for the dying. What would you like to do to develop your skills and abilities in this area of nursing care?

Further Reading

Dickinson, D., Johnson, M. and Katz, J.S. (eds) (2000) *Death, Dying and Bereavement*, 2nd edn. Sage, London. This book provides a useful collection of papers and articles, including cultural and ethical issues.

Hill, S. (1977) *In the Springtime of the Year*. Penguin, London. This is a useful novel as it explores how two people experience different reactions to grief, neither fully understanding the other.

Lewis, C.S. (1961) *A Grief Observed*. Faber & Faber, London. The story of the philosopher and writer, well known for his Narnia books. Lewis writes movingly of his feelings following the death of his wife. You might also like to watch the film *Shadowlands*, which is meant to recount the journey experienced by Lewis and his wife as she becomes ill and ultimately dies.

Nyatanga, B. (2001) *Why is it so Difficult to Die?* Mark Allen, Dinton Quay. A useful book for health-care professionals, exploring many aspects of death and loss.

Payne, S., Seymour, J. and Ingleton, C. (eds) (2004) *Palliative Care Nursing; Principles and Evidence for Practice*. Maidenhead, Open University Press. A comprehensive textbook covering a diverse range of palliative care topics.

References

Aries, P. (1981) *The Hour of Our Death*. Knopf, New York.

Barclay, S. (2001) Palliative care for non-cancer patients: a UK perspective from primary care. In Addington-Hall, J.M. and Higginson, I.J. (eds) *Palliative Care for Non-cancer Patients*. Oxford University Press, Oxford.

Buckman, R. (1998) Communication in palliative care: a practical guide. In Doyle, D., Hanks, G. and Macdonald, N. (eds) *Oxford Textbook of Palliative Medicine*. Oxford University Press, Oxford.

Clark, D. (1993) *The Future for Palliative Care: Issues of Policy and Practice*. Open University Press, Buckingham.

Collick, E. (1986) *Through Grief: The Bereavement Journey*. Darton, Longman & Todd, London.

Cooke, H. (2000) *When Someone Dies: A Practical Guide to Holistic Care at the End of Life*. Butterworth-Heinemann, Oxford.

Davies, B. and O'Berle, K. (1990) Dimensions of the supportive role of the nurse in palliative care. *Oncology Nurses Forum* 17: 87–94.

Davis, B.D., Cowley, S.A. and Ryland, R.K. (1996) The effects of terminal illness on patients and their carers. *Journal of Advanced Nursing* 23: 512–20.

DoH (Department of Health) (1999) *Our Healthier Nation*. DoH, London.

Dougherty, L. and Lister, S. (eds) (2004) *Royal Marsden Hospital Manual of Clinical Nursing Procedures*, 5th edn. Blackwell, Oxford.

Ellershaw, J. and Wilkinson, S. (eds) (2003) *Care of the Dying: A Pathway to Excellence*. Oxford University Press, Oxford.

Faull, C., Carter, Y. and Woof, R. (eds) (1998) *Handbook of Palliative Care*. Blackwell, Oxford.

Finlay, I. (1995) The management of other frequently encountered symptoms. In Penson, J. and Fisher, R. (eds) *Palliative Care for People with Cancer*. Edward Arnold, London.

Freud, S. (1917) *Mourning and Melancholia*. Standard edition, vol. XIV, 1957. Hogarth Press, London.

Glaser, B.G. and Strauss, A.L. (1968) *Time for Dying*. Aldine Press, Chicago.

Goodall, A., Darge, T. and Bell, G. (1994) *The Bereavement Training Manual*. Winslow, Bicester.

Henley, A. (1986) *Good Practice in Hospital Care for Dying Patients*. King's Fund, London.

Hospice Information Service (2001) *Palliative Care Facts and Figures*. www. hospiceinformation.co.uk.

Jarrett, M and Maslin-Prothero, S. (2004) Communication, the patient and the palliative care team. In Payne, S., Seymour, J. and Ingleton, C. (eds) *Palliative Care Nursing: Principles and Evidence for Practice*. Maidenhead, Open University Press.

Kellehear, A. (2000) Spirituality and palliative care: a model of needs. *Palliative Medicine* **14**: 149–55.

Klass, D., Silverman, P.R. and Nickman, S.L. (1996) *Continuing Bonds: New Understandings of Grief*. Taylor & Francis, London.

Komaromy, C., Siddell, M. and Katz, J. (2000) The quality of terminal care in residential and nursing homes. *International Journal of Palliative Nursing* **6**: 192–200.

Kubler-Ross, E. (1969) *On Death and Dying*. Macmillan, New York.

Lewis, C.S. (1961) *A Grief Observed*. Faber & Faber, London.

Macmillan Cancer Relief (2005) *Gold Standard Framework* http://www.macmillan.org.uk/healthprofessionals/disppage.asp?id=2062.

Morgan, J.D. (1995) Living our dying and our grieving: historical and cultural attitudes. In Wass, H. and Neimeyer, R.A. (eds) *Dying: Facing the Facts*, 3rd edn. Taylor & Francis, Washington.

Narayanasamy, A. (2001) *Spiritual Care: A Practical Guide for Nurses and Health Care Practitioners*, 2nd edn. Mark Allen, Dinton Quay.

NHSE (NHS Executive) (1996) *A Policy Framework for Commissioning Cancer Services: Palliative Care Services*. NHS Executive, London.

NICE (National Institute for Clinical Excellence) (2004) *Guidance on Cancer Services: Improving Supportive and Palliative Care for Adults with Cancer. The Manual*. NICE, London.

ONS (Office of National Statistics) (1997) *Mortality Statistics: England & Wales 1996, General*. Stationery Office, London.

Parkes, C.M. (1996) *Bereavement: Studies of Grief in Adult Life*. Routledge, London.

Rinpoche, S. (1992) *The Tibetan Book of Living and Dying*. Rider, London.

Rosenblatt, P.C. (1997) Grief in small-scale societies. In Parkes, C.M., Laungani, P. and Young, B. (eds) *Death and Bereavement Across Cultures*. Routledge, London.

Rubin, S.S. (1993) The death of a child. In Stroebe, M., Stroebe, W. and Hansson R.O. (eds) *Handbook of Bereavement: Theory, Research and Intervention*. Cambridge University Press, Cambridge.

Saunders, C. (1978) *The Management of Terminal Illness*. Arnold, London.

Seedhouse, D. (1997) *Health Promotion: Philosophy, Prejudice and Practice*. John Wiley & Sons, London.

Stoll, R. (1989) The essence of spirituality. In Carson, V. (ed.) *Spiritual Dimensions of Nursing Practice*. W.B. Saunders, Philadelphia.

Stroebe, M. and Schut, H. (1999) The dual process model of coping with bereavement: rationale and description. *Death Studies* **23**: 197–224.

Townsend, J., Frank, A.O., Fermont, D., Dyer, S., Karran, O., Walgrove, A. and Piper, M. (1990) Terminal cancer care and patients' preference for place of death: a prospective study. *British Medical Journal* **310**: 415–17.

Veatch, R.M. (1995) The definition of death: problems for public policy. In Wass, H. and Neimeyer, R.A. (eds) *Dying: Facing the Facts*, 3rd edn. Taylor & Francis, London.

Victor, C.R. (2000) Health policy and services for dying people and their carers. In Dickenson, D., Johnson, M. and Katz, J.S. (eds) *Death, Dying and Bereavement*, 2nd edn. Sage, London.

Walter, T. (1997) The ideology and organisation of spiritual care: three approaches. *Palliative Medicine* **11**: 21–30.

Walter, T. (1999) *On Bereavement: The Culture of Grief*. Open University Press, Buckingham.

Wilson, M. (1975) *Health is for People*. Darton, Longman & Todd, London.

Worden, W.J. (1983) *Grief Counselling and Grief Therapy*. Tavistock, London.

WHO (World Health Organization) (2005a) *WHO Definition of Palliative Care*. http://who. int/cancer/palliative/definition/en/.

WHO (World Health Organization) (2005b) *WHO Pain Ladder*. http://who.int/cancer/palliative/painladder/en/index.html.

Yalom, I.D. (1980) *Existential Psychotherapy*. Basic Books, New York.

Useful Websites

www.pallcare.info Palliative Care Matters
Links to current issues in palliative care

www.bbc.co.uk Contains excellent pages on palliative care, ethical issues and bereavement

www.ncpc.org.uk National Council for Palliative Care
Features relevant and trusted links on a wide range of related topics

www.macmillan.org.uk Macmillan Cancer Support
A charity that works to improve the lives of people affected by cancer

www.who.int/cancer/palliative/definition/en Definition of Palliative Care from the World Health Organization

11 Wound Management

Contents

- A Professional Perspective
- The Healing Process
- Factors Affecting Wound Healing
- Complications of Wound Healing
- The Optimum Environment for Healing

- Care-planning in Wound Management
- Chapter Summary
- Test Yourself!
- Further Reading
- References

Learning Outcomes

The purpose of this chapter is to explore the prevention of pressure ulcers and the nursing management of wounds. At the end of this chapter, you should be able to:

- Define the terms 'wound' and 'pressure ulcer'

- Discuss the use of risk assessment tools in your current area of work

- Identify the different grades of pressure ulcer

- Discuss ways in which pressure ulcers can be prevented

- Outline the stages of the healing process

- Discuss the factors affecting wound healing

- Describe the optimum environment for wound healing

- Describe how each stage of the nursing process may facilitate the nursing management of wounds

- Identify different types of dressing and other wound management strategies and discuss their appropriateness for different wounds and stages of healing.

The chapter contains a number of activities that will help to deepen your understanding of this complex topic. Some of these activities require you to access and read more specialist textbooks in anatomy and physiology or wound management.

■ A Professional Perspective

Tissue viability, including **pressure ulcer** prevention, and wound management are high-profile areas of nursing activity that fall clearly within the domain of the professionally qualified nurse. They are important in terms of both patient comfort and care and the financial strain placed upon service providers (Cullum and Dealey, 1996).

All nurses are expected to seek out best evidence and apply it in their everyday practice (DoH, 2000) Evidence-based education and clinical guidelines, such as those developed by NICE (2003), and benchmarking processes, such as those outlined in *Essence of Care* (DoH, 2003), are key elements in establishing sound, client-focused, evidence-based practice. You may have noticed journal articles and websites concerned with tissue viability and wound management, and you may be familiar with multidisciplinary associations such as the Wound Care Society, the Tissue Viability Society and the European Pressure Ulcer Advisory Panel (EPUAP). Many NHS Trusts employ clinical nurse specialists for tissue viability, with the distinct remit of managing and coordinating care, teaching and research in wound management and pressure ulcer prevention. It is, however, important to remember that this area of nursing practice is one that most, if not all, practitioners will encounter, both pre- and postqualification.

Accountability in wound management

Inherent in the concept of professionalism is the notion of service and with this the 'duty of care' that is entered into during practice, for which the professional practitioner is held accountable (Carpenter, 1993; NMC, 2004). Whenever a professional nurse assesses, plans, implements or evaluates a care intervention, a duty of care arises. The nurse can be held to account for the knowledge base upon which such an intervention is founded and must be able to demonstrate practice within the limits of such knowledge (NMC, 2004).

The duty of care defines the minimum standard of practice that a patient can expect. In professional nursing practice, this is informed by the Code of Profes-

tissue viability
the sustained health, growth and repair of body tissues

pressure ulcer
'an area of tissue death caused by pressure distorting the capillaries and cutting off the blood supply for a critical length of time' (Bliss, 1990, p. 65). 'The critical determinants of pressure ulcers are believed to be intensity and duration of applied pressure. Extrinsic and intrinsic factors influence tissue tolerance' (Cullum and Clark, 1992, p. 427)

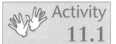

Activity 11.1

Visit the European Pressure Ulcer Advisory Panel website at www.epuap.com to review its contents and identify any additional relevant websites. Download any potentially useful information.

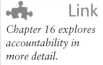

Link

Chapter 16 explores accountability in more detail.

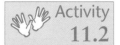

Activity
11.2
Find out if any
clinical audits of
pressure ulcers or
wound manage-
ment practice are
undertaken in your
current placement.
What audits are
carried out? How
frequently are they
done? Where are
the results recorded
and how is action
taken?

clinical audit

a process for measuring
outcomes of care and
levels of performance
against explicit criteria,
with the aim of
improving the quality
of care

**evidence-based
practice**

the conscientious, explicit
and judicious use of
current best evidence in
making decisions about
the care of individuals
(Sackett et al., 1996)

sional Conduct (NMC, 2004) as well as national standards such as *The Patient's Charter* (DoH, 1991), professional guidelines (Nelson, 1997) and local policies, guidelines, protocols and procedures. If the duty of care is breached, it is possible that a case of negligence may be brought against either the service provider (organisation) or the individual practitioner accountable for the nursing care involved.

Accountability and responsibility are similar concepts that are often confused. A distinction can be made in that in order to be held accountable for something, you must have authority over it. This means that you must be in a position to make a decision about a particular course of action. If you are not in such a position, it is your responsibility to say so.

Clinical governance, a government policy initiative, helps to provide a framework for professional effectiveness and accountability in all aspects of healthcare provision (DoH, 2000). We can consider wound management in terms of the clinical governance framework, as illustrated in Table 11.1.

Table 11.1 Clinical governance framework

Key elements of the clinical governance framework	Relationship to wound management and pressure ulcer prevention
Evidence-based practice	Ensuring that wound management interventions and pressure ulcer prevention strategies are based on best evidence
Clinical effectiveness	Ensuring that we do the 'right things, for the right people, with the right knowledge and skills and at the right time'
Risk management	Ensuring that we assess all possible risks and plan care to minimise these Ensuring that we learn from adverse events to prevent future problems
Monitoring clinical practice	Ensuring that we undertake regular clinical audits of pressure ulcer prevention and wound management practice, using published guidelines as benchmarking tools
Continuing professional development	Ensuring that we keep our knowledge and skills up to date with current developments
Professional self-regulation	Ensuring that we are always able to account for our practice
Dissemination of good practice	Ensuring that we learn from and share examples of good practice with other members of the interprofessional team

Link
*Chapter 16 also deals
with clinical gover-
nance.*

What is a wound?

Having identified tissue viability and wound management as regular nursing activities, and highlighted the importance of accountability in wound management, the next step is to examine what is meant by the term 'wound' and identify the different types that may be encountered.

Any kind of breach in the integrity of the skin or underlying tissues is commonly described as a wound. Wounds can be classified according to how they were caused, whether they are acute or chronic, how deep they are, the stage of healing, or the method by which they are expected to heal. Examples of how these classifications may be interlinked are illustrated in Table 11.2. The three modes of healing are discussed later in the chapter.

Table 11.2 Examples of wound classification

Description of wound	Cause	Expected mode of healing	Acute or chronic
Surgical excision	Removal of skin and underlying tissues during surgery	Secondary intention	Acute
Surgical incision	Precise cut made during surgery	Primary or delayed primary intention	Acute
Burn	Thermal, electrical or chemical	Secondary intention	Acute
Laceration (cut)	Trauma	Primary intention	Acute
Abrasion (graze)	Trauma	Secondary intention	Acute
Puncture (stab wound)	Trauma	Primary or secondary intention	Acute
Venous ulcer	Pathology (intrinsic), for example chronic venous insufficiency	Secondary intention	Chronic
Arterial ulcer	Pathology (intrinsic), for example atherosclerosis	Secondary intention	Chronic
Diabetic ulcer	Pathology (intrinsic), for example diabetes	Secondary intention	Chronic
Pressure ulcer	Pathology (extrinsic), for example pressure, friction or shearing	Secondary intention	Chronic
Fungating wound	Pathology (intrinsic), for example carcinoma	Neither	Chronic
Infected wound	Pathology (intrinsic), for example abscess or gross contaminant	Secondary or tertiary intention	Acute or chronic

Activity 11.3

What types of wound have you seen in practice? Using Table 11.2, try to identify the cause and mode of healing of each type. Discuss with your mentor the differences in management of acute and chronic wounds.

atherosclerosis

the thickening and calcification of the arteries and narrowing of their lumens that occurs as a result of the deposition of fatty substances (plaques) along the arterial walls

Assessing the risk

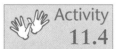

Activity 11.4

Find out which pressure ulcer risk assessment tool is in use where you work. What risk factors are included in it? Compare it to the Waterlow scale illustrated in Table 11.3. Ask your clinical mentor the following: How are the risk assessment tools used? How often is each assessment carried out? Who carries it out? How are the results documented and acted upon? How is the client involved in this?

A number of wounds, particularly chronic wounds, are associated with underlying pathology: for example, venous ulcers are often caused by chronic venous insufficiency, arterial ulcers by peripheral vascular disease, fungating wounds by carcinoma and pressure ulcers either by pressure, shearing or friction. The likelihood of certain wounds developing as a result of an underlying pathology can be assessed and there are a number of risk assessment tools available to assist nurses and other health professionals in their clinical judgement. However, the validity of many of the tools is still questionable and they should not be used in isolation. They include pressure ulcer risk assessment tools, such as the Braden scale (Bergstrom et al., 1987) and Waterlow scale (2005), and diabetic foot ulcer risk assessment tools (Farndon et al., 2001). See Table 11.3 for an example of a risk assessment scale. Once a patient has been identified as vulnerable, preventive measures should be put in place.

Table 11.3 An example of a pressure risk assessment tool: the Waterlow scale

WATERLOW PRESSURE ULCER PREVENTION/TREATMENT POLICY
RING SCORES IN TABLE, ADD TOTAL. MORE THAN 1 SCORE/CATEGORY CAN BE USED

BUILD/WEIGHT FOR HEIGHT	♦	SKIN TYPE VISUAL RISK AREAS	♦	SEX AGE	♦	MALNUTRITION SCREENING TOOL (MST) (Nutrition Vol.15, No.6 1999 - Australia			
AVERAGE		HEALTHY	0	MALE	1	A - HAS PATIENT LOST WEIGHT RECENTLY		B - WEIGHT LOSS SCORE	
BMI = 20-24.9	0	TISSUE PAPER	1	FEMALE	2	YES - GO TO B		0.5 - 5kg = 1	
ABOVE AVERAGE		DRY	1	14 - 49	1	NO - GO TO C		5 - 10kg = 2	
BMI = 25-29.9	1	OEDEMATOUS	1	50 - 64	2	UNSURE - GO TO C AND		10 - 15kg = 3	
OBESE		CLAMMY, PYREXIA	1	65 - 74	3	SCORE 2		> 15kg = 4	
BMI > 30	2	DISCOLOURED GRADE 1	2	75 - 80	4			unsure = 2	
BELOW AVERAGE		BROKEN/SPOTS GRADE 2-4	3	81 +	5	C - PATIENT EATING POORLY OR LACK OF APPETITE		NUTRITION SCORE If > 2 refer for nutrition assessment / intervention	
BMI < 20	3					'NO' = 0; 'YES' SCORE = 1			
BMI=Wt(Kg)/Ht (m)²									

CONTINENCE	♦	MOBILITY	♦	SPECIAL RISKS				
COMPLETE/ CATHETERISED	0	FULLY	0	**TISSUE MALNUTRITION**	♦	**NEUROLOGICAL DEFICIT**		♦
URINE INCONT.	1	RESTLESS/FIDGETY	1					
FAECAL INCONT.	2	APATHETIC	2	TERMINAL CACHEXIA	8	DIABETES, MS, CVA		4-6
URINARY + FAECAL INCONTINENCE	3	RESTRICTED	3	MULTIPLE ORGAN FAILURE	8	MOTOR/SENSORY		4-6
		BEDBOUND e.g. TRACTION	4	SINGLE ORGAN FAILURE (RESP, RENAL, CARDIAC,)	5	PARAPLEGIA (MAX OF 6)		4-6
SCORE		CHAIRBOUND e.g. WHEELCHAIR	5	PERIPHERAL VASCULAR DISEASE	5	**MAJOR SURGERY or TRAUMA**		
10+ AT RISK				ANAEMIA (Hb < 8)	2	ORTHOPAEDIC/SPINAL		5
15+ HIGH RISK				SMOKING	1	ON TABLE > 2 HR#		5
20+ VERY HIGH RISK						ON TABLE > 6 HR#		8
				MEDICATION - CYTOTOXICS, LONG TERM/HIGH DOSE STEROIDS, ANTI-INFLAMMATORY MAX OF 4				

Scores can be discounted after 48 hours provided patient is recovering normally

© J Waterlow 1985 Revised 2005*
Obtainable from the Nook, Stoke Road, Henlade TAUNTON TA3 5LX
* The 2005 revision incorporates the research undertaken by Queensland Health.

www.judy-waterlow.co.uk

REMEMBER **TISSUE DAMAGE MAY START PRIOR TO ADMISSION, IN CASUALTY. A SEATED PATIENT IS AT RISK**
ASSESSMENT (See Over) IF THE PATIENT FALLS INTO ANY OF THE RISK CATEGORIES, THEN PREVENTATIVE NURSING IS
REQUIRED A COMBINATION OF GOOD NURSING TECHNIQUES AND PREVENTATIVE AIDS WILL BE NECESSARY
<u>ALL ACTIONS MUST BE DOCUMENTED</u>

PREVENTION PRESSURE REDUCING AIDS		**Skin Care**	General hygiene, NO rubbing, cover with an appropriate dressing
Special Mattress/beds:	10+ Overlays or specialist foam mattresses.		
	15+ Alternating pressure overlays, mattresses and bed systems	**WOUND GUIDELINES**	
	20+ Bed systems: Fluidised bead, low air loss and alternating pressure mattresses	**Assessment**	odour, exudate, measure/photograph position
	Note: Preventative aids cover a wide spectrum of specialist features. Efficacy should be judged, if possible, on the basis of independent evidence.	**WOUND CLASSIFICATION - EPUAP**	
		GRADE 1	Discolouration of intact skin not affected by light finger pressure (non-blanching erythema)
Cushions:	No person should sit in a wheelchair without some form of cushioning. If nothing else is available - use the person's own pillow. (Consider infection risk)		This may be difficult to identify in darkly pigmented skin
	10+ 100mm foam cushion	**GRADE 2**	Partial thickness skin loss or damage involving epidermis and/or dermis
	15+ Specialist Gell and/or foam cushion		
	20+ Specialised cushion, adjustable to individual person.		The pressure ulcer is superficial and presents clinically as an abrasion, blister or shallow crater
Bed clothing:	Avoid plastic draw sheets, inco pads and tightly tucked in sheet/sheet covers, especially when using specialist bed and mattress overlay systems	**GRADE 3**	Full thickness skin loss involving damage of subcutaneous tissue but not extending to the underlying fascia
	Use duvet - plus vapour permeable membrane.		The pressure ulcer presents clinically as a deep crater with or without undermining of adjacent tissue
NURSING CARE		**GRADE 4**	Full thickness skin loss with extensive destruction and necrosis extending to underlying tissue.
General	HAND WASHING, frequent changes of position, lying, sitting. Use of pillows		
Pain	Appropriate pain control		
Nutrition	High protein, vitamins and minerals		
Patient Handling	Correct lifting technique - hoists - monkey poles Transfer devices	**Dressing Guide**	Use Local dressings formulary and/or www.worldwidewounds.com
Patient Comfort Aids	Real Sheepskin - bed cradle		
Operating Table			
Theatre/A&E Trolley	100mm(4ins) cover plus adequate protection	IF TREATMENT IS REQUIRED, FIRST REMOVE PRESSURE	

Source: Reprinted with the permission of Waterlow, www.judy-waterlow.co.uk

■ The Healing Process

The ability to support the maintenance of tissue viability, prevent pressure ulcers and manage wounds effectively is underpinned by a sound understanding of the structure and function of normal, healthy skin and the normal healing process. Normal wound healing is a complex, well-coordinated, multiphase process. The phases of this process are usually described separately to facilitate understanding, but it is important to remember that each phase overlaps with the next, often running concurrently, and each phase may vary in duration, be reversed or become static in certain circumstances. There may also be evidence of the different phases of healing within the same wound.

The phases of wound healing

Four main phases have been identified and these are discussed in more detail.

Haemostasis

Haemostasis involves wound contraction, which decreases the surface area of the wound, vasoconstriction and the formation of a clot to reduce bleeding and exposure to contaminants. This process is part of the physiological response to blood **extravasation.** Platelets are activated by exposure to extravascular collagen,

extravasation
leakage of fluid from a
blood vessel

releasing growth factors that stimulate tissue regeneration, and then become sticky and aggregate, getting trapped in a fibrin mesh, which forms the bulk of the clot.

Inflammatory phase

The inflammatory phase usually occurs over three to seven days and is initiated by the release of chemical mediators, such as histamine and **prostaglandins**, which attract neutrophils, monocytes and fibroblasts to the injured area by a process called **chemotaxis**. These mediators cause blood vessels to become more permeable and to vasodilate, allowing **wound exudate**, containing protein, nutrients and growth factors, to leak out of the capillaries and bathe the injured area. This inflammatory response is a normal response to injury and is not to be confused with infection. This phase is delayed in patients who are immunosuppressed or have infected wounds.

The primary functions of this phase are:

- *To combat potential infective organisms*: neutrophils are activated in the inflammatory response and clear the site of contaminating organisms, aided by the phagocytic action of the macrophages
- *To cleanse the area of debris*: monocytes enter the area and transform into activated macrophages to clear the debris through phagocytosis. This debris is often seen as creamy yellow **slough**, particularly in chronic wounds
- *To initiate* **angiogenesis** *and* **collagen synthesis**: macrophages stimulate the production of a variety of angiogenic **growth factors and cytokines** such as interleukin. This process initiates the growth of capillary buds (angiogenesis) as well as the regrowth of sympathetic nerve fibres. The process of angiogenesis is stimulated by a hypoxic environment. Fibroblasts, activated by these mediators, migrate to the wound site, initiating the early stages of the proliferative phase.

Proliferative phase

The proliferative phase of the wound healing process occurs over a variable time span and is characterised by the formation of **granulation tissue**, which has a dense network of capillaries, fibroblasts and collagen fibres. The fibroblasts produce an **extracellular matrix**, which is a framework of collagen fibres, elastin and proteoglycans, anchored by fibronectin, that support and sustain the products of angiogenesis. The successful progress of this phase is dependent upon the oxygen and nutrient supply.

The growth of capillary buds forming a network of loops within the wound is crucial to the level of oxygen available during the proliferative phase, as fibroblast activity is sensitive to oxygen supply. These capillary buds give granulation tissue its characteristic knobbly or granular appearance.

---

prostaglandins

hormone-like substances that affect vasomotor and smooth muscle tone, capillary permeability, platelet aggregation, endocrine and exocrine functions and the nervous system

chemotaxis

a response involving movement towards or away from a chemical stimulus

wound exudate

a translucent, yellow-tinged fluid, rich in proteins and antibodies, produced during the inflammatory phase of the healing process

slough

soft dead tissue resulting from injury or inflammation

angiogenesis

the production or growth of new blood vessels

collagen synthesis

the production of supportive, protein-based, fibrous connective tissue

growth factors and cytokines

small molecular weight proteins that regulate cell proliferation

granulation tissue

red, moist, fragile connective tissue that is characteristic of the proliferative phase of the healing process

extracellular matrix

a gel-like matrix produced by fibroblasts, composed of various polysaccharides, collagen fibres and water

Two other major processes occur concurrently within the proliferative phase of wound healing – epithelialisation and contraction. The granulation tissue filling the wound bed is gradually resurfaced by epithelial cells, which migrate in from the wound margins or regenerate as 'islands' from hair follicles or glands. Epithelial cells regenerate and migrate by sliding over one another across the wound surface, and their eventual contact with one another inhibits further migration. This process is facilitated by a moist, warm and oxygenated environment. The process of contraction, initiated during the inflammatory phase, is largely controlled by the activity of myofibroblasts (which develop from fibroblasts) that reduces the surface area of the wound. Granulation, contraction and epithelialisation mark the completion of the proliferative phase.

Maturation phase

The final maturation phase in the wound healing process is concerned with the remodelling and strengthening of the collagen fibres within the wound. The collagen produced during earlier stages is relatively soft, type III collagen, which is deposited fairly randomly during granulation, resulting in a low tensile strength (about 25 per cent of normal tissue) in the newly healed wound. During maturation, this is replaced with stronger type I collagen, which is organised through cross-linking of the collagen fibres into bundles lying at right angles to the wound margins. This increases the tensile strength of the wound to about 80 per cent of normal tissue: it will never become as strong as uninjured tissue. This ongoing process, facilitated by the activity of fibroblasts and characterised by a gradual reduction in vascularity of the wound site, shrinkage and paling of the scar tissue, can continue over a number of years.

Modes of healing

It is common to refer to the healing process as occurring by one of three modes: primary intention, secondary intention or tertiary intention, and these are now discussed.

Primary intention

Healing by primary intention occurs in wounds where there has been little or no tissue loss and the skin edges can be brought together, usually by sutures, staples or glue, to ensure an absence of dead space in the wound. The four phases of wound healing occur, but there is little granulation tissue produced and minimal wound contraction, epithelial cells migrating along the suture line. Remodelling of the collagen fibres in scar tissue takes place, as previously described, and there is usually minimal defect. Most surgical wounds and lacerations (cuts) heal by primary intention.

Secondary intention

Healing by secondary intention refers to wounds where there has been tissue loss and the skin edges remain apart. Again, the wound will progress through all four phases of healing, but it will be necessary for the wound bed to fill with granulation tissue, to become resurfaced with epithelium and to contract before and during scar formation. Pressure ulcers, leg ulcers, burns and abrasions (grazes) are all examples of wounds that will heal by secondary intention.

Tertiary intention

pus
_____

characteristic fluid composed of exudate, dead tissue debris, macrophages and bacteria

Healing by tertiary intention or delayed primary closure is where a wound that may be infected or contaminated is left open to facilitate the drainage of **pus** and the formation of granulation tissue. When the complicating factor has been excluded, the wound can be surgically closed and healing by primary intention can take place.

■ Factors Affecting Wound Healing

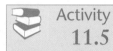

Activity
11.5

Consider Figure 11.1. Try to explain how each factor affects wound healing and note how they are interrelated. Now read Chapters 4 and 5 of Bale and Jones (1997). Try to identify how the factors affecting wound healing are reflected in the nursing care of infants, children and adolescents, and how this may differ from the nursing care of adults. How may assessment of skin differ for patients with darkly pigmented skin? See Bethell (2005).

Wounds do not heal in isolation, and it is important to consider the whole person, by completing a holistic assessment, which should aim to identify any existing or potential problems that will adversely affect wound healing. The numerous factors to be considered during an assessment are illustrated in Figure 11.1. and include local, systemic and contextual factors. Some of the key factors are discussed here. By reviewing each element, the nurse will be able to develop an effective wound care strategy.

Nutrition

Good nutrition is essential for wound healing. There is a relationship between protein-energy malnutrition and delayed healing, reduced tensile strength, infection and the development of pressure ulcers. There is also evidence, in a recent Cochrane review, that nutritional supplements reduce the number of new pressure ulcers (Langer et al., 2003). Proteins are essential for collagen synthesis, angiogenesis and cell reconstruction (Wells, 1994). They contribute to osmotic equilibrium and the immune response and are a source of energy. Low blood protein levels (measured in terms of serum albumin) and negative nitrogen balance have been linked to impaired wound healing and increased vulnerability to pressure ulcers (Green et al., 1999).

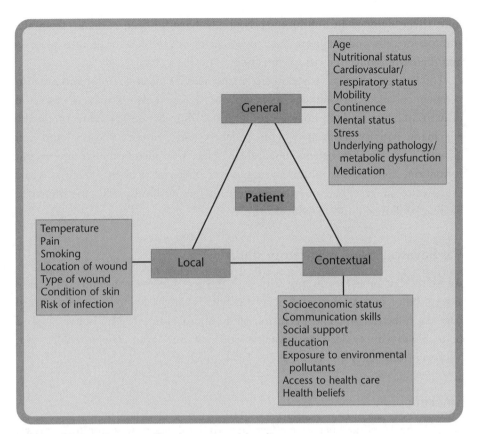

Figure 11.1 ● Factors affecting wound healing

Lipids, provided from the dietary fat intake, are vital components of cell membranes. Dietary fat is also the largest source of energy, required for wound healing, as well as providing a source of fat-soluble vitamins. Essential polyunsaturated fatty acids (**PUFA**) are precursors of prostaglandins and hence have a role in the inflammatory process. There is some evidence that PUFA improve wound healing (Declair, 1997) and reduce wound infection (Gottschlich et al., 1990).

Carbohydrate, in the form of glucose, is the primary energy substrate required for cellular metabolism. If glucose from carbohydrate is unavailable, amino acids will be oxidised to meet the energy requirements of healing, thus depleting the pool of amino acids available for reconstruction and tissue repair.

Vitamin C is involved in the metabolism of many amino acids and is required for the synthesis of collagen and cross-linking collagen fibres, facilitating the **hydroxylation** of proline and lysine, which are essential components of collagen (Lewis and Harding, 1993). Iron (as well as providing the primary component of haemoglobin, which facilitates the transport of oxygen in the bloodstream) is a co-factor in this process. Vitamin C and vitamin E, strong antioxidants, also

PUFA

simple lipids, including the omega-3 fatty acids

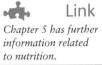 Link
Chapter 5 has further information related to nutrition.

hydroxylation

the formation or addition of a hydroxyl (OH) group

limit tissue damage by inhibiting potentially harmful **free radicals** from the surfaces of cells and facilitate the movement of white blood cells into wounds and therefore reduce the risk of infection.

The B vitamins are involved in enzymatic activity (as co-factors) and are also active in collagen cross-linkage, as is vitamin A, which also influences epithelial growth and acts on lymphocyte proliferation. Zinc is another co-factor in the enzymatic activity associated with collagen and protein synthesis and cell growth. Zinc also has beneficial stabilising effects on membrane structures and formation, and has an inhibitory action on bacterial growth. There is some evidence to suggest that, in patients with low serum levels, oral zinc improves healing (Wilkinson and Hawke, 1998).

Cardiovascular and respiratory status

Link

Chapter 7 has further information related to cardiovascular and respiratory status.

Anything that interferes in any way with oxygen delivery will tend to increase susceptibility to infection and delay healing. There is an inverse relationship between infection risk and perfusion (Jensen and Hunt, 1991). Ischaemia and poor blood supply lead to unstable collagen and poor re-epithelialisation. Venous insufficiency can result in venous leg ulcers.

Smoking

Nicotine has a marked negative effect on peripheral blood flow, immune activity, epithelialisation and contraction, and carbon monoxide reduces the available oxygen (Siana and Gottrup, 1992). This will lead to delayed healing.

Pathophysiology

Poorly controlled diabetes mellitus impairs glucose metabolism, which retards healing and increases the risk of infection, as insulin is essential for fibroblast activity and hyperglycaemia interferes with macrophage activity, collagen synthesis and re-epithelialisation (Barbul and Purtill, 1994).

Age

Wound healing complications are more common in the elderly, due to the body's reduced capacity to repair and slower cellular activity. The elderly are also more likely to have an associated pathology or be undernourished.

Pain

Pain can have a detrimental effect on recovery and healing. The European

Wound Management Association, in a position paper on pain, stated that dressing removal, especially if adherent to new tissue, has been identified as the most painful experience associated with a wound (EWMA, 2002). Pain needs to be assessed in terms of intensity, duration and frequency and the effect it is having on the patient's mental state.

> **Link**
>
> *Chapter 7 also discusses pain.*

Stress

Stress is implicated in poor healing due to reduced efficiency of the immune response. Carers of relatives with Alzheimer's took significantly longer to heal from a punch biopsy, compared to other carers (Kiecolt-Glaser et al., 1995).

■ Complications of Wound Healing

There are occasions when the wound healing process is interrupted and healing does not progress as anticipated. Some commonly observed complications in the wound healing process are now discussed.

Infection

Infection can significantly delay healing and increase hospital stay. Nearly all wounds are **contaminated** and many are **colonised** but this will not affect the healing process – indeed many chronic wounds can tolerate high levels of bacteria and still heal normally – but an overwhelming number of bacteria (10^5 organisms per gram of tissue) will result in a clinical **infection**, interfering with the healing process by prolonging the inflammatory phase and depleting resources (Robson, 1997). This is generally characterised by localised cellulitis (heat, swelling, redness and pain) and an increase in wound exudate (often purulent in nature). In chronic wounds, cellulitis may be absent and other signs, such as a darkening in the appearance of granulation tissue, a change in pain or odour, may be the only indicators. When a chronic wound appears to stop improving and is not healing, it may be because it is **critically colonised**.

contaminated
contain bacteria that are multiplying

colonised
contain multiplying bacteria where there is no host reaction

infection
multiplication of bacteria in tissue with an associated host reaction

critically colonised
contains high levels of bacteria and is unresponsive to treatment, although no clinical signs of infection (Davis, 1998)

Dehiscence

'Dehiscence' is the term used to refer to the 'splitting' open of a closed surgical wound. If the collagen fibres that have been laid down are not strong enough to withstand the internal and external tensions applied to the wound, the newly formed layers of the wound will separate. The dehiscence of a wound is often associated with infection and/or the presence of a haematoma. The dehisced wound may be left to heal by secondary intention, which will significantly increase the time to heal and the risk of complications.

Haematoma

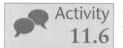

Activity 11.6

Can you think of certain measures that could be taken to prevent any of these complications of healing? Discuss your ideas with your colleagues.

Haematoma is the name given to a localised collection of blood and plasma trapped within the skin or an organ, which can become a breeding ground for bacteria and interfere in collagen deposition.

Haemorrhage

Primary haemorrhage (severe blood loss during surgery) and intermediary haemorrhage (severe blood loss immediately following surgery) can affect wound strength by interfering with the function of the fibroblasts. Secondary haemorrhage (blood loss up to 10 days postoperatively) commonly results in haematoma formation and subsequent infection.

Abnormal healing

Abnormal healing is characterised by abnormalities in scar tissue formation and includes:

- *Hypertrophic scarring:* common in young patients. A large amount of scar tissue is laid down along the incision line, resulting in a raised, fibrous wound site
- *Keloid scarring:* more common in patients with heavily pigmented skin. Again, a large amount of scar tissue continues to be laid down, but in this case the scar tissue infiltrates the surrounding skin, resulting in bulbous growths over and around the wound site
- *Overgranulation:* can occur when granulation tissue progresses beyond the normal wound bed (Dunford, 1999). It is often associated with a prolonged inflammatory phase and results in delayed re-epithelialisation
- *Contractures:* hypercontraction of the wound during the maturation phase can result in excessive shortening of the associated muscle tissue, which, combined with the presence of fibrous scar tissue, inhibits muscular extension
- *Malignant disease:* because of the intense cellular activity within a wound, there is the potential for chronic wounds to undergo malignant change. Failure to heal over an extended period of time can be associated with such a process.

The Optimum Environment for Healing

Wound bed preparation, through the creation of an optimum environment for wound healing, is essential. Careful planning is required to choose the most appropriate wound care products and to involve the patients wherever possible to increase compliance with treatment. One glance through a hospital formulary or a look around a modern treatment room will give an indication of the numerous products currently available to facilitate wound management. Such an array can create a certain amount of confusion when deciding which product will be best suited to which wound. In order to avoid this situation, it is important to make a thorough assessment of the patient and their wound (see Casebox 11.1 below), and plan the best wound care strategy. Basic principles of wound care include cleansing or debridement, management of exudate, and moist, interactive healing (Miller and Glover, 1999). Morgan (2004) described the characteristics of an 'ideal dressing', which would provide the optimum environment at the wound–dressing interface, although few, if any, of the dressings available conform to every criterion.

The characteristics of this ideal dressing are:

- *Moist:* research conducted over 40 years ago (Winter, 1962) indicated that re-epithelialisation was enhanced when a moist environment was maintained, both within the wound bed and at the wound–dressing interface. This means that the body must be well hydrated and dressings should promote high humidity
- *Free from excess exudate:* although wound exudate, containing white cells, nutrients and growth factors, is essential to moist wound healing, excess wound exudate will interfere with the healing process, contributing to wound bed oedema. It will also leak on to the surrounding skin, resulting in the **maceration** of healthy tissue, as well as providing a potential entry portal for infective organisms

  maceration
  the softening and detexturising of tissues due to prolonged exposure to moistness

- *Protected from bacterial contamination:* the wound requires a physical barrier, and thought must be given to potential sources of infection. Strike-through of exudate allows the passage of bacteria in and out of the wound
- *Protected from particulate or toxic contamination:* foreign bodies, such as fibres or granulomas, can act as a focus for bacteria. Again, a physical barrier is required that will not shed fibres into the wound
- *Thermally insulated:* the length of time a dressing stays on a wound between changes is an important factor. Not only should any dressing used maintain a stable temperature, but also practices such as frequent, unnecessary exposure of the wound, the use of cold cleansing solutions and changes in the ambient temperature must be avoided, as any persistent drop in temperature will lead to vasoconstriction, reduced cellular activity for several hours and shift the **oxygen dissociation curve** to the left, resulting in a decrease in the amount of oxygen delivered to the tissues (Morgan, 1994). Wounds heal more slowly in cold environments: if skin temperature drops from 20°C to 12°C, tensile strength reduces by 20 per cent.

  oxygen dissociation curve
  the plotted curve that demonstrates the release of oxygen from haemoglobin in capillaries into the interstitial fluid in areas of low oxygen tension

- *Well perfused:* gaseous exchange may take place at the wound–dressing interface, but it is more important that there is a good blood supply to ensure that the oxygen and nutrient demands of the wound are met, as well as removing waste products from the wound site
- *Protected from mechanical trauma:* new epithelial cells and capillary buds are extremely delicate and can be easily damaged during dressing changes (especially if the dressing material adheres to the wound surface or the surface is rubbed during wound cleansing). Studies have shown that these cells can also be damaged by the use of antiseptic solutions, for example hypochlorite (Leaper, 1996). Thus, the environment must be assessed for potential hazards that could cause further trauma
- *Undisturbed:* frequent dressing changes, however 'wound environmentally friendly' the dressings are, will interfere with the healing process and may be associated with an increase in pain.

As well as promoting the optimum environment for wound healing, the 'ideal dressing' should be cost-effective, perform in such a way as to maximise the achievement of treatment objectives, be acceptable to patients and carers and be readily available in both hospital and community settings.

Different types of dressing vary in terms of their suitability to absorb exudate, aid debridement, facilitate granulation or re-epithelialisation, and reduce infection or odour. Not all dressings of a similar type have the same characteristics and you will need guidance in making the best choice. There are a large number of different dressings available (see Table 11.4) and new ones are constantly being added to the formulary (Morgan, 2004). Many Trusts have developed their own wound formulary or guidelines. Table 11.5 is an example of wound management guidelines that can help the nurse in her decision-making.

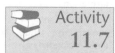

Activity 11.7

Find a copy of Morgan (2004) or your pharmacy department's formulary of wound management products. Note that the dressings listed are divided into groups, for example hydrocolloids. Identify the particular characteristics of as many groups as you can and compare them with the elements described in the text. See if you can identify an example (by trade name) for each group.

Table 11.4 Generic types of wound dressings

Modern wound dressings	Examples
Foams	Lyofoam® (SSL), Allevyn® (S&N)
Hydrocellular	Allevyn® compression (S&N)
Hydrogels	Purilon Gel® (Coloplast), Intrasite Gel® (S&N), Geliperm®
Semi-permeable films	Opsite® (S&N), Tegaderm® (3M)
Hydrocolloids	Comfeel® (coloplast), Granuflex® (ConvaTec)
Alginates	Sorbsan® (Maersk), Kaltostat® (ConvaTec), Algisite M® (S&N)
Fibre-hydrocolloids	Aquacel® (ConvaTec)
Low-adherent	N.A Ultra® (J&J), Mepitel® (Molnlycke)
Silver dressings	Avance® (SSL), Acticoat® (S&N), Arglaes® (Maersk)

Table 11.5 Wound management guidelines

Exudate	Size	Appearance of wound					
		Necrotic (eschar)	Sloughy	Granulating	Epithelialising	Infected	Fungating
Non/low	Shallow	*Enzymatic debridement* Consider surgical debridement	**Hydrogel** **Hydrocolloid** *Larval therapy*	**Hydrocolloid** **Polyurethane foam** N.A. dressing Silicone dressing	Semi-permeable film Extra-thin hydrocolloid N.A. dressing Silicone dressing Polyurethane foam	**Iodine** **Antibacterial gel (anaerobic)** *Semi-permeable film with silver* Seek wound care specialist opinion	**Silicone dressing** **Antibacterial gel** **Deodorising pad**
Medium/high	Shallow	**Hydrogel** *Enzymatic debridement* Consider surgical debridement	**Hydrocolloid** **Hydrogel** **Alginate wafer** **Polyurethane foam** **Hydropolymer** *Larval therapy*	**Hydrocolloid** **Alginate wafer** **Polyurethane foam** **Hydropolymer**	**Hydrocolloid** **Alginate wafer**	**Antibacterial gel** **Hydrogel** **Iodine** **Deodorising pad** Seek wound care specialist opinion	**Antibacterial gel** **Polyurethane foam** **Deodorising pad**
Medium/high	Cavity		**Hydrogel** **Alginate rope** **Fibre-hydrocolloid** *Vacuum-assisted closure (VAC)* *Larval therapy* *Hydrocellular*	**Hydrogel** **Polyurethane foam** **Alginate rope** **Fibre-hydrocolloid** *Hydrocellular*		**Antibacterial gel** **Hydrogel** **Fibre-hydrocolloid** **Deodorising pad** *Cadexamer iodine* Seek wound care specialist opinion	**Fibre-hydrocolloid** **Alginate** **Antibacterial gel** **Deodorising pad** Seek wound care specialist opinion

Notes:
- Wound products in bold available from pharmacy direct.
- Wound products in italics available via tissue viability nurse specialist or on consultant request.
- Before selecting product, refer to Wound Information Sheet for specific information and warnings about the product.
- Remember to assess your patient before choosing a wound care product.
- Please contact the tissue viability nurse specialist for further advice or assistance.

Source: Adapted from Jackson and Creevy (2001).

There are also a growing number of non-dressing alternatives for managing wounds. Larval therapy uses sterile maggots on sloughy, infected or critically colonised wounds to aid debridement. Manuka honey has antibacterial and anti-inflammatory properties and appears to aid healing in a wide range of wounds (Molan, 1999). The use of negative pressure through vacuum-assisted closure has stimulated angiogenesis and growth of granulation tissue, controlled oedema at the wound bed and hence reduced healing time (Collier, 1997).

Care-planning in Wound Management

> **Link**
>
> *Chapter 1 explains the nursing process in detail.*

As you will have discovered from working through Chapter 1, one of the most effective methods for designing a programme of care interventions is the nursing process. The five stages of the nursing process form the framework for a systematic and holistic review of nursing care, based around a problem-solving approach. One of the benefits of adopting a systematic approach such as this is that you will be able to demonstrate clearly through documentation not only the decision-making processes involved in designing care interventions, but also – and most importantly – the effectiveness of those interventions.

A good way of exploring care planning in detail is to use a client profile. The profile described in Casebox 11.1 forms the basis for the following detailed analysis of planning care in wound management.

Casebox 11.1

Mr Hartley is a frail, elderly gentleman of 84 years, who is a widower. He has arterial disease and type II diabetes mellitus and has had two toes on his left foot amputated. He now lives in a residential home but maintains regular contact with his family. Mr Hartley is able to get around fairly independently, using a walking frame, but sometimes needs help to get out of the chair. He is a friendly gentleman who enjoys the company of others. Mr Hartley normally smokes 20–40 cigarettes a day.

Mr Hartley has been admitted to hospital for the management of pressure ulcers that have developed over his **ischial tuberosities**. On admission to hospital, he appears slightly agitated but interested to find out about his new surroundings. As the ambulance crew transfer Mr Hartley into bed, he winces several times but quickly regains his composure. He is rather pale and drawn and his clothes appear loose. There is a damp patch where he has been sitting on the ambulance trolley.

Mr Hartley sets about organising his belongings; he has an assortment of sweets as well as toiletries, cigarettes and lighter. He moves around the bed, reaching over to pull the locker nearer and places an old wedding photo next to his water jug and then flops back, looking tired. A nurse arrives to see how he is settling in.

ischial tuberosities

the bony protuberances present on the ischium (the curved bone that forms the base of each half of the pelvis), commonly known as the 'sitting bones'

Wound assessment

Morison (2000) suggests that a holistic assessment taking into account environmental and social factors should form the foundation of any wound management strategy. A number of frameworks exist for wound assessment. In order to design a comprehensive wound management programme for Mr Hartley, it will be necessary to use a framework or model to identify any actual or potential problems and state the related nursing diagnoses.

The following is a wound assessment framework (Morison et al., 2004):

- General physical condition
- Mental state
- Mobility
- Nutritional status
- Continence
- Concurrent disease
- Cardiovascular status
- Pain
- Skin
- Risk assessment.

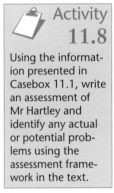

Activity 11.8

Using the information presented in Casebox 11.1, write an assessment of Mr Hartley and identify any actual or potential problems using the assessment framework in the text.

Having completed Activity 11.8, you will probably have identified the problems described below.

General physical condition

Although Mr Hartley has a slight degree of disability associated with the amputation of two of his toes, he demonstrates a reasonable level of independence. He does not appear to have any difficulty breathing, either at rest or on exertion. However, he seems to tire easily and is rather pale and drawn.

Actual problem
Mr Hartley appears tired and pale.

Mental state

Mr Hartley is alert and oriented. He appears happy to participate in conversation with the nursing staff. He is aware of his immediate needs and takes steps to meet them independently. No actual or potential problems have been identified.

Mobility

Mr Hartley's mobility is slightly limited. He uses a walking frame to move about but can get himself around the bed. He can transfer from one surface to another fairly independently.

Actual problem

- Mr Hartley will be subject to pressure while sitting or in bed.

Potential problems

- Mr Hartley might experience fatigue because of the effort he puts into moving around the bed, and this may lead to unrelieved pressure while in bed
- He may have a reduced ability to manoeuvre his walking frame because of the unfamiliar surroundings
- There is a risk of injury (to either Mr Hartley or the staff) while facilitating movement and manual handling.

Nutritional status

Mr Hartley is pale and drawn and his clothes seem loose. He is a type II diabetic. The presence of pressure ulcers means that he requires additional protein and vitamins in his diet to ensure wound healing.

Actual problems

- Mr Hartley appears to have lost weight
- He has enhanced protein, vitamin and mineral requirements.

Potential problem

- Mr Hartley may develop poor diabetic control, which may lead to an increased infection risk and delayed wound healing.

Continence

Mr Hartley may be suffering from urinary incontinence.

Actual problems

- Mr Hartley may have urinary incontinence
- He is slow to get to the toilet independently.

Potential problems

- Mr Hartley may suffer skin excoriation from leakage of urine and his wound may be contaminated by leaking urine
- He may suffer from constipation as a result of immobility.

Concurrent disease

Mr Hartley suffers from type II diabetes mellitus. No actual problems have been identified.

Potential problem

- Poor control of diabetes is associated with impaired wound healing.

Cardiovascular status

Mr Hartley has arterial disease, which has led to the amputation of two toes on his left leg. He is also a heavy smoker, with no apparent intention of giving up. This will further compromise his cardiovascular system.

Actual problem

- Arterial disease implies an impaired blood flow to wound sites and impaired healing. Mr Hartley is a smoker; smoking exacerbates the effects of cardio-vascular disease as well as being a causative factor for it. It is also a health and safety hazard while Mr Hartley is in hospital.

Potential problems

- Smoking is associated with impaired healing
- Mr Hartley may suffer withdrawal symptoms if he reduces or eliminates his nicotine intake
- Further deterioration of his cardiovascular system will lead to multisystem failure.

Pain

Although Mr Hartley did not verbally complain of any pain, his facial expressions during manual handling indicate that he might be experiencing some pain.

Actual problems

- Mr Hartley is not voicing his experience of pain
- Pain is often associated with stress and anxiety that will delay healing.

Potential problems

- Mr Hartley appears slightly agitated and may be frightened, but may be reluctant to cause a fuss
- It may be difficult to assess the level and nature of his pain and the effectiveness of any interventions
- Increasing pain may further limit Mr Hartley's mobility.

Skin

Mr Hartley has pressure ulcers over his ischial tuberosities. It is unclear how many wounds are present or what their status is. There is insufficient information to clearly describe the problems at this stage.

Risk assessment

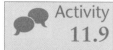

Activity 11.9

Having conducted your initial assessment of Mr Hartley, now review your assessment and identify any additional information required, specifying how you would obtain this.

Mr Hartley has been admitted with pressure injuries and is therefore at risk of developing additional wounds. There is, however, insufficient information to complete a full risk assessment at this stage.

You may be surprised at how much information can be gathered from the careful reading of a client profile, but certain areas need clarification so that problems can be better identified. You will now need to take into account the factors affecting wound healing described in Figure 11.1 above, to enhance the data you have already gathered.

Now tackle Activity 11.9. Your answer may include the following.

General physical condition

You will want to know more about Mr Hartley's respiratory status. Does he have a cough or a wheeze? Are there any signs of cyanosis? Has Mr Hartley recently suffered from any chest infections? Does he have a history of respiratory disease? What is his general state of well-being?

Mental state

Although Mr Hartley appears to be adjusting well to the situation, you will need to observe and listen carefully to detect any signs of distress or disorientation. Be aware of the reactions of visitors: are they at all concerned about Mr Hartley's behaviour?

Mobility

Link

Chapter 9 has more information on mobility issues.

It is necessary to assess the extent of Mr Hartley's mobility and identify what types of aid to mobility and manual handling may be required. A thorough assessment of mobility can only be effected by direct observation of Mr Hartley over a period of time (minimum 24 hours) and will need to be repeated regularly.

Continence

Link

Chapter 6 has more information related to continence.

You will need to establish if Mr Hartley is suffering from urinary incontinence and, if so, how long he has been suffering from it. In order to promote continence and prevent constipation, you will need to establish Mr Hartley's normal bladder and bowel habit. A continence chart can be used to assess this.

Nutritional status

It is important to use a nutritional screening tool, such as MUST (Elia, 2003) to identify if Mr Hartley is undernourished or is at risk of protein-energy malnutrition. This will include weight and calculation of his body mass index, in addition to recent weight loss. You should ask Mr Hartley if he can remember what he has eaten and drunk over the past 24 hours and what his favourite foods are and try to establish the reason for his ill-fitting clothes. You will also need to establish how much he understands about diet and diabetes. There are a number of nutritional guidelines for pressure ulcer prevention that you can use to help in your assessment, such as the EPUAP one (Clark et al., 2004).

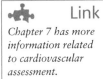

Link

Chapter 5 looks at some factors to consider when assessing nutritional status.

Concurrent disease

In order to enhance your information relating to Mr Hartley's diabetes, it will be necessary to establish a pattern of blood glucose level over a period of time, starting with a baseline level on admission. You will also need to know whether Mr Hartley is excreting glucose in his urine. It is important to establish whether he is taking any medication to control his diabetes and whether this has been taken regularly, as prescribed.

Cardiovascular status

The extent of any arterial disease present and Mr Hartley's understanding of his condition and prognosis should be clarified. You will need to establish the possibility of negotiating a reduction in the number of cigarettes he smokes. Is he willing to give them up for a trial period? How does he feel about this?

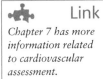

Link

Chapter 7 has more information related to cardiovascular assessment.

Pain

You will need to establish whether Mr Hartley is experiencing pain and, if so, its nature, intensity, location, duration and precipitating factors (for example movement or wound dressing changes). You will also need to ascertain Mr Hartley's feelings about pain control and prevention.

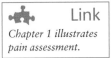

Link

Chapter 1 illustrates pain assessment.

Skin

Assess the quality of the skin in terms of hydration, elasticity, colour, temperature and integrity. Establish exactly how and where the integrity of the skin has been breached, assessing each wound individually and recording:

- *Wound site:* anatomical location
- *Wound dimensions:* measure wound surface area by tracing around the edge of the wound or by recording length/width and depth. Photographs are often used to record wound size

- *Pressure ulcer grading:* a numerical value relating to their severity (Reid and Morison, 1994; EPUAP, 1998) (see Chart 11.1 for classification of pressure ulcers)

necrotic
dead, devitalised tissue

eschar
dead tissue, characterised by its dry, crusty, black appearance, which adheres to the wound bed

- *Wound bed status:* the percentage of wound bed occupied by **necrotic tissue** (**eschar**), slough, granulation tissue and epithelial tissue. You may also aim to establish the stage of wound healing and presence of oedema (although this is not always possible)
- *Exudate:* is the level high, medium or low? Is it increasing or decreasing? Is the exudate purulent or bloodstained?
- *Infection:* are there any signs or symptoms to indicate a wound infection?
- *Odour:* present/absent?
- *Edge of wound:* is it well defined? Is it raised or rolled? Is there any undermining of surrounding area?
- *Surrounding skin:* is it intact? Well perfused? Macerated? Inflamed? Eczematous? Oedematous?
- *Expected mode of healing.*

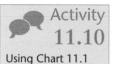

Activity 11.10

Using Chart 11.1 and the wound assessment outlined in the text, assess the wound of a patient with a pressure ulcer. How easy was it to assess the grade of pressure ulcer? How did you assess the size of the wound? Where are wound details documented?

Chart 11.1 ● Classification of pressure ulcers

- Grade 1: non-blanching erythema of intact skin, discoloration of the skin, warmth, oedema, induration or hardness may also be used as indicators, particularly on individuals with darker skin
- Grade 2: partial thickness skin loss involving epidermis, dermis, or both. The ulcer is superficial and presents clinically as an abrasion or blister
- Grade 3: full thickness skin loss involving damage to, or necrosis of, subcutaneous tissue that may extend down to, but not through, underlying fascia
- Grade 4: extensive destruction, tissue necrosis, or damage to muscle, bone or supporting structures, with or without full thickness skin loss

Source: Adapted from EPUAP (1998).

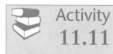

Activity 11.11

Try to locate the quality standard(s) for the prevention and management of pressure injuries in your workplace. How many of these assessment criteria are reflected within them?

Pressure ulcer risk assessment

Use a risk assessment tool, such as the Braden scale (Bergstrom et al., 1987) or Waterlow scale (Waterlow, 2005; Table 11.3 above) to provide a framework for professional judgement when assessing Mr Hartley's level of risk of further pressure injury. The initial risk assessment must be completed as soon as possible after admission so that preventive measures can be taken. Some areas have particular quality standards relating to the prevention and management of pressure injury, and these will often specify the timeframe within which risk assessment should take place, for example *Essence of Care* benchmarks (DoH, 2003).

There are a number of national and international pressure ulcer prevention guidelines now available, such as those developed by NICE (2003) or the European Pressure Ulcer Advisory Panel (EPUAP, 1998).

Assessment in wound management can be summarised thus:

- Assessment is an ongoing process
- Actual and potential problems are identified, to formulate a nursing diagnosis and provide the knowledge base for planning care interventions
- The client is recognised as the primary source of information and secondary sources of information include relatives, carers, friends, other members of the multidisciplinary team, documentation and electronically stored data
- The primary aim is to assess the client and his or her environment in terms of conduciveness to wound healing
- The secondary aim is to establish and record wound status, including any factors that may complicate or impair the healing process
- A risk assessment should form part of the process.

Planning nursing care

You will now be ready to enter the planning stage of the nursing process. It is important to ensure that, whenever possible, you involve the client in agreeing the broad aims, setting objectives and identifying appropriate interventions. You will now be starting to understand the complexity of nursing care in wound management. The interventions that relate directly to the wound itself form only part of a range of activities that are vital to supporting wound management. Chart 11.2 describes Mr Hartley's wound status on admission to hospital. It is now possible to design a nursing care plan for the management of this wound, based upon your assessment and informed by a sound knowledge base of the principles of wound management. Following the previously outlined stages, the plan of care will develop as follows.

Identifying the broad aim will be carried out in conjunction with Mr Hartley, asking him what he hopes will be the outcome of his stay in hospital and to what extent he is willing to participate in his care and carefully establishing how realistic these hopes may be. In this case, the broad aim may be identified as:

To create a local environment that will be conducive to and promote wound healing. The expected outcome is that the necrotic tissue and slough will be removed and there will be formation of granulation tissue.

Chart 11.2 ● Mr Hartley's wound status on admission to hospital

Wound 1
- Cavity wound, located over left ischial tuberosity
- Diameter 6 cm, depth 6 cm
- Pressure ulcer grading of 4 – full thickness skin loss with extensive destruction and tissue necrosis, extending to underlying bone, tendon or joint capsule
- Wound bed composed of 70 per cent slough, 30 per cent necrotic eschar
- Moderate exudate level
- No signs of clinical infection or odour
- Well-defined edge with undermining for 2 cm to the left of wound
- Surrounding skin excoriated and poorly perfused
- Expected mode of healing – secondary intention

Specific objectives negotiated with Mr Hartley will include:

autolysis

the natural breakdown of dead, or foreign, organic material by leucocytes and rehydration

- Relieving pressure to prevent further development of pressure ulcers
- Debriding the wound to encourage the **autolysis** of necrotic tissue and slough and its removal from the wound bed
- Controlling exudate to avoid leakage
- Protecting the wound from contamination to prevent infection
- Protecting the surrounding skin to prevent further breakdown.

Next, *appropriate interventions* should be devised. Having already established that each objective is a statement of intention, or a 'what we want to do', the next step involves designing nursing interventions, the 'how we are going to do it'. This can be done by reviewing each objective and identifying what action needs to be taken and what resources might be required.

Here are two examples of interventions:

1. *Specific objective:* Relieving pressure to prevent further development of pressure ulcers
   Nursing intervention:
   - Install an alternating pressure or constant low pressure device and chair cushion
   - Encourage Mr Hartley to move from side to side at regular intervals, to redistribute weight while in bed, and support position using the 30 degree tilt (Clark, 1998) and pillows, if appropriate
   - Limit sitting times

- Mr Hartley may not be able to get out of bed unaided if an alternating pressure system is used and will need assistance
- Mr Hartley to agree to participate and use the prescribed equipment
- Record interventions on a repositioning chart (refer to NICE guidelines, 2003).

2. *Specific objective:* Protecting the surrounding skin to prevent further breakdown

   Nursing intervention:

   - Wash and dry surrounding skin sparingly, if contaminated, to avoid removing natural skin barriers
   - Avoid friction and shearing to skin by use of appropriate manual handling techniques
   - Choose a skin barrier to protect the skin from further excoriation, which may be caused by proteolytic enzymes in the exudate digesting the corneal layers of the skin.

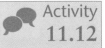

Activity 11.12

Review your assessment for Mr Hartley. Select one of the actual problems identified and discuss how care may be planned, explaining how each nursing intervention will affect wound healing and identifying which other members of the interprofessional team may be involved.

Implementing care

The implementation stage of any wound management plan is critical in that:

- You ensure that planned care is given
- You actively involve the client and other members of the interprofessional team
- You record which elements of the care plan have been carried out, when and by whom
- You begin to evaluate as you implement care, noting the length of time taken to complete an intervention, the ease with which it was undertaken, the degree to which the client was able (or willing) to participate, any associated teaching activities and any changes that occurred while you were implementing care.

If we examine the implementation of the three specific objectives in Mr Hartley's care plan – debriding the wound, controlling exudate and protecting the wound from contamination – we can take a step-by-step approach to analysing how this intervention may be implemented:

1. On admission, the dressing in place is found to be unsuitable, that is, it does not conform to the criteria for an ideal dressing. It is therefore necessary to implement the planned nursing intervention.
2. Select the appropriate dressing, using the data from your wound assessment and the hospital wound formulary, documenting the selection and giving a rationale, for example:

Activity 11.13

Select any one of Mr Hartley's other specific objectives and, following the framework illustrated in the example in the text, design a nursing intervention to enable you to meet that objective. Work through this activity with the support of your clinical mentor.

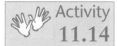

Activity 11.14

With your clinical mentor, and following the local guidelines for aseptic technique, select a hydrogel and a polyurethane foam dressing from the treatment room of your clinical area. Prepare everything you would need to implement the wound dressing element of Mr Hartley's care plan.

Hydrogel selected to instil into wound bed to rehydrate the wound and promote the removal of necrotic tissue by autolytic debridement. Adhesive foam dressing selected to cover the hydrogel in the wound bed, to absorb excess exudate and protect the wound from contamination.

3. Explain the use of the dressing to Mr Hartley, giving him an opportunity to examine the dressing and ask any questions.
4. Prepare Mr Hartley for the dressing to be applied. Encourage him to participate and make any comments throughout the dressing change (for example to describe any pain or suggest ways in which he may assist).
5. Prepare for the dressing change following local guidelines for aseptic technique.
6. Decide if the wound needs to be cleansed to remove any loose debris and particulate matter in the wound bed. Select an appropriate cleanser (such as normal saline) and use to irrigate the wound bed (Pudner, 1997).
7. Instil the hydrogel into the cavity of the wound.
8. Apply the dressing according to the manufacturer's instructions and ensure it is firmly in place.
9. Clear the area. Ensure Mr Hartley is comfortable and give him an opportunity to comment or ask any questions.
10. Document the episode as soon as possible.

Link

Chapter 1 identifies ways of evaluating nursing care.

Evaluation of care

By focusing and reflecting on what is happening, both during and after the implementation of a nursing intervention, and then recording your findings, the nursing documentation not only serves as a record of events, but also becomes a dynamic, working tool. The description of interactions between client and nurse will provide additional information. This may lead to further assessment or revisions to the care planned, if relevant.

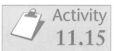

Activity 11.15

Consider the wound dressing element of Mr Hartley's wound management plan. List any possible information you might acquire from Mr Hartley and your observations. Describe how you might revise the care plan as a result of your findings. Discuss this with your clinical mentor.

The key to success in making a care plan a 'working' document is your ability to evaluate the effectiveness of the nursing interventions you have designed. In the management of wounds, you will need to:

- Review the factors affecting wound healing
- Review the wound status
- Evaluate the agreed nursing interventions.

■ Chapter Summary

The effective nursing management of wounds and the prevention of pressure ulcers is a complex area of activity involving integrated and systematic assessment, the identification of problems, and the planning, implementation and evaluation of nursing interventions. This chapter has given you an overview of the elements underpinning the principles of wound healing and management, highlighting the importance of ongoing, evidence-based education to inform decision-making in practice, the value of reflection as a way of evaluating your experiences, the wide range of tools, frameworks and guidelines available to assist in making a professional judgement and the central role of the nurse in managing care.

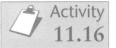

Activity 11.16

There are a wide range of resources and evidence available concerning wound care. Undertake an internet search using the search field 'wound management'. Make a note of the search engine used (how efficient was it?) and the search field (how productive was it?; did you need to widen or reduce it?). Post your findings on the student notice board or discuss at your next learning group tutorial and invite comments.

Test Yourself!

1. What are the main causes of pressure ulcers?

2. What preventive measures can be taken to avoid the development of pressure ulcers?

3. What are the four main phases of wound healing?

4. The factors affecting wound healing have been described in terms of local, systemic and contextual. How many of these factors can you list?

5. What are the criteria identified to provide the optimum environment for wound healing?

6. What specific wound characteristics would you include in your assessment of the patient?

■ References

Bale, S. and Jones, V. (1997) *Wound Care Nursing: A Patient-centred Approach*. Baillière Tindall, London.

Barbul, A. and Purtill, W. (1994) Nutrition in wound healing. *Clinical Dermatology* **12**: 133–40.

Bergstrom, N., Braden, B., Laguzza, A. and Holman, V. (1987) The Braden scale for predicting pressure sore risk. *Nursing Research* **36**: 205–10.

Bethell, E. (2005) Wound care for patients with darkly pigmented skin. *Nursing Standard* **20**(4): 41–9.

Bliss, M. (1990) Geriatric medicine. In Bader, D.L. (ed.) *Pressure Sores: Clinical Practice and Scientific Approach*. Macmillan, Basingstoke – now Palgrave Macmillan.

Carpenter, D. (1993) Key working and primary nursing: accountability and professional practice. In Giddey, M. and Wright, H. (eds) *Mental Health Nursing: From First Principles to Professional Practice*. Chapman & Hall, London.

Clark, M. (1998) Repositioning to prevent pressure sores: what is the evidence? *Nursing Standard* **13**(3): 58–64.

Clark, M., Schols, J., Benati, G., Jackson, P., Engfer, M., Langer, G., Kerry, B. and Colin, D. (2004) Pressure ulcers and nutrition: a new European guideline. *Journal of Wound Care* **13**(7): 267–72.

Collier, M. (1997) Know-how: a guide to vacuum-assisted-closure. *Nursing Times* suppl. January.

Cullum, N. and Clark, M. (1992) Intrinsic factors associated with pressure sores in elderly people. *Journal of Advanced Nursing* **17**(4): 427–31.

Cullum, N. and Dealey, C. (1996) Presentation given to the all party group on skin at the House of Commons. *Journal of Tissue Viability* **6**(1): 20–3.

Davis, E. (1998) Education, microbiology and chronic wounds. *Journal of Wound Care* **7**(6): 272–4.

Declair, V. (1997) The usefulness of topical application of essential fatty acids to prevent pressure ulcers. *Ostomy/Wound Management* **43**(5): 48–54.

DoH (Department of Health) (1991) *The Patient's Charter*. Stationery Office, London.

DoH (Department of Health) (2000) *The NHS Plan*. Stationery Office, London.

DoH (Department of Health) (2003) *Essence of Care: Patient-focused Benchmarks for Clinical Governance*. Stationery Office, London

Dunford, C. (1999) Hypergranulation tissue. *Journal of Wound Care* **8**(10): 506–7.

Elia, M. (2003) *The MUST Report*. BAPEN, Redditch.

EPUAP (European Pressure Ulcer Advisory Panel) (1998) *Pressure Ulcer Prevention Guidelines*. EPUAP, Oxford.

EWMA (European Wound Management Association) (2002) *Position Statement on Pain at Wound Dressing Changes*. Medical Education Partnership, London.

Farndon, L., Henderson, M. and Wright, V. (2001) Conflict to consensus: development of a regional risk assessment tool. *Diabetic Foot* **4**(1): 35–42.

Green, S., Winterberg, H., Franks, P., Moffatt, C., Eberhardie, C. and McLaren S. (1999) Dietary intake of adults, with and without pressure sores, receiving community nursing services. *Journal of Wound Care* **8**(7): 325–30.

Gottschlich, M., Jenkins, M. and Warden, G. (1990) Differential effects of 3 enteral dietary regimens on selected outcome variables in burn patients. *Journal of Parenteral and Enteral Nutrition* **14**: 225–34.

Jackson, P. and Creevy, J. (2001) Wound management guidelines used in Southampton University Hospital Trust. Personal communication.

Jensen, J. and Hunt, T.K. (1991) The wound healing curve as a practical teaching device. *Surgery, Gynecology and Obstetrics* **173**(1): 63–4.

Kiecolt-Glaser, J., Marucha, P., Mercado, A., Malarkey, W. and Glaser, R. (1995) Slowing of wound healing by psychological stress. *Lancet* **346**(8984): 1194–6.

Langer, G., Schloemer, G., Knerr, A., Kuss, O. and Behrens, J. (2003) Nutritional interventions for preventing and treating pressure ulcers. *Cochrane Database of Systematic Reviews*, issue 4.

Leaper, D. (1996) Antiseptics in wound healing. *Nursing Times* **92**(39): 63–8.

Lewis, B.K. and Harding, K.G. (1993) Nutritional intake and wound healing in elderly people. *Journal of Wound Care* **2**(4): 227–9.

Miller, M. and Glover, D. (1999) *Wound Management*. NT Books, London.

Molan, P. (1999) The role of honey in the management of wounds. *Journal of Wound Care* **8**(8): 415–18.

Morgan, D.A. (2004) *The Formulary of Wound Management Products*. Euromed Communications, Haslemere.

Morison, M. (2000) *The Prevention and Treatment of Pressure Ulcers*. C.V. Mosby, London.

Morison, M., Ovington, L. and Wilkie, K. (2004) *Chronic Wound Care: A Problem-based Learning Approach*. Mosby, Edinburgh.

Nelson, E.A. (1997) Consensus statements. *Journal of Wound Care* **6**(3): 107.

NICE (National Institute for Clinical Excellence) (2003) *Clinical Guideline: Pressure Ulcer Prevention*. http://www.nice.org.uk/pdf/clinicalguidelinepressuresoreguidancenice.pdf.

NMC (Nursing and Midwifery Council) (2004) *The NMC Code of Professional Conduct: Standards for Conduct, Performance and Ethics*. NMC, London.

Pudner, R. (1997) Wound cleansing. *Journal of Community Nursing* **11**(7): 30–6.

Reid, J. and Morison, M.A. (1994) Towards a consensus: classification of pressure sores. *Journal of Wound Care* **13**(3): 157–60.

Robson, M. (1997) Wound infection. *Surgical Clinics of North America* **77**(3): 637–50.

Sackett, D., Rosenburg, W. and Muir Gray, J. (1996) Evidence-based practice: what it is and what it isn't. *British Medical Journal* **312**(7023): 71–2.

Siana, J. and Gottrup, F. (1992) The effects of smoking on tissue function. *Journal of Wound Care* **1**(2): 37–41.

Waterlow, J. (1988) Calculating the risk. *Nursing Times* **38**(9): 58–60.

Waterlow, J. (2005) *Pressure Ulcer Prevention Manual*. Waterlow, Taunton.

Wells, L. (1994) At the front-line of care. *Professional Nurse* **9**(8): 525–30.

Wilkinson, E.A.J. and Hawke, C. (1998) Oral zinc for arterial and venous leg ulcers. *Cochrane Database of Systematic Reviews*, issue 4.

Winter, G. (1962) Formation of the scab and the rate of epithelialisation of superficial wounds in the skin of the domestic pig. *Nature* **193**: 293–4.

◼ Useful Websites

www.epuap.com European Pressure Ulcer Advisory Panel

www.ewma.org European Wound Management Association

www.tvs.org.uk Tissue Viability Society

www.woundcaresociety.org Wound Care Society

www.worldwidewounds.com Worldwide Wounds (*Electronic Wound Care Journal*)

www.cochranewounds.org Cochrane Wounds Group

www.medicaledu.com Wound Care Information Network

Professional Issues

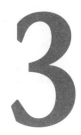

12

Understanding Ourselves

Contents

- Self-concept
- Self-awareness
- Self and Sources of Stress
- Factors Affecting Stress

- Attitudes
- Chapter Summary
- Test Yourself!
- References

Learning Outcomes

The main aim of this chapter is for all those working within the health and social care profession to gain an understanding of the importance of self-awareness. After reading the chapter, you should have a greater understanding of:

- Self-concept: the development of self-concept, models of self and self-awareness

- Stress: models of stress and modifiers of stress

- Attitudes: attitude formation and the relevance of attitudes for health-care practice.

This chapter is about good practice. The main thrust is on developing a sense of empathy; understanding one's own motives for behaviour in order to understand others; to be able to step out of one's own frame of reference and to see the world from the other's perspective, being at one and remaining separate.

'Understanding ourselves' is an important goal for those who work with people. It is not possible to truly **empathise** with another without an understanding of the motives and drives underpinning your own behaviour. Self-awareness is an essential quality for nurses and social care workers to be able to function in an effective and therapeutic way.

empathise
to understand and imagine another person's feelings

The self is a private world that may in everyday life need little exploration, and there are circumstances in which an exploration of understanding the self may seem like a luxury, if not an indulgence. Do the homeless, the hungry or those in war-torn areas of the globe need to understand their motivation for their behaviour? Abraham Maslow's (1968) model of the self may help to understand the relevance of the self-concept in context.

Maslow's hierarchy of needs (Figure 12.1) is a framework that orders the needs of life. It predicts that there is an order in which needs have to be satisfied to enable individuals to reach their full potential. The lower levels identify the requirement to satisfy physical needs such as hunger and warmth, with a progression through needs such as love and esteem to aesthetics and the final need of self-actualisation (Maslow, 1968). Maslow's theory of growth and development will be further discussed later in this chapter.

Maslow's hierarchy of needs
a pyramid with basic needs (physical, safety) at the lower levels, which the person has to satisfy before progressing to achieve higher order needs (love, esteem, cognitive, aesthetic), culminating in self-actualisation at the pinnacle

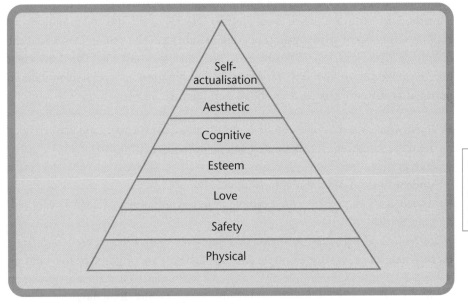

Figure 12.1 ● Maslow's hierarchy of needs

Link
Chapter 5 provides more information on satisfying the basic need for food.

All professionals and care workers need to understand what it is to be a professional carer; to understand self-motivations that underpin the choice to care and to be able to disentangle self thoughts and emotions from those of the people in receipt of care. The nature of caring dictates that the people with

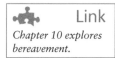

Link

Chapter 10 explores bereavement.

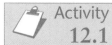

Activity
12.1

Before reading on, try this brief exercise. Write down 20 answers to the following question: 'Who am I?'

---

self-concept

the knowledge that a person has about him- or herself

whom nurses and carers have the most intimate contact are the most vulnerable people. If assumptions about behaviour are based one's own past experience and feelings, it may be doing patients a grave disservice. When a nurse is faced with the death of a patient and grieving relatives, for example, is her distress a sharing of those people's distress and loss, or has it more to do with unresolved issues of grief or mortality in her own life? Thus, an understanding of self thoughts, feelings and behaviour is essential for nurses and other care professionals to reach their maximum potential as carers.

■ Self-concept

Self-concept is the knowledge that a person has about himself. It is information chiefly acquired by interactions with others (Baron and Byrne, 1997). It is a schema, an organised set of beliefs and feelings that are self-referent. The self-concept influences how we process information about the external social world and its relationships to 'me'. The schema holds information about motives, emotions, self-evaluations, abilities and so on, and we access this self-schema every time we use self-referent information (Baron and Byrne, 1997).

Research into the self-concept frequently uses the 'Who am I?' approach, sometimes known as Gordon's phenomenological approach (Gordon, 1968), as a method of study. Rentsch and Heffner (1994) used this methodology to explore self-concept with a group of student subjects. The researchers asked the question, 'Who am I?' of 230 subjects. Their analysis confirmed Gordon's eight broad categories of the self, reflecting a combination of social identity and personal attributes. These are (Rentsch and Heffner, 1994):

- *Existential aspects:* for example I am unique, I am special, I am attractive
- *Self-determination:* for example I can achieve my educational goals
- *Interpersonal attributes:* for example myself in relation to others, I am a student nurse, I am a daughter/son
- *Ascribed characteristics:* for example I am a woman/man, I am 19 years old, I am British
- *Interests and activities:* for example I enjoy football, I like dogs
- *Internalised beliefs:* for example I am a socialist, I am opposed to fox-hunting
- *Self-awareness:* for example my beliefs are well integrated, I am a good person
- *Social differentiation:* for example I am poor, wealthy, I am gay.

The self-concept is, however, more than the sum of the answers to 'Who am I?' The schema for self contains information about the individual's past experiences, it encompasses memories and expectations of the future. Baron and Byrne (1997) maintain that the self is the sum of everything a person knows and what he imagines he can be.

To conceptualise this schema as a fixed structure is, however, misleading as there is change over time: the self-concept alters with life events and new learning. It may be that it is vulnerable to change in a short period of time, for example if a woman loses her job, her self-concept will undergo a redefinition from being a person who is employed to one who is unemployed. The opposite can of course occur when a person gains employment, passes a driving test or achieves a goal. The concept of self is therefore not a rigid **percept** but one that is fluid and vulnerable to change.

It is important to understand the effects of change and why this change to the self-image occurs, because a failure to do so may lead to psychological discomfort as the person resists the redefinition of or addition to self-knowledge. Change can be threatening, particularly if it is enforced rather than chosen.

percept

an object or phenomenon that is perceived

Development of self-concept

The sense of self develops as a function of growing older. The child learns about the environment and her relationship to the people and objects within that environment by being in the world. The child learns that she is a separate entity within the world rather than symbiotic with the caregiver and the external world. She learns that objects exist independently of her, that is, the child comes to understand that when she cannot see a toy, it still remains in the world rather than no longer existing. Similarly, the child learns that she exists independently of her environment and that she can act and have an effect on the world, particularly on other people. As a result of interactions with caregivers, friends, teachers and so on, children learn about an 'I' separate from other people and objects (Mischel, 1986). Consequently, they establish a **self-schema**. In early infancy, this is knowledge about the self existing as an independent entity, but as the child matures, the schema enlarges. During middle childhood, there is a shift in the self-descriptors from concrete, physical descriptions to social comparisons and psychological descriptors (Brooks-Gun and Paikoff, 1992). Montemeyer and Eisen (1977) asked a group of 10–18-year-olds to answer the question 'Who am I?' They found that, with age, there was an increase in the use of self, ideology and belief references, and a decrease in physical categories as descriptors.

Activity 12.2

Ask a few children to answer the question 'Who am I?' What descriptors do children use?

self-schema

your mental representation of understanding about yourself

Erikson's theory of personality development

One theoretical framework that places the establishment of the self-schema within a developmental context is Erikson's eight-stage psychosocial theory of development (Erikson, 1959). Each stage has a task of transition or crisis, the resolution of each crisis influencing the subsequent stages. The task is to resolve the conflict between two opposing choices and to balance in favour of a positive or negative outcome. A positive resolution will result in the acquisition of an

Erikson's theory of personality development

at each of the eight stages of development, from the first years of life to the ageing years, there are special issues that must be confronted before personal development can succeed. His ideas were developed from psychoanalytic theory

adaptive strength that will sustain the individual's progress through the next stage of life span development. Each life crisis gives the individual more knowledge about the world and his relationship to it (Erikson, 1959). These are the eight stages:

- *Stage 1 – Trust versus mistrust*
  Trust is about learning what to expect from the world. This is not just that the world is a safe place with consistency and nurturing, but also that dangerous people can be trusted to be dangerous. Irregularity and inconsistency will, however, lead to mistrust, and the child experiences anxiety and insecurity
  Adaptive strength: Hope

- *Stage 2 – Autonomy versus shame and doubt*
  This is a stage of gaining mastery over the world and, particularly for the young child, over the body. If the child is encouraged to explore his body, there will be a growth of self-confidence, enabling an exploration of the physical and social worlds. If constantly criticised, the child will feel ashamed and come to doubt himself
  Adaptive strength: Will

- *Stage 3 – Initiative versus guilt*
  The child will begin to ask questions to further his knowledge and skills, realising that he has some influence over his environment and the people in it. The child may become successful at manipulating his surroundings, but if reaching out to the world is met with disapproval and reproof, the child will feel inept, resulting in an emerging sense of guilt
  Adaptive strength: Purpose

- *Stage 4 – Industry versus inferiority*
  The child is learning about accomplishment and task completion. A sense of industry will feed a sense of achievement, whereas failure to complete or accomplish will result in a sense of inferiority, which may be lifelong
  Adaptive strength: Competence

- *Stage 5 – Identity versus role confusion*
  This was viewed by Erikson as a crucial stage of development. **Identity** is a structure within an organised set of values and beliefs about oneself. These may be expressed in a variety of ways, for example occupation, politics, religion and relationships. Erikson maintains that an integrated identity cannot occur before adolescence because of immature cognitive, physical and social development, but a failure to integrate during this stage will result in role confusion
  Adaptive strength: Fidelity

- *Stage 6 – Intimacy versus isolation*
  This stage presents the young adult with the task of forming intimate relationships with others. It encompasses a sense of connectedness, a fusion of

one's identity with someone else's, safe in the belief that you will retain your sense of self intact. The opposing resolution is isolation, a feeling that occurs when a person is threatened by the behaviour of others
Adaptive strength: Love

- *Stage 7 – Generativity versus self-absorption*
  The positive aspect of this task is **generativity**: an interest in the next gener- | **generativity**
  ation. The primary interest is in nurturing offspring but, for those without | an interest in the next generation
  offspring, energy may be directed into creative and altruistic concerns. The
  opposite of this outwardly directed interest is self-absorption, an indulging of
  the self as though it were a child, one's one and only child
  Adaptive strength: Care
- *Stage 8 – Integrity versus despair*
  This is the final life task in which the individual is faced with integrating the
  life cycle, an acceptance of one's life as being one's own responsibility
  Adaptive strength: Wisdom.

Erikson's theory outlines a framework of growth and development that is inevitable and irresistible. Erikson (1959) hypothesised a ground plan for growth, each stage having its time of ascendancy until all aspects of personality are fully developed to form an integrated personality.

Resolution in a negative direction means that individuals become restricted in their development and fail to benefit from the adaptive strength associated with each life task. Working with the vulnerable, nurses need to have insight into the self, some understanding of how life tasks have been resolved. Nurses need to access their own thoughts, feelings and motivations for behaviour to be able to have an awareness of how they may respond to the thoughts, feelings and behaviour of others. There is an acknowledgement within the field of health care that nurses and care workers need to demonstrate positive regard; nurses aim to promote a sense of value in their patients, but to be successful, there is a need to have an understanding of one's own values, attitudes, thoughts and feelings. Nurses need to be comfortable with themselves before they can begin to understand others.

■ Self-awareness

Rawlinson (1990) defines **self-awareness** as: 'bringing into consciousness | **self-awareness**
[those] various aspects of our understanding of ourselves'. The 'various aspects' | the condition of being able to analyse the
refer to the components of self. Rawlinson (1990) differentiates self-awareness | motives for one's
from self-consciousness, which, rather than being a constructive appreciation of | behaviour
the self, is a concern for others' perception of our own self. Self-awareness is a
condition of being able to analyse the motives underlying one's own behaviour.
Most of the time people act and interact, giving scant attention to why, the focus

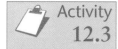
Activity 12.3

What does it mean to be self-aware? Reflect on this question and jot down your thoughts.

being the consequences or achievement of goals. Self-awareness is the antithesis of self-consciousness, the latter being a concern with others' opinions and the former a concern with the motives for and effectiveness of one's behaviour.

A model of self that illustrates the importance of self-awareness in the growth and development of a confident, effective person is the Johari window (Luft and Ingham, 1955). This model is depicted as a window with four panes, each representing a facet of the self (Figure 12.2). The Johari window is useful in understanding the nature of self-awareness. The aim is to enlarge the public self. The more comfortable we are with what others know about us, the easier it is to understand pain at times of change for ourselves and for others. But this is just one model of self; others offer different frameworks in which to strive for self-knowledge. The four facets of the self in the Johari window are each discussed in turn.

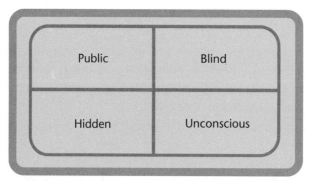

Figure 12.2 ● The Johari window: four facets of the self

The public self

public self

the things we know about ourselves and are comfortable for others to know

The **public self** is that information which we know about ourselves and are happy for others to know. This may include name, occupation and marital status. It may also include age (although some people prefer to keep their age a secret), background and personal details. If, for example, I meet anyone from Norfolk, I am, as a person who lived there for many years and has happy memories from that time, immediately prepared, indeed keen, to share my experiences of living there with that person. This is a way of interacting with others that allows me a sharing of common experiences and knowledge with someone I may not know but with whom I share a part of my self-concept, that is, someone who knows and likes Norfolk. This then is public knowledge; it is not a secret, as I am prepared to share it with anyone. These exchanges are not only interactions that we are prepared to be known by, but also a means of validating beliefs and opinions and affirming the status of 'person'.

The blind self

The **blind self** is knowledge known to others but not known to the self. It is an area of knowledge that can be threatening. What is it that others are not telling us? It could be that a woman's dress is tucked in the back of her knickers or that a man's fly is undone. More often, however, it is the psychological, behavioural or social equivalent. The 'other' is able to form a totally different perspective on our behaviour, habits and mannerisms of which we are totally unaware. Do you know what you look like from the back view? Do you know what your walk looks like? Others may find our presence pleasing but, conversely, they may find it unpleasant. The more information that we are given about the blind self, the greater the degree of self-awareness that is allowed to develop. If I am given information about my behaviour of which I have previously been unaware, I have the choice to change or continue, with the knowledge of the effect that this behaviour may have on others.

Giving an example of knowledge in the blind self is not easy, as I do not know what others know about me to which I am not privy. When I was sister in a day hospital, however, I was asked by a member of staff whether I would be willing to allow a health-care support worker to be flexible with her time as she had family problems. As part of my self-image was kind and caring, I had no hesitation in agreeing, provided that the day hospital was safe for patients and the care was delivered as it should be. I was curious to know why this woman had not asked me herself. The reply from the staff nurse to this query was that I was unapproachable. This came as new knowledge to me and challenged my existing self-concept as a kind, caring and considerate manager. Now, I could have responded in two ways. First, I could have been defensive. When the self-concept is threatened or challenged, there is a shift to mobilise defence strategies to protect the status quo. Hostility is one means of defence: I could have become angry, projecting my feelings of threat on to the other person. A second response is to accept that this was how I appeared to this member of staff and the person on whose behalf she was speaking. These two responses are discussed below.

Defensive response

A **defence mechanism** is a protective strategy employed when the self is under threat. When information is seen as threatening, the self rallies a defence mechanism to maintain equilibrium. The psychodynamic view proposes that the human organism is unable to tolerate anxiety, and we deal with this state by developing defence strategies that protect against this painful state. Defence mechanisms arise from the unconscious as a way of distorting reality in order to exclude feelings of anxiety from consciousness (Pervin, 1984). Being given information about yourself that is unacceptable will produce a state of anxiety, and

blind self

things known about us by others, but not known to us

Link

Chapter 13 outlines how an incident of this kind would respond to a structured approach.

defence mechanism

a protective strategy employed when the self is under threat

one way of dealing with this is projection. Projection occurs when internal, unacceptable feelings are projected externally; thus, feelings of internal hostility are projected outwards, so that you think the other person is being hostile. In the example above, I held the view that I was an approachable manager, but this view was under threat. A hostile response would have shifted this internal hostility from the self externally to the staff nurse, invalidating her opinion.

Acceptance

An alternative approach is to acknowledge the state of anxiety produced by this incongruous information, and if you choose to do so, this gives you the opportunity to alter the image of self conveyed to the world. By accepting the 'other's' perspective, not necessarily as truth but as a valid opinion, there is a growth in self-awareness. So in my example, I could not accept the truth of being unapproachable, but I did accept that this was how I was perceived by others.

The hidden self

hidden self

the things we hide from others

The **hidden self** is the part of the self that is hidden from public gaze. This corner of the window hides that of which we are ashamed, frightened and embarrassed; here lie unacceptable thoughts and feelings. A disclosure of information from this area is threatening and can elicit great anxiety. As an example of the hidden self, we can draw on the literature on carers. Caring for a dependent relative can be a pleasure and enjoyable: it can bring meaning to life and a new perspective to a relationship. However, it is not unusual for carers to feel hostile and angry towards their charges. Admitting that we have these thoughts is a frightening exercise. The dependent person cannot help being ill or disabled; the crying, sleepless baby is vulnerable and helpless. Disclosing feelings of bitterness, resentment, anger and hostility may bring criticism and hostility on the carers themselves, the logic being that, 'If I admit that I feel like hitting X, I will be reviled and ostracised.'

Yet the reality may be that, by disclosing these fears, the person will find warmth, understanding and support. Revealing secrets may bring a realisation that others feel like you do and behave like you do, and that the behaviour, thoughts and feelings that leave you feeling guilty and ashamed are common to others in a similar situation. It is no accident that self-help groups are a popular means of offering support for people caring for dependent relatives. Affiliation with other people in a position similar to our own is an effective way of easing anxiety and lessening our sense of isolation. These groups provide a forum for people to disclose unacceptable thoughts and feelings, facilitating a growth in understanding of the self as carer. There are times when this hidden part of the self needs help to facilitate disclosure, but accepting this part of the self-concept helps the individual to feel more comfortable with the self and as such enables a growth in self-understanding.

The unconscious self

The **unconscious self** is an interesting but enigmatic area of the self. This is knowledge not known to the self or others, and the question 'Does it exist?' has to be asked. The psychodynamic theory of personality maintains that the unconscious drives behaviour and can be revealed by free association and within dreams. However, the antithesis of this is the behavioural perspective. If it cannot be observed, it cannot be studied, but behaviour can be observed and can therefore be attributed to the consequences of action. This is not necessarily to deny the unconscious but to deny the validity of being able to say that the unconscious is a cause of behaviour. Wittgenstein maintained that when an individual looks inside himself, he finds a beetle in a box, a beetle that only he can see and touch (Humphrey, 1984). We all have a beetle, but I do not know what your beetle is like and you have no access to mine. Therefore what can I say about how your beetle influences your behaviour? If so little of this section of the window is available to the world, the unconscious is a territory to be explored only by the intrepid and with experienced, expert guidance (Humphrey, 1984).

unconscious self
things not known to ourselves or others

Maslow's hierarchy of needs

Maslow's hierarchy is usually depicted as a pyramid with basic needs, such as safety and hunger, forming the base and self-actualisation forming the pinnacle (see Figure 12.1 above). A more appropriate view, however, may be to see this structure in terms of a more fluid model. Maslow viewed basic needs as drives that, when they were met, enabled a move to a higher level of need. However, not everyone chooses to move beyond a particular level of need and it may be that the rigidity of Maslow's framework provides a safe boundary for the self-concept. But, choosing to move on to a greater fulfilment of need is to expand self-knowledge, broaden experience and move towards a greater understanding of the courage and anxieties of others.

Rogers' model of self

Rogers' model of self consists of all the knowledge that we have about the self, all the constituents of 'I' or 'me' (Atkinson et al., 1993). The three dominant features of this model are the *real self*, the *ideal self* and *self-esteem*. Rogers

Rogers' model of self
developed from explorations of individuals' subjective understanding of their 'self', consisting of 'I' or 'me'

maintained that we tend to interpret events in the world in relation to the self. We all have a percept of how we are in the world, an image of the self and its relationship to others, objects and events. This image is modelled on the ideal self, the goal for which we strive, the perfect, the self without flaw. The difference between the image we have of the self and the ideal self is the measure of **self-esteem**, the worth that we attribute to the self. This self-image and level of self-esteem are not, however, necessarily a true reflection of the real self. It is possible for people who outwardly appear successful and competent to have low self-esteem and define their self-concept as inadequate. This may be because people set themselves goals that are too high or unachievable, a consequence of which may be, for some, a need for therapy to assist with the attainment of psychological well-being (Atkinson et al., 1993).

self-esteem

confidence and value in one's own worth or abilities

Self and Sources of Stress

When the self-concept is threatened, the resulting discomfort is a manifestation of **stress**, so the relationship between stress and the self-concept needs to be explored in order to achieve a better understanding of the self.

Selye (1980) maintains that stress suffers from being too well known and too little understood. Nursing is a pressurised occupation. Nurses are put under the pressures of time and limited resources, while daily facing the pressures of others' pain, discomfort and distress, with little time to acknowledge the effect that this may be having on their own emotions and self-concept. Self-esteem has certainly been implicated as a factor influencing our perception of stress. Stress occurs when the demands of the situation exceed an individual's personal resources, and whereas a degree of stress is thought to be useful in motivating us to action, there needs to be an awareness of how to maintain a balance between what is motivating (the degree of arousal necessary for the successful performance of a task) and arousal that exceeds the optimum level for effective performance. The experience of the latter is stress, which is unpleasant and anxiety-provoking.

stress

a state of mental, emotional or physical tension, pressure and strain

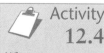

Activity 12.4

What causes you stress? Draw two columns, heading one 'Positive' and the other 'Negative'. List your answers according to whether you find the stressor motivating or threatening.

Models of stress

Stimulus-based model

A simple model of stress is the stimulus-based model, which characterises the environment as providing a stressor and the person as experiencing stress or strain. But although this may offer a description, it does not elucidate the process by which people find themselves under pressure.

Response-based model

The response model offers a more detailed approach to understanding stress. The environment is the source of the stressor or stimulus, and the person's stress is the response. Selye (1980) conceptualised this as a non-specific response to excessive demands on individual coping resources. Selye believed that the response did not depend on the nature of the stressor and that the response was a protective mechanism (Cox, 1978). There are three identifiable stages to the response syndrome that form the **general adaptation syndrome (GAS)**.

General adaptation syndrome (GAS)
response to stress characterised by three stages: the alarm reaction, the resistance stage and exhaustion

Alarm reaction

This stage is related to a high level of physical arousal, which causes the release of adrenaline. It is during this initial stage that the organism's susceptibility to the specific stressor increases, and if the severity of the response is great enough, death may ensue. With less severe stressors but prolonged exposure, however, pituitary/adrenocorticotrophic hormones are released within the body, and the resistance stage of the GAS is initiated.

Resistance stage

During this stage, physical arousal remains high. Adaptation occurs as the parasympathetic nervous system attempts to counteract the effects of the sympathetic nervous system. The organism is therefore able to resist the debilitating effects of the stressor, although the threshold for eliciting the stress response has been lowered for further encounters with this specific threat or other non-specific stressors.

Exhaustion

If exposure continues, the final stage of the GAS is entered, that of exhaustion. Hormone reserves are depleted, fatigue results and the felt experience of this stage is frequently that of depression.

Interactional model

The **interactional** model incorporates the stress response model with the demand placed on the individual and the subjective perception of that demand. There is an acknowledgement that the consequences of coping strategies will influence the perception of felt stress and that this provides feedback for future action when faced with a similar threat. Cox and Mackay (1978) proposed the man–environment transaction model, which they describe as eclectic, drawing on stimulus and response models. This model explicitly identifies that a stress system is an individual perceptual phenomenon (Cox, 1978).

interaction
refers to the interaction between man and environment

The man–environment model has five identifiable stages:

1. Actual capability and demand.
2. Perceived capability and demand.
3. Psychophysiological changes.
4. Consequences of coping responses.
5. Feedback.

The last component is a particularly important feature of this model, because it is the feedback the individual receives from the environment that determines the degree of felt stress and the perceived effectiveness of coping strategies.

Information-processing model

The information-processing model emphasises the importance of cognitive and attentional factors. The individual selectively attends to stimuli and will interpret information as stressful or otherwise by comparing it with past experience (Figure 12.3).

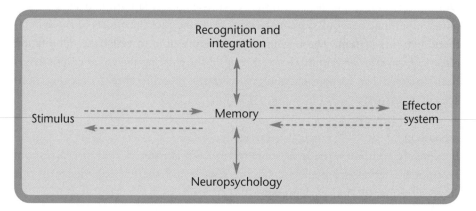

Figure 12.3 ● Information-processing model of stress

Memory and decision-making therefore play a role in the processing of stimuli, and cognitive appraisal will elicit emotions, such as anxiety, anger, fear and sadness, previously associated with similar situations. This model proposes that stressors and stress responses can only be so if the individual's perception of the situation is that a threat exists. This view is in line with the premise that what one individual perceives as a threat, another may view as a challenge. Why is it that one individual will succumb to the debilitating effects of stress, manifest in illnesses such as peptic ulcers, coronary artery disease and depression, whereas another person in the same circumstances thrives on the motivation of the environment? Kobasa (1979) identifies challenge as a characteristic of the hardy personality, an individual whose susceptibility to illness is less than that of others who may perceive life events as stressful and have less than effective coping strategies.

Link

Chapters 14 and 15 deal with teams, which may influence the level of stress we feel.

■ Factors Affecting Stress

What acts as a source of stress will vary from one individual to another, but there are some events and encounters that have a shared effect; it is the interpretation of these as either a threat or a challenge that differs. The stressful life events model describes events as sources of stress (Holmes and Rahe, 1967). Holmes and Rahe's social readjustment rating scale was the outcome of research that asked people to rate the degree to which they found life events stressful. The resulting list covers a whole range of general life experiences such as the death of a spouse, marriage, childbirth, moving house, Christmas and going on holiday. But is the experience of a desirable event the same as that of one with negative consequences or connotations? Is the stress of preparing for Christmas a similar experience to that of losing a job? Although there may be emotional strain associated with positive events, there is an expectation of reward that provides a different perspective from that of events that may have negative connotations. Why is it, then, that people vary in their response to events and encounters? There are several possible factors influencing this appraisal including personality, social support and emotions, and these are now discussed.

Personality

It seems that some people are predisposed to experience life events as stressful (Watson and Clarke, 1984); some individuals have a predisposition to negative affectivity, expressing distress and discomfort across a variety of situations rather than responding to specific situations. The corollary of this is the person who is predisposed to interpret demanding events as challenging and is able to cope effectively. Kobasa (1979) described this personality type as a hardy personality.

The hardy personality has three constructs:

- *Challenge:* a willingness to accept change and to face novel situations as opportunities for growth and development
- *Commitment:* the tendency to involve oneself in whatever situations or events one encounters
- *Control:* the belief that one has influence over life events and the assumption of personal responsibility for those events.

Hardy individuals are mentally and physically healthier than others. They seem to appraise events more favourably than other individuals and have more effective coping strategies than non-hardy personality types.

Social support

Social support is the perceived comfort derived from a social network that includes significant others, family, friends, community organisations and professional practitioners. There are four broad types of social support:

1. *Emotional:* this is an expression of empathy, caring and concern towards a person. It provides a sense of belonging and being loved at times of stress.
2. *Esteem:* this support is expressed through positive regard. Esteem support enables the development of a sense of worth and competence.
3. *Tangible/instrumental:* this is support that comes from practical help. It may manifest itself in any way, from the loan of money to someone doing the shopping or housework, or helping with personal care. This is the support given by someone when individuals are unable to perform a task or activity themselves.
4. *Informational:* this support is derived from advice, direction, suggestion and feedback. This support is manifest as information that allows an individual to make an informed appraisal or decision.

Link

Chapters 14 and 15 deal with teams, which can be a useful source of social support.

Social support reduces the stress that people experience. Stress has been demonstrated to have detrimental effects on health, and social support has been shown to be protective against these adverse effects.

So how does social support protect against ill-health? Two theories have been proposed:

- The *buffering hypothesis* proposes that a good supportive network has a protective effect at times of high stress (Cohen and Hoberman, 1983)
- The *direct effect hypothesis* maintains that social support is beneficial regardless of the amount of stress experienced, influencing the appraisal of events as stressful or challenging (Cobb, 1976).

Emotions

Negative events have a greater potential than positive events to be interpreted as stressful, and our emotions will influence the appraisal of a situation. Common emotions associated with stress are fear and anger, whereas a similar event associated with a pleasant emotion may not be interpreted as stressful. If while travelling we are, for example, aroused to anger by delays, our interpretation may be that the journey is stressful, but if the delay in the journey is perceived as an opportunity for time out from a busy schedule, the journey may be described as pleasant.

Recognising stress in ourselves, being able to identify the feelings that indicate stress, is important as the effect that this has on our behaviour within the clinical area will affect the patients for whom we are caring. Similarly, we need to have an understanding of what our patients may be experiencing, not so that we are in position to say, 'Yes, I know how you're feeling and this is how I deal with it' or to be able to evaluate someone else's experience, but so that we, as nurses, can empathise with our patients and provide the support that may be necessary to reduce the adverse effects of their experiences.

We need to have some understanding of how stress can affect behaviour in order to understand our patients' behaviour. This may enable us to anticipate times when stress may be heightened and when it may be at a minimum. An understanding of how people may appraise a situation as stressful needs to be part of the nurse's repertoire of skills in order to provide care most effectively. Being there for people when the need for support is at its most pressing is one of the most valuable skills of caring. The practice of nursing requires prioritisation when delivering care and being able to anticipate possible stress for patients when making these judgements.

So, making judgements about patients' affect, behaviour and cognition requires skill in empathy and analysis. An understanding of the self is essential to begin the process of analysis. We need to understand our thoughts and feelings in order to tease out the rationale for the actions and reactions of self and others. We also need to have an understanding of attitudes in order to be able to suspend our subjective evaluations and account for the evaluative judgements of others, so it is to an examination of attitudes that we now turn.

■ Attitudes

As we grow from infancy to adulthood, we are influenced by a variety of different pressures from parents, family, friends, school and the media. These pressures form the basis of our **attitudes**, beliefs and opinions. Attitudes reflect our values, the worth we attribute to events, people and objects. Sharing values is a way of building relationships; we seem to have a natural rapport with those who share our perspective. The way we dress, the music we like, the political beliefs we hold all contribute to the development of friendships. But when we nurse, we cannot be that selective. Indeed, all human life is to be found in the health-care context. Nurses are charged with being genuine, being warm and demonstrating unconditional positive regard; these are Rogers' core conditions necessary to effect change within a therapeutic relationship (Rogers, 1959). How easy is it though for these conditions to exist? There are times when we are, as nurses, required to suspend judgement in order to give our undivided attention. In some cases, this is not difficult, but, in others, our attitudes, beliefs and opinions may block our ability to

attitude
the sum of one's beliefs and opinions

enter the 'other's' world perspective and give care at an optimum level. Making the effort to know someone's background may make the difference between treating someone as an object in receipt of a service and a person who requires nursing care.

Casebox 12.1

Thomas was a patient on a male medical ward. He had been diagnosed with **Parkinson's disease**. I met Thomas when I was working with a student nurse in my role as a clinical teacher. Thomas was sitting in the day room but wanted to return to his bed to rest. The student nurse and I helped Thomas to return to his bed; he walked part of the way but when this became too much, we completed the journey with the aid of a wheelchair. Thomas was in a great deal of distress with the rigidity and discomfort of his condition. When he was on the bed, he had several demands regarding how to make him comfortable but,

after a few minutes, we were able to leave him.

My debriefing with the student nurse was revealing. She told me that she did not like this patient. He was bad tempered and uncooperative. He could do more for himself than he did do; she said he was lazy. Her diatribe shocked me; when this young woman looked at Thomas she saw 'a grumpy, lazy, difficult old man', not an experienced individual, an ex-sailor who had spent part of his national service in Palestine helping to shape world history. This man had been on the last ship to leave Palestine when the British mandate left Palestine and

now, here he was, a patient on a medical ward, who was losing his independence in a battle he couldn't win against Parkinson's disease, and with it his dignity and his identity.

Of course, my role was to enable this student to change her perspective; to convey to her that like and dislike were not relevant concepts in the realm of patient care. My job was to help this student to begin to develop a sense of empathy, enter into Thomas's frame of reference, see the world through his eyes, and understand him as a person with a history and not just a bad patient with difficult demands.

Parkinson's disease

a slow progressive neurological disorder with resting tremor, muscle rigidity and weakness, shuffling gait and a mask-like appearance

As an illustration of this point, let us consider the experience of the student nurse asked to care for a man with Parkinson's disease described in Casebox 12.1. Thomas had a reputation among the nurses for being difficult. The student nurse said she did not like him because, 'You can't like everyone, can you?' This statement requires challenging and analysis in the context of nursing care. When we acknowledge likes and dislikes, we are expressing an attitude. On what are these judgements based? Sometimes they are based on only limited information: our interactions with the patients and possibly the comments of our colleagues. Knowledge can be inaccurate and incomplete, and, as nurses, we need to be prepared to alter our opinions, to allow our knowledge of our patients to be fluid and flexible. How is this achieved? By being non-judgemental. A person-centred approach to care, an approach that starts with the patient before any judgements or decisions, is more likely to facilitate a rapport that will contribute to reducing the impact of the stress of being a patient.

Thomas, the gentleman with Parkinson's disease, had been admitted for a review of his condition. He was slow when mobile and dependent when in bed. He had the typical mask-like expression seen in patients with Parkinson's disease and demonstrated the on/off syndrome when walking. He was perceived by the nurses as demanding because, when he asked for assistance, he was time-consuming and appeared ungrateful for the help. The nurses found him difficult to please, and he always insisted on having things done strictly his way. The student nurse interpreted his behaviour as difficult and hostile, and the consequence was that she judged him as an unpleasant man.

This may of course have been an accurate judgement, but an alternative explanation is that here was a man angry and frustrated at his loss of independence. Thomas was pedantic about his needs; he wanted his way because he was no longer able to perform, without help from another person, activities that most of us take for granted. This patient's expectation was that others would substitute what he would like to do for himself. This nurse needed to develop her skill of empathy to see the world from his perspective. Nurses need to listen to the patients' stories – most people have a story if we can make the right connection – and see beyond the label of 'difficult to understand'. As nurses, if we label our patients as we do our friends and acquaintances, we fail to acknowledge the meaning of our profession, the meaning of care.

> **Link**
> *Chapter 13 describes how this scenario would benefit from a structured, thoughtful approach.*

Part of this process is to understand attitudes, how they are formed and how they can be changed. Attitudes influence behaviour, and as such we need to have an insight into the effect of our own attitudes on our nursing practice. We also need to consider our patients' attitudes and how these may be influencing their compliance with treatment and their thoughts and feelings about being in a vulnerable, dependent position.

There are three components of an attitude:

1. *Affective:* the feelings held towards an object or event that is to some degree either positive or negative. This is the component that represents our likes and dislikes.
2. *Behavioural:* the observable translation of an attitude. If feelings are positive, we develop an approach tendency or behaviour that increases contact with the object or causes us to engage with that situation. If our feelings are negative, we tend to develop avoidance tendencies or behaviours that distance us from the object or event.
3. *Cognitive:* the rational part of the attitude, defining the object or situation towards which the attitude is directed. This encompasses people and groups, and consists of knowledge about the object or situation even though this knowledge may be incomplete.

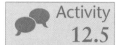

Activity 12.5

What is your opinion of smoking? How did you form this opinion? What do you think about people who smoke? What do you think about people who do not smoke?

This three-component model of attitudes is useful in trying to make sense of our experience, but it is based on the assumption that all three components are consistent. If, for example, we hold positive beliefs about an object or event, this should elicit positive feelings and an approach tendency. But is this always the case? Try Activity 12.5.

Your opinion about smoking may be influenced by whether your parents smoked, whether your friends, the people with whom you wish to affiliate, smoke and whether you smoke. Perhaps you think that smoking in moderation is OK and that people who do not smoke are prudish and boring. You may, however, believe that smoking is a health hazard not just for those who smoke, but also for those of us who have to inhale the smoke from others' cigarettes, making smokers selfish and antisocial, if not downright dangerous. It may be that you hold strong beliefs about smoking because of your experience of its effect on someone you know, or you may have beliefs about smoking but not to such an extent that you object to others smoking in your presence.

An alternative model is the expectancy value model. This proposes that we hold attitudes according to what we expect of an object or event and the degree to which this event or object will contribute to our goals and values.

Attitudes are formed by both direct and indirect methods. Direct experiences tend to produce more accurate knowledge on which to form judgements, but indirect methods also have a great influence. These include vicarious experience as well as what others, for example parents, peer group, schools and the media, say and do.

Changing attitudes can be a difficult task, but it does have real relevance for nurses as it is people's attitudes towards health behaviours that influence risky health behaviours and whether they are likely to modify any behaviour that will lessen their susceptibility to ill-health. The relationship between the patient and the nurse can be an important factor in changing a person's attitudes. Some of the factors that contribute to a change in attitude include:

- Trust
- Like and dislike
- Credibility
- Perceived attractiveness
- Individual beliefs
- Self-esteem.

In other words, the relationship between the nurse and patient is important in influencing patients' attitudes. This highlights the importance of the nurse developing interpersonal skills and understanding how to establish and build a rapport.

What happens when our behaviour is inconsistent with our beliefs? When we behave in a way that is contrary to our beliefs, we are left with a feeling of psychological discomfort described as **cognitive dissonance**. This discomfort may arise, for example, when a person who smokes firmly holds the belief that it is harmful to the self and others, or one who drives a car on a regular basis believes that this is a major form of pollution and therefore also harmful. Any behaviour that counteracts our beliefs can lead to a feeling of discomfort, which we try to reduce. Individuals, on the whole, strive for cognitive consistency. As nurses, an understanding of self and the motives underlying behaviour can lead to an attitude change and a greater degree of objectivity when making an assessment of the patients in our care.

cognitive dissonance
a state of tension that occurs when an individual holds two or more thoughts/beliefs that are psychologically inconsistent

A further issue that needs to be addressed in a discussion of attitudes is that of **prejudice**. Prejudice arises from a faulty generalisation directed towards a specific person or group of people because they are members of a particular group. A prejudice ignores qualities or characteristics that would negate our opinion, and whereas prejudice is generally thought of as being negative, we may equally well ignore negative qualities as well as positive ones (Oliver and Hyde, 1993). If, as nurses, we believe that people who are short-tempered and particular in the way in which their needs are met are difficult patients, we will adopt a prejudicial approach to people who fit these criteria. The cognitive component of prejudice is more commonly known as a **stereotype**. One definition of a stereotype is that it is a type of shorthand, a way of understanding without having to go to first principles each time we wish to communicate or understand an event or situation. The knowledge that we hold about the world is organised into schemata, clumps of knowledge that include stereotypes, but by using this shorthand in our professional life, we exclude a great deal of knowledge and information about people that will enrich our understanding and enhance our nursing care.

prejudice
the combination of negative beliefs, attitudes and discriminatory behaviour towards those in a particular target group

stereotype
a form of cultural shorthand; shared knowledge or information about an object or event

The student nurse described above who said she did not like Thomas, the gentleman with Parkinson's disease, had adopted an attitude about this patient based on her belief about how patients should behave and possibly about the nature of Parkinson's disease. This also suggests, however, that her knowledge about the condition was incomplete, and that her attitude towards the patient's behaviour was limited and prejudicial. Knowledge should be acquired as this student progresses through her training. Will an increase in knowledge widen her understanding? The expectation is that it will, and that it will, in turn, influence her attitude to patients with Parkinson's disease who remain expressionless, unable to give the usual feedback that helps us to understand our impact on another person.

Will this increase in knowledge also help to develop the individual's understanding of her action and reaction to patients who may be having difficulty coming to terms with a redefinition of self from independent to dependent? This requires an analysis not just of knowledge in terms of generalising neutral facts to the subjective human experience, but also of the nurse's own thoughts, feelings and behaviours.

■ Chapter Summary

This chapter attempts to explain why it is important for nurses and other health and social care professionals to have an understanding of the self. It covers issues of the self-concept and its development, self-awareness, stress, attitudes and prejudice. Nurses need to have an understanding of the self in order to enable a greater understanding of the people for whom they care. A knowledge of the self will promote empathy by a growth in self-awareness and an insight into the factors that may threaten the self-concept, such as stress and prejudice. By understanding our own motivations for behaviour, our own responses to stress, the origins of attitudes and prejudices, we will better understand those of the people for whom we care.

Test Yourself!

1. Define the self-concept.

2. What is the difference between being self-aware and being self-conscious?

3. Can you define stress?

4. List the factors that may modify the impact of stress.

5. What are attitudes?

6. Why is it important for nurses to have an understanding of attitude change?

7. What are some of the factors in the nurse–patient relationship that contribute to attitude change?

■ References

Atkinson, R., Atkinson, R., Smith E. and Bem, D. (1993) *Introduction to Psychology*, 11th edn. Harcourt Brace Jovanovich, Fort Worth, TX.

Baron, R. and Byrne, D. (1997) *Social Psychology*, 8th edn. Allyn & Bacon, Boston.

Brooks-Gun, J. and Paikoff, R.L. (1992) Changes in self feelings during the transition towards adolescence. In McGurk, H. (ed.) *Childhood Social Development, Contemporary Perspectives*. LEA, London.

Cobb, S. (1976) Social support as a moderator of life stress. *Psychosomatic Medicine* **38**: 300–14.

Cohen, S. and Hoberman, H.M. (1983) Positive life events and social supports as buffers of life change stress. *Journal of Applied Social Psychology* **13**: 99–125.

Cox, T. (ed.) (1978) *Stress*. Macmillan, London.

Cox, T. and McKay, C. (1978) Stress at work. In Cox, T. (ed.) *Stress*. Macmillan, London.

Erikson, E. (1959) *Identity and the Life Cycle*. International University Press, London.

Gordon, C. (1968) Self-concept: configurations of content. In Gordon, C. and Gergen, K.J. (eds) *The Self in Social Interaction*, vol. I: *Classic Contemporary Perspectives*. John Wiley & Sons, New York.

Holmes, T. and Rahe, R. (1967) The social readjustment rating scale. *Journal of Psycho-somatic Research* **11**: 213–18.

Humphrey, N. (1984) *Consciousness Regained: Chapters in the Development of Mind*. Oxford University Press, Oxford.

Kobasa, S. (1979) Stressful life events, personality and health. An inquiry into hardiness. *Journal of Personality and Social Psychology* **37**: 1–11.

Luft, J. and Ingham, H. (1955) *The Johari Window: A Graphic Model for Interpersonal Relationships*. National Press, New York.

Maslow, A. (1968) *Toward a Psychology of Being*. Van Nostrand Rheinhold, New York.

Mischel, W. (1986) *Introduction to Personality*, 4th edn. Holt, Rinehart & Winston, Fort Worth, TX.

Montemeyer, R. and Eisen, M. (1977) The development of self-conception from childhood to adolescence. *Development Psychology* **13**(4): 314–19.

Pervin, L. (1984) *Personality: Theory and Research*, 4th edn. John Wiley & Sons, London.

Oliver, M.B. and Hyde, J.S. (1993) Gender differences in sexuality: a meta analysis. *Psychological Bulletin* **114**: 29–51.

Rawlinson, J. (1990) Self awareness: conceptual influences, contribution to nursing, and approaches to attainment. *Nurse Education Today* **10**: 111–17.

Rentsch, J.R. and Heffner, T.S. (1994) Assessing self-concept: analysis of Gordon's coding scheme using 'Who am I?' responses. *Journal of Social Behaviour and Personality* **9**(1): 283–300.

Rogers, C. (1959) A theory of therapy, personality and interpersonal relationships as developed in the client centred framework. In Koch, S. (ed.) *Psychology: A Study of Science*, vol 3: *Formulations of the Person and the Social Context*. McGraw-Hill, New York.

Selye, H. (1980) The stress concept today. In Kutash, I.L and Schlesinger, L.B. (eds) *Handbook on Stress and Anxiety*. Jossey-Bass, San Francisco.

Watson, D. and Clark, L.A. (1984) Negative affectivity: the disposition to experience aversive emotional states. *Psychological Bulletin* **96**: 465–90.

◼ Useful Websites

www.nelh.nhs.uk National Electronic Library for Health Programme
Works with NHS Libraries to develop a digital library for NHS staff, patients and the public

MELANIE JASPER

13 Developing Skills for Reflective Practice

Contents

- What is Reflective Practice?
- The Reflective Practitioner
- Skills for Beginning Reflective Practice
- Choosing an Experience to Reflect on
- Reflective Processes
- Using Models and Frameworks to Guide Reflective Activity
- Reflective Learning in the Practice Environment
- Recording your Reflective Work
- Chapter Summary
- Test Yourself!
- References

Learning Outcomes

This chapter explores ways in which we can learn from our experiences and develop reflective skills that help us to make decisions about the best form of care to give to our patients. Reflective practice is one of the key ways that practitioners work as professionals – a hallmark of which is lifelong learning and development. For reflective practice to be used to its optimum effect, the skills need to be developed and learnt as part of the way nursing and midwifery is learnt. At the end of this chapter, you should be able to:

- Identify and discuss the key features of reflective practice
- Discuss the significance of reflective learning for professional practice
- Use reflective processes as ways of learning from your experiences
- Identify ways in which reflective learning has become part of your practice as a student practitioner
- Justify action taken as a result of reflection
- Identify learning opportunities in the practice environment
- Write reflectively in order to identify your learning and devise action plans
- Compile a portfolio utilising evidence and reflective writing to demonstrate the achievement of your objectives and learning outcomes.

What is Reflective Practice?

It is probably true to say that the main way we learn throughout our lives is through learning from experiences. Most of the time we do not consciously think about our learning, we just file the experience away in our heads and probably subconsciously avoid or repeat actions and ways of doing things as a result. Sometimes, though, these subconscious thoughts find their way into our conscious mind and we are aware of them. How many times have you caught yourself thinking 'I did that last time and it worked really well, so I'll try it again.' And, on the other hand, 'I tried that last time, and what a mess that turned out to be, so let's try something different.'

These two outcomes are the essence of **reflective practice** – first, we learn to think consciously about our actions and evaluate them, and repeat those that are successful and eliminate those that are not. Secondly, reflective practice is about taking some sort of action – it is not simply about thinking things over in some way. Of course, we all use some form of reflection every day to ensure that we link our past experiences with what we are planning to do now, or in the future. Try Activity 13.1 to see how you already use reflection in your work.

Very little that we do is unrelated to things we have done in the past. We tend to momentarily recall, even if subconsciously, experiences we have had that are similar to the ones we are faced with in the present. We build up, over time, a reservoir of **paradigm cases** (Benner, 1984) or examples of each type of case and then draw on these to inform our current action. Hence, the name 'reflective practice'. Reflective practice is about how we practise as a result of our reflective activity. It is not reflection alone, as practice is about *doing* something as a result of the learning that has taken place during reflection. It can be summarised by using the ERA (experience–reflection–action) cycle described by Jasper (2003) in Figure 13.1.

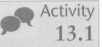

Activity 13.1

Think yourself back to your last day in clinical practice and identify a task you undertook. What did you do? How did you do it? Why did you do it that way? Had you done this task before? If so, what knowledge and skill did you draw on from that time which you used to inform this time? If not, what related knowledge and skill did you draw on that helped you with this task? Did you do anything differently as a result of the development of your knowledge and skills?

reflective practice
_____
professional practice guided by structured reflection on feelings, experience and empathy in order to make practice robust and enhance learning

paradigm cases
_____
examples of patterns, particular perspectives that inform meaning and action

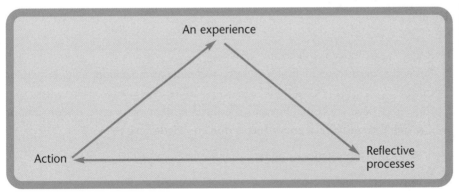

Figure 13.1 ● The ERA cycle (Jasper, 2003, with permission from Nelson Thornes)

Although this is a cycle, because action taken as a result of reflection will result in a different understanding and perspective being taken about something, it is important to see it as an eternal triangle. If one element of the triangle is removed, the concept itself ceases to exist. This is significant for the idea of reflective practice, in that if reflection on an experience does not result in action being taken – or a change in the behaviour of the person reflecting – then clearly it is not reflective *practice* that is happening. You might be *practising reflection*, that is, thinking about things that have happened to you, but this is not the same as *practising reflectively*, which involves the conscious use of reflection to inform practice. Practice itself always involves some sort of action, a 'repeated exercise to improve a skill, action as opposed to theory'.

Much of the learning that a student practitioner does is within the practice environment, yet there are no formal strategies, as when you are learning in a classroom or learning from books or the internet, that ensure you revisit the knowledge or skill and 'embed' it as part of you. Classroom or book learning often involves repetition, or consideration of what you are learning, so that it is remembered.

But, of course, being a practitioner involves a great deal more than simply remembering knowledge – it is about transferring that knowledge into action, about the 'practising' of being a practitioner. The consequences therefore of not knowing or understanding what you are doing as a practitioner are far-reaching in terms of the harm that you might do to someone in your care. Reflective practice, and developing the skills of constantly practising reflectively, go in some ways to helping practitioners to avoid making mistakes and helps to ensure that actions taken can always be justified and explained against the practitioner's experience and evidence base. This is just one of the reasons why practitioners need to practice reflectively. Jasper (2003, p. 5) suggests others, as summarised in Figure 13.2.

In sum, however, these probably boil down to three main purposes of reflective practice:

1. Reflective practice is a learning activity.
2. Reflective practice contributes to improvements and developments in patient care.
3. Reflective practice contributes to the development of practice theory about nursing and midwifery and informs our knowledge base.

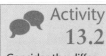

Activity 13.2

Consider the different learning and teaching methods that you use as a student in university. Invariably, a lecture providing knowledge about a subject will be followed by seminar or group discussion work to consider the subject so that the key points are reinforced. How does this reinforcement happen with the other types of learning experiences you may have: reading books and journal articles; practical work in a skills laboratory; web-based learning; educational visits; practice placements.

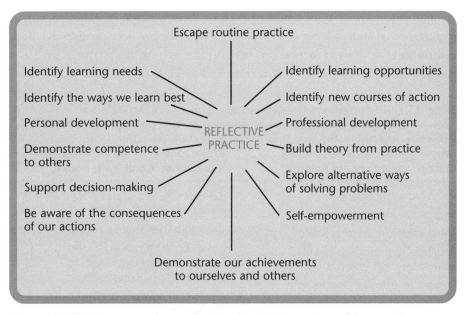

Figure 13.2 ● Reasons why professional practitioners need to practise reflectively (adapted from Jasper, 2003)

■ The Reflective Practitioner

Professional practice is a complicated business. Nurses and midwives are registered with a professional body, the Nursing and Midwifery Council (NMC), upon qualification, and from that time become accountable for their actions as practitioners. It is therefore important that they continue to develop the knowledge base for their practice and expand the range of skills and experiences that enable them to develop beyond the basic level of competence and safe practice that qualification certifies.

However, it would be unrealistic to think that all practitioners continue to study in the formal way that involves the working towards qualifications or accredited learning that happens at the preregistration stage. While many will inevitably return to formal learning opportunities to extend their qualifications, they also need to find ways of recognising and using the learning opportunities in their practice environment and to expand and develop their practice for the benefit of their clients. In fact, Schön (1983) suggests that this is the primary way that all professionals work in action, as professional practice becomes a cycle of drawing on previous knowledge, considering its application for the problem at hand, and testing out new ideas and variations to find one that fits this new situation.

Schön (1983) identified two main types of reflection that professionals use in their everyday practice – reflection-in-action and reflection-on-action. A

Link

Chapter 16 explores the responsibilities of being a registered practitioner and what it means to be professionally accountable.

comparison of the characteristics of each of these is made in Table 13.1. It is important to distinguish between these types of reflection because although both contribute to reflective practice, it is mainly reflection-on-action that is used as a learning strategy because of its conscious and deliberative nature.

Table 13.1 Characteristics of reflection-in-action and reflection-on-action

Reflection-in-action – the way that people think and theorise about practice while they are doing it	Reflection-on-action – conscious exploration of an event to discover more about it and learn from it
Perceived as automatic	Retrospective – it occurs after the event has happened
Seen as an unconscious activity	Conscious, deliberative activity
Often called 'intuitive' practice	It is a cognitive process involving analysis, interpretation and recombination of information
Results from a combination of knowledge, skills and practice	It results in new perspectives being taken on the event
Difficult to articulate and explore	It acknowledges the knowledge being used and results in knowledge deficits being identified
	Active process of transforming experience into knowledge
	Contributes to the development of practice theory

Reflection-in-action

reflection-in-action

reflection on an event as it is being experienced

Reflection-in-action is more than simply 'thinking-while-doing'. According to Schön (1983), reflection-in-action has two components – thinking about the action that is being taken, and thinking about the knowledge that is contributing to that action. Schön (1983) describes the combination of these as 'knowing-in-action', but emphasises that for most of the time the practitioner uses this subconsciously. In other words, the practitioner is constantly reacting to the stimuli of the practical situation and scanning her knowledge and experience base for the paradigm cases identified by Benner (1984), which she can compare to the present situation and then take action. Schön (1983) considered that thought and action were inseparable, they are two parts of the same process of reflection-in-action. This process usually happens so rapidly that it is unconscious, that is, practitioners are not aware of doing it unless something happens to make them stop and think or challenge what they are doing. It is then that it becomes a learning activity.

Of course, reflection-in-action depends entirely on the bank of experience that each person carries in their head. As a result, it is often seen as the characteristic way that advanced practitioners, or experts, practise, rather than the way that beginning practitioners function in the practice setting. But, anyone who has practical experience will begin to draw on their memory of paradigm cases once they have developed confidence in certain abilities and their knowledge base. Try Activity 13.3 for an illustration of this.

Probably the most important aspect of reflection-in-action for the student nurse or midwife is learning to recognise when you are doing it and to take note of what is happening. This is significant, because it means that we are constantly aware of our practice, we are selecting from alternatives and challenging the ways in which practice occurs. This helps to guard against routinised practice that can be seen to have characterised nursing and midwifery in the past (Walsh and Ford, 1989).

It also enables you to note areas for your future development – whether this means extending your formal knowledge, discussing what happened with your mentor or considering, by yourself or with others, whether there are different ways in which that situation could be approached in the future.

Reflection-on-action

When you carry forward these examples for further work, they become **reflection-on-action**, which takes place away from the arena of the experience and after the event itself. This allows you to put all your concentration into exploring the event that has happened from all perspectives and using it as a stimulus for your own learning. It is the development of strategies for reflection-on-action that will enable you to become a reflective practitioner, as well as helping you to make the most of the experiences you encounter in the practice setting. It is also these skills that, once embedded in the way you practise, will stay with you throughout your professional career and enable you to be a 'lifelong learner' in practice.

■ Skills for Beginning Reflective Practice

While to some extent being reflective is part of being human, Atkins and Murphy (1993) suggest that there are certain underlying skills needed for the development and use of reflective practice, and for reflection to be successful as a strategy for learning. They define these as:

- self-awareness
- description
- critical analysis
- synthesis
- evaluation.

We will now discuss these five skills in more detail.

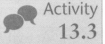

Activity 13.3

Think back to your last day in practice and mentally run though the day. Can you remember:

- Things that you did automatically, without having to think about them
- Occasions where you found yourself thinking through what you were doing and questioning whether you were doing the right things
- Asking yourself whether you could do anything differently
- Questioning, in your head, the knowledge you were drawing on
- Referring back to similar situations that you had already dealt with.

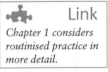

Link

Chapter 1 considers routinised practice in more detail.

reflection-on-action

in-depth reflection on an event after it has finished

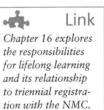

Link

Chapter 16 explores the responsibilities for lifelong learning and its relationship to triennial registration with the NMC.

Self-awareness

Atkins (2004, p. 29) says that 'to be self-aware is to be conscious of one's character, including beliefs, values, qualities, strengths and limitations. It is about knowing oneself.' Self-awareness enables practitioners to look at themselves and the part they play in human interactions, honestly, and acknowledge the roles they played. The notion of honesty is probably the key to self-awareness, because if we are not able to stand back and own our actions, words and thoughts, it is unlikely that we will develop into reflective practitioners, who are able to explore their role, their knowledge and understanding, and their actions in any given event. To some extent, self-awareness is linked with maturity (but not necessarily chronological age) and the ways in which we have been encouraged to take responsibility for our own actions in the past. It is also dependent on whether we have been encouraged to understand ourselves as an individual and recognise, for instance, what our fundamental beliefs and values are, what our beliefs and values about nursing are, and what our beliefs and values about ourselves are.

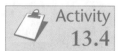

Activity 13.4

Complete the following:

- The three values I hold most strongly are …
- I believe nursing/midwifery to be …
- The three attributes in other people that I value most are …
- The three things I dislike about myself most are …
- The three things I dislike most in others are …
- My understanding of professional practice is …

Description

The key to successful reflection is the ability to describe an experience – accurately identifying its key characteristics and without expressing a judgement – so that someone else can recognise and understand it. This may be verbally or in writing.

Good description takes a lot of practice, as it is tempting to stray away from an objective account into subjective observations or demonstrative language. It is also easy, until you have practised a great deal, to be side-tracked from the central features of the experience and end up a long way from where you started. Atkins (2004, p. 33) suggests that 'the account contains the following key elements: significant background factors (the context), the events as they unfolded in the situation, what you were thinking at the time, what you were feeling at the time, and the outcome of the situation.' Particularly difficult is recounting the personal emotive aspects of the event, without imposing some judgement at the same time.

The purpose of the description is to provide you with the substance to reflect on. This must come from your own experiences and arise from your own actions in practice if it is to be meaningful in helping you to learn from the experience. The description also needs to relate to your own actions, as opposed to assigning meaning to the actions of others.

Critical analysis

critical analysis

making considered judgements about strengths and weaknesses

Critical analysis involves, firstly, being able to break down an experience into its component parts, and then to make judgements about the strengths and weaknesses of them. Being 'critical' does not mean finding fault with something. It involves considering, in an objective way, good parts of an experience, what went well, for example, or what part you played in the experience that was effective; and then identifying those parts that could have been done better, or areas where you consider you need further development. This is where the attribute of self-awareness really comes into play, as it involves taking an honest, sometimes critical look at our part in an experience. Atkins (2004, pp. 36–7) suggests that being critically analytical involves:

- Identifying and illuminating existing knowledge of relevance to the situation
- Exploring feelings about the situation and the influence of these
- Identifying and challenging assumptions made
- Imagining and exploring alternative courses of action (after Brookfield, 1987).

Identifying existing knowledge

The theoretical knowledge that we acquire in our preregistration education, or even in post-qualifying courses, underpins the decisions that we take on a daily basis. Often, we are not aware of accessing that knowledge, but consider it as part and parcel of the way we practise. However, knowledge develops at a rapid rate, and there is always new evidence being published that needs to be taken into account when deciding on the most appropriate care for our patients.

Reflective practice often involves exploring the knowledge that we used when making decisions and taking action, thus it is important to be able to identify that knowledge and how we used it.

Having completed Activity 13.5, depending on the experience you selected, you may find that you have a longer list in one box than another, and this will always happen, dependent upon the types of experience you explore. What this exercise shows us is that we inevitably have to draw on a range of sources of knowledge (Carper, 1978) to inform our practice, and rarely simply use one source of knowledge. This is illustrated in Chart 13.1.

Link

Chapter 16 explores the concept of evidence-based practice in clinical decision-making.

Activity 13.5

Select one of the experiences you identified in Activity 13.3. Divide a piece of paper into four and head each section with the following: Theoretical or scientific knowledge, Ethical or moral knowledge, Personal knowledge, and The 'art' of nursing. Think about the experience you have identified, considering the types of knowledge you used to inform that experience. Write these down under the headings.

Chart 13.1 ● Analysing an experience to identify the sources of knowledge that inform it

Description of the experience: Dawn was caring for Arthur, an 80-year-old man suffering from the end stages of bowel cancer. He and his wife had decided they wanted him to end his days in his own home. The care being provided was palliative, as Arthur was unconscious and surrounded by his family – his wife, two sons and daughters-in-law. Dawn was aware that Arthur would die soon, probably in the next hour. She had supported Arthur and his family as a visiting Macmillan nurse since his diagnosis and referral to the service via the hospice. She considered her role as having several aspects in terms of caring for the dying, unconscious patient and maintaining his dignity at the end of his life. However, her role also included caring for the family at this time, offering support with compassion and sensitivity.

Theoretical or scientific knowledge	*Ethical or moral knowledge*
● The dying processes ● Bereavement theory ● Physical care of the dying patient ● Physical care of the unconscious patient	● Understanding the legal parameters of what professionals are able to do when helping people at the end of their lives ● The principles of beneficence, non-maleficence, confidentiality and informed consent ● The NMC Code of Professional Conduct ● A cultural understanding of right and wrong
Personal knowledge	*The 'art' of nursing*
● Being a person and understanding the importance of personal dignity to all people ● Being a daughter and watching her father die ● Experience of caring for other dying patients	● Professional experience as a Macmillan nurse caring for other patients in similar circumstances ● Being with the patient and their family at this distressing time ● 'Knowing', by experience, that the time of death was approaching and how to support the family at this time

beneficence

promotion of what is best for the patient/client

non-maleficence

avoiding harm

Exploring feelings related to the situation

Feelings and the emotional components of an experience are as important as the actions taken and the outcomes that result. Sometimes, though, these are the most difficult to express to others, or even to own for oneself. Often, we choose to reflect on painful experiences, or those that have made us uncomfortable, and it is essential to explore these experiences for the roots of these feelings and why they are important to us. Conversely, we may reflect on good experiences that invoked positive emotions, particularly when something went very well or resulted in a positive outcome. Again, it is important to identify these emotions and seek out the source of these so that we can attempt to reinforce these activities and plan to be successful.

Identifying and challenging assumptions

Much of modern health-care practice is built upon the successes of the past – what worked or didn't work in other people's experiences. As a result, it is easy for caring activities to become 'custom and practice' or part of the culture of a clinical area. How often have you asked a question about something, only to be told 'it's the way we've always done it.' Being critical involves being willing to explore these 'taken-for-granted' ideas, practices and assumptions and maintaining an open mind about the ways in which things are decided and done. Sometimes this is not a comfortable process, as it involves challenging the status quo, and often challenging those in authority at the same time.

Imagining and exploring alternative courses of action

Again, key to this stage is the ability to retain an open mind and be willing to accept that there may be another way of doing something, even if it has 'always been done like that'. This involves being willing to think creatively and 'outside the box'.

Synthesis

Synthesis means recombining the individual elements of something, often in a different way and informed by the critical analysis that has gone on, in order to take a new perspective, or see new things as a result. This is combined with new sources of information and knowledge, such as in the approach of evidence-based practice. It involves professional creativity, and should result in the optimum care for each one of our patients as individuals.

Evaluation

Finally, a prerequisite for reflective practice is the ability to make a judgement about something, or to 'give it a value'. This is exactly what evaluation is – judging the value of something. Thus it means that a practitioner must be able to form their own opinions about the standards of care and whether care can be improved by changes to practice.

The idea of reflection suggests a solitary and independent activity, largely in the hands and under the control of the reflector themselves. However, within a professional capacity, and as a strategy for learning, the skills of reflection need support and facilitation if they are to be as successful as any other learning strategy. Hence, within your programme of study, it is likely that you will receive formal teaching regarding reflection within the university, as well as help in

Activity 13.6

Look back on the list of skills that Atkins and Murphy (1993) identify as being prerequisite for reflective practice. How confident are you that you have these skills, and which ones do you feel require more development. Who can you get to help you to develop these?

developing these skills in the practice environment from your mentors and supervisors. You will also have opportunities to practise reflection in group activities and in one-to-one supervision sessions with your mentor. As a result, you will slowly develop these skills until they become an automatic part of the ways in which you also practise.

■ Choosing an Experience to Reflect on

critical incidents

making considered judgements about significant incidents that provide opportunities to learn

Experiences that you reflect on in a formal way for the purpose of learning are often referred to as **critical incidents**. This doesn't mean that they are great big dramatic events, or necessarily important to other people. What matters is that the incident or experience is important to you, and has meaning for you in some way. This may be because what happened was extraordinary or unusual and sticks in your mind for some reason. It may have been a really good experience that made you feel happy or confident, or you felt you did a good job. Other experiences that stand out are often those with less good outcomes, or as Atkins and Murphy (1993, p. 1189) suggest, arise from 'an awareness of uncomfortable feelings or thoughts. This stems from a realisation that, in a situation, the knowledge one was applying was not sufficient in itself to explain what was happening in that unique situation.'

It is worth remembering that for the majority of the time, for the majority of our lives, things go well. Indeed, if you think back over the past week, how many times can you remember when things went wrong? Yes, they might not have gone as you expected, but how often does the way things work need to go exactly as you had imagined or planned for? Actually, there are usually many ways in which events might go, none of them necessarily being better than others as long as an acceptable outcome is achieved. This is the foundation for the notion of learning from your experiences – it is by using reflection that we learn to move away from fixed ways of thinking, to think creatively and find different ways of tackling problems, so moving practice forward.

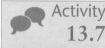

Activity 13.7

Think back over the past two shifts you worked in practice. What stands out in your mind? These events are probably just the sort of critical incidents that could be used as material for reflective learning.

Hence, it is important to view all types of experience as opportunities for learning, and to embrace those events that caused us 'uncomfortable feelings or thoughts' simply as ways in which we can explore and develop our practice. These might well be the stimulus for expanding our knowledge base for practice, or for seeking help with areas of practice that we are having difficulty mastering. The key to responsible and accountable practice is for us to recognise the limits of our knowledge and competence in order to provide safe practice for our patients and clients. Hence, using examples of knowledge deficit and developing the skills of reflective practice as a tool within professional practice are vital to being a registered practitioner. Chart 13.2 lists some examples of experiences that can be used as critical incidents as a basis for reflective practice.

Chart 13.2 ● Examples of critical incidents

- The first time a particular skill is practised: such as feeding or bathing a patient, giving an injection, delivering your first baby
- The first time a new learning environment is experienced: for example a new ward placement; nursing in the home or general practice surgery; encountering patients and clients in hospital departments such as outpatients, clinics or for diagnostic tests
- Witnessing new events: for example a cardiac arrest; a chest drain being inserted; a baby being born by instrumental or operative delivery
- Events which have gone well for you: such as getting a good grade for an assignment; where you have made a difference to the outcome for a patient; where you have changed the course of something; the first time you carry out actions without direct supervision
- Events that you have found challenging: such as dealing with anxious, violent or aggressive patients; giving bad news to patients, or supporting them after others have done this; dealing with patients who you felt powerless to help; dealing with conflict with other members of staff
- Events that have made you feel uncomfortable: for example witnessing poor or dangerous care; events where you feel you could have acted differently; events that made you question your ambition to be a nurse or midwife; situations in which you felt you were unfairly treated
- Events that you cannot get out of your head for some reason: these events provide a rich source of material for reflection, because exploring them to uncover the reasons why they are sticking in your mind often provides a great deal of personal insight

■ Reflective Processes

Having ensured that you are familiar with the skills needed for reflective practice, we can now move on to exploring the processes that reflective practice involves. There are many models and frameworks suggested that provide a structured approach for reflective practice. These essentially build on Kolb's (1984) experiential learning cycle, a four-stage process starting with *observation* and going through the stages of *reflection* leading to *concept development/theorising*, and resulting in an *action*. Kolb's four stages, when applied to a practitioner's situation, can be extended into six stages, all of which are included within the majority of published frameworks or those that you might be asked to use by your lecturers or supervisors. These stages are summarised in Chart 13.3.

Chart 13.3 ● Stages in reflective processes used in reflective practice

- *Stage one – Selecting an event to reflect on*
  Any experience that is complete enough in itself to be described as a separate entity can be used. This is often referred to as a critical incident. It is important to select this carefully, depending on what it is you want to learn from the experience, who is likely to be party to your reflections, and whether there may be consequences from it, especially in professional terms. Similarly, if you are discussing this with others, are you likely to need consent from any third party involved in the event

- *Stage two – Observing and describing the experience*
  This provides the raw material for your reflective activity by giving a full description of what happened, including the context of the experience. Different frameworks or models will ask you to structure this in a different way, depending on the type of outcome you want to achieve. One useful way of doing this is to answer the questions who, where, when, what, why and how? Writing an incident down may give you a different description to verbally describing it

- *Stage three – Analysing the experience*
  This involves breaking down the experience into component parts. Useful questions at this stage are the why and how? You will be forming conclusions about the experience at this stage, using evaluative skills, and may designate different parts as 'good' or 'bad'. At this stage, you may start to perceive the situation differently, and possibly see your role in it in a different light

- *Stage four – Interpreting the experience*
  Here you widen out your analysis to consider the experience in the light of other knowledge. At this stage, you may choose to focus on different aspects of the experience and concentrate on those that seem most important. You will start to get explanations at this stage, and may bring in theoretical knowledge or other wider experiences to consider this experience through

- *Stage five – Exploring alternatives*
  Having thoroughly explored the experience itself, you can now move on to consider whether other courses of action could have happened, which would have resulted in a different ending to the experience. Remember, the purpose of this activity is to learn from this experience; simply validating what you or someone else actually did is not necessarily going to help you learn anything. This stage may be uncomfortable as it asks you to step outside your normal frames of reference and take different viewpoints

● *Stage six – Framing action*

  This where you need to commit to some sort of action, for example you may resolve to go and talk about the experience with someone else, go to the library to increase your knowledge base, or perhaps change your practice in some way. At this stage, it is worth considering what you would do differently if the situation, or something similar, happened again. You may see this as an opportunity to engage in practice development activities in the area in which you are working

Source: Adapted from Jasper (2003).

You will notice from Chart 13.3 that you are asked, as you move through the stages, to try to think outside the ways you normally think. At first, this is challenging, and when doing this initially, it often helps to work with someone else who can ask you questions and draw you along avenues that you wouldn't normally go down. As with any learning strategy, the amount you learn is often directly related to the amount of effort put in and the amount of commitment you give it. Learning by reflection is not necessarily easy, nor is it comfortable, as it involves us in reconsidering and exploring some of the fundamental ways in which we see and understand the world, and questioning those. It also asks us to consider our actions and relationships with others, and to look at the ways we interact with people, often asking ourselves whether what we did was appropriate or could have been done differently. Reflective learning is probably the only learning strategy that uses your own experiences as the raw material in this way, and the only strategy that actively engages you in exploring your own actions, feelings and consequences as part of the learning experience. This is why Atkins (2004) suggests that anyone engaging in reflection as learning needs to have self-awareness and a degree of insight and acceptance of responsibility for their own actions before starting out on this road.

Reflective learning has entered professional practice as a learning strategy because of the move of nursing and midwifery education into higher education. The ability of 'critical thinking' is expected of any person who graduates from higher education, and has been recognised as one of the essential attributes of those engaged in independent professional practice. Using reflective processes to develop critical thinking abilities will help you to become a critical thinker. When starting out on reflective activity, it is often helpful to use a reflective framework, or model, that has been specifically designed to draw you through the stages of the reflective processes.

The following section gives a brief overview of a few of the frameworks available for use by students for reflection.

■ Using Models and Frameworks to Guide Reflective Activity

All frameworks for reflective activity are designed with differing underpinning beliefs and values, and with different purposes in mind. Hence, it is important to be able to select a suitable framework for the type of reflection you want to engage in, the purposes you are using it for, and the outcomes you want to achieve. As a student practitioner, it is likely that you have been given at least one framework to use within your programme. This will have been selected because it fits with the philosophy that underpins the programme and reflects other elements of the course itself, such as the practice assessment you undergo, or the teaching strategies that are fundamental to helping you to acquire the knowledge and skills you will need as a registered practitioner. This section, then, does not provide an 'off-the-shelf' package using one author's reflective framework; rather, it presents some criteria that you might use to select a framework for use if you are in the position of being able to do so.

As you will have deduced, we use reflective strategies for many different reasons, but these can be grouped into three main purposes:

- As a learning strategy: to identify our knowledge base, or deficit
- To improve patient care
- To develop practice and practice theory.

Although each may arise from the other, in that if our knowledge about something improves, then this will be translated into more evidence-based care and therefore develop practice, using one framework all the time will not necessarily enable us to achieve all these aims. These criteria, then, as outcomes of your reflective activity, can be used for selecting a framework to use.

As a student, learning is likely to be the primary purpose for reflection. This will also increase your knowledge base. Therefore it is useful to identify and use a framework that has its origins in particular educational beliefs and values. As professional practitioners, we are all adults and beyond the pedagogy associated with school learning, so we require a framework that respects us as independent learners and recognises the individual nature of our experiences. Hence, we might look to frameworks for reflection that arise from the **andragogical** paradigm identified by Carl Rogers (1983), which value the self-direction of the learner and tap into their own motivation and urgency to learn. This is reflected in Gibbs' (1988) reflective cycle, which focuses essentially on the experiences of the individual as central to learning and results in an action plan that relates to the person's own self-development. Gibbs' 'reflective learning cycle' is probably the one most commonly used in health-care professional education at present, and is considered

andragogical

adult learning – recognises that adults' learning style is different from that of children – adults are predisposed to seeking knowledge as self-motivators and independent learners

user-friendly because it can be used at any stage of a practitioner's career, from student to advanced practitioner. It incorporates the six stages of the reflective process, but focuses initially on the emotions of the person who is the reflector, developing an understanding of the experience from this. This framework is useful, therefore, for a student who wants to identify their learning and knowledge as a result of experiences, but who also wants to develop an action plan arising from these. Chart 13.4 provides the stages of this framework.

Activity 13.8

Use Gibbs' framework to work through an experience you have had. You can either think this through, write it down or use it verbally with another person.

Chart 13.4 ● A worked example using Gibbs' reflective framework

- Description – what happened?
- Feelings – what were you thinking and feeling?
- Evaluation – what was good and bad about the experience?
- Analysis – what sense can you make of the situation?
- Conclusion – what else could you have done?
- Action plan – what would you do if this situation arises again?

Similar to Gibbs' model is a framework that arose from Atkins and Murphy's (1993) original work, which again uses the reflector's feelings as the vehicle for exploration of an event. The specific stages used in this framework are:

- Being aware of uncomfortable feelings or thoughts
- Describing the situation, including thoughts and feelings
- Analysing the feelings and knowledge relevant to the situation
- Evaluating the relevance of the knowledge
- Identifying any new learning that has occurred
- Putting it into action.

It must be noted that this work arose from a literature review of the concept of reflective practice at the time – a view that has developed and moved on since that time. This is particularly so in relation to the stimulus for reflective activity, which is generally accepted as having moved on from 'being aware of uncomfortable feelings' to any critical incident that is complete enough in itself to be described in full. This moves the emphasis from discomfort as the only source of reflective activity, and has been responsible for the wider acceptance of the methods of reflection entering the mainstream learning and teaching strategies in nursing and midwifery as well as in other health-care professions.

Although all reflective frameworks will increase the understanding of the practitioner about their situation and result in learning, one framework that originally focused specifically on uncovering and understanding the knowledge being used in a particular situation is Johns' model of 'structured reflection'.

This model arose from one of the first nursing development units and has been developed and refined continuously since the early 1990s. The 13th version was published in 2000, and adapted in Johns' book *Guided Reflection: Advancing Practice* in 2002. This framework uses a series of questions and prompts to guide the reflector through re-experiencing the event. These questions relate to:

- Identifying significant issues
- Exploring feelings
- Consequences of actions taken
- The role and feelings of others
- The underpinning knowledge used
- Comparing the situation with previous ones
- Current feelings about the experience
- The individual moving forward from the experience.

What has occurred in the development of this framework is firstly its apparent complexity, but also a subtle change in its focus towards outcomes for patients as well as for the practice of the individual nurse. Although Johns' framework appears more complicated than that of Gibbs, the complexity lies in the detailed way the reflector is drawn through the list of cues, rather than it being a difficult or complex framework to grasp. What is required, however, is a paper copy of the cue questions on hand to act as that guide, whereas Gibbs' framework is easy to remember once you are familiar with it and it can be carried in your head for spontaneous verbal reflection.

Another framework, focusing not so much on learning but development, is that presented by Holm and Stephenson (1994) as a 'practitioner's framework'. While this has been published, it was originally devised by the practitioners, when they were students themselves, to guide their own practice. Again, and similar to Johns', it asks specific and focused questions as opposed to the more generalised ones used by Gibbs, and Atkins and Murphy. The questions ask about the role the person took in an incident; the actions taken; how the situation could have been improved for all concerned; what changes could be made; learning; new knowledge; broader issues such as ethical or social that have arisen.

This framework presents not only the main questions, but follow-up questions that invite the reflectors to explore their experiences more fully and ask questions they perhaps would not have thought of themselves. While models and frameworks that look more complicated may initially be off-putting to students, they have the advantage of presenting an easy-to-follow structure that aids the reflector through the reflective processes in a particular way. This is a definite bonus for beginning reflectors, as it takes practice, and some courage, to ask oneself difficult questions, particularly if we don't like the idea of the answer!

One model that looks more simple than any of the others is the original work of Borton (1970). It is another developmental model, encouraging the reflector to consider the experience from whatever viewpoint or focus they want to take to achieve their own outcomes. It is structured through three question stems:

- *What ... ?* Questions that describe the situation such as: what happened? What did I do? What did others do? What did I feel ?
- *So what ... ?* Questions that invite the reflector to look behind the experience and explore the knowledge and theory base and her personal understanding of the situation, resulting in a personal theory. These might be: so what evidence informed my decisions? So what was I trying to achieve? So what experiences have I had previously that contribute to my understanding of the situation?
- *Now what ... ?* Questions that encourage the reflector to plan active interventions based on the theory developed such as: now what am I going to do? Now what do I need to find out? Now what needs to change?

This is the only one of the frameworks that asks the reflector to commit to action, rather than it remaining hypothetical. It is extremely easy for reflectors to use at all stages in their development as reflective practitioners, provided they are confident enough to devise their own questions based on what they want to achieve. In many ways though, these are also its weaknesses, as it is dependent upon the reflector, or the person acting as the questioner, to ask the questions that will challenge the reflector sufficiently.

A note of caution has to be made here, in that it is always worth finding out more about the origins of a framework before using a shorthand version presented in this way. The original references for all these have been provided. In the case of Borton's framework, however, which is significantly older than the rest, I'd like to signpost the reader to Rolfe et al.'s (2001) discussion and development of this model, which also incorporates some of the strategies of the other frameworks presented here to make it more user-friendly for the reflector.

> **Activity**
> **13.9**
> Consider the frameworks presented here. Which of these appeals to you most? Why is this?

■ Reflective Learning in the Practice Environment

Most of the opportunities for learning from practice will be found in the practice environment, and this practical experience will make up 50 per cent of your course. It is therefore extremely important for you to devise strategies that will make the most of the opportunities available and to gain the maximum knowledge and skill from your placements. It is worth taking some time to prepare for your placements so that you know what it is you need to get out of them and how you might do this.

Preparing for a placement

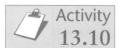

Activity 13.10

Make a list of what you need to achieve by the end of your next clinical placement. Review this list in terms of outcomes almost achieved, those that are part achieved, and those that are completely new to you.

As already identified, all our experiences are built on what we already know. So, no matter what stage you are at in your course, you will have some experiences as the basic building blocks. So your first reflective activity when preparing for a new placement needs to be a review of your last placement, your practice assessment documents and your learning outcomes, to assess what it is you need to achieve in your new placement. It is likely that you will also have theoretical assignments to complete during your placement, so these need to be counted in with the learning outcomes from practice over the time period.

If you have completed Activity 13.10, you will be beginning to realise where you need to put the most effort in over the next few months, and the amount of work that needs to be done. Part of this work is to identify the learning experiences in the clinical environment that will help you to achieve your outcomes, and, if you are lucky, will provide the material for a theoretical assignment.

It is also worth reflecting on the sorts of opportunities that your next placement will offer so that you can maximise these in fulfilling your learning objectives. Find out as much about the placement area as you can before you arrive for your first shift. It may be worth making a preliminary visit and meeting your supervisor informally. Many areas provide information booklets about the type of work that goes on in the area, the types of patient received and the conditions treated. Similarly, midwifery areas differ in the services they offer to their clients – even if you are returning to a similar sort of area to one you have worked in before, the experience will offer a different philosophy of care, different customs and practices and different ways of doing things that you will need to adjust to.

Taking a positive-action approach to learning

You will have given yourself a head start in achieving your objectives if you have completed the tasks in the previous section. The next involves planning to use the opportunities you have identified to the full. This may involve keeping some sort of clinical log or diary to ensure that you record your activity, and then selecting from this as an aide-memoire when doing reflective activity that will help you learn from your experiences. Similarly, you can take an active part in organising your learning by ensuring that you know what is going on in the environment on a daily basis and are in the right place at the right time to experience activities. Finally, it is worth discussing with your supervisor, at an early stage in the placement, what it is you need to complete, and what you'd like to experience, as part of this time.

Using others to support your learning

Not only is there a wealth of learning opportunities in the clinical environment, there is also a large pool of different people who can contribute to your learning. In most clinical environments, you will be working as part of an interprofessional team of health-care professionals, each of whom take a different approach and bring a different perspective to patient care. So, it is not just the nurses and midwives who will be able to support your learning, but also the allied health professionals, medical staff and supporting staff such as chaplains, social workers, clinical psychologists and others.

Primarily, though, you will be working under the direction of your own supervisor, whose role it is to ensure that you have a range of learning experiences and opportunities to enable you to fulfil your learning needs. It is your supervisor's responsibility to help you to practise and develop reflective skills in relation to the clinical experiences you have with them in order to begin your own reflective practice. Therefore, it is important for you to use this person to maximum effect and take up any opportunities offered for reflective work. This may be through prearranged clinical supervision meetings, but it is more likely that these opportunities will arrive ad hoc during your shift, and it will take effort from both of you to ensure that you reflect informally whenever the opportunity arises.

Reflective dialogues are one of the main ways that you will be learning through other people. This may be through clinical supervision sessions, which are planned and structured in some way, or informal occurrences that happen opportunely when there is an event worthy of developing reflectively. It is not only qualified practitioners who will help you in this way, very often you learn as much by working reflectively with your student colleagues. In particular, colleagues are useful for practising reflection using a reflective framework, as the more you do this, the more you will become comfortable with the technique and it will be part of the way you practise. Try to take the opportunity, when talking over your experiences, of suggesting that you talk through it in a structured way. Working in pairs, one can be the reflector, the other the facilitator. It is the latter's role to ensure that the reflector stays within the framework's structure when talking about their experience. After an agreed time period, swap roles, giving the other person the same amount of time to work through their experience. The facilitator has the responsibility of ensuring that the reflective cycle is completed, that is, some sort of action is planned and the other person is committed to taking that action.

Self-directed reflective learning in the clinical environment

There are various simple strategies that you can use to ensure that you make the most of what the clinical environment has to offer. A quick and simple way to use reflection daily is to get into the habit of reviewing the day and identifying what has happened to you and what you have learnt. Although this is a superficial activity, as with all reflective work, it is likely to lead to other things. For instance, if you use a technique called 'three-a-day' (outlined in Chart 13.5), you will give yourself plenty of material to reflect on, especially if you focus the 'three' on particular areas of knowledge or skills.

Chart 13.5 ● Using the three-a-day reflective technique

The three-a-day technique is simply a way of focusing your thoughts back over a particular time period. You can choose to focus on anything, but the trick is to identify the 'top' three of those. Several examples are given below, but for this to be of most use to you, it is worth getting into the habit of creating your own foci. These might arise from your knowledge or skills needs or your learning outcomes, for instance. Or you might need to give your confidence a bit of a boost, or perhaps, if you are doing well, to identify your weaknesses that could do with some work. Some examples are:

● Three things that went well today are ...
● Three things that I enjoyed today are ...
● Three things that I learnt today are ...
● Three skills that I used today are ...
● Three things that I am good at are ...
● Three things that I find difficult are ...
● Three drugs that I am familiar with are ...
● Three people who I admire as role models are ...
● Three people who I don't admire are ...

This list is endless!
However, the key to this activity is not really the answers you gave, but what you then go on and do with these answers. For instance, look back to the last two sentences about people you may or may not admire. Having identified these people, you might like to think about why you admire them, or not; what it is about the way they conduct their practice that makes them a role model; what it is you can learn from them, or decide to avoid, from having observed them.
Getting into the habit of using this technique every day is a simple way of learning reflectively from practice. You may then decide to pick on one of these experiences as a focus for more formal reflective activity using a reflective framework. With practice, you can do this mentally, arriving at new perspectives or defining courses of action that you will take as a result of your experience.

Another way to use reflection on a regular basis is to make the effort to write up or discuss at least one critical incident each week using a reflective framework. If you write these and keep them in your portfolio, this will not only provide you with regular practice of reflective learning techniques and develop your skills, it will also give you a dynamic record and evidence of your experiences and development in practice, and provide material for theoretical assignments.

Finally, always keep your eye on the future, both short and long term. Developing the habit of periodically reviewing your learning outcomes and your progress towards meeting them will ensure that you identify any deficits along the way and have time to plan to rectify them. As with the reflective frameworks that work through asking questions, try to develop the habit of continually questioning yourself.

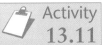

Activity 13.11

Take a few minutes to review the opportunities and ideas presented in this section and jot down some examples for each one that you could use during your own placements.

Recording your Reflective Work

Most of the reflective work you do will be informal, within the workplace, either by yourself or with others, or by yourself away from the workplace. However, many university programmes now require formalised reflective activity to be demonstrated, either within written assignments or as components within a portfolio. Even if you are not required, as part of your course, to write reflectively, it is certainly worth considering doing this in a reflective journal or log, to enhance the value of the experiences you have in practice (Jasper, 2004) and as a self-directed learning strategy.

Written reflection is a different strategy to verbal or informal mental reflection and often results in different outcomes. This is partly because of the particular features of reflective writing, as identified by Jasper (2003):

- We always write for a purpose – it is not random activity but is deliberate
- Reflective writing takes place in the first person – it is impossible to put ourselves at the centre of our writing if it isn't
- Writing requires us to order our thoughts – whatever we use to do this, a structured framework or one devised by ourselves, all writing has some sort of order to it
- Writing creates a permanent record that we can return to again and again and view differently each time
- Writing helps to develop our creativity by enabling us to see connections between previously disparate items of information
- Writing enhances our analytical ability by helping us to break things down
- Writing reflectively helps us to be critical thinkers as we explore alternatives and weigh different ways of perceiving things
- Writing can be used to develop new understanding and knowledge.

Writing reflectively does not need to take the same form all the time, although you may be required to use a specific format within your course.

Most common, in terms of reflective writing as a student, is likely to be the recording and analysis of critical incidents, and the use of reflective reviews at specific periods in your course.

Critical incident analysis

It is usual for students to be asked to use a framework to analyse a critical incident in a written format, to provide the practice of using a structure to analyse a problem. In many ways, this is no different to using, for instance, the nursing process to assess patient needs, diagnose nursing care, plan and implement a care strategy and evaluate it once delivered. The frameworks simply provide you with a way of structuring and ordering your writing in a certain way, while giving emphasis to particular elements of it. Any of the frameworks presented in this chapter can be used in this way. However, as you become more confident in your reflective activity, you may find that you want to adapt frameworks to suit the purpose of your reflection, or even to create your own in the way Holm and Stephenson (1994) did.

> **Link**
> *Chapter 1 details the nursing process.*

Reflective reviews

Reflective reviews differ from critical incident analysis in that they take a wider look at an experience, a series of experiences or over a period of time. For instance, you might be asked to evaluate your learning within a specific placement, or to review your progress towards a set of learning outcomes. The simplest way of doing this is to start off with the learning outcomes as a framework, and then construct a discussion showing how your experiences demonstrate your achievements. But many people will want to develop more creative ways of doing this, by focusing on one particular patient's case history, for instance, and linking skill and knowledge developments and achievements to that. While there is no one way to write reflective reviews, it is important that the central feature of them is reflective learning and practice, thus they need to demonstrate how learning has been achieved through reflective processes. This will inevitably involve self-critique and evaluation, showing that you are working towards the self-assessment and evaluation of your own practice required of a registered practitioner.

Using reflective writing in portfolios

In creating a permanent record through reflective writing, you will be beginning to produce evidence that can be used within a portfolio to demonstrate your achievements. In many courses, portfolios are used to collect evidence for practice assessment and to demonstrate your competence at each stage of your course. Sometimes portfolios will be used as module assessments, to create and reflect on evidence of specified learning outcomes and experiences that demonstrate the understanding of theory and its application to the student's practice. Finally, on completion of your course, you will need to keep an ongoing professional portfolio to demonstrate your competence as a practitioner for the purposes of triennial registration with the NMC. A summary of the uses that may be made of portfolios is presented in Table 13.2.

Table 13.2 Uses of portfolios

	As a student	As a practitioner
Public use	● For coursework assessment ● For assessment of your practice competences ● To collect evidence of your achievements ● For use in applying for your first post as a qualified practitioner	● To fulfil the NMC's PREP requirements for continuing professional development for triennial registration ● To demonstrate to others your accountability for your competence as a practitioner ● As part of the annual employee appraisal process ● As part of the interview process for selection onto a course ● As part of selection process for a new job ● To keep together evidence of your ongoing development, for example records of attendance at conferences and study days, independent reading and so on
Private use	● As a self-directed learning strategy ● As a learning strategy to compile an ongoing record of your development ● To keep a record of your experiences ● To work through your experiences reflectively as a learning strategy	● As part of lifelong learning, using your experiences as the focus for development ● To work through experiences in practice in order to learn from them

At the very minimum, a portfolio is a collection of artefacts that presents a picture of you as a practitioner. In your professional career, it will be collected for a specific purpose and to demonstrate certain things – this may be while you are a student, where the parameters will be closely specified for you, or it may be for the NMC's purposes in verifying standards for postregistration education and practice (PREP).

> **Link**
>
> *Chapter 16 explores the NMC's PREP requirements in more detail.*

However, you may decide to widen the contents and use of your portfolio and incorporate within in it a reflective journal or log, or any of the reflective work that you do while you are on placement. It is important to remember that a portfolio is a private document and belongs to you. No one can make you show it, in its entirety, to anyone else. Where it becomes a public document, open to the scrutiny of others, is where it forms part of a course of study, or may be requested by the NMC for audit purposes, and the only parts that you need to show, and can select from, are those specified in an agreement – such as the assessment criteria of your course, or the requirements of the NMC. Even so, you can select what is contained within your portfolio, and can remove parts of it if you want to, making sure that what remains and is open to scrutiny will do you no harm in a public arena. Many practitioners use reflective writing to explore events in practice that they find disturbing or maybe do not reflect on themselves in a particularly good light. It would be naive for those practitioners to leave these sorts of writing in their portfolios.

The purpose of the majority of portfolios is to demonstrate your achieve-ments – whether this be against specified learning outcomes as a student, or to demonstrate accountable competent practice as a registered practitioner.

Using personal development plans

Personal development plans (PDPs) are increasingly being used within higher education to enable students to plan and focus their learning activities. These are therefore ideal for incorporating within reflective practice, because they demand an element of forward planning and identification of both your learning needs and the achievements that need to result during your course of study. It is possible that these will even be the start of your reflective activity, as they often contain action plans to be completed, and review stages throughout your course to enable you to evaluate your progress towards your goals.

The range of PDPs available is vast, as they are usually designed to meet the needs of a specific institution or course, hence it is not appropriate to explore these in detail here, because if you are required to use them, you will be intro-duced to them as part of your programme. Similarly, many employers now require all their employers to have a PDP that is reviewed annually at perform-ance review. These serve the purpose of helping the employee to consider their own future within the organisation, or their own career, and plan a strategy that will contribute to their personal and professional development.

■ Chapter Summary

This chapter has presented the basic elements of reflective practice as a requisite component of professional practice. Indeed, if these are acquired by every preregistration student throughout their three years of studying for the professional register, it will contribute considerably to the standards of practice and quality of care experienced by our service users. Equally as important, developing the skills of reflective practice empowers the practitioner in making judgements and supporting their decision-making, resulting in the development of practice theory and a knowledge base that derives from practice experiences. These skills are just a beginning, however; following course completion, it is likely that the majority of the learning and development that you do will arise from practising as a reflective practitioner. So, not only are these skills important to ensure our patient's quality of care, they are significant for every individual practitioner in gaining the most out of their working lives.

Test Yourself!

1. What is reflective practice and what are its components?

2. Why do professionals need to practise reflectively?

3. What is the difference between reflection-in-action and reflection-on-action?

4. What are the six stages of reflective processes?

5. How might models and frameworks of reflection help you to reflect?

6. What criteria would you use in choosing a model of reflection?

7. How can you maximise the learning opportunities in the clinical environment by using reflective techniques and practice?

8. How is writing reflectively different from reflecting in other ways?

■ Further Reading

Bulman, C. and Schutz, S. (eds) (2004) *Reflective Practice in Nursing*. Blackwell Publishing, Oxford.

Jasper, M.A. (2003) *Beginning Reflective Practice*. Nelson Thornes, Cheltenham.

■ References

Atkins, S. (2004) Developing underlying skills in the move towards reflective practice. In Bulman, C. and Schutz, S. (eds) *Reflective Practice in Nursing*. Blackwell Publishing, Oxford.

Atkins, S. and Murphy, K. (1993) Reflection: a review of the literature. *Journal of Advanced Nursing* **18**: 1188–92.

Benner, P. (1984) *From Novice to Expert*. Addison-Wesley, Menlo Park, CA.

Borton T. (1970) *Reach, Touch, Teach*. McGraw-Hill, London.

Brookfield, S.D. (1987) *Developing Critical Thinkers: Challenging Adults to Explore Alternative Ways of Thinking and Acting*. Open University Press, Milton Keynes.

Carper, B. (1978) Fundamental patterns of knowing in nursing. *Advances in Nursing Science* **1**: 13–23.

Gibbs, G. (1988) *Learning by Doing: a Guide to Teaching and Learning Methods*. Further Education Unit, Oxford Polytechnic, Oxford.

Holm, D. and Stephenson, S. (1994) Reflection – a student's perspective. In Palmer, A., Burns, S. and Bulman, C. (eds) *Reflective Practice in Nursing*. Blackwell Scientific, Oxford.

Jasper, M.A. (2003) *Beginning Reflective Practice*. Nelson Thornes, Cheltenham.

Jasper, M. (2004) Using journals and diaries within reflective practice. In Bulman, C. and Schutz, S. (eds) *Reflective Practice in Nursing*. Blackwell Publishing, Oxford.

Johns, C. (2002) *Guided Reflection: Advancing Practice*. Blackwell Publishing, Oxford.

Kolb, D. (1984) *Experiential Learning as the Science of Learning and Development*. Prentice Hall, Englewood Cliffs, NJ.

Rogers, C. (1983) *Freedom to Learn for the 80s*. Merrill, Columbus.

Rolfe, G., Freshwater, D. and Jasper, M. (2001) *Critical Reflection for Nursing and the Helping Professions: a User's Guide*. Palgrave – now Palgrave Macmillan, Basingstoke.

Schön, D. (1983) *The Reflective Practitioner*. Temple Smith, London.

Walsh, M. and Ford, P. (1989) *Nursing Rituals: Research and Rational Actions*. Butterworth Heinemann, Oxford.

PHIL RUSSELL

Chapter

14

Social Behaviour and Professional Interactions

Contents

- Therapeutic Communication
- Core Qualities
- Therapeutic Skills
- Working Together: People in Groups
- Being in Control rather than Controlling

- Chapter Summary
- Test Yourself!
- Further Reading
- References

Learning Outcomes

This chapter is concerned with one-to-one and group interactions. After reading through it, you should be able to:

- Describe the core qualities of therapeutic communication

- Identify six therapeutic interventions and suggest ways in which these might be implemented in your practice

- Describe the difference between primary and secondary groups

- Describe the interdependence of team, task and individual needs

- Discuss the importance of assertiveness to nursing practice

- Describe the process for refusing requests and handling criticism

- Reflect on further areas of study to enhance your own therapeutic communication skills.

This chapter begins by examining therapeutic communication, or the therapeutic use of self. It explores the meaning of these terms, before asking what qualities are required to enhance communication beyond just conveying information. It then examines in more detail some of the tools available to start the process of developing good therapeutic skills that can be used with patients, families and colleagues.

Nurses seldom work in isolation but are more usually part of a specific group or team. Groups tend to have their own dynamics, and an understanding of how groups function can help in developing happier and more efficient teamwork. Nurses may work with a variety of diverse groups, for example support groups for patients, therapy groups, commonly found in mental health settings, and families, which form a special kind of group. Some of the issues important to group dynamics will be examined. What constitutes a group? What sort of group are you likely to encounter? What is the role of nurses as group members? What makes effective teams and good leaders?

Lastly, this chapter will examine a more specific aspect of interaction, building on some of the issues raised earlier in the chapter. Nurses are at the forefront of care and have an important role in liaising with an extremely wide range of people. In doing so, they sometimes have to deal with difficult situations. This section will examine how, through developing assertiveness, nurses can develop greater self-confidence and work more effectively towards positive working relationships and patient outcomes.

therapeutic

aiding an individual's well-being

Throughout this chapter, the term 'nurse' will be used for the person who is the provider of the **therapeutic** communication. The nurse may be from any branch – mental health, learning difficulties or adult nursing. The terms 'client' and 'patient' are often used interchangeably, some branches using the term 'client' more freely than others. To avoid any confusion, the recipient of the therapeutic exchange will be referred to here as the client.

Finally, this chapter is not intended to be a training manual or a comprehensive guide to social interactions. Instead, it offers some signposts on which to base further study, investigation and development.

■ Therapeutic Communication

therapeutic communication

purposeful communication aimed at enhancing an individual's well-being

The term **therapeutic communication** has been chosen rather than 'interpersonal skills' or 'counselling'. We all use interpersonal skills all the time whenever we are relating to another person, sometimes constructively, sometimes destructively. To be therapeutic, however, means to aid the well-being of an individual; thus, therapeutic communication has the intention of assisting or helping others.

There is evidence to suggest that the communication exchange between nurses and clients, including relatives, is not always as good as it might be (Ley,

1988; Brereton, 1995). There are many diverse and complex reasons for this. Perhaps the fact that we are all communicating all the time results in a feeling that we do not need to learn how to do something we have been doing all our lives: it seems to be common sense. Perhaps nurses have become complacent about communication. Furthermore, there is a tendency for some nurses to see themselves as people of action rather than words. Many nurses are not comfortable unless they are 'doing', a stance influenced by the ethos of today's clinical environment and the pressures of work. Hewison (1995) found support for the fact that many nurse–client interactions continue to be task oriented, routinised and often superficial.

Nevertheless, nurses do express a desire to communicate well with clients; Buckroyd (1987) found that paediatric nurses wanted to be able to help children in distress but often felt ill equipped to deal with these emotional and difficult interactions. Skilled therapeutic interventions can, as Nichols (1989) points out, minimise the psychological morbidity associated with ill-health, and nurses are ideally placed to provide this kind of care to clients. Therapeutic communication is an essential and central aspect of nursing whichever branch nurses specialise in.

The NHS Knowledge and Skills Framework (KSF) sets communication as its first core dimension (DoH, 2004). The purpose of the NHS KSF is to define and describe the essential components of communication that NHS staff need to apply in their work if they are to deliver quality care. Within the communication dimension, there are four levels:

1. Communicate with a limited range of people on day-to-day matters.
2. Communicate with a range of people on a range of matters.
3. Develop and maintain communication with people about difficult matters and/or in difficult situations.
4. Develop and maintain communication with people on complex matters, issues and ideas and/or in complex situations (DoH, 2004).

> **Activity 14.1**
>
> Try to think of some scenarios that would be applicable to each of the levels of the communication core dimensions.

Some of these will be explored in this chapter but the next section will focus primarily on the core qualities that underpin therapeutic communication and some of the skills that can assist in the process and practice of therapeutic communication.

■ Core Qualities

Three particular qualities have been identified as playing an important part in any therapeutic alliance:

1. Empathic understanding.

congruence

a matching of inner feelings and outer behaviour

2. Genuineness, or **congruence**.

3. Unconditional acceptance.

The requirement for these attributes was first identified in the context of counselling by Carl Rogers, the father of person-centred therapy. Rogers identified these three qualities as being necessary and sufficient to enable constructive personality change (Rogers, 1957). In other words, no other forms of therapeutic intervention are needed. This approach has had a considerable influence on nursing because of the control it gives back to clients, empowering them to make their own decisions and enabling their psychological growth. Nurses are, however, rarely in a position to use these interventions exclusively – to do so risks ignoring many other helpful strategies (Burnard, 1995) – but the three core qualities are considered to be important components in the therapeutic relationship and lay the foundation on which other skills and strategies can be built. They are thus worthy of further explanation.

Empathic understanding

empathic understanding

the ability to perceive accurately the feelings of another person and to communicate this understanding to him or her

Empathic understanding is essentially a sensitivity for *what* another person is feeling but not for *how* he or she is feeling. You can never feel exactly the same as other people, as their construction of the world will always differ from yours in some way. You can, however, be sensitive to what they are feeling and convey this to them in a way that helps them to feel someone has a valid insight into their world: they feel understood. Rogers (1980) describes empathy as 'a way of being with another person, entering into their world, communicating their sensings'. Nevertheless, it remains a difficult concept to understand and practise, as it is more than just a communication process.

Egan (2002) defines two types of empathy: 'primary empathy' and 'advanced empathy'. The former is much more straightforward, although not necessarily simple. It involves listening carefully to what clients are saying and responding in a way that indicates an understanding of what they are saying from their perspective. The latter is a deeper kind of empathy, more akin to reading between the lines, picking up not only what the client says, but also what lies behind it. As Rogers (1980) suggests, it is 'sensing meanings of which the client is scarcely aware'. This might usefully be compared with being a musician. Some musicians can read the score and play the notes in the correct sequence, but the highly skilled musician sees behind and beyond the notes, understanding the full expression of the music as intended by the composer. Developing these sensitivities appears to come more easily to some than others, but empathic understanding can be enriched with careful reflection on how you respond to clients. What is not required is some sort of phoney understanding. It is important to be genuine.

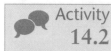

Activity 14.2

Think of someone you know well, and, in your mind, try to become that person. As that person, write a character sketch of yourself. In other words, try to see yourself through someone else's eyes.

Genuineness

Genuineness is about being open and honest, and is sometimes referred to as 'congruence' or 'authenticity'. This is not to suggest that carers are being dishonest, but it is possible to be deceived about your feelings towards others. The professional mask often worn by nurses can distort the way of being with a client. Genuineness is less to do with telling untruths and more to do with having an openness, an attitude that conveys congruence between what you are thinking and feeling, and what you are saying. It is not hiding behind a uniform or a professional role: the very process of professionalisation can result in taking on a role that hides the self. Unfortunately, such a lack of genuineness often shines through to clients like a bright light, causing them to withdraw into themselves. Egan (1994) offers some guidance on developing an attitude of genuineness:

genuineness
the ability to show oneself without putting on a façade

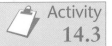 **Link**
Chapter 12 looks at the development of self-concept and self-awareness.

- *Not overemphasising the helping role:* and thus avoiding being patronising and condescending
- *Being spontaneous:* this is not the same as overtly expressing all your current feelings, but it does mean not being afraid to express them when appropriate
- *Not being defensive:* as a nurse, you will not always find that you are able to help, but getting to know your own strengths and weaknesses will enable you to be less defensive
- *Being open:* when appropriate, do not be afraid to use your own life experience (see Nelson-Jones, 1997, for guidance on appropriate self-disclosure).

Much of being genuine is about having a better understanding of ourselves. Activity 14.3 and Figure 14.1 will give you some insight into your own experiences. If, for example, you have experienced a loss, this might help you to understand a client better, but it might also make you less tolerant of an angry client who reminds you of your own undealt-with anger.

Activity 14.3

Draw a timeline similar to the one in Figure 14.1 and identify the positive and negative influences in your life. Think about how these events have helped to mould and create you, and how they might influence your relationship with your clients.

```
POSITIVE

Start school (5)    Sister born (6)    Happy holiday (11)    Passes A levels (16)
- - - - - - - - - - - - - - - - - - - - - - - - - - - - - - - - - - - - - - - - - - -
Mum in hospital (7)    Had big argument with Dad (12)    Grandparent died (17)

NEGATIVE
```

Figure 14.1 ● Example of a timeline (with age in brackets)

Unconditional acceptance

Unconditional acceptance or 'unconditional positive regard' is a frequently misunderstood quality. It can appear as if you must like everyone, regardless of what they have or have not done or who they are. Indeed, if you accept the statements above about genuineness, pretending that you like everyone means that you are not being genuine. Unconditional acceptance, however, is about accepting clients as fellow humans entitled to care and respect, which is not the same as liking them as you do your friends or accepting their behaviour and value systems, which may be at odds with your own. As Mearns (1994) comments, 'Don't confuse unconditional positive regard with liking.' You may not like certain individuals, or their behaviour, but it is not for you to judge them, especially from your position as a carer. Developing the skill of acceptance depends very much on your ability to accept yourself. These are not easy qualities to cultivate or execute, although some nurses will find this easier than others. What is of concern is the way in which individuals often assume that they possess these qualities just because they have read about them, as if they develop through some osmotic process. These are, however, qualities that take time to develop and must be practised. In reality, they are never fully available to us, so we can only aspire to them. One way to start the process of developing them is to begin reflecting on our interactions with clients and colleagues.

Link

Chapter 13 provides some guidelines on how to reflect on your practice.

These core qualities form an important element in developing a person-centred approach to care. This approach is one that holds the needs of the individual central and represents a shift in the view we hold of caring practices (Ford and McCormack, 2000). Talerico (2003) suggests that the key features of a person-centred approach are:

- Knowing the person as an individual and being responsive to individuals and family characteristics
- Providing care that is meaningful to the person in ways that respect the individual's values, preferences and needs
- Viewing care recipients as biopsychosocial human beings
- Fostering development of consistent and trusting care-giving relationships
- Emphasising freedom of choice and individually defined, reasonable risk taking
- Promoting physical and emotional comfort
- Appropriately involving the person's family, friends and social network.

These key features represent a whole philosophy of care and do not only relate to communication, but communication itself must adopt an approach that puts the patient and family at the centre of care. The following framework provides a valuable toolkit and is based on a humanistic approach that values a person's unique needs and preferences.

▨ Therapeutic Skills

Heron (2001) has devised a simple but comprehensive model for therapeutic communication that is referred to as 'six-category intervention analysis'. Within the six primary categories lie a wide range of more specific interventions; although the categories are considered to be exhaustive, the interventions are not and have the capacity for great flexibility. Heron (2001) emphasises that the categories are not a model of counselling but instead a set of analytical and behavioural tools. Many of the interventions are not uniquely identified by Heron, but he provides an effective framework, within which all six interventions, including those related to giving information and advice, can be used in one-to-one interactions. Figure 14.2 illustrates the six categories.

The first three categories – confronting, informative and prescriptive – are authoritative, in that the nurse is taking greater responsibility for guiding the client's responses. The other three interventions – catalytic, cathartic and supportive – are facilitative, that is, the authority remains primarily with the client. No single intervention is more important than any other, and none of the interventions seeks to control or take autonomy away from the client. Instead the emphasis is on developing an enabling relationship in which clients can explore their own worlds and make appropriate decisions for themselves.

Activity 14.4

Make a list of clients who might be difficult to accept because their value system, beliefs or behaviours are different from your own, for example a drug addict. Think of a client or someone you know who you do not really like. Write down five positive qualities about that person. Discuss with a colleague how you might better manage working with a client you do not like or whose values and behaviour are opposite to your own.

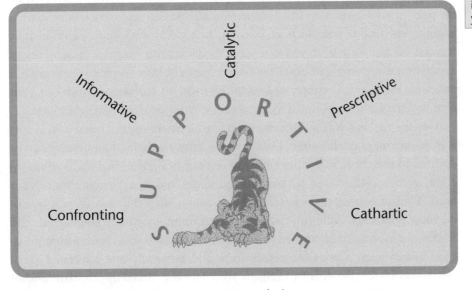

Figure 14.2 ● Six-category intervention analysis (after Heron, 2001)

Catalytic category

Although there is no hierarchy to the six categories, the catalytic category will be outlined first because it probably contains the most frequently used interventions. Heron describes **catalytic interventions** in terms of learning and problem-solving. These interventions enable clients to explore their thoughts and feelings, thus gaining insight and enabling them to be in a better position to make decisions about their future. The skill lies in effective listening and responding in ways that help clients to move on, but at their own pace and with their own agenda. This category requires the nurse to identify which intervention from the toolkit is most appropriate for assisting clients in this exploration.

The following interventions will be outlined here: listening; simple and selective reflection; paraphrasing; open and closed questions; logical and empathic building; and checking for understanding.

catalytic interventions

a set of basic interventions that assist the client with self-discovery and learning

Listening

Before you can listen to others, it is important to give the individuals concerned your full and free attention. This can be difficult if there is much going on in the immediate environment and your mind is focused on other issues. Stevens (1971) suggests that we have three zones of awareness; a *fantasy zone*, an *inside zone* and an *outside zone*. When your awareness is on fantasy, you are conscious of your thoughts and images, for example you may be trying to interpret what the person has just said or thinking about your own past or future agendas. When your awareness is inside, you are aware of your own inner sensations: as you sit reading this book, you may be aware of your eyes straining to read the words on the page. If your awareness lies outside, you are focused on external events, what is going on outside you, such as listening to a client with your attention fully focused on him or her. If you can learn to distinguish between these zones of awareness, it is possible to use them more effectively, thus keeping your focus out and with the client, fleetingly changing the focus to fantasy to check out your own thoughts and occasionally being aware of your own internal sensations.

One way in which you can demonstrate your attention and interest in clients is by giving them quality time. Even if this is only a couple of minutes, it can be devoted to the client as quality time rather than being a rushed and haphazard event, with you distracted by your surroundings and what is going on in your head. This, of course, takes practice, but giving quality time to others is one of the most important skills you can offer. In addition, your body language should convey the message that you are listening with interest to the client. Maintaining good eye contact, a relaxed open posture and a friendly and interested facial expression invites the client to talk to you. The occasional appropriate nod of the head indicates that you are listening and interested. Once you are giving clients your full attention, it is necessary to demonstrate that you are trying to understand their world from their frame of reference. In other words, you are being empathic rather than imposing your world, values, beliefs or judgements on the client.

Simple and selective reflection

Simple reflection, sometimes known as 'echoing', is helpful when the client appears stuck. It involves repeating the last word or few words back to the client with the same intensity of expression used by the client. The client may, for example, end the sentence saying, 'and I feel very unhappy'; you respond, 'You feel very unhappy', and the client is encouraged to continue the story, 'Yes, ever since …'. The difficulty in using this intervention is in deciding when it is appropriate and beneficial, as inappropriate use will simply annoy the client.

Selective reflection is similar, involving listening carefully for issues that seem to stand out as being significant and then feeding them back to the client without changing the content: 'You commented a moment ago about how angry you were with your mother.' This gives the client the opportunity to continue to develop this theme. Care must be taken not to direct the client down avenues of your own choosing rather than of the client's choice. It is easy to think that you know what the client's problem is, but in reality you will often be misguided in your assumption. In both simple and selective reflection, you should be listening for the emotionally charged words the client uses.

Paraphrasing

Paraphrasing is one way of conveying to clients that you have listened to them and have tried to grasp an understanding of what they are saying to you. When paraphrasing, you rephrase what the client has said in your own words. An example of this type of intervention might be:

Client: I'm very worried about my daughter. This problem has been going on for so long, I wonder if she will ever be the same again.

Nurse: It seems like there is no end to your daughter's problem and you're worried she will never be the little girl you used to know.

Open and closed questions

These **dichotomous** interventions are relatively simple but take practice to master. Open questions invite an open answer, whereas a closed question

dichotomous
divided into two separate groups

invites a closed answer. As an example of a closed question, 'Do you have pain?' invites a yes or no response, whereas 'How are you feeling?' invites a response much more of the client's choosing. Although it is rather simplistic, the 'who', 'what', 'where', 'when' and 'how' questions tend to elicit a more open response. The important word to be remembered here is 'invites': a closed question may instead receive an open response and an open question a closed one.

These questions are more appropriately seen as lying on a continuum of being more or less open; the more open they are, the greater the opportunity for client self-direction. The compulsive helper who tends to try to maintain control of the interaction more frequently asks closed questions. They can, however, be useful in eliciting specific information such as a name or telephone number. 'Why' questions should be used cautiously as they may alienate clients by forcing them to introspect inappropriately. After all, if they knew 'why', they would very often not need help.

Logical and empathic building

Logical building helps to develop a scaffolding for the client by bringing together salient points from the dialogue. Clients are often confused and appear to be rambling as they try to express their feelings; the nurse can assist by periodically marshalling the various points into some coherent order. For example, you might say, 'It seems as if these are your main concerns, Mr Jones. You are worried about how you will cope if you return to work and about who will take care of the children.'

Empathic building is rather like reading between the lines. As you carefully listen to what the client is saying, you are attempting to understand the feeling behind the words. It is important to use other cues such as tone of voice, eye contact and facial expressions to help you to understand what the client might be experiencing. Your empathic understanding is then relayed to the client in the form of a statement: 'It sounds as if you are really hurting about …' or 'You are really frightened because …'.

Checking for understanding

It is very important to check periodically that you are, as fully as possible, understanding what the client is saying. This is especially important if you feel that you are becoming confused or if the client is giving contradictory messages. Clarifying the situation can prevent much misunderstanding and helps you to stay within the client's frame of reference.

Cathartic category

As a baby and during infancy, the tendency is to spontaneously give vent to emotions, be they of joy, grief, anger or fear. As you grow older, the responses become modified through modelling, learning or choice, as you decide the best way to master life. You learn perhaps that it is wrong to cry and bad to express anger, that to be fearful might show weakness, or even that it is *not OK* to have fun and enjoy yourself. This may make it difficult to express yourself, particularly at times of crisis. The difficulty with helping others with their emotions is that you may not yet have come to understand your own repressed emotional world. It is one thing to intellectualise and say to the client that it is OK to cry, but if you are sitting there feeling uncomfortable with your own emotions, this may well be conveyed to the client. It is also unhelpful to coerce someone into expressing emotions, such as insisting on a bereaved person crying. Given time, space and permission, clients can choose when and how they want to express their emotions.

Working with emotions can be difficult and often requires specific training, but becoming more responsive to people's emotional needs does not require in-depth training. What it does require, however, is for you to become sensitive to your own emotions and those of your clients. The angry client may awaken memories of an angry parent in your life, or a dying client may provoke memories of an earlier loss. What makes you laugh, cry or get angry? Do you close down your emotions because it is easier that way and you stand less chance of getting hurt? The best way to help clients with their emotions is to be accepting of them and give them permission – permission to be angry parents when they find out that their new baby has learning difficulties, permission to be afraid when they find out they have multiple sclerosis or cancer, permission to cry when old hurts are uncovered in a group therapy session, permission to feel relief when someone they love dies, as their loved one has been released from suffering and they themselves from the burden of caring.

Touching, eye contact, listening, being with someone and giving permission are all ways of using **cathartic interventions**, but it is also important to be conscious of the cultural perspective. Touch may not be acceptable in some cultures, and eye contact may offend. Do not be afraid to check these things out. Does your eye contact cause the client to withdraw or become more responsive? Ask whether clients would like you to hold their hand.

cathartic interventions

interventions that seek to enable clients to let go of painful emotions including anger, fear, love and grief, thus releasing tension that has built up within them

confronting interventions

interventions that directly challenge and heighten the client's awareness of restrictive attitudes, beliefs or behaviours of which he or she may be unaware

Confronting category

Confronting interventions are involved with informing clients of what they are unaware of. Because of the nature of confrontation, the intervention may be received by clients with some degree of shock as they come face to face with issues that they were either not aware of or not acknowledging. For the nurse, the process of confrontation can also be uncomfortable. He or she is to some extent making an informed judgement that the client will benefit from the confrontation, but the nurse's fear of being wrong or managing the confrontation poorly can lead to anxiety about how to deliver the information. Furthermore, the nurse may become aware of feelings related to previous confrontations in his or her own life. These anxieties can lead the nurse to avoid the issue and 'beat around the bush' or alternatively take a very direct and heavy-handed approach. A more appropriate approach is to take control of these inner feelings and get the confrontation right in order to convey the confrontation clearly and supportively.

What sorts of issue might be seen as confrontations? There are many potential examples, such as breaking bad news or raising awareness of attitudes and behaviours. The examples below give some indication of how confrontations can be used:

- In a group session, John appears to avoid talking about his feelings:
  'You have explained what you were thinking John, but what is it you are feeling?'
- Mr Patel does not appear to be taking responsibility for looking after his recently fashioned colostomy:
  'I notice you are always asking nurse Radley to change your colostomy bag.'
- Fasia is a young woman with Down's syndrome who is preparing for her first job:
  'Fasia, are you aware that whenever someone speaks to you, you look away?'
  (The nurse demonstrates what Fasia may be unaware of)
- You notice that the parents of three-month-old Stephanie, admitted with a chest infection, are irregular visitors:
  'It seems you are unable to visit Stephanie very often.'

Breaking bad news is a further example of a confronting intervention. Maguire and Faulkner (1993) make the point that you cannot soften the impact of bad news, as it remains bad news however it is broken, but you can break the news in a way that is supportive and gives the client a chance to absorb what is happening. There is insufficient space here to discuss in detail the problems of breaking bad news, but the following (Buckman, 1993) are useful guidelines:

Link

Chapter 10 deals with end-of-life issues.

- Prepare clients for the news, offering them privacy and ensuring that they are sitting down
- Inform them that you have bad news, and then give them the facts in a simple, informative and unambiguous manner

- Allow them time to take in the news, giving them the choice of being alone or having someone remain with them
- Finally, be supportive throughout the interaction and offer follow-up help.

Informative category

Why do you need to give information? Clients clearly require information so that they can understand their illness or health problem. Without information, they are left groundless and are not in a position to make reasoned decisions about their care. It is important that information is given to help clients to understand and maintain control rather than this just being a duty of the health-care professional. It appears that most people want information about their illness, even if it is bad news (Ley, 1988). It also seems that clients are reluctant to seek out information in health-care settings, often being afraid of wasting nurses' time, being unsure of whom or what to ask, or sometimes not being sure whether they can ask for information. It therefore falls to the health-care professional to ensure that quality information is delivered appropriately and in the client's best interest.

Informative interventions are often seen as the easiest to master. Most people feel that they are capable of providing information, but it is perhaps this confidence itself that results in a poor delivery of information. Although clients want and need information, it must be delivered at the right level, in the right quantity and at the right time. Too many clients fail to understand the information given to them or forget what they have been told, especially if it is bad news (Ley, 1988). You may be able to remember occasions on which a lecture has been overloaded with information or delivered at a depth or in a manner that leaves you confused. The good lecture provides the right information, at the right depth and at the right time in the course, perhaps leaving you to find something out for yourself. This last aspect is often important in mental health nursing, where you may wish to encourage clients to find out some information for themselves and take responsibility for doing so.

informative interventions

interventions that seek to impart new knowledge, information and meaning that are relevant to the client's needs

Prescriptive category

Prescriptive interventions, such as suggesting a course of action the client might take, attempt to redirect the client's behaviour. One pitfall of this intervention is that it can be too prescriptive, thus removing control from the client. What health-care professionals believe is in the clients' best interests does not always relate to how clients themselves see the situation. Nevertheless, the nurse is in possession of much knowledge and may feel that a certain action really will be best for the client, therefore suggesting, recommending or proposing some

prescriptive interventions

interventions that seek to suggest, advise or propose ideas to the client

action to the client and leaving the situation open for its acceptance or rejection. On other occasions, the nurse may be even more consultative, suggesting a number of options to clients and discussing these in a way that gives them maximum control and choice. At other times, the nurse may be very directive, for example when stopping a diabetic client accidentally overdosing with an insulin injection.

Link

Chapter 4 discusses safety issues.

Supportive category

supportive interventions

interventions encompassing an attitude of mind that unconditionally affirms the worth and value of the client

Supportive interventions underpin the use of all other interventions. Whatever intervention is being used, it should be used in such a way that supports the individual and is not in any way destructive. Heron (2001) identifies three ways of using interventions. The first is a valid way that is appropriate to the needs of the client. In other words, it is the correct intervention delivered in the right way, at the right time and in the correct manner. The second interventional style is degenerative, in which, despite good intentions, intervention is used poorly because of a lack of skill, experience, self-awareness or a combination of all three. Finally comes a perverted intervention in which the intervention is used in a deliberately perverse way, to the detriment of the client.

Link

Chapter 12 looks at the development of self-awareness.

Although the supportive category underpins all other categories, it is also a category in its own right. The interventions it encompasses involve the affirmation of others, being with them and demonstrating in a genuine way a care and concern for them. It may involve appropriate touch or appropriate self-disclosure. You demonstrate support for your clients when you willingly do things for them, when you greet them welcomingly and celebrate their achievements, however small these may appear to be. This should be conveyed in an unpatronising manner, and you must resist becoming overly nurturing, which may deny clients their independence. The three core conditions of empathy, being genuine and offering unconditional acceptance are central to the supportive category.

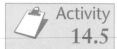

Activity 14.5

For each of the six categories discussed above, give two or three examples of how you might constructively use them when interacting with actual clients or colleagues with whom you have worked.

The above interventions provide a useful framework within which therapeutic communication can be developed. What has been presented here is an outline on which you can build. All the interventions can be developed and extended, requiring practitioners to research their use and practise their application if they are to be successfully employed.

■ Working Together: People in Groups

As social animals, people tend to live in groups or be members of a group. There are a whole variety of different groups to which you might belong: you probably belong to a family, have a group of friends, perhaps belong to a club and maybe are a member of an organisation such as the Royal College of Nursing. You will belong to a large group called 'nurses', you may be a committee member, you are part of a work group in your clinical area and, as a student, you are part of a particular intake. Other groups you may come across may be study groups, rehabilitation groups and therapy groups. Nursing often involves working with a specific group or 'team' of nurses. They also form part of a larger group of health-care professionals that work together as the interdisciplinary team. A team is a group of people that have a common goal and need to work cooperatively to achieve that goal. The more effective the teamwork, the better the client care and the greater the satisfaction with your work role.

Belonging to a group has many benefits, such as a feeling of belonging, having a shared identity and the benefits of the support you receive from the group. There is a degree of security from being part of a group in which attitudes and values are similar and in which learning can take place. There is, however, also some cost to belonging to a group. You are expected to conform, and you may feel that you are surrendering some of your own personal identity.

The study of groups has interested psychologists and sociologists for a long time and has generated considerable research. This section will confine itself to some of the core issues of groups as a platform for further study.

What is a group?

Most people have a common concept of what a group is, and few of the examples above will be difficult for readers to identify as groups. It should also be evident that groups are diverse and can vary considerably in their size and function, some being more formal than others. Because of this, definitions are not always helpful, and it is more productive to focus on some of the central characteristics of groups than on definitions. A principal feature of a group is that individuals believe themselves to be members of the group, there being some degree of interdependence and interaction.

Groups can be divided into primary and secondary groups. Secondary groups are usually considered to be larger, and their members have less direct contact. The hospital in which you work is a larger group, and you may never have contact with many of its members. Nursing as a profession is a large secondary group, as is a political party.

Primary groups tend to be closer and more intimate, all the members having face-to-face contact. Such groups might be family groups, friendship groups or small work groups. If you belong to a group, you probably have some expectations of that group, for example the way in which members are likely to behave, some of the attitudes you might expect them to hold and perhaps a code of conduct, be it explicit or implied. Nurses will be expected to have an attitude of

Activity 14.6

Think of all the groups you belong to, both in and out of work. Choose two or three of these and consider what role you play in the group. Make a list of all the people that might go to make up a interdisciplinary team in your area of practice.

norm

a shared way of
behaving and thinking

anomie

lack of the usual social
and ethical standards

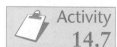

Activity 14.7

Make a list of the
norms for your clin-
ical area. A simple
example may be
whether or not you
wear a uniform.
What might be the
consequences if the
group ignored
these norms?

caring and working in a manner that is in the best interests of the client. These expectations are known as **norms** and are attained through observation, experience and learning. Although there is invariably a degree of flexibility, it is also expected that all members of the group will more or less conform to these norms. Without some conformity, it would be difficult to operate in a social world. We would be left with a sense of **anomie**, bewilderment, with no frame of reference. Imagine what would happen if, each time you came to work, your group of nursing colleagues behaved radically differently, one day caring, the next not, sometimes wearing a uniform and sometimes casual clothes.

The group you work with in your clinical area is a formal primary group, and this group will have established a set of informal norms and expectations related to the group's behaviour. The degree to which members of the group uphold these norms is an indication of the cohesiveness of the group. The hierarchy may impose other, more formal norms, and it would be expected that these would be adhered to. Needless to say, these two sets of norms may on occasions clash, causing some discontent.

Leadership of groups

Various research studies have identified different styles of leadership and their effectiveness (Lewin et al., 1939; Sayles, 1966; Fielder, 1971). These styles reflect the divide between being *autocratic*, when one person makes the decisions; *democratic*, when a consensus of opinion is sought; *person-centred*, in which the leader places greatest emphasis on people; and *task-centred*, in which the focus is on completing the task. These dimensions are probably best viewed as a continuum rather than as definitive styles of leadership. Good leaders, although they may have a predominant style, will adjust their leadership according to the situation (Bass, 1990). It is, for example, often important to be autocratic in a cardiac arrest situation, everyone needing to know exactly who is in charge and what needs to be done. On other occasions, such as when deciding on a new policy, a more democratic, person-centred style may be more productive, allowing for open discussion and the sharing of ideas.

Leaders may be emergent, elected or appointed. *Emergent* leaders are common in crisis situations or when no leader has previously been identified; *elected* leaders are common in political situations or on committees. In the case of a clinical area, there is usually an *appointed* leader, someone given the position because of his or her skills and qualifications. Although you may currently be a student, you will in due course become a staff nurse and will be expected to have some responsibility as an appointed leader.

When a group come together to achieve a common goal, they are usually referred to as a team and Adair (1988) identifies three broad areas of need to be considered by the leader in order to maintain good teamwork. These are the *team*, the *task* and the *individual*, each being equally important and interrelated, as shown in Figure 14.3. These three areas are now discussed in more detail.

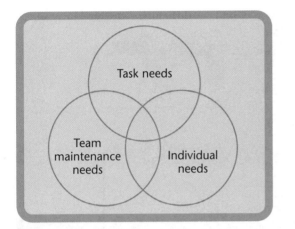

Figure 14.3 ● Three circles model (after Adair, 1988)

Maintaining the team

A team is made up of individuals and as such takes on its own personality distinct from that of its individual members. One of the responsibilities of the leader is to form a cohesive team that will go forward together to meet the agreed objective without diminishing the individuality of its members. One of the difficulties often expressed by new staff nurses is how to effect an appropriate distance from the team, one that is neither overfamiliar nor too distant. Adair (1988) suggests that distance should be emphasised if the nurse was known to the staff before adopting the new position, if the nurse feels that staff are becoming overfamiliar and taking advantage of the situation, or when the leader is responsible for implementing unpopular decisions. Distance should be minimised when trying to establish and build trust, and if all members are roughly equal in knowledge and experience. The assertiveness skills referred to in the next section of this chapter should help in this respect.

Groups or teams take time to establish, and Tuckman (1965) suggests that as groups develop, they pass through a series of stages. Being aware of these stages can help in understanding the progress of a group, and you may be able to identify some of these stages in relation to your group of students and how they have changed since commencing training. The four stages of forming, storming, norming and performing are shown in Figure 14.4. This process is most clearly seen in the smaller groups that come together to achieve a given purpose, the groups and subgroups formed during nurse training being good examples of

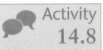

Activity 14.8

Think of a particular task you might want to achieve as a team, such as implementing a new ward procedure. Using Figure 14.3 above, blank out the Task circle. How will this influence achieving your objective? Now blank out the Team circle. How will this influence reaching your goal? Finally, blank out the Individual circle and carry out the same exercise.

these. However, many other groups, such as the group you work with in the clinical area, go through similar stages, and this is often cyclical in nature as the environment and personalities change.

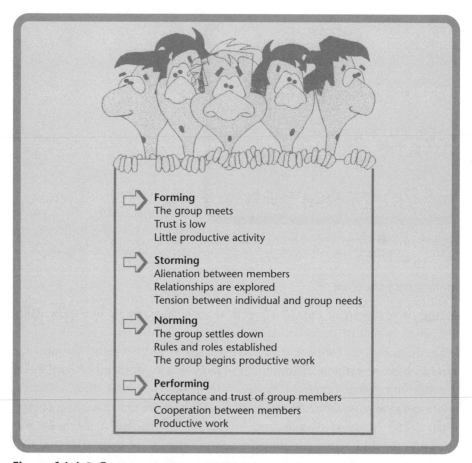

Forming
The group meets
Trust is low
Little productive activity

Storming
Alienation between members
Relationships are explored
Tension between individual and group needs

Norming
The group settles down
Rules and roles established
The group begins productive work

Performing
Acceptance and trust of group members
Cooperation between members
Productive work

Figure 14.4 ● Group processes (after Tuckman, 1965)

Maintaining the task

The task is the objective to be achieved by the group. Such objectives may be varied, from the day-to-day care of individuals to establishing new **protocols** for working practices. The success of such endeavours may depend heavily on the team working together and will require clearly defined objectives. Imagine working with a team and trying to achieve some ill-defined goal. This will not only be inefficient, but also frustrating for the team members. When all the team members understand what is required of them and what their role is in achieving the aim, morale and enthusiasm for the task will remain high.

protocols
_____
regulations or patterns
of working

Maintaining the individual

All groups consist of individuals and as such have individual needs and individual skills. The leader must be careful not to undermine these needs but to encompass them; in this way, individuals can be valued and their skills used to maximum effect within the group. Meeting members' needs may be as simple as ensuring regular meal breaks or valuing them as individuals, providing security, trust and a sense of autonomy.

Leaders do not always of course select their own team members, and some members will need more support than others. Harkins (1987) has identified a phenomenon called 'social loafing' in which some members of the group may do as little work as they can get away with. It is a bit like one member of a tug-of-war team appearing to pull but in fact not exerting any effort at all, the task then becoming far harder for the other members. By identifying each person's role, encouraging and monitoring progress, and encouraging group support, social loafing can be minimised.

■ Being in Control rather than Controlling

Assertiveness is sometimes confused with aggressiveness, arrogance and getting one's own way. It is not, however, about controlling others but about being in control of yourself. It is about respecting yourself and others, recognising that you have rights, including the right to be listened to, while remembering that others also have the same rights. It is about good, positive and equitable communication and negotiation so that both people in the interaction feel respected. It is working towards a win–win situation rather than a win–lose or lose–lose scenario. Some people find that being assertive comes quite naturally to them, others feel less confident and sometimes intimidated, whereas others become aggressive.

assertiveness
a positive way of behaving in relationships, based on honesty, openness and a respect for all parties

There are many reasons why people behave in the way they do, often related to learned behaviour during childhood. Some of the gendered messages commonly conveyed by parents, teachers and the media are shown in Table 14.1.

Table 14.1 Gendered behaviour messages

Male	Female
Be strong	Be gentle
Be successful at any cost	Be kind
Don't let people walk over you	Don't argue
Don't be weak	It is wrong to be angry
Stand up for yourself	It is selfish to think of yourself
Be in control	

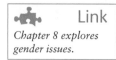

Link

Chapter 8 explores gender issues.

transactional analysis

a theory of personality and an approach to communication that promotes personal growth and change

Activity 14.9

Try to identify situations in which you find it easy to be assertive and ones in which you find it difficult. Ask yourself what it is about these situations that makes it easier or harder.

Those in the first column have traditionally been the messages conveyed to boys and those in the second column the messages to girls. Men traditionally strive to win and see compromise or giving in as weakness and failure. Women have tended to acquiesce, being afraid to speak out, especially on their own behalf. The young are often told not to answer back, to have respect for authority, but although this may be valid, what they are not told is how to be heard while still being respectful to others, whoever the others may be. The messages in both columns may of course apply to either sex, and not all women become passive or all men aggressive.

The 'I'm OK, you're OK quadrangle', taken from **transactional analysis** and shown in Figure 14.5, gives us a picture of the different ways in which people may have learned to respond as a result of childhood experiences. In quadrant 1, the aggressive person does not really care about the rights or feelings of the other person: the 'I'm all right Jack' syndrome. In quadrant 2, the person puts himself down; he may be fearful of hurting or offending others and tends to believe that others are better, echoing the 'children should be seen and not heard' approach. This person may be liked but not respected, or may be seen as weak and used by others. In quadrant 3, the person is deceitful. He may be complimentary to others or full of excuses and apologies; before you know where you are, you are doing something for him that you did not really want to do. You suddenly feel cheated and not quite sure how you got into that situation. The assertive person, shown in quadrant 4, cares about both himself and others. He speaks clearly about his wants and needs in an unambiguous way but also listens to the needs and wants of others. Although some people's behaviour very obviously matches one of these quadrants, it is more common to take something from each of the four quadrants. It is more usual for us to be able to be assertive in some situations and not others. Some people are assertive at home or with their friends and relations but not assertive at work. Others may be assertive at work but struggle to be assertive in their private lives.

1. AGGRESSIVE I'm OK but you are not OK	2. SUBMISSIVE/PASSIVE I'm not OK but you are OK
3. MANIPULATIVE I'm OK and I'll let you think you're OK but really I don't believe you are	4. ASSERTIVE I'm OK and you're OK

Figure 14.5 ● The I'm OK, you're OK quadrangle

Why assertiveness?

Although assertiveness is important for any group, nurses have been identified as a group that finds being assertive difficult (McCartan and Hargie, 1990). This might be attributable to being a profession whose principal purpose is to care for others. Furthermore, nursing has historically had a tradition of duty and subservience. Becoming more assertive is, however, important for two main reasons. The first is to promote mental health, in that non-assertive behaviour can lead to being pushed aside and not listened to, or to being labelled aggressive. Indeed, these have been some of the common stereotypical portrayals of nurses: the submissive, dutiful carer or the dominant, matronly figure. Both these approaches can lead to increased stress and loss of confidence for the nurse, whereas being assertive earns respect from others and an increase in self-confidence.

Second, being assertive is important for the sake of those for whom the nurse is caring and for colleagues and staff working alongside the nurse. It enables the nurse to be in a position to be an advocate for the client, whether in relation to a client's direct care or indirectly by challenging working practices. Staff working relationships can be one of the greatest stresses for health-care workers, but by caring for one another, by being open and respectful, working relationships will be enhanced. Hargie et al. (1994, p. 273) identify seven functions of assertiveness that will help individuals to:

- Ensure that their personal rights are not violated
- Withstand unreasonable requests from others
- Make reasonable requests of others
- Deal effectively with unreasonable refusals from others
- Change the behaviour of others towards them
- Avoid unnecessary aggressive conflicts
- Confidently, and openly, communicate their position on any issue.

Enhancing your assertiveness skills

There are five principles central to being assertive:

1. *Listen carefully to what the other person has to say*: this immediately shows some respect for the other person's opinion and feelings. Furthermore, you have the information you need rather than defensively jumping to conclusions.
2. *Say what you think and feel*: your feelings and thoughts are as important and relevant as anyone else's. You have the right to be heard.
3. *If appropriate, say what you want to happen*: without this, the other person is left guessing what you want. It is important here to be specific.

4. *Be persistent:* do not be side-tracked or wrong-footed but stay with the issue in hand, repeating it if necessary until the issue has been satisfactorily addressed.

5. *Be prepared to compromise:* this must be done from a position of choice to bring about a satisfactory conclusion for all involved rather than because of coercion or 'just for a quiet life'.

Non-verbal communication

non-verbal communication

communicating without the use of spoken language, for example by gestures, body posture and facial expression

In addition to these central aspects, it is important to project yourself in a positive manner, using your body language and **non-verbal communication**. It is no good saying the right things if your body language does not complement your words. Birdwhistell (1970) estimates that up to 70 per cent of social interactions are conveyed via a non-verbal channel; therefore, if your non-verbal communication conveys aggression or passivity, that is what the receiver will be aware of, no matter what you are saying.

Positive communication requires positive non-verbal communication. It is of course important to take into account cultural differences in body language, in which eye contact, proximity and touch may be very different. In principle, eye contact should be direct and appropriate rather than aggressive staring or passive avoidance. Good eye contact demonstrates that you are interested in the other person and have nothing to hide. An individual's personal space is also important. We usually stand closest to those with whom we are most intimate and furthest away during normal social encounters (Hall, 1966). Standing inappropriately close can be threatening, whereas standing too far off can be interpreted as withdrawing. Your posture should be upright and open, with an absence of any gestures that could be interpreted as being aggressive, such as finger-pointing, folded arms or the hands on the hips. The tone of voice should be firm but relaxed and gentle. A good understanding of non-verbal communication can enhance interactions, and it is worthwhile taking the time to consider how you use non-verbal communication and to observe how others use it.

Assertiveness techniques

Two aspects of assertiveness will be outlined here – saying no to a request or demand and managing criticism – both of which can be potentially difficult to manage.

Saying no

Saying no can be particularly difficult for some people. It often raises old anxieties, reminders of when people have said no to us, particularly as children.

There is often an underlying fear of hurting or offending others. Furthermore, if you say no, they may not like you, and the feeling of rejection can be painful and frightening. Simply agreeing to a request when you do not want to can, however, mean being taken for granted and used by others. It can also mean not respecting the other person's ability to accept the refusal. Remember that you have the right to say no without feeling guilty. It is the request rather than the person that is being turned down. Nevertheless, some people do seem to have difficulty in understanding that no means no, so unfortunately it is sometimes necessary to be persistent and explicit in saying no.

Before saying no, take time to consider the request. You may, for example, say, 'Can I come back to you in five minutes?' or 'Can I consult my diary before I give you an answer?' If you really do want to say no, say it clearly and unambiguously. You do not have to give a reason, but if it helps, then do so, providing that it does not undermine your decision. Remember that it is your choice whether to say yes or no. It is the act of choosing that is so important; you do not then feel that you have been railroaded into a decision or have backed down when you really wanted to say no. Once you have made your decision, you must stick to it; two techniques can help in sticking to the point.

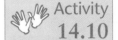

Activity 14.10

If you find it difficult to use your voice assertively, choose a range of scenarios and try verbalising your response to yourself until you get a feel for the right manner and tone of voice. If possible, stand up and speak into a tape-recorder.

The broken record

This really is just repeating what you have already said. If, for example, your manager asks you to do an extra shift but you already have a prior appointment, you may, after careful consideration, say, 'No, I can't do that shift; I have already made other arrangements.' But your manager persists. You can respond by saying, 'As I said, I have made other arrangements and I am not able to do that shift.' Remember that this should not be conveyed in an aggressive manner but in a firm and respectful one. In some cases, it may be necessary to repeat yourself several times to reinforce the message, and you should try to use some of the same words each time so that you do not become diverted.

Fielding the response

This is in some ways similar to the above, but it involves a summarising technique as well as sticking to and repeating your statement. This summarising can be important because it conveys to others that you have heard them and understand their point of view. In the following example, you acknowledge the other person's difficulty and indicate that you would be willing to help if you could, but you also make it clear that you have needs of your own and these, too, should be respected: 'No, I can't work that shift. I realise that you are short of nurses for this shift and if I could help I would, but as I have said, I have made other arrangements.'

Managing criticism

Managing criticism is included here because nurses, along with many other professionals, receive criticism as part of their everyday lives. Criticism can be positive if handled well but a source of hurt and anger if it is not constructively imparted. Given constructively, criticism can help you to reflect on your practice and, if appropriate, modify and enhance it.

There are basically three possible responses to criticism. First, the criticism may be *invalid*, in which case you can reject it. Second, it can be *valid*, in which case you can accept it. Third, it can be *partly valid*, in which case you can accept the valid aspects and reject the invalid ones (Bond, 1986). Before any judgement can be made, you must, however, listen to the criticism. Do not reject it immediately; if necessary, ask for time to think about what you have been told.

Some examples may help to illustrate the three responses.

1. **Invalid**
   Staff nurse to student: 'You don't attend any of the ward rounds.'
   Student: 'I do; in fact I have been on every ward round that has taken place when I have been on duty.'
2. **Valid**
   Staff nurse to student: 'Nurse Kahn, you have forgotten to attend to Mrs Walmsley's dressing.'
   Student: 'Yes I have, I'm sorry. I will go and do it as soon as I have finished this.'
3. **Partially valid**
   Staff nurse to student: 'Nurse Reid, you're always late for these meetings.'
   Student: 'I am late for this meeting and I apologise, but in fact I have been here on time for all the other meetings.'

Fogging

A useful technique to use when you feel that you are being attacked is that of fogging. Fogging tends to slow the other person down and gives you time to formulate a response. There is often an expectation on the part of the person attacking you that you will immediately disagree, but if you agree in part with what they are saying, this tends to draw them from their critical parental stance to a more adult one. An example may help to illustrate this. After you have been in the difficult situation of breaking bad news to a client, the charge nurse sees the client crying and appears to blame you: 'What have you said to Ms Bland? You have obviously upset her.' You might respond by saying, 'Yes, she is very upset; I have just explained to her ...'. Here, you are not agreeing that it is your fault, but you do agree that Ms Bland is upset. The scene is then set for more constructive dialogue to take place between you and the charge nurse.

Conclusion

The very notion of assertiveness can alienate some people. This may be because of their misunderstanding of assertiveness or because of their observations of people who claim to have been on an assertiveness course. It is, in essence, just good, caring communication, communication that respects one's autonomy and the autonomy of others. The techniques involved in being assertive are relatively straightforward, but changing your behaviour may be less easy. Assertiveness training rarely addresses the archaic reasons why you as an individual communicate the way you do. This is not to say that you cannot improve your communication skills through being assertive, but this needs to be carried out alongside developing your own self-awareness. It may, however, take time and practice to adjust the way in which you present yourself. Taking small steps in situations you can cope with will be more rewarding than trying to change overnight. Use your reflective practice to examine your own behaviour, and consider situations in which you were assertive and those in which you wish you had been more assertive.

■ Chapter Summary

In the author's recent experience, a client who was about to die commented that the nurse caring for him seemed to have chosen the wrong profession. It was not her knowledge or technical skills that concerned him but the poor way in which she communicated with him and the other clients around him. Fortunately, there are many examples of good communication to counter this rather sad tale. Clients need more than scientific intervention as part of their care. During your nurse education, you will learn many facts and gain expertise that will undoubtedly be of benefit to the clients in your care. Whatever your chosen branch, your skills must include an expertise in open and caring communication with clients, families and colleagues; without this, you will be failing in your duty of care. It is possible to enhance your communication style and develop good therapeutic communication skills supported by research-based theory. This chapter has only allowed a glimpse into the world of social and professional interactions but provides a basis for further study, reflection and practice.

Test Yourself!

1. Name the three core qualities that are necessary for personal growth and change.

2. Name the six categories of Heron's six-category intervention analysis and give examples of how these may be used in your area of practice.

3. Give five interventions that could be used in the catalytic category.

4. List seven members of the interdisciplinary team in your area of practice.

5. Describe what is meant by a 'primary group' and a 'secondary group'. Give two examples of each.

6. Describe the elements of the three circles model.

7. What are the four stages that Tuckman suggests groups move through as they establish themselves?

8. There are four ways to respond in an interaction, one of which is by being manipulative. What are the other three?

9. What are the five principal stages of being assertive?

10. Criticisms may be 'invalid', 'valid' or 'partially valid'. What are the recommended methods of responding to these types of criticism?

11. How are you going to develop the themes described in this chapter?

■ Further Reading

The following books will help to develop the themes referred to in this chapter.

The core conditions

Mearns, D. and Thorne, B. (1988) *Person-centred Counselling in Action*. Sage, London.

Rogers, C.R. (1980) *A Way of Being*. Houghton Mifflin, New York.

Therapeutic interventions

Culley, S. (1991) *Integrative Counselling* Skills. Sage, London.

Heron, J. (1990) *Helping the Client: A Creative Practical Guide*. Sage, London.

Adair, J. (1988) *Effective Leadership*. Pan Books, London.

Niven, N. and Robinson, J. (1994) *The Psychology of Nursing Care*. Macmillan – now Palgrave Macmillan, Basingstoke.

Assertiveness

Bond, M. (1986) *Stress and Self-awareness: A Guide for Nurses*. Heinemann Nursing, London.

Other useful texts

Buckman, R. (1993) *How To Break Bad News*. Papermac, London.

Hargie, O., Saunders, C. and Dickson, D. (1994) *Social Skills in Interpersonal Communication*, 3rd edn. Routledge, London.

Nelson-Jones, R. (1997) *Practical Counselling and Helping Skills*, 4th edn. Cassell Educational, London.

Stewart, W. (2001) *An A–Z of Counselling Theory and Practice*. Nelson Thornes, Cheltenham.

■ References

Adair, J. (1988) *Effective Leadership*. Pan Books, London.

Bass, B.M. (1990) *Handbook of Leadership: Theory, Research and Managerial Applications*, 3rd edn. Collier-Macmillan, London.

Birdwhistell, R.L. (1970) *Kinesics and Context*. University of Pennsylvania Press, Philadelphia.

Bond, M. (1986) *Stress and Self-awareness: A Guide for Nurses*. Heinemann Nursing, London.

Brereton, M.L. (1995) Communication in nursing: the theory–practice relationship. *Journal of Advanced Nursing* **21**: 314–24.

Buckman, R. (1993) *How to Break Bad News*. Papermac, London.

Buckroyd, J. (1987) The nurse as counsellor. *Nursing Times* **83**: 42–4.

Burnard, P. (1995) Implications of client-centred counselling for nursing practice. *Nursing Times* **91**(26): 35–7.

DoH (Department of Health) (2004) *Agenda for Change Project Team, The NHS Knowledge and Skills Framework and the Development Review Process*, appendix 2, core dimension 1: Communication. DoH, London.

Egan, G. (1994) *The Skilled Helper*, 5th edn. Brooks-Cole, Monterey, CA.

Egan, G. (2002) *The Skilled Helper*, 7th edn. Brooks-Cole, Monterey, CA.

Fielder, F.E. (1971) Validation and extension of the contingency model of leadership effectiveness: a review of empirical findings. *Psychological Bulletin* **76**: 128–48.

Ford, P. and McCormack, B. (2000). Keeping the person in the centre of nursing. *Nursing Standard* **14**(46): 40–4.

Hall, E.T. (1966) *The Silent Language*. Doubleday, New York.

Hargie, O., Saunders, C. and Dickson, D. (1994) *Social Skills in Interpersonal Communication*, 3rd edn. Routledge, London.

Harkins, S. (1987) Social loafing and social facilitation. *Journal of Experimental Social Psychology* **23**: 1–18.

Heron, J. (2001) *Helping the Client: A Creative Practical Guide*. Sage, London.

Hewison, A. (1995) Nurses' power in interaction with patients. *Journal of Advanced Nursing* **21**: 75–82.

Lewin, K., Lippitt, R. and White, R. (1939) Patterns of aggressive behaviour in experimentally created 'social climates'. *Journal of Social Psychology* **10**: 271–99.

Ley, P. (1988) *Communicating with Patients*. Croom Helm, London.

McCartan, P.J. and Hargie, O. (1990) Assessing assertive behaviour in student nurses: a comparison of assertion measures. *Journal of Advanced Nursing* **15**: 1370–6.

Maguire, P. and Faulkner, A. (1993) Communicating with cancer patients: 1. Handling bad news and difficult questions. In Dickenson, D. and Johnson, M. (eds) *Death, Dying and Bereavement*. Sage, London.

Mearns, D. (1994) *Developing Person-centred Counselling*. Sage, London.

Nelson-Jones, R. (1997) *Practical Counselling and Helping Skills*, 4th edn. Cassell Educational, London.

Nichols, K.A. (1989) Institutional versus client-centred care in general hospitals. In Broome, K.A. (ed.) *Health Psychology: Processes and Applications*. Chapman & Hall, London.

Rogers, C.R. (1957) The necessary and sufficient conditions of therapeutic personality change. *Journal of Consulting Psychology* **21**(2): 95–103.

Rogers, C.R. (1980) *A Way of Being*. Houghton Mifflin, New York.

Sayles, S.M. (1966) Supervisory style and productivity: review and theory. *Personnel Psychology* **19**(3): 275–86.

Stevens, J.O. (1971) *Awareness: Exploring, Experimenting, Experiencing*. Real People Press, Moab, UT.

Tuckman, B.W. (1965) Development sequence in small groups. *Psychological Bulletin* **63**(6): 384–99.

Talerico, K.M. (2003) Person-centered care: an important approach for 21st century health care. *Journal of Psychosocial Nursing & Mental Health Services* **41**(11): 12–16.

Useful Websites

www.skillscascade.com/index.htm SkillsCascade
The site contains a range of resources to promote and support the teaching of communication skills in health care. It has been set up by East Anglia Communications skills cascade and contains some really useful guidance on communication

www.infed.org/thinkers/et-rogers.htm#intro Infed on Carl Rogers
Although based around Carl Rogers' influence on education, this site gives some good background to Carl Rogers and outlines the core conditions

www.dh.gov.uk/Home/fs/en The Department of Health
Have a look at the National Service Framework for Older People and in particular person-centred practice. Go to the DoH home page and type 'older people NSF', then follow the links

www.businessballs.com Business Balls
This site, designed for people in business, has an excellent range of information useful for anyone wanting to explore communication, assertiveness and groups

JANET McCRAY

Nursing Practice in an Interprofessional Context

Contents

- What is Interprofessionalism?
- Moves towards Interprofessional Practice
- Teamwork
- Working in Teams
- Responses to Teamworking
- Chapter Summary
- Test Yourself!
- References

Learning Outcomes

At the end of this chapter, the reader will be able to:

- Define the term 'interprofessional practice'
- Identify elements of good and bad practice in teamwork settings
- Highlight different professionals' contributions to teamwork
- Describe the role of the primary health-care team
- Discuss the challenges that the primary health-care team presents to different professionals
- Plan methods of working in practice that will support effective interprofessional teamwork
- Consider the ethical issues that interprofessional practice may create.

■ What is Interprofessionalism?

Interprofessional is the term most recently used to describe professionals from different disciplines working together. The definition suggests that these professionals are working in collaboration to achieve the same goals for the client, patient or service user. Interprofessional practice can occur in a range of settings, from that of the acute medical ward to community support for older people.

Other terms are also used in place of and in preference to interprofessional: Leathard (2003) notes that, in health care, **multidisciplinary** and interdisciplinary have commonly been used to describe practice. Leathard cites Marshall et al. (1979), who define multidisciplinary practice as the work of a group of individuals with different training backgrounds, for example nursing, medicine, occupational therapy, health visiting and social work, who share common objectives but make a different but complementary contribution. Interdisciplinary has been described by Payne (2000) as work 'where professional groups make adaptations to their role, to take account of and interact with the roles of others'. The term 'multi-agency' is also used to describe the involvement of a range of services and professionals in the delivery of health and social care to an individual. To help the reader, the term 'interprofessional' will be used when describing teamwork that involves working towards the same goal for patients or clients.

Transdisciplinary teamwork (Garner and Orelove, 1994) may be a more radical form of practice. It can include working across ordinary professional boundaries to meet the needs of the client or service user. A nurse in the field of learning disability may, for example, give advice on housing or welfare benefits to a young man, although, in day-to-day practice, this would usually be the role of the social worker.

Two key features of interprofessional practice are teamwork and collaboration. Thus, the concept of interprofessional practice may be interpreted in a range of ways, which will be explored in this chapter.

■ Moves towards Interprofessional Practice

Link

Chapter 3 reviews how government policy is enacted.

Over the past 30 years, changes in the delivery of health and social care have placed a different emphasis on the role and work of professionals. These changes have been created by government policy and concerns about the cost and focus of health and welfare provision. In addition, the developing role of some professional groups and the need to respond in order not to undermine the provision of services has required a new look at practice. Advances in technology that have reduced the time spent in hospital, in addition to the deinstitutionalisation movement, have placed an emphasis on care in the community. This has had an impact on more vocal and questioning consumers and service user groups seeking an understanding of, or participation in, decisions about the treatment and services offered, together with welfare rights. These changes have not occurred in isolation: all can be attributed to one or more of the factors identified. Because this chapter explores interprofessional work, it may be worth reviewing each of these elements separately.

Government policy and the focus of health and welfare provision

Moves to introduce general management structures created by the Griffiths Report (DoH, 1983) refocused the activity and roles of professionals within the NHS, one of the greatest changes being the movement of nurses and clinicians into general management. A second change was the division of the functions of delivering and purchasing care, Owens and Petch (1995) explaining this move as an attempt by the government to control budgets and resources. These changes also occurred in social care and formed part of the NHS and Community Care Act 1990. The separation of the functions of purchasing and providing health and social care was also to influence general practice and the role of the GP. In addition, it offered social workers and nurses new opportunities to support other groups with long-term needs, for example people with learning disability.

The ongoing implementation of the White Paper *The New NHS: Modern, Dependable* (DoH, 1997) and *The NHS Plan* (DoH, 2000a), together with *Primary Care, General Practice and the NHS Plan* (DoH, 2001a), has confirmed the emphasis on primary health care, with the creation of primary care Trusts (PCTs). PCTs are responsible for consulting with local communities on healthcare needs as well as commissioning the health care needed from a range of services, for example acute health care. Such changes will continue to affect the way in which professionals work together and will create different partnerships and relationships for practice. The government sees PCTs as being pivotal in achieving changes in public health, as set out in the document *From Vision to Reality* (DoH, 2001b).

In practice, this means new roles for some professionals. In primary care, for example, practice nurses may take on the responsibility for managing specific elements of chronic disease management, a role traditionally undertaken by the GP. Equally, the caring for people who have a terminal illness in their own homes may now be undertaken by community or district nurses.

In other sectors of health care, interprofessional working continues to be an essential part of the NHS's modernisation agenda, as seen with cancer services, where patient outcomes may be more positive if support is offered in an interprofessional context (Audit Commission/Commission for Health Improvement, 2001).

Role expansion

The Greenhalgh Report (Greenhalgh and Company, 1994) reviewed the role of junior doctors and recommended the reduction of their weekly working hours. One response to this initiative has been that of a broader role for nurses. The document *The Scope of Professional Practice* (UKCC (now NMC) 1992) had already identified several areas in which nurses could take on broader and more autonomous roles, for example nurse prescribing and nurse practitioner roles within community hospitals and nurse-led clinics.

The NHS and Community Care Act 1990 also created alterations in the provision of long-term care, which have resulted in a closer working relationship between nurses and social workers, while massive changes in the provision of social care continue, with emphasis on person-centred provision. The Green Paper on social care, *Independence, Well-being and Choice* (DoH, 2005a), if accepted after consultation and in Parliament, will further change the nature of professional and interprofessional relationships. The implementation of the new general medical services (GMS) contract has changed the practice role of GPs and nurses (BMA, 2003), while the NHS Knowledge and Skills Framework (KSF) brings other priorities, including skills, into interprofessional collaboration (DoH, 2004a).

Finally, there has been a blurring of the boundaries between health visitors, district nurses and community nurses, although with emphasis on developing specific areas of expertise. All this means a greater emphasis on teamwork and multiprofessional cooperation, because clinical work that lay in the domain of the GP or hospital-based doctor is now being transferred to other professionals.

Changes in service provision

Link

Chapter 3 expands upon the issue of deinstitutionalisation.

As technology and approaches to treatment have changed, some patients and clients are spending less time in acute hospital settings. Many people are discharged and supported by community or district nurses in their own homes, the majority of care being provided by family members. Running parallel to these developments has been the deinstitutionalisation movement for those who are older or have a learning disability or mental health need.

The transition from institution to community care has seen a change in role for the professional groups of nurses, occupational therapists, psychologists and speech therapists, which has been compounded by an increasing emphasis on voluntary and independent sector provision in the community. Work that might once have been undertaken by qualified professionals may now be carried out by support workers or vocationally trained employees.

In contrast, professional roles have become more specific because of the different types of support required in community settings. At the same time, the cost of some roles has been questioned and the need for a professionally qualified individual has been challenged. Interwoven throughout these changes has been an increased demand for interprofessional collaboration in order to coordinate service delivery in the community.

The rights of service users, clients and patients

The recognition of the changing position of service users with regard to the services offered has gained momentum. An acknowledgement of fragmented services and a need to create a seamless service have built the foundation for change. Responses from service user groups now occur through patients forums overseen by the Commission for Patient and Public Involvement, set up in 2003. Such activity sets the scene for a partnership between the service user and professional, as well as a greater input into decision-making on the use of resources. This change in position of the service user or client has meant that the involvement of a large number of professionals in their specific care group is no longer accepted, and greater collaboration within and across professional teams will be needed in order to minimise this and ensure access to the appropriate services.

Why interprofessionalism is important to nurses

For nurses practising in a range of health-care and social care settings, the need for collaboration to meet service user needs will be a priority, and working together with other professionals will be part of everyday practice. In order to make sense of interprofessional working and enhance its success, it is necessary to have a clear picture of how nursing practice in the interprofessional team has evolved over time and what factors have impinged upon its success. A greater understanding of the role of other professional groups may be gained by thinking about interprofessional practice, which may give nurses greater confidence in collaboration.

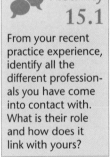

Activity
15.1

From your recent practice experience, identify all the different professionals you have come into contact with. What is their role and how does it link with yours?

■ Teamwork

When interprofessional or multidisciplinary work is described, it is usually a function of **teamwork**. Definitions have been explored and developed over a number of decades. The World Health Organization (WHO, 1984) describes a team as:

teamwork

a group of identified professionals working together to achieve a specific outcome or set of outcomes

> A group who share a common health goal and common objectives determined by community needs, to the achievement of which each member of the team contributes, in accordance with his or her competence and skill and in coordination with the function of others.

Similarly, Rubin and Beckhard (1972) describe it thus: 'a team is a group of people who make different contributions towards the achievement of a common goal.' Others would offer a three-strand definition: belonging and being part of something successful; synergy, a common objective or purpose; and being able to achieve more collectively than as individuals outside the teamwork setting.

Collaboration

collaboration

a term to describe working together. The use of the term 'collaboration' often suggests that there may be conflict present and that the work may at times be difficult

Collaboration can be defined as 'work across boundaries, work with difference' (Loxley, 1997); successful collaboration depending on team members having clear ideas about what they hope to achieve. These ideas should be clear not just to the individual team members, but also to all those contributing to the team activity. Equally, team members should be working to meet the same goals or objectives for patients.

Effective collaboration requires mutual support and the space for disagreement or the exploration of different views to take place. Part of the process of collaboration is deciding when it is needed and when individual team members can make autonomous decisions. In emergency situations, for example, there may be limited time for collaboration, but this does not stop collaboration occurring in emergency or crisis intervention work. Instead, team members may need to develop protocols or guidelines that take into account the decision-making process so that these guidelines can be followed in difficult situations or circumstances.

Factors affecting teamwork

From the definition, the route to teamwork may seem straightforward, although in reality it is a more complicated process. Many factors can influence the ability of a team to practise effective cooperation, all these occurring in the changing context of health and social care practice. Important among these factors are financial constraints, team support, endorsement and professional boundaries.

Financial constraints

When budgets and resources are constrained, the issues of cost and who will foot the bill for intervention can create tension within teams. Practitioners at ground level often wish to work collaboratively to solve problems with service users, but the managers who hold the budgets may be constrained and less able to be facilitative, perhaps placing restrictions on the amount of collaboration that takes place.

Team support

A key factor in team development is that of coordination, and resources may once again influence the level of support. Teams need accountable individuals to help the problem-solving process and take practice-focused solutions forward. These individuals may be identified as leaders or coordinators. Those teams lacking leadership or coordination are not as likely to achieve effective outcomes for clients. As a result, the cost in terms of an individual leader's time has to be met. Equally, teams require a physical environment in which to meet, as well as scheduled time to discuss problems, evaluate progress and plan future developments. All these have both obvious and hidden cost implications.

Endorsing teamwork

Team members need to be able to see the benefits of a team-based model of care. When professionals are under pressure to maintain their current workload, finding time for additional means of collaborating and reviewing their current practice may seem yet another, somewhat onerous task. The lynchpin of good practice may thus be evaluation, as this enables team members to consider the effectiveness of their intervention and whether it has achieved the outcome that was anticipated. Balancing the results of the intervention against the time and cost involved may help team members to decide on the relevance of the team activity they have undertaken. Team members may need to consider the best use of their time together and set priorities, all of which may change following review. As teams work together over a longer period of time, they may be able to make decisions more swiftly, but ongoing evaluation may help them to decide whether such teamwork processes ensure the best outcomes for patients.

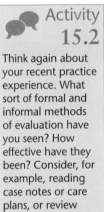

Activity 15.2

Think again about your recent practice experience. What sort of formal and informal methods of evaluation have you seen? How effective have they been? Consider, for example, reading case notes or care plans, or review meetings within social care agencies.

Professional boundaries

For teamwork to be centred on clear outcomes for service users and patients, team members need to be clear about the nature of their role within the team and what the boundaries of that role are. In other words, they need to ask what their professional role is, and where it ends and becomes the responsibility of a different professional. Hudson (1999) notes the significance of professional boundaries and the need for clarity with regard to professional roles and models of care, for example which practice activity is defined as core and to be taken on by all members, and which is seen as specific and thus the role of one discipline. Do differing approaches to practice, for example the medical versus the social model of care, impact on collaboration? Without clarifying the roles, team members may drift towards a common ground, which means that some areas of practice can be neglected.

The changing role of the registered nurse for people with learning disabilities (RNLD) illustrates this. In practice, RNLDs may be the leaders of care, when there is physical long-term care to be provided for a person with learning disabilities. However, other professionals working in primary care may not know about the RNLD role or how to access these nurses and may also have statutory responsibility for meeting the needs of this group of people, as in the case of social workers. Consequently, people with learning disabilities and their families may miss out on a significant resource, and other professionals who could gain from the experience and knowledge of an RNLD might also remain uninformed. McCray's research (2003) has shown that health-care relationships are only one aspect of the role of the RNLD and collaboration with social workers and social work teams and other professional groups was also important. However, it is how this collaboration across disciplines takes place that will impact on the final outcomes for people with learning disabilities and their families.

A lack of clarity about the content and nature of other professions' roles can create significant barriers to good practice. These need to be overcome or acknowledged by both those working in teams and those coordinating them. Other elements under the heading of professional socialisation can also inhibit or sustain good working practices.

Professional socialisation

Individuals' socialisation into and integration within a specific professional group may impact upon their ability to work within an interprofessional team. When a person enters a career pathway with the intention of registering as a professional nurse, for example, a key element of the process is that of **professional socialisation** into the role. This may include guidelines on what clothing to wear in practice, the particular skills and competences learnt in the common foundation programme and the way in which the client or patient is described, all manifesting themselves in how the learner develops the role or identity of a nurse. Similar processes will occur in all professional groups, a consequence being that when teamwork is practised, such factors may impinge on team integration. Some specific elements of professional socialisation are language, personal, professional and interprofessional values, ethics and status.

Language

A vocabulary of terminology and abbreviations is used continuously within each professional group to communicate information, and the language involved may be unique to that profession. When teamwork is undertaken, the meaning of particular words and expressions will need clarification. If clarity is not sought,

---

professional socialisation

the process of taking on a set of values and an identity that are associated with and underpin a particular profession

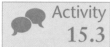

Activity
15.3

Think about your first weeks of nurse education. What activities formed part of the socialisation process? Were you aware of this process at the time?

assumptions may be made about the meaning of specific language and actions, one result being conflict or conflicting views when language is interpreted in different ways by those who do not belong to that particular professional group.

Personal values

A **value** is something that individuals hold at the centre of their being. Values are developed over time and from experience, and personal values may reflect an individual's culture, moral stance or lifestyle. Values may be a product of age or historical tradition. Such values may be translated into action through the development of specific views or attitudes, either positive or negative. Values held may suggest that all individuals have the right to the same opportunities, for example that all people with learning disability should be part of ordinary community life. In this case, attitudes, shown in terms of behaviour for example, could be acting as an independent advocate for an individual when the person needs help with communicating his wishes. In contrast, attitudes may remain observable only in terms of how positively or negatively an individual views a person or situation.

value
something that an individual holds at the centre of his or her being, developed over time and from experience

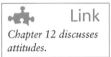
Link
Chapter 12 discusses attitudes.

Professional values

In addition to personal values, individuals who participate in professional education may also develop a further set of values, and there may be assumptions made within teams about the values of the different professional groups. All are working towards similar goals for the service user, ideally in partnership with that person, but values may in reality be different. Social work may, for example, be concerned with interprofessional practice and achieving outcomes for service users based on a recognition of oppression and inequality in society, and the care plan or care management assessment set in place might reflect this. Equally, physiotherapists may be focused on physiological factors that inhibit good health for service users. In working towards collaborative practice, discussion based on values and what they mean to individual professions may work towards an understanding of professional action. If values are ignored, however, this may lead to greater tension in teams (Braye and Preston-Shoot, 1994).

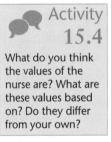
Activity
15.4
What do you think the values of the nurse are? What are these values based on? Do they differ from your own?

Link
Chapter 1 discusses care planning.

Interprofessional values

Loxley (1997) describes the core values of interprofessional work as trust and sharing. She uses the word **utilitarian**, that is, being or having practical worth, to endorse their validity in teamwork. Essential components of trust and sharing are that they must remain two-way. This means not only relying on people's commitment to the team's purpose or task, but also taking on the team members' beliefs in themselves as being able to deliver the goods or take on the

utilitarian
a solution that aims for the greater good, one which has a practical outcome

role, and meeting these expectations. Achieving the ability to trust others and to share practice with them will require confidence and a clear understanding of one's own professional role, which may become more complex when individuals are of a different status.

Ethics

Interprofessional practice may bring to the fore ethical dilemmas in the practice setting. Sheppard (1996), for example, describes potential areas of conflict between professions. GPs will have as their highest priority respect for the life of the patient, whereas a social worker's major concern will be the wishes of the clients themselves. This could lead to conflict over issues regarding the clinical treatment of individuals, particularly if they are already unwell or have a mental illness or learning disability. Child protection work can also create ethical dilemmas if the needs of the child conflict with those of other family members at home. Nurses too can be involved in a range of complex situations, for example when planning discharge for older people. There may be a difference between the wishes of the older person in question and the family members. The older person may wish to go home, whereas the hospital consultant may think a nursing home more appropriate. As a nurse, whose wishes do you act upon?

Status

For teams to work effectively, mutual trust and a respect for all members' contributions to the team are required. This trust is achieved partly by having a greater understanding of the key role of other professional groups and acknowledging the differences and similarities in language, values and models of practice used by other professions. The team coordinator or leader should facilitate this process as a model for teamwork is developed.

Nurses have traditionally been seen as semi-autonomous practitioners working to guidelines drawn up by medical staff; doctors have been seen as making autonomous clinical decisions and advising other members of the health-care and social care teams on practice. Speech therapists and physiotherapists, although autonomous practitioners, work largely on an individual basis with clients, advising on specific areas of intervention. Because of these differences, power and status may become an issue when teamwork is undertaken. Doctors, for example, may have difficulty taking advice from other health-care professionals, whereas nurses may lack the confidence to advise or provide information related to a specific area of practice. Social workers' views of good practice in mental health services may clash with a more medically oriented response from a consultant psychiatrist. All this can influence the way in which teams function and create future stress for team members.

Good practice in teamwork

At this point, nursing practice in an interprofessional context may seem complex and to be avoided at all costs! Nevertheless, having realistic expectations of teamwork may help the nurse to prepare for practice with greater confidence and maintain a focus on what is significant to the outcomes for the client or service user. Some reasons for this are as follows.

Knowledge

Knowledge that identifies some probable causes of friction within the teamwork setting can help to make sense of difficulties and begin to shape the problem-solving process, in other words to help the practitioner to find a workable solution to the situation. Because of the knowledge held, an acceptance of team members' differences and different contributions to teamwork can gradually lead to mutual trust. This will in turn contribute towards a working environment in which it is safe to air conflict or state different opinions. A further spin-off will be the prevention of isolation and an increased willingness to share information.

Methods of practice intervention

The responses to a client's or service user's needs may differ across a range of different professionals. A medical model approach may favour giving information and a course of treatment to individuals; this model may be used by doctors. Some nurses may also adopt an information-giving role. In contrast, other professionals may seek a more partnership-based model of practice, seen for example, as Oliver (1996) suggests, where the professional is viewed as a resource to be used by the particular service user. In other words, the individual service user will direct the professional's approach, personally requesting specific information, action and responses. This approach is developing within social work and care management-type roles and is explored in the service development part of the Green Paper on social care (DoH, 2005a). The different models of practice of different professional groups can lead to an inconsistency of information for the service user and cause greater confusion. The teamwork process should, however, provide a framework within which issues such as what information should be given and the level of commitment required by each professional are clearly stated and agreed.

Pritchard (1995) adopts Bruce's (1980) 'teamwork for presentation' matrix to identify stages of team cooperation (Table 15.1). Pritchard's matrix illustrates the steps leading to the committed team by describing cooperation in a range of teamwork activities. The main use of this tool has been in the assessment or diagnosis of a team's current position. Here it is used to give an example of what could be achieved within the teamwork setting. Moreover, as Pritchard (1995) notes, there is a need to link teamwork performance to outcomes for service users and, as such, to begin to meet need.

Table 15.1 Stages of team cooperation

| Activity | Level of commitment | | |
	Nominal	Convenient	Committed
Team goal-setting	No explicit goals	Follow doctors' orders	Shared explicit goals
Role perceptions	Stereotypes common	Some understanding	Roles clearly understood
Professional status	Wide differences	Differences inhibit cooperation	Differences ignored
Referral of patients	To agency rather than individual professionals	Referral by delegation	Easy two-way referral and open access
Interaction within team	Very little and irregular interaction	Some interaction	Close regular interaction, formal and informal
Mutual trust	Lacking	Guarded	Strong and developing
Communication failure	Often	Sometimes	Rare
Confidentiality	A problem	Problems partly solved	Not a problem
Advice to patients	Inconsistent	Poor coordination	Consistent
Preventive care	Not possible	Possible	Optimum conditions

Source: Modified from Bruce (1980).

Meeting need

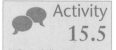

Activity 15.5

What skills are required to share differing opinions with others? How can these be used?

Link

Chapter 12 provides more information on teamworking.

In a team where conflict is aired and individual members feel safe to share differing views, steps can be taken towards clear mutual goals. These can help the teamwork forward, preventing obstruction and avoiding difficult issues. Payne (2000) suggest that, as a starting point to meeting need, the team must be able to identify agreed objectives and be able to articulate and resolve differences. Finally, the team must be able to manage interpersonal issues – how the team feel about each other – and make a commitment to teamwork. In learning to manage all these factors, the needs of service users or clients can remain central to the team's purpose.

■ Working in Teams

So far this chapter has reviewed some of the factors that can affect teamwork, these being generic in setting and content. In this section, the role of the primary health-care team will be explored to provide a specific example of teamwork and multiprofessional practice.

What is the primary health-care team?

In the foreword to the summary of the White Paper *Primary Care: Delivering the Future* (DoH, 1996), **primary health care** was described as 'the NHS most people see – the NHS of the family doctor and their team, community nurses, therapists as well as pharmacists, dentists and optometrists'. It will also include midwives, district nurses and health visitors. Since the implementation of the White Paper *The New NHS: Modern, Dependable* (DoH, 1997), the role of the primary health-care team (PHCT) has continued to develop and grow: traditional teams based around health centres may now include counsellors and mental health nurses, and social workers will be involved in areas such as child protection and provision for older people. Plans set in place by the 1996 White Paper have reviewed and expanded the role of the nurse in learning further skills, such as prescribing medication. Equally, the role of the practice nurse has expanded to take on referrals from people who would ordinarily have seen their GP. In addition, the new strategy for people with learning disabilities, *Valuing People* (DoH, 2001c), highlights the relationship between the PHCT and other services in meeting the ongoing health-care needs of this group of people as one means of preventing social exclusion.

primary health care

the continuing health and social welfare care offered appropriately to individuals in need living in private households

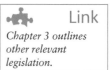

Link

Chapter 3 outlines other relevant legislation.

How it has evolved

Jeffereys (1995) wrote that, as a result of the *Family Doctors Charter* (BMA, 1965) in 1966, arrangements were set in place for positive community-based practice. This charter established a positive role for non-hospital-based medicine, a structure for interprofessional work being instigated. Jeffereys identified the elements of this structure as allowances for GPs who worked together on one site, and promoting the employment of receptionists and practice nurses, by providing reimbursement for their services, and offering interest-free loans for more modern premises. The Health Services and Public Health Act 1968 endorsed a health-promotion role for general practice that involved the prevention of ill-health and support for families. Thus, the role of the primary health-care team gradually emerged.

Further changes were to occur in the 1980s as the Conservative government set about cutting the increasing public expenditure. Pietroni (1994) reported that the White Paper *Priorities for Health and Social Services in England* (DHSS, 1976) and the *NHS Management Inquiry* (DoH, 1983) resulted in the NHS and Community Care Act 1990. The Act placed further responsibilities

Link

Chapter 3 has more information on changing health-care policies.

for care within the primary health-care team, making it the first point of call for all referrals. The introduction of the GMS contract (BMA, 2003) has changed the way in which GPs are funded and their quality and performance measured in relation to specific targets for the nations health. These developments maintain the place of the GP at the centre of decision-making within the PHCT, although, increasingly, other professionals, such as practice nurses, might take on the assessment and management role of patients with chronic diseases such as diabetes. Chart 15.1 highlights the key developments within primary health-care nursing practice.

Chart 15.1 ● Key developments in primary health-care nursing

District nursing

1970s   Introduction of attachment schemes
          District nurses based at GP practices. Established primary health-care teams

1972   Report of the Committee on Nursing made recommendations for formal post-basic education, which became law in 1979

1974   Royal College of General Practitioners (RCGP) published *Nursing in General Practice in the Reorganised NHS*

1990s   Extended role of the district nurse may include the prescribing of medication, previously the task of the GP
          Review of educational requirements of the role as part of the English National Board specialist pathway curricula

2000s   As professionals in primary care trusts, guidance in the delivery of the NHS plan (DoH, 2002)

● Further development of prescribing role with potential for selection and training as independent prescribers
● Support for development of palliative care role as part of *The NHS Cancer Plan* (DoH, 2001)
● The NHS KSF (DoH, 2004a) and *Agenda for Change* (DoH, 2004b) offer transparent criteria for professional role development.

Practice nursing

1970s   Nurses attached to GP practice

1986   Cumberlege Report, *Neighbourhood Nursing: A Focus for Care* (DHSS, 1986), recommended development of the nurse practitioner role – taking on direct referrals to ease the pressure on GPs

1987   Government rejected these plans

1990s   Role of practice nurses under review

1996   White Paper *Primary Care: Delivering the Future* (DoH, 1996) advocates major changes to practice nurse education and role within the primary health-care team

1998   Configuration of primary care groups may mean changes in the practice nurse role

2000s   As primary care Trust professionals, opportunity to develop specialist clinical skills in primary care settings (DoH, 2003)

- Change in role and responsibility created by the GMS contract offers opportunity for further specialism (DoH, 2003)
- Potential outcome of the NHS KSF (DoH, 2004a) and *Agenda for Change* (DoH, 2004b) for this group of nurses not yet fully developed, although may offer positive development opportunities (McCray, 2005).

Health visiting

1976   Court Report identified the health visitor as a major agent of prevention in family work (Orr, 1975)

1970s   Central Council for the Education and Training of Health Visitors
and   continued to assess the role of the health visitor, especially when the
80s   focus on child protection and children at risk increased

1980   Standing conference on health visitor education, A Time to Learn, looked at the changing role of health visiting

1990s   Role still unclear. Purchaser concern with cost of health visitor intervention

1998   Configuration of primary care groups may mean changes in the role of the health visitor

2000s   The NHS KSF (DoH, 2004a) and *Agenda for Change* (DoH, 2004b) offer transparent criteria for professional role development in primary care Trusts

- Green Paper on children's services, *Every Child Matters* (DoH, 2005b), may further develop collaborative role. Health visitors could be employed in newly configured children's trusts.

Quality services in the community

As part of the NHS modernisation agenda, the PHCT is continuing to face the challenge of effective teamwork and the need to develop further professional roles. The government's aim to achieve a seamless service remains, in order that clients and patients are not seen by a vast number of different professionals and to prevent their continual assessment and attendance at different clinics. An emphasis on developing primary health care remains a top priority, the principles of good primary care, shown in Figure 15.1 below, being highlighted with regard to quality. In addition, one of the key functions of primary care groups will be that of **clinical governance**, ensuring that effective, high-quality care is offered to a specific population.

clinical governance

a comprehensive method of determining the quality of provision of service, focusing on professional accountability, audit, patient or client perception of the service and value for money

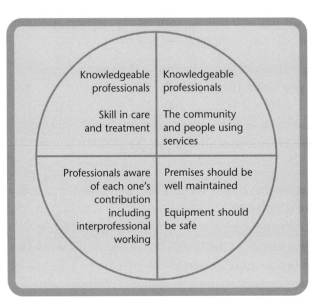

Figure 15.1 ● **Principles of good primary care** (adapted from DoH, 1996)

Role of the professional within the primary health-care team

There are still decisions to be made about further extended roles for nurses and how these will contribute to the PHCT. Equally, the need to use resources effectively remains an issue. Also unanswered is why there is still an ongoing need to re-emphasise interprofessional teamwork when PHCTs have been in existence for more than 25 years. Teamwork should be seen as an essential part of working together, yet some gaps still exist. Some broad reasons for the difficulties encountered in teamwork were raised earlier in the chapter. If we look specifically at PHCTs, all the factors identified may inhibit good practice, but at this point it is worth looking at some further constraints on teamwork within PHCTs:

● *Location:* It is probable that the core members of the PHCT are situated on one site within a local health centre. Other professionals, such as social workers, who provide an input to the team may, however, be based at different locations. As a consequence, they may miss out on informal contact and lines of communication

- *Team size:* A range of individual professionals may be involved in providing services, and the size and extent of this may impact on team development. Too large a team may prevent clear and focused discussion and inhibit the decision-making process. Examples of this may be seen in the child protection and mental health services
- *Payment:* Individual professionals working as part of the PHCT will be employed on different rates of pay and conditions of service. This could lead to a feeling of resentment among some team members
- *Resource management:* Responsibility for practice and performance may not be clearly identified. In some teams, GPs may be the decision-makers when funding for services is allocated. In contrast, practice nurses and other nurse practitioners may have limited financial or budgetary control. Although individual practitioners may see themselves as autonomous, issues such as payment and access to resources can lead to an inequality of status, and, as a consequence, individual contributors to teamwork may be seen as being of more or less value.

In the changing climate of primary care, in which GPs may have greater financial autonomy, the position of other professionals may be under greater scrutiny, for example when making decisions about the effectiveness of the input of various professionals and, in doing so, questioning roles and performance. Part of this process may lead to a narrowing down of certain roles and a limited input of some professionals to primary health-care teams. Such activities may restrict good teamwork.

Moving towards cooperation

The place of interprofessional work currently remains uncertain. Pockets of good practice are observable, but mutual cooperation and the desires of service users can be in conflict with government policy, the way in which funding mechanisms operate and the struggle for power of some professional groups (Figure 15.2). The National Service Framework (NSF) for Older People (DoH, 2001d) set out under standard 2 – person-centred care – the need for health and social care agencies to provide a single assessment process by April 2004. However, as Glasby (2004) notes, this has not been straightforward and there are a number of key areas that require change, one of which is that of partnership working, which still remains problematic.

> **Link**
> Chapters 2, 3 and 18 have further information related to NSFs.

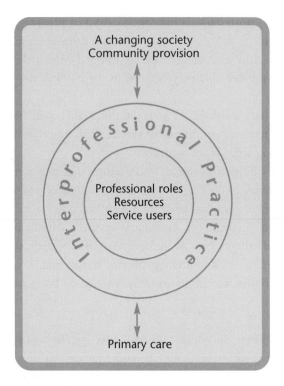

Figure 15.2 ● Factors affecting interprofessional work

■ Responses to Teamworking

Research and reports

A considerable amount of research and evaluation has been undertaken in the area of teamwork in primary health and social care. In the 1980s, many of the findings of studies focusing on primary health-care settings were negative, and the reluctance to collaborate of some specific professional groups, such as doctors, is well documented. More recently, however, the value of interprofessional work has become the focus of research and evaluation. Most of the work published emphasises the positive responses to collaboration across different professional groups. As the body of research grows, along with an increasing amount of research funding for such projects, it is likely that effective mechanisms for change will be identified and implemented. A significant number of reports have been published that focus on the value of collaboration, and how to collaborate more effectively. These include:

● *A Fruitful Partnership: Effective Partnership Working* (Audit Commission, 1998)

- *Partnership in Action: New Opportunities for Joint Working between Health and Social Services* (DoH, 1998)
- *Taking your Partners: Using Opportunities for Interagency Partnership in Mental Health* (Sainsbury Centre for Mental Health, 2000)
- *Towards a Common Cause – a Compact for Care: Inspection of Local Authority Social Services and Voluntary Sector Working Relationships* (DoH, 2000b)
- *Securing Better Mental Health for Older Adults* (DoH, 2005c).

Educational developments

Education has been one response to the interprofessional agenda. Providers of educational programmes have seen educational activity as a route to a greater understanding of the professional roles of others. Most of the activity that has occurred has been at postregistration or post-qualifying level. Individual professionals have come together to share units of study, an emphasis on problem-solving having been developed during the 1990s. Loxley (1997) reproduces a table from the Centre for the Advancement of Interprofessional Education (1996) that gives a detailed review of the coordinating bodies and their activities.

A number of universities and schools of medicine, social work and nursing are also developing units or forums for the development of interprofessional practice initiatives, notably the New Generation project between the Universities of Southampton and Portsmouth. A range of online networks are also available and these are given at the end of the chapter.

Interprofessionalism as a 'theory' for practice

Many of the elements that form interprofessional practice have been brought together in this chapter. Much of this has centred upon teamwork and collaboration, and a review of roles and professional boundaries. We have seen how the developments in community care have created many of these changes. In reality, interprofessionalism has been seen as a set of skills or competences, rather than a whole new way of informing practice, with a theoretical underpinning. For example, from what knowledge base does interprofessional work come? Loxley (1997) suggests that assumptions are made about what knowledge from a certain discipline might be helpful but that this has not been investigated or studied in a coherent way. It is largely driven by what services need, and because of this, a sound theoretical framework has not yet developed.

A number of academics and practitioners are beginning to study and build a theory for interprofessional practice. As this develops, it is possible that those professionals who have been reluctant to make interprofessional practice a priority may begin to participate.

Personal responses

Link

Chapter 13 describes an approach to thinking about individual responses in a structured and useful way.

The moves forward outlined above tackle complex issues at a societal service and organisational level. An individual in practice can still, however, begin to create change. For a nurse practising in a interprofessional setting, thinking about individual responses to teamwork and reflecting on their cause or foundation may be helpful. Observing professionals who hold effective team member skills may also provide ideas for the development of personal knowledge and skills.

From this perspective, individual methods of working that can help effective teamwork can be shaped. Part of this exercise should include an active consideration of the role of service users in the process.

■ Chapter Summary

The route to interprofessional practice is a complex one. At times, the agendas of government, service managers, professionals and service users seem to be in conflict, but positive examples can nevertheless be seen in practice. As practitioners, educationalists and service managers design the organisational structures needed to develop further multiprofessional work, professionals can build on their skills in collaboration. The interface of health and social care delivery can then become a positive one.

Test Yourself!

1. What does the term 'interprofessional practice' mean?

2. Provide examples from your own experience of good and bad teamwork.

3. How do different professionals contribute to teamworking?

4. What challenges does working in a PHCT create for the nurse?

■ References

Audit Commission (1998) *A Fruitful Partnership: Effective Partnership Working.* Audit Commission, London.

Audit Commission/Commission for Health Improvement (2001) *NHS Cancer Care in England and Wales.* Audit Commission, London.

BMA (British Medical Association) (1965) *Family Doctors Charter: A Charter for the Family Doctor Service.* BMA, London.

BMA (British Medical Association) (2003) *Investing in General Practice: The New General Services Contract.* British Medical Association/National Health Service Confederation, London.

Braye, S. and Preston-Shoot, M. (1994) *Empowering Practice in Social Care.* Open University Press, Buckingham.

Bruce, N. (1980) *Teamwork for Preventative Care.* Research Studies Press/John Wiley & Sons, Chichester.

Centre for the Advancement of Interprofessional Education (1996) *National Coordinating Bodies and their Interests.* CAIPE, London.

DHSS (Department of Health and Social Security) (1976) *Priorities for Health and Personal Social Services in England.* HMSO, London.

DHSS (Department of Health and Social Security) (1986) *Community Nursing Review. Neighborhood Nursing – A Focus for Care* (Cumberlege Report). HMSO, London.

DoH (Department of Health) (1983) *NHS Management Inquiry* (Griffiths Report). HMSO, London.

DoH (Department of Health) (1990) *Caring for People. Community Care in the Next Decade and Beyond.* HMSO, London.

DoH (Department of Health) (1996) *Primary Care: Delivering the Future.* HMSO, London.

DoH (Department of Health) (1997) *The New NHS: Modern, Dependable.* Stationery Office, Norwich.

DoH (Department of Health) (1998) *Partnership in Action: New Opportunities for Joint Working between Health and Social Services.* A discussion document. HMSO, London.

DoH (Department of Health) (2000a) *The NHS Plan.* Stationery Office, Norwich.

DoH (Department of Health) (2000b) *Towards a Common Cause – a Compact for Care: Inspection of Local Authority Social Services and Voluntary Sector Working Relationships.* Stationery Office, Norwich.

DoH (Department of Health) (2001a) *Primary Care, General Practice and the NHS Plan.* Stationery Office, Norwich.

DoH (Department of Health) (2001b) *From Vision to Reality.* Stationery Office, Norwich.

DoH (Department of Health) (2001c) *Valuing People. A New Strategy for Learning Disability in the 21st Century.* Stationery Office, Norwich.

DoH (Department of Health) (2001d) *The National Service Framework for Older People.* Stationery Office, Norwich.

DoH (Department of Health) (2001e) *The NHS Cancer Plan: Education and Support for District and Community Nurses in the Principles and Practice of Palliative Care Education Initiatives Funded under the Programme.* Stationery Office, Norwich.

DoH (Department of Health) (2002) *Liberating the Talents: Helping PCTs and Nurses to Deliver the NHS Plan.* Stationery Office, Norwich.

DoH (Department of Health) (2003) *Practitioners with a Special Interest in Primary Care: Implementing a Service for Nurses with a Special Interest in the Programme: Liberating the Talents.* Stationery Office, London.

DoH (Department of Health) (2004a) *The National Health Service, Knowledge and Skills Framework and the Development Review Process* (draft document). Stationery Office, London.

DoH (Department of Health) (2004b) A*genda for Change Proposed Agreement: Sept 2004* (final draft). Stationery Office London.

DoH (Department of Health) (2005a) *Independence, Well being and Choice: Our Vision for the Future of Social Care in England.* Green Paper. Stationery Office, London.

DoH (Department of Health) (2005b) *Every Child Matters.* Green Paper. Stationery Office, London.

DoH (Department of Health) (2005c) *Securing Better Mental Health for Older Adults.* Stationery office, London.

Garner, H.G. and Orelove, F.P. (1994) *Teamwork in Human Services. Models and Application across the Life Span.* Butterworth Heinemann, Boston.

Gilmour, M., Bruce, N. and Hunt, M. (1974) *The Work of the Nursing Team in General Practice.* Council for the Education and Training of Health Visitors, London.

Glasby, J. (2004) Social services and the single assessment process. *Journal of Interprofessional Care* **18**(2): 129–39.

Greenhalgh and Company (1994) *The Interface between Junior Doctors and Nurses: A Research Study for the Department of Health.* HMSO, London.

Hudson, B. (1999) Primary health care and social care: working across professional boundaries. *Managing Community Care* **7**(1): 15–22.

Jeffereys, M. (1995) Primary health care. In Owens, P., Carrier, C. and Horder, J. (eds) *Interprofessional Issues in Community and Primary Health Care.* Macmillan – now Palgrave Macmillan, Basingstoke.

Leathard, A. (2003) *Interprofessional Collaboration: From Policy to Practice in Health and Social Care.* Brunner & Routledge, Hove.

Loxley, A. (1997) *Collaboration in Health and Welfare.* Jessica Kingsley, London.

Marshall, M., Preston, M., Scott, E. and Wincott, P. (eds) (1979) *Teamwork For and Against: An Appraisal of Multidisciplinary Practice.* British Association of Social Workers, London.

McCray, J. (2003) Leading interprofessional practice: a conceptual framework to support practitioners in the field of learning disability. *Journal of Nursing Management* **11**: 387–95.

McCray, J. (2005) Personal and people development for practice nurses. *BMJ ELearning.*

Oliver, M. (1996) *Social Work. Disabled People and Disabling Environments.* Jessica Kingsley, London.

Orr, J. (1975) Health visiting in the UK. In Hockey, L. (ed.) *Primary Care Nursing.* Churchill Livingstone, London.

Owens, P. and Petch, H. (1995) Professionals and management. In Owens, P., Carrier, J. and Horder, J. (eds) *Interprofessional Issues in Community and Primary Health Care.* Macmillan – now Palgrave Macmillan, Basingstoke.

Payne, M. (2000) *Teamwork and Multiprofessional Care.* Palgrave – now Palgrave Macmillan, Basingstoke.

Pietroni, P. (1994) Interprofessional teamwork. In Leatherhead, A. (ed.) *Going Inter-professional*. London, Routledge.

Pritchard, P. (1995) Learning to work effectively in teams. In Owens, P., Carrier, J. and Horder, J. (eds) *Interprofessional Issues in Community and Primary Health Care*. Macmillan – now Palgrave Macmillan, Basingstoke.

RCGP (Royal College of General Practitioners) (1974) *Nursing in General Practice in the Reorganised NHS*. RCGP, London.

Rubin, I.R. and Beckhard, R. (1972) Factors influencing the effectiveness of health teams. *Millbank Memorial Fund Quarterly* **50**(3): 317–37.

Sainsbury Centre for Mental Health (2000) *Taking your Partners: Using Opportunities for Interagency Partnership in Mental Health*. Sainsbury Centre for Mental Health, London.

Sheppard, M. (1996) Primary care roles and relationships. In Watkins, M., Hervey, N., Carson, J. and Ritter, S. (eds) *Collaborative Community Mental Health Care*. Arnold, London.

UKCC (United Kingdom Central Council for Nursing, Midwifery and Health Visiting) (1992) *The Scope of Professional Practice*. UKCC (now NMC), London.

WHO (World Health Organization) (1984) *Glossary of Terms Used in the Health for All Series*. WHO, Geneva.

◾ Useful Websites

www.caipe.org.uk Centre for the Advancement of Interprofessional Education (CAIPE)

www.kingsfund.org.uk King's Fund

www.health-homerton.ac.uk/ipl/home University of Cambridge Interprofessional learning portal

16

Challenges to Professional Practice

Contents

- Defining Professional Practice
- The Responsibilities of Professional Practice
- Philosophies and Ideologies
- Quality
- Clinical Governance
- Models and Frameworks of Care

- Evidence-based Practice
- Lifelong Learning
- Where to Next?
- Chapter Summary
- Test Yourself!
- References

Learning Outcomes

The aim of this chapter is to start you thinking about some of the issues that influence the ways in which nurses operate as registered practitioners to manage and deliver nursing care. At the end of the chapter, you should be able to:

- Define professional practice and discuss the responsibilities involved

- Understand *The NMC Code of Professional Conduct: Standards for Conduct, Performance and Ethics* in relation to your own roles and responsibilities as a student, with particular reference to accountability, informed consent and the Freedom of Information Act

- Describe the role that personal, organisational and professional beliefs and values play in underpinning practice

- Identify the influence of philosophies and frameworks of care in nursing practice

- Discuss the significance of quality assessment, standards and the role of clinical governance in evaluating nursing care

- Identify your own responsibilities for evidence-based practice and lifelong learning.

By the time you reach the end of the common foundation programme, you will have gained some confidence in clinical skills, experienced a range of placements aimed at broadening your perceptions of nursing and your clients, and developed a theoretical foundation on which to build the more specialised theory of your chosen branch of nursing. The issues raised in this chapter can be seen as challenges that nurses have addressed in an effort to move from an occupation dominated and directed by medical practitioners, to one with a developing knowledge and skill base of its own, which has a direct influence on client care. All these subjects will be addressed in more detail in your branch studies and are merely touched upon here in terms of raising your awareness of what the responsibilities of being a **registered practitioner** are.

registered practitioner
a nurse, midwife or health visitor who is registered on the professional register with the NMC

The issues to be considered are:

- Defining professional practice
- The responsibilities of professional practice
  - The NMC Code of Professional Conduct (NMC, 2004a)
  - Accountability
  - Informed consent
  - The Freedom of Information Act
- Philosophies and ideologies (beliefs and values)
- Quality
- Clinical governance and research governance
- A knowledge base for nursing – models and frameworks of care
- Evidence-based practice
- Lifelong learning.

Before addressing the theoretical issues, however, it is worth taking time to consider just what we mean by 'professional practice'.

■ Defining Professional Practice

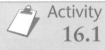

Activity 16.1

Take a few minutes to think back over your experiences to date and note down the expectations you would have of any person you consulted as a professional, for example a lawyer, a doctor or an architect.

The debate over whether or not nursing is a profession has been raging for over 20 years, and each of us has our own views on it (for an overview of this, see Cronin and Rawlings-Anderson, 2004). The whole issue is largely a sterile one that has little impact on the way in which nurses practise nursing; what is far more important for nursing students is how we choose for ourselves what constitutes 'professional' behaviour and how we enact that in our practice. So perhaps the best place to start this chapter is by identifying what we mean by professional practice. Try Activity 16.1.

Some of the issues you identified probably relate to such things as:

- The knowledge people have
- Their professional qualifications or evidence of belonging to a professional body or organisation that licenses or registers them to practise
- The skill they exhibit in their practice
- Their conduct, for example the way in which they dress, their manner, how they treat you, the respect they show you and the confidence they have in their ability to help you
- A recommendation from other people or the fact that they are recognised for their particular expertise.

Hence we all carry with us a personal view of what professional practice is.

Superimposed on this will be external definitions that arise from the professional bodies governing the people who they license to practise, for example codes of practice, and criteria established by government policies. Similarly, there may be expectations of professional practice that derive from employers and contracts of employment.

Moloney (1992) suggests that the set of attributes displayed by people in professional practice can be seen as 'professionalism' and that they relate essentially to the attitudes and attributes they display. The first of these is that a profession is indeed 'practised' or engaged in rather than being a theoretical activity. Other attitudes may be a commitment to work and an orientation towards service rather than personal profit. Similarly, there may be a requirement for accountable practice that is based on evidence and an inherent motivation for learning and the development of a knowledge base. These arise, as we have seen, from a multitude of sources, the first being the values adopted by the profession and outlined by its professional body.

■ The Responsibilities of Professional Practice

Link

Chapter 3 describes in greater detail the regulation of the professions.

The Nursing and Midwifery Council (NMC) was established in 2002 as the regulatory body for nurses, midwives and health visitors. This body superseded the United Kingdom Central Council for Nursing, Midwifery and Health Visiting (UKCC) and the previous four National Boards that held responsibility for standards of education for practice.

The core function of the NMC is 'to establish and improve standards of nursing and midwifery care in order to serve and protect the public' (www.nmc-uk.org). The powers of the NMC were set out in the Nursing and Midwifery Order 2001. Its key tasks are to:

- Maintain a register listing all nurses and midwives
- Set standards and guidelines for nursing and midwifery education, practice and conduct
- Provide advice on professional standards
- Provide quality assurance in nursing and midwifery education
- Set standards and provide guidance for local supervising authorities for midwives
- Consider allegations of misconduct or unfitness to practice due to ill-health (www.nmc-uk.org).

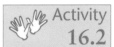

Activity 16.2

Access and review the contents of the new NMC website www.nmc-uk.org. Note any information about the revised Code of Professional Conduct. Discuss your findings with your practice-based mentor or study group.

In order to carry out these tasks, the NMC publishes guidance for professionals, employers and the public detailing the standards of practice that professionals are expected to achieve.

The most significant of these for student nurses are probably the NMC Code of Professional Conduct (NMC, 2004a) and *An NMC Guide for Students of Nursing and Midwifery* (NMC, 2002). Other recent publications that might be of interest are listed in Table 16.1.

Table 16.1 NMC publications of interest to students

Title	Date of publication
Fitness for Practice Summary	17/10/2001
Guide for Students of Nursing and Midwifery	1/04/2002
Guidelines for Records and Record-keeping	1/01/2005
Guidelines for the Administration of Medicines	16/08/2004
Midwives Rules and Standards	2/08/2004
Perceptions of the Scope of Professional Practice	1/01/2000
Practitioner–client Relationships and the Prevention of Abuse	1/04/2002
The PREP Handbook	1/08/2004
The NMC Code of Professional Conduct: Standards for Conduct, Performance and Ethics	8/12/2004

Note: All these are available online at www.nmc-uk.org.

The purpose of the Code of Professional Conduct (2004a) is to:

- Inform the professions of the standard of professional conduct required of them in the exercise of their professional accountability and practice
- Inform the public, other professions and employers of the standard of professional conduct they can expect of a registered practitioner.

The Code states that, as a registered nurse, midwife or specialist community public health nurse, you must:

- Protect and support the health of individual patients and clients
- Protect and support the health of the wider community
- Act in such a way that justifies the trust and confidence the public have in you
- Uphold and enhance the good reputation of the professions.

Chart 16.1 shows the responsibilities placed on practitioners by the Code of Professional Conduct.

Chart 16.1 ● Code of Professional Conduct

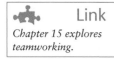 **Link**

Chapter 15 explores teamworking.

As a professional nurse or midwife, you are personally accountable for your practice. In caring for patients and clients, you must:
- Respect the patient or client as an individual
- Obtain consent before you give any treatment or care
- Cooperate with others in the team
- Protect confidential information
- Maintain your professional knowledge and competence
- Be trustworthy
- Act to identify and minimise risk to patients and clients
In addition, the NMC recommends that a practitioner has professional indemnity insurance.

Source: NMC (2004a). Available at www.nmc-uk.org.

As well as taking on the professional regulatory role of the UKCC in terms of accountability in practice and determining standards for practice, the NMC is responsible for two significant aspects of quality assurance in the education of nurses, midwives and specialist community public health nurses (formerly referred to as health visitors):

- Setting standards for preregistration education and also for those education programmes leading to a recordable qualification (that is, one that is entered on the register of practice)
- Monitoring the quality of all education programmes leading to registerable or recordable qualifications.

The NMC quality assurance framework incorporates, together with the Higher Education Funding Council Quality Assurance Agency (QAA), elements of institutional approval, approval in principle, validation, annual monitoring, periodic review and subject review. To achieve this, the NMC works in partnership with:

- Education purchasers – strategic health boards and workforce confederations
- Quality assurance organisations such as the Healthcare Commission and the QAA
- Service providers, both NHS and independent
- Higher education institutions
- Multiprofessional regulatory bodies such as the General Medical Council, Health Professions Council and General Social Care Council.

One of the most significant issues to have been highlighted by the UKCC, which has been transferred to the NMC, in terms of standards of professional practice and professionalism, is that of accountability (Watson, 1992).

What is accountability?

The NMC define being accountable as 'responsible for something or to someone' (NMC, 2004a, p. 13). Although we tend to talk in terms of professional responsibility, there are in fact four different types of **accountability** that can be identified for registered nurses, midwives and specialist community public health nurses:

accountability

being answerable for one's actions

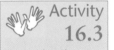

Activity 16.3

Try to identify examples from your own life that would fit under each type of accountability listed in the text.

1. Professional accountability.
2. Accountability to the employer under a contract of employment.
3. Accountability to the patient under existing law provision.
4. Accountability to the profession under the Nurses, Midwives and Health Visitors Act 1979.

Thus, although we usually focus on the latter in terms of professional issues, it is important to remember that nurses, as individual members of society, need to be accountable in terms of the expectations of any other member of society, that is, they cannot commit a criminal act and expect to be defended by a professional code.

Features of professional accountability

Professional accountability assumes that the practitioner is a member of a profession, accepting the status, rights and responsibilities that this brings and thus using one's professional judgement and being answerable for it. Jacobs (2004) suggests that the core of a nurse's accountability is the personal accountability assumed by the individual, enshrined within the Code of Professional Conduct. This professional accountability means that nurses are legally accountable for their work and can be removed from the professional register for unpro-

professional accountability

being answerable to the NMC for decisions made and actions taken in the course of practice

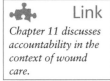

Link

Chapter 11 discusses accountability in the context of wound care.

fessional behaviour that breaches the Code of Professional Conduct (NMC, 2004a). We can identify two features of it – decision-making and an obligation to explain and justify any actions taken.

As a nurse, you are privileged to be allowed to make decisions about areas of care based on your knowledge, skills and experience. The NMC suggests that

> professional accountability involves weighing up the interests of patients, using (your) professional judgment and skills to make a decision and enabling you to account for the decision you make. (NMC, 2002, p. 3)

These will quite often be life-saving decisions or decisions that have a huge potential impact on your clients: think, for example, of the responsibility underlying a health visitor's decision to refer a suspected case of child abuse to the social services department. Practitioners are imbued with the power to make decisions because they are recognised as being competent in their area of practice and their clients trust them to act in their best interests, that is, nurses have a *duty of care* to those they care for. Conversely, however, lies the expectation that all practitioners will, if asked, be able to justify the basis on which they made their decisions. This implies that there is both a right and a duty attached to professional accountability. In recognising the nurse's autonomy, there is a concomitant responsibility to act in the best interests of the client.

Student nurses and accountability

As the NMC makes clear, students can never be professionally accountable because they are not entered on the professional register; it is the registered practitioner with whom the student is working who is professionally responsible for the consequences of a student's actions or omissions (NMC, 2002). But students may be held to account by their university or in law. A registered nurse may, for example, delegate the task of giving an intramuscular injection to a student. The student is accountable for not causing harm to the patient and should therefore not give the injection if he or she does not feel competent to do so. The registered nurse, however, retains the professional accountability in terms of ensuring that the correct drug and dosage are administered and for ensuring that the student is, in the registered nurse's opinion, competent to administer the drug. Thus, students may be given responsibility by qualified nurses who themselves retain accountability. If students have doubts about their own competence, but carry on and give injections and cause harm to the patient, they may be accountable in law for their actions.

The NMC (2002) outline certain expectations of students in terms of their conduct within a professional context:

Link

Chapter 4 outlines the technique of intramuscular injection.

- To respect the wishes of patients at all times
- That the student introduces themselves accurately at all times when speaking to patients either directly or by telephone
- That the student accepts appropriate responsibility in the absence of a mentor, supervisor or other registered practitioner; but does not participate in any procedure for which they have not been fully prepared and in which they are not adequately supervised
- To respect patient confidentiality with reference to the NMC *Guidelines for Records and Record-keeping* (NMC, 2005).

The nurse's role in obtaining informed consent

For a long time, the nurse's role in informed consent has been vague and confused, both in legal terms and in practice, but it was clarified in 2001 with the publication of the *Reference Guide to Consent for Examination or Treatment* (DoH, 2001a) as part of the strategies outlined in the government White Paper *Good Practice in Consent* (DoH, 2001b). This is summarised in Chart 16.2. The 12 key points clarify the need to obtain consent for *anything* that is done to patients, the issues surrounding obtaining consent for children, who is responsible for obtaining consent, the notions of competence to give consent and rights to refusal of treatment.

Chart 16.2 ● The law in England: 12 key points on consent

1. Before you examine, treat or care for competent adult patients you must obtain their consent.
2. Adults are always assumed to be competent unless demonstrated otherwise. If you have doubts about their competence, the question to ask is 'can this patient understand and weigh up the information needed to make this decision?' Unexpected decisions do not prove the patient is incompetent, but may indicate a need for further information or explanation.
3. Patients may be competent to make some health-care decisions, even if they are not competent to make others.
4. Giving and obtaining consent is usually a process, not a one-off event. Patients can change their minds and withdraw consent at any time. If there is any doubt, you should always check that the patient still consents to your caring for or treating them.
5. Before examining, treating or caring for a child, you must also seek consent. Young people aged 16 and 17 are presumed to have the competence to give consent for themselves. Younger children who understand fully what is involved in the proposed procedure can also give consent (although their parents will ideally be involved). In other

cases, someone with parental responsibility must give consent on the child's behalf, unless they cannot be reached in an emergency. If a competent child consents to treatment, a parent cannot override that consent. Legally, a parent can consent if a competent child refuses, but it is likely that taking such a serious step will be rare.

6. It is always best for the person actually treating the patient to seek the patient's consent. However, you may seek consent on behalf of colleagues if you are capable of performing the procedure in question, or if you have been specially trained to seek consent for that procedure.

7. Patients need sufficient information before they can decide whether to give their consent, for example information about the benefits and risks of proposed treatment, and alternative treatments. If the patient is not offered as much information as they reasonably need to make their decision, and in a form they can understand, their consent may not be valid.

8. Consent must be given voluntarily: not under any form of duress or undue influence from health professionals, family or friends.

9. Consent can be written, oral or non-verbal. A signature on a consent form does not itself prove the consent is valid – the point of the form is to record the patient's decision, and also increasingly the discussions that have taken place. Your Trust or organisation may have a policy setting out when you need to obtain written consent.

10. Competent adults are entitled to refuse treatment, even where it would clearly benefit their health. The only exception to this rule is where the treatment is for a mental disorder and the patient is detained under the Mental Health Act 1983. A competent pregnant woman may refuse any treatment, even if this would be detrimental to the fetus.

11. No one can give consent on behalf of an incompetent adult. However, you may still treat such a patient if the treatment would be in their best interests. 'Best interests' go wider than best medical interests, to include factors such as the wishes and beliefs of the patient when competent, their current wishes, their general well-being and their spiritual and religious welfare. People close to the patient may be able to give you information on some of these factors. Where the patient has never been competent, relatives, carers and friends may be best placed to advise on the patient's needs and preferences.

12. If an incompetent patient has clearly indicated in the past, while competent, that they would refuse treatment in certain circumstances (an 'advance refusal'), and those circumstances arise, you must abide by that refusal.

Source: DoH (2001b).

The public are becoming more informed about their rights within health care and also more litigious in pursuing infringements of those rights through the legal justice system. At the same time as publishing guidance for professionals in terms of obtaining consent, the government offered a series of guides for different patient groups – adults, children and young people, people with learning difficulties, parents, and relatives and carers (all available on the Department of Health website www.dh.gov.uk) to ensure that patients are aware of their rights.

Nurses are in a vulnerable position with regard to their accountability to both the patient and those who may be directing the patient's care; this is often the case when nurses are carrying out treatments and procedures under the instruction of others. It is easy to assume that consent has been obtained by others, but the guidelines suggest that it is the responsibility of the person giving the treatment to obtain that consent. This must, of course, be documented and recorded in the patient's notes.

Essential parts of accountability are making contemporaneous and accurate records of nursing care and the consequences for clients if they have not been given the care they require. Health-care records are increasingly being written and stored on computers, so it is worth spending some time considering the implications of computer-held records for nurses.

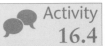

**Activity
16.4**

Think back to your last clinical day. Make a list of the patients you cared for and what you did for them. Consider the 12 points in Chart 16.2 against the care you were involved in. For each thing you did, consider whether consent was necessary, whether you or someone else gained that consent, and how this was done. Are there any lessons to be learnt from this?

The use of computers

Using computer facilities in record maintenance and care-planning can be a definite advantage to the profession, providing that clear guidelines for practice are established. Issues that need to be considered before implementing any system on a large scale are:

● The acquisition and storage of client-related data
● The compilation of a database of nursing care practices, including the generation of alternatives
● Accountability for individualised care plans
● The maintenance of records
● Confidentiality, security and access.

Freedom of Information Act 2000

The Freedom of Information Act 2000 followed the Data Protection Act in order to give people a general right of access to information held by or on behalf of public authorities, and to promote a culture of openness and accountability in public sector bodies. People have access to information held by public bodies in two ways:

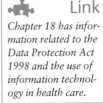

Link

Chapter 18 has information related to the Data Protection Act 1998 and the use of information technology in health care.

1. Through publication schemes – to make certain information available as described by the public body, for instance NHS Trusts, universities and local councils.
2. General right of access – people have a right to make a request for any information held by a public authority and the authority has to comply with the Act by responding. This right came into force on 1 January 2005.

As a student professional practitioner, you need to understand the publication schemes of the placements where you gain your experiences, and what your role is if a member of the public approaches you with a request for information under the Act. These cannot, of course, be presented here, as they will be specific to the organisation you are working with.

The principles on which these two pieces of public legislation are founded derive from society's beliefs about people's rights and responsibilities when living within it, arising from a concern to promote fairness and equality. Similarly, each profession in society is founded on a set of beliefs and principles that underpin how it relates to society and how its members practise. It is to this subject that we now turn.

■ Philosophies and Ideologies

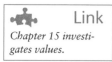
Link
Chapter 15 investigates values.

These principles can be seen as philosophies and ideologies.

Philosophies are sets of beliefs and values that guide the way in which we operate in the world, while ideologies are sets of ideas, assumptions and images that help people to make sense of society and provide individuals with distinctive social identities.

Personal beliefs and values

We all practise from a belief and value system that has arisen from our own personal experiences of life and what we have encountered. Jasper (1996) suggests that personal beliefs and values arise from the following sources:

Activity 16.5

Take a few minutes to list the beliefs and values that you hold that made you want to become a nurse. Can you attribute any of these to Jasper's sources?

● Our religious beliefs and moral upbringing
● Our ethnic origins
● Our educational opportunities
● Our social class
● The environment in which we grew up
● Our life experiences.

In addition to these personal life experiences, we accumulate various other beliefs and values that are accommodated into the way we practise as nurses.

You will have already encountered different ways of looking at the world from your nursing education, from the practitioners and educationalists with whom you work, and from your reading. You will have developed particular ways of looking at things that direct the way in which you give care. Think, for example, about concepts that you have met, such as 'holistic care', 'individualised care' or 'reflective practice', or even about the difference between your ideas of what nursing is now compared with what you thought it would be when you started your nursing education.

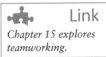
Link
Chapter 13 contains details of reflective practice.

In addition to these beliefs and values, you will also have been exposed to professional ones as defined by the NMC and illustrated in Chart 16.2 above. Such professional codes of conduct clearly identify the standards of practice that are expected from practitioners and provide them with a baseline of values and beliefs deemed appropriate at that particular time. Indeed, the NMC possesses the power to sanction any practitioners who contravene the code, even in their personal lives. The beliefs and values of professional codes are absorbed into the individual belief and value system of the practitioner. Thus, anyone calling themselves a nurse, midwife or specialist community public health nurse is assumed to behave in the way expected of a registered practitioner, as set out in the Code of Professional Conduct (NMC, 2004a).

The final sources of influence on your personal beliefs and values are those arising from your employing organisation and from wider societal issues such as government policy relating to health and social care. These sources of beliefs are likely to change, or be modified, at an even more rapid rate than those arising from educational or professional philosophies because they will be subject to political influences and trends, for example the impact that the introduction of the internal market has had on the provision of infertility treatment by the NHS or the decisions taken in some health authorities to restrict access to health care depending on the age of the client.

Link
Chapter 3 contains more information on the internal market.

Wright (1986) suggests that the combination of these sources of values and beliefs can be regarded as a personal philosophy that is used to shape our practice and education, provide motivation, prompt research and set our management style.

Nursing philosophies and mission statements

As nurses, we tend to work in teams to provide nursing care. The care delivered by a team of nurses working together will be directed by our beliefs and values in the same way that our own style of nursing is.

Link
Chapter 15 explores teamworking.

The word 'philosophy' in nursing tends to refer to a way of doing things that is underpinned by a written statement of beliefs and values. Mawdsley (1991) sees a nursing philosophy as:

an invaluable tool which directs and influences patient care. It is a series of beliefs, values and outlooks that can be developed in any area concerned with patient care, with the purpose of demonstrating what nurses feel their particular specialty should be achieving both for patients and nursing staff. Often, these philosophies are turned into 'mission statements' for the clinical area that they serve, and reflect those written for the organisation as a whole.

For a philosophy to be a true representation of the care delivered by a team, there are two key elements that it must contain. First, it must be an agreed statement that reflects the shared perceptions, beliefs and values of all those concerned. Second, it must be related to their own practice and have practical applications. Johns (1991) identifies the value of a philosophy when he says:

> Staff who share a common positive belief about nursing, within the context of their workplace, are more likely to give consistent and congruent care for the benefit of their patients.

A *nursing philosophy* is therefore:

- A statement of intent and belief
- An explanation of how and why things are done
- A statement of the purpose of the organisation and individuals
- A statement of the ideas behind our behaviour and actions
- A reflection of members' ideals and ideas for nursing, which should be endorsed by their peers
- An outlook that should include the future, expectations and reflection
- A consideration of the role of nursing.

A *written philosophy* includes:

- What you do
- Why you do it
- What you value and why
- What is important and why
- The uniqueness of your practice or ward and so on
- The qualities offered.

Although written philosophies tend to be the end result of values' clarification and teamwork, they mark just one stage in the overall process of developing nursing knowledge, a process that begins when nurses start to think about what they are doing and why. Creating a philosophy of care for a clinical area, or being able to articulate your own philosophy, sets the baseline for thinking

Activity 16.6

All clinical areas providing placements are required to have a nursing philosophy. Think back to your last placement. Were you introduced to the philosophy? How was its relationship to care explained? Look again at the six components of a written philosophy. How successful is your example in covering these? To what extent are the characteristics of a philosophy present? Does your example really reflect the nursing care given in that clinical area?

about and making connections between our knowledge base, our skills and our experience, and for considering how these can be taken forward.

The success of a philosophy as a working document for a clinical area will often depend on the way in which it was devised in the first place. If it is meant to reflect the combined values of the area or team to which it relates, it is essential that those people were involved in developing it. Described below are two approaches to philosophy development.

The top-down approach

In this case, the philosophy tends to be imposed by the managerial system and is a reflection of organisational beliefs, which are not necessarily applicable to the nursing care. As a result, the philosophy may become a paper exercise, the components not being shared by the nurses, who lack any ownership or motivation to use it within their practice. This, however, may not necessarily be the case, because when organisations adopt change, responsibility and accountability are delegated downwards. Many nurses are using broad policy statements created within an organisation and developing their own philosophies from them, incorporating the beliefs and values of their own nursing environment. These are fine as broad statements, but they do not necessarily relate to the specific environment of nursing in which teams of nurses are working and, although helpful as value statements, are not necessarily useful as operational policies.

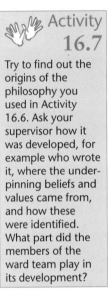

Activity 16.7

Try to find out the origins of the philosophy you used in Activity 16.6. Ask your supervisor how it was developed, for example who wrote it, where the underpinning beliefs and values came from, and how these were identified. What part did the members of the ward team play in its development?

The bottom-up approach

In this case, it is the people who will have to use the philosophy who are involved in writing it. Philosophies developed in this way tend to include the 'how, what, when, why, who and where' of practice, which can then be used as a way of directing and delivering care within a specific environment.

Purposes of a philosophy

Practical application

It can now be seen that a nursing philosophy must, if it is to be effective, have practical application to a specific area and must reflect the practices that currently occur. It should stimulate the nurses to reflect on their practice in terms of being able to justify the nursing care delivered and learning from their experiences. The philosophy can also be used to teach nursing care to students or other types of worker, and can form the basis of the development of nursing care in that area.

Facilitating teamwork

Link

Chapter 15 looks further at values and beliefs in team-working.

Similarly, a philosophy as a working document will facilitate teamwork, as all members of the team will share common values and beliefs that have been made explicit and open. A published philosophy may even be used to recruit new members of the clinical team, as it can be used to advertise the beliefs and values underpinning care to potential applicants and form the basis of exploring whether a person will fit into the ward team. A philosophy will also encourage continuity of care while the client is being looked after in that clinical area and enable a smooth transfer to other areas or upon discharge.

Setting a baseline for the development of quality and standards in practice

standards of care

these usually identify the minimum standard to which an aspect of care is expected to conform and provide the criteria against which the quality of care can be measured

quality of care

the measure of the standard of care used to evaluate the services being delivered. The term 'quality' needs to be accompanied by an adjective describing the standard to be achieved, for example 'high'-quality care

It seems logical to assume that if a philosophy for a clinical area has been agreed by the team working in it, it will serve as a starting point for setting the **standards of care** and assessing the **quality of care** delivered. If the philosophy identifies your beliefs and values, and these are translated into the way in which you work and what you intend to provide, you have already set some standards to be achieved. The quality of your care can be measured by finding ways of evaluating the outcome of care against your original intentions.

■ Quality

On the surface, this aspect is very simple, but let us take some time to think about what we mean by quality. Quality is a nebulous term that means different things to different people. One problem lies in the necessity to qualify the term with a value word such as 'high' or 'low' in order to give it some meaning. It is, for example, clearly meaningless to talk about 'quality' care without defining the standard of quality you are aiming for – 'quality' could refer to anything.

Another problem relates to who defines the quality. Think, for example, of the values that you might attribute to high-quality care in giving a blanket bath. You might identify privacy, time, skilled staff and other issues relating to assessing the condition of your client and completing the task in a certain length of time. Your client may well, however, look for different measures of quality such as being embarrassed, keeping warm or feeling clean in the way they would like to feel clean. Your ward manager may well, on the other hand, think of good-quality procedures as relating to completing the work schedule, meeting the client's needs as identified in the care plan and complying with the treatment schedule.

It is important, therefore, where any measurement or assessment of quality is attempted, to ask several overarching questions about what it is that is being attempted.

What is being assessed?

This evolves from the definition of quality that is in operation, organisational needs, externally imposed criteria such as government targets and the beliefs and values that underpin the model of quality being used. Koch (1994) suggests that there have previously been three generations of quality evaluation: measurement oriented, objective oriented and judgement oriented:

- *Measurement-oriented approach:* boundaries or quality criteria are selected by the health-care professionals and data are collected in statistical terms. Examples of this are the waiting times of clients attending a particular outpatient department and the wound infection rate following a specific surgical procedure
- *Objective-oriented approach:* this uses observational techniques to assess the strengths and weaknesses of care against stated objectives. Many of the well-known quality audit tools, such as Phaneuf's audit of documentary records (Phaneuf, 1976), use this approach
- *Judgement-oriented technique:* involves the evaluation of care against standards set by 'experts', usually in the form of quality assurance committees. Approaches within this category often have a dual purpose in terms of quantifiable standards of practice and the marketing of services as labels such as 'excellent' or 'poor' are awarded. A recent initiative of this type is the assessment of nursing outcomes (Higgins et al., 1992; Griffiths, 1995), which relates the outcome achieved to the process used to achieve it. Benchmarking against 'best identified practice' is another example of this type of approach.

These three categories of approach share the characteristics of the standards being set by health-care experts, thus ignoring client-generated concerns, and of being of a quantifiable nature, data being collected by a disinterested observer (Koch, 1994). They might not, however, suit the purposes of nurses wanting to evaluate the quality of their own work, especially as few of these approaches involve client-generated issues relating to the everyday care received. Koch (1994) suggests that this can be achieved by using a fourth-generation approach to the evaluation of quality that is negotiation oriented, involving a skilled negotiator who acts as facilitator in setting the agenda for quality among all the stakeholders.

> **Link**
>
> *Chapter 13 outlines a way of performing a structured and thoughtful review of your care activities.*

Another approach to involving clients in assessing the quality of care has been the development of client satisfaction schedules (Bond and Thomas, 1992; Avis et al., 1995; Simpson et al., 1995). These have the advantage of enabling the clients' perspectives to be drawn into the quality debate and often use **qualitative approaches** to data-gathering, which generate material relating to clients' expe-

qualitative research approaches

approaches that use in-depth and holistic methods through the collection of narrative data and a flexible design

quantitative research approaches

approaches to investigating phenomena that lend themselves to precise measurement and quantification, often involving a rigorous and controlled design

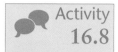

Activity 16.8

Think of a recent encounter with a client in which you worked independently in directly delivering care. Describe the scene in as much detail as possible. What was the main purpose of this interaction? What other purposes might there have been? Describe your part in the interaction. Did your actions or interventions achieve the original purposes? How do you know this? Can you think of any other ways to evaluate the effectiveness of your interaction? As a result of this interaction, what have you learnt about the quality of care that you gave?

riences, rather than **quantitative approaches**, which rely on objective statistics yet do not describe subjective experiences. Thus, when exploring quality assessment in your own area of practice, it is important to be able to identify exactly what you are assessing. This leads to the next question: What purpose you are assessing it for?

Although you have probably not yet had to think very much about the quality of care that you deliver because you have been closely supervised in clinical practice, you will, as you move into your branch studies, need to make such decisions and clarify the purpose of evaluating that quality for your own personal and professional development. This is where the skills of reflective practice that you met in Chapter 13 will be useful to you. Now refer to Activity 16.8.

This activity highlights one purpose of quality assessment – meeting individual practitioners' needs to ensure their own high-quality care. Many other purposes can, however, be identified if you refer back to the beginning of this section. These are listed briefly below and can be a stimulus to further reading as you go through your branch studies. Quality may be assessed in order to:

- Ensure value for money
- Attract funding for a service
- Demonstrate target achievements
- Audit a service
- Award training status to a clinical area
- Verify that standards of practice are being achieved
- Publicise a service
- Provide new business or services.

The next question that needs to be addressed is: What structure will the approach take? This is not the place to outline the strategies available for assessing quality; suffice it to say that there is a whole range of approaches depending on what it is you want to assess and the purpose of your assessment. These also change with policy and practice development, and with the need to respond to ever-changing governmental policies.

■ Clinical Governance

The NHS has been subject to numerous reviews since its inception, many of which have attempted, either implicitly or explicitly, to address concerns relating to the quality of the service provided. Approaches such as total quality management, quality circles, continuous quality improvement, the King's Fund initiative, Investors in People, re-engineering, the dynamic standard-setting system and medical/clinical audit, to name but a few, have been among the quality initiatives employed in the past. But this begs the question: 'If we have been down this road before, why do we appear to be making a return journey?'

Recent key concerns emerging appear to be responsibility and accountability for quality of performance. The introduction of the clinical governance framework can be described as a direct response to these concerns.

What is clinical governance?

In autumn 1997, the New Labour government produced the first of a series of key documents setting out the agenda for health care into the next century. The notion of clinical governance (DoH, 1997, emphases added) was thus introduced:

> The Government requires every NHS trust to embrace the concept of Clinical Governance, so that *quality* is at the core, both of their *responsibilities* as *organisations*, and of each of their staff as *individual professionals*

with clinical governance being defined as

> a framework through which NHS organisations are accountable for continuously improving the quality of their services and safe-guarding high standards of care by creating an environment in which excellence in clinical care will flourish. (DoH, 1998)

The strategies described and implemented over the succeeding years ensured that, for the first time, all health-care organisations have a statutory duty to seek quality improvement through clinical governance. A line of accountability was drawn, identifying individual responsibility for ensuring organisational performance, in terms of not only sound financial management, but also the integration of existing quality assurance and performance monitoring systems into a framework for continuous quality improvement. The chief executive or chair of the governing body was to be 'the accountable officer' and NHS Trusts were required to produce their first clinical governance reports in spring 2000, with annual monitoring. These documents are published in the public domain, encouraging openness and emphasising accountability.

In addition to this, a statutory body, the Commission for Health Improvement (later renamed the Commission for Health Audit and Improvement, and now superseded by the Healthcare Commission), was set up with powers to scrutinise, support, investigate, police and inquire, backed by the legal duty of quality imposed on every organisation. Quality assurance and improvement are no longer 'optional extras' but a statutory obligation.

The stated aim of clinical governance (DoH, 1998) is seductive and deceptively simple:

Safeguarding high standards of care by creating an environment in which excellence in clinical care will flourish.

The reality is, however, rather more complex, requiring a change in culture that could in some cases almost be described as a paradigm shift. Organisations, and the individuals who comprise them, will face a number of developmental challenges.

The following could be described as prerequisites for clinical governance:

- A supportive culture, nurturing integrity and honesty
- A consensus regarding the meaning of the concepts underpinning clinical governance
- Time to do 'it'
- Clearly defined lines of accountability within the organisation: who is responsible for what and when? Who holds the decision-making authority and is therefore accountable for discharging a responsibility?
- Leadership across all professional groups
- Robust communication and record-keeping systems
- Mechanisms to support clinical supervision/peer review and critical reflection for all professional (and, increasingly, non-professional) groups.

Elements of clinical governance

It is increasingly apparent that clinical governance is a framework within which a number of existing systems and processes are integrated. The key elements of the clinical governance framework can be summarised as:

- Education
- Continuing professional development
- Clinical audit (multiprofessional)
- Evidence-based practice
- Clinical effectiveness
- Clinical risk assessment, management and reduction
- Improving practice
- Defining outcomes of care, treatment or therapy
- Collecting high-quality clinical data
- Monitoring clinical practice
- The systematic dissemination of 'best practice', both within and outside the organisation

- Professional self-regulation
- Service user involvement.

These key elements can also be described in a series of logical (albeit overlapping) groupings (Figure. 16.1).

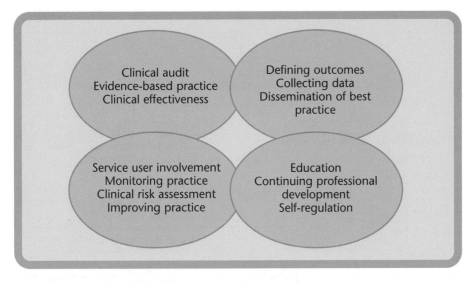

Figure 16.1 ● The clinical governance framework

Many, if not all, of these systems and processes already exist in one form or other. In some areas, they are well defined, in others, they operate in an ineffective, piecemeal fashion. The challenge posed by clinical governance is to develop these systems to an uncommonly sophisticated level of integration. This will be characterised by moving away from a culture of self-protection and blame to one of self-regulation and learning through experience. It will include progress from a position of isolation and professional tribalism to one of collaboration and interprofessional teamworking. The challenge will incorporate moving from practice based upon tradition, ritual, folklore and personal preference to practice that is centred around expert professional judgement, which is itself informed by sound, appropriate evidence, critical analytical and reflective skills.

Organisational systems and processes will need to transform from being isolated 'pockets' of activity to being an integrated, coherent framework with the service user firmly located at the centre. The design of service provision will be the vehicle for achieving excellence in care, whether this is operationalising health improvement plans within specific, nationally agreed performance frameworks or enhancing individual quality of life and well-being in chronic, life-limiting or terminal conditions. Exemplars in practice will be recognised and systematically disseminated. Complaints and risk management systems will be

Link

Chapter 15 contains explanations of interprofessional teamworking.

Activity 16.9

Look again at Figures 16.1 and 16.2. Which elements of the clinical governance framework do you think have the greatest impact on each part of the clinical governance cycle and why?

used to identify and analyse problems so that they too can become part of the 'flow of information' feeding into the quality improvement cycle that lies at the heart of clinical governance (Figure 16.2). Unlike other cycles, the clinical governance cycle can be broken into at any point. The challenge is to ensure that, no matter where the cycle is entered, all the components are engaged (Severs, 1998).

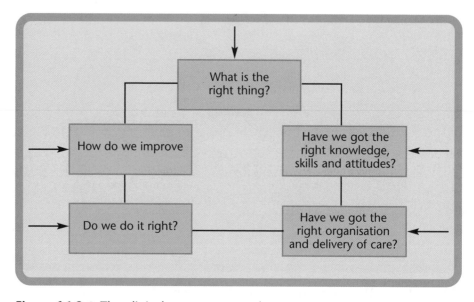

Figure 16.2 ● The clinical governance cycle

Research governance

The latest addition to the notion of health-care governance has been an emphasis on public protection through the *Research Governance Framework for Health and Social Care* (DoH, 2001c). This framework has been designed to ensure that all research involving patients, service users, care professionals or volunteers or their organs, tissues or data meets certain standards ethically, in terms of quality, and in terms of its design and conduct. This includes independent reviewing procedures, strategies for the informed consent of participants, the protection of patient data and an assessment and reduction of the element of risk involved. In short, the framework:

● Sets standards
● Defines mechanisms to deliver standards
● Describes monitoring and assessment arrangements
● Improves research quality and safeguards the public by:
    ● Enhancing ethical and scientific quality
    ● Promoting good practice

- Reducing adverse incidents and ensuring lessons are learned
- Preventing poor performance and misconduct
- Is intended for those who:
  - Participate in research
  - Host research in their organisation
  - Fund research projects or infrastructure
  - Manage research
  - Undertake research
- Is designed for managers and staff, in all professional groups, no matter how senior or junior (DoH, 2001c, p. 2).

This has implications for nursing and midwifery students in terms of both their own academic work for their programme of study, and their role with patients and users of the health service who are taking part in research.

At an individual level, all research projects carried out by health and social care students must have ethical approval from their university. They may also need to go to their local research ethics committee if they involve service users and patients in their study. For this reason, to prevent clinical areas becoming overwhelmed by the amount of research being undertaken, and to ensure that the research is worthwhile and likely to contribute to the knowledge base, most undergraduate programmes do not allow their students to undertake empirical primary research. Ethical approval processes involve the research proposal being scrutinised by a panel of experts to ensure that it meets the standards required.

Students may, during their clinical experiences, be involved in the delivery of care to patients who are taking part in research studies. These may include trialing new drugs or experimental procedures, and it is important that the patients are supported in their understanding of the study, including their rights in terms of giving informed consent and their right to withdraw at any time. Students need to understand these rights, and their role as advocate for the patient.

All these issues have a direct link to the philosophy of care that has been created for the clinical area. This philosophy sets the baseline for determining the focus that quality assessment will take and relates directly to the standards of care to be achieved.

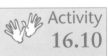

Activity 16.10

Gather together from your clinical area as many examples as you can in an attempt to assess the quality of care being provided. Consider such aspects as a tracking form for client care, the presence of written standards for procedures, the evaluation of care against the written philosophy and the collection of statistics relating to bed occupancy.

■ Models and Frameworks of Care

Another purpose of a nursing philosophy is to underpin the model of nursing that is used to direct care in the clinical area.

One of the major challenges that nurses have faced in the quest for professional practice is the development of a knowledge base that can be seen to relate specifically to nursing. Prior to the 1950s, there was very little theory that could be seen to be exclusively concerned with the ways in which nurses practised in a specific capacity. Since that time, and related in particular to the move of nursing education into American and latterly British universities, nurse theorists have attempted to identify a nursing knowledge base that is separate or built eclectically from other foundations of theory. Some authors, usually from outside nursing, argue that there is no specific knowledge that can be seen to belong to nursing, and they therefore justify the designation of nursing as a semiprofession. Others suggest that there is no such thing as a knowledge base belonging to any particular profession, rather, it is the special combination of the way in which knowledge from different sources is collected together and used to underpin practice that provides the focus of a profession. In addition, although nursing is still in the infant stages of creating nursing knowledge, this has developed effectively over the past 60 years, as the growth in academic journals of nursing will testify. The creation of models of nursing was one of the first attempts at creating a knowledge base specific to nursing in this way.

What is a model?

Link

Chapter 1 has more information related to models.

Wright (1990) defines a nursing model as:

> a collection of ideas, knowledge and values about nursing which determines the way nurses, as individuals and groups, work with their patients or clients.

Models therefore:

> help nurses to organise their thinking about nursing and then set about their practice in an orderly and logical way.

Hence the primary purpose of a model is to help nurses to understand nursing from a particular viewpoint and use that to direct their care. But what do we mean by a model? In everyday life, a model is often seen in a physical way, as with a model house, boat or aeroplane. Although it does not contain all the elements or components of the real thing, it acts as a representation of that thing. So how does this help us with models of nursing? Models of nursing also act as a representation of reality but from a particular viewpoint: nursing models describe, or represent, nursing from the viewpoint of the writer and present different ways of looking at or understanding nursing. Nursing models are thus abstract models that help us to make sense of the way in which nursing happens.

These models do not have to be published, formal models written by theorists: each one of us has our own informal model that we carry around in our head. These comprise individual collections of ideas about nursing, socialised behaviour and experience from both nursing and life, and determine a great deal of nursing care as they form the basis of the way in which each nurse practises. Although these informal models are obviously important to the individual, there are certain problems associated with individuals practising their own model rather than one that is shared by others in the team. Informal models are usually value laden and are not necessarily based on commonly held values. In a way, they are 'secret' models, but at the same time we seem to make the assumption that everyone else shares our values.

Formal models occur, however, when the values, beliefs and ways of working are made explicit and shared by the team of nurses in the clinical area. They enable groups of nurses to think about, and carry out, nursing in a fairly similar way, with clear objectives for the delivery of care because the model purports to represent the nursing care to be achieved by that team.

Over the past 60 years, many models have been created that claim to represent the reality of nursing. Although most of these originate in the USA, the most commonly used model in practice in the UK, the activities of daily living (ADL) model (now known as activities of living model), was devised by Roper et al. in Edinburgh in the 1980s. The ADL model was developed from Virginia Henderson's description of what nursing does in helping clients with 14 activities of living (Henderson, 1966). These were refined by Roper et al. (1980) as an educational model to help students to learn about nursing. Other models have different origins and therefore are developed and structured around different beliefs and values and ways of viewing the world. It is important to emphasise that nursing theorists do not claim that the view of the world and nursing they propose is the only view – rather that these different views are proposed in order to provide professionals with alternative perspectives on nursing and the delivery of nursing care. The notion of nursing theory therefore is to help nurses to develop and expand a 'toolkit' of knowledge and skills that enables them to offer the most appropriate care for their individual patients.

When you reach the end of your common foundation programme, it is important to identify just what nursing is to you, as you will, from then on, increasingly be called on to defend your own practice as a nurse. It is important to make the link between nursing being a special discipline in its own right, having a specific knowledge base, and the role that theory generation will play in that. We need to have evidence on which to base our practice, and there is little purpose for theory if it does not relate in some way to practice. We need to know what to do and why we do it, one of the purposes of theory being to enable us to practise from an informed basis. After all, that is why you are undertaking an educational programme in preparation for registered practice rather than working as an unqualified member of staff. But what are the other purposes of theory?

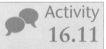

Activity
16.11

What knowledge base does nursing share with other disciplines? Think here about both the practical and theoretical components of your course and try to identify the disciplinary base that informs each one. What makes nursing different from other disciplines, that is, what is special about nursing? Where does the knowledge come from that informs the 'special' nursing components? Where does nursing theory come from? What is the purpose of nursing theory?

Purposes of theories

There are many purposes to which theories are put, one overall reason being to make scientific findings meaningful and generalisable. In nursing, the main purpose must be to enhance nursing practice. Subsidiary purposes include:

- The provision of knowledge
- Enhancing nursing's power by developing the knowledge base
- Explaining and predicting previously unexplained events
- The stimulation of new discoveries
- Aiding decision-making
- The support of professional autonomy in practice, education and research.

Finally, it is worth thinking about your own personal development in relation to being able to select the appropriate nursing action. Although much of the theoretical work that you have undertaken so far is based on learning facts and skills, you must remember that your critical powers are also being developed. It is important to see theory in a developmental light, in terms of how being able to discuss and differentiate, evaluate and justify helps your critical thinking.

■ Evidence-based Practice

A recent development in healthcare has been the notion of evidence-based practice, which depends on practitioners' ability to discern and chose from available evidence in their field, marry this with their own expertise, and make independent judgements based on the combination of the two. Mulhall (1998, p. 5) says that 'evidence-based care concerns the incorporation of evidence from research, clinical expertise and patient preferences into decisions about the health care of individual patients', suggesting that sources of evidence are multiple. Furthermore, Hewitt-Taylor (2002, p. 48) adds that 'the type of information used to generate an evidence-base for practice should be decided according to how appropriate each form of evidence is for the issue in question, and the availability of evidence', supporting the rather obvious notion that evidence for practice is wide ranging.

Evidence-based practice is often confused with research-based practice, in which only research findings are perceived as evidence, thus narrowing the types of evidence available for practitioners to only those generated from research. Indeed, some types of evidence are regarded as better than others, resulting in the development of a 'hierarchy of evidence', where sources of evidence, and the way it has been generated, are considered when choosing the rationality of the evidence on which decisions are to be made. A whole industry has been built up around the notion of robust evidence, in part led by the Cochrane Database and the NHS

Centre for Research and Dissemination. Unsurprisingly, they put their evidence, arising from the systematic review of research studies in different areas, as being at the top of such a hierarchy, with large-scale, well-designed primary studies, random controlled trials and other controlled studies following on behind. Then come large-scale primary studies using other methodologies, followed by descriptive studies and reports (including national and local standards, guidelines, customer surveys, support groups) and, finally, the opinions and experiences of respected authorities based on clinical experience and professional consensus.

The implicit assumption behind a hierarchy imposes a higher value on some as opposed to others, resulting in confusion for practitioners attempting to differentiate between 'good' and 'poor' evidence. However, the narrow definition of 'evidence' as research based was not originally intended. Sackett et al. (1996, p. 311) define evidence-based medicine as:

> the conscientious, explicit and judicious use of current best evidence in making decisions about the care of individual patients. The practice of evidence-based medicine means integrating individual clinical expertise with the best available external clinical evidence from systematic research. By individual expertise we mean the proficiency and judgment that individual clinicians acquire through clinical experience and clinical practice.

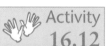

Activity 16.12

Select one of the activities that you did recently when caring for a patient. What was the evidence base that you used when carrying this out. How did this evidence inform your care?

This gives weighting to both the clinical expertise and experience of the practitioner by suggesting that evidence alone is insufficient for decision-making – it is the *combination* of best evidence with clinical expertise that leads to evidence-based practice.

As accountable practitioners, even as students, it is important that you constantly update your knowledge and feed this into the sources you use to decide on the best courses of action for your patients and clients. In turn, the experiences that you have in your practice will contribute to your knowledge base and enable you to develop your own 'evidence' for practice in the future.

■ Lifelong Learning

Being a professional practitioner in today's world of constantly changing knowledge and skills requires each individual to continuously update their practice through lifelong learning.

One of the main functions of the old UKCC was the maintenance of a 'live' register of qualified nurses, midwives and health visitors, with one of its objectives being to determine an education and training policy and programme to ensure that nurses, midwives and health visitors who are trained and registered meet the needs of society in the 1990s and beyond.

In order to achieve this objective, the UKCC established a set of training rules and for the first time included a statement of the outcomes of training. While clarifying and developing initial training for registration, the UKCC also developed a policy for the standards of post-qualifying education under the heading 'post-registration education and practice' (PREP). The UKCC provided practitioners with *The PREP Handbook* (UKCC, 2001, now NMC, 2004b), which consolidated all the previous guidance, provided details of the continuing professional development (CPD) standard that was to be achieved and clarified the definitions used.

There are two separate standards that affect a practitioner's registration, one relating to practice and one to CPD. When completing your notification to practise for triennial registration, you are signing to confirm that you:

- Have worked in some capacity by virtue of your registration for a minimum of 100 days (750 hours) during the previous five years or undertaken a return to practice course (practice standard)
- Will undertake a minimum of five days (35 hours) CPD over the three-year period and record this in your personal portfolio, and make this available to the NMC for audit purposes if required to do so.

These standards have been framed to ensure that the public can have the confidence that every registered nurse, midwife or specialist community public health nurse is competent and safe to practise using evidence-based care. If you look at these carefully, however, you will see that they are the *minimum* expected of a practitioner. In fact, most practitioners will achieve far more than these requirements by attending study days or taking further qualifications.

Lifelong learning is not simply about increasing one's knowledge – it is about how this is used to inform practice, incorporating critical analytical skills and reflective practice that enables the practitioner to respond to the individual needs of their patients through patient-centred care. It is thus every practitioner's responsibility to learn and develop their practice throughout their lifetime.

■ Chapter Summary

This chapter has introduced many of the issues that you will meet in greater depth in the remainder of your course. What ties all these issues together is the need for you to adopt the mantle of being a professional, registered nurse, with the accompanying privileges and responsibilities that this entails. On emerging fully qualified from the branch programme, you will be expected to have adopted a professional ethos, to be competent and accountable for your practice, and to have acquired the necessary knowledge, skills and experience to give you professional authority.

Learning, however, does not, and cannot, stop on qualification. Quite apart from the NMC's requirements for triennial registration, you will, as a qualified practitioner, need to be able to provide evidence-based practice. In order to do this, you will continue to practise academic skills and will direct your own learning so that you can deliver care of the quality that you want to achieve. Courses for registration are only the beginning of a long and exciting journey but you will have acquired the skills needed for lifelong learning. During the remainder of your course, you will consolidate those skills and this will enable you to take more responsibility for your own personal and professional development.

Test Yourself!

1. (a) What is meant by professional practice?
   (b) What are the responsibilities associated with professional practice?

2. (a) What is meant by the NMC Code of Professional Conduct?
   (b) What are your roles and responsibility, as a student, under the Code of Professional Conduct?
   (c) What is your accountability as a student nurse?
   (d) How does this differ from the accountability of a registered practitioner?
   (e) What does 'informed consent' mean? When is it needed, who can give it and who can obtain it?

3. How do beliefs and values influence nursing care?

4. (a) Why is quality assessment important in professional care?
   (b) What impact will the introduction of clinical governance have on nursing care?

5. How do models of care influence the care that a client receives?

6. Why is it necessary for registered practitioners to practise from a contemporaneous knowledge base?

■ Further Reading

On accountability

Tilley, S. and Watson, R. (2004) *Accountability in Nursing and Midwifery*. Blackwell Publishing, Oxford.

On clinical governance

McSherry, R. and Pearce, P. (2002) *Clinical Governance: a Guide to Implementation for Healthcare Professionals.* Blackwell Science, Oxford

Wright, J. and Hill, P. (2003) *Clinical Governance.* Churchill Livingstone, Edinburgh.

■ References

Avis, M., Bond, M. and Arthur, A. (1995) Satisfying solutions? A review of some unresolved issues in the measurement of patient satisfaction. *Journal of Advanced Nursing* **22**(2): 316–22.

Bond, S. and Thomas, L.H. (1992) Measuring patients' satisfaction with nursing care. *Journal of Advanced Nursing* **17**(1): 52–63.

Cronin, P. and Rawlings-Anderson, K. (2004) *Knowledge for Contemporary Nursing Practice.* Mosby, Edinburgh.

DoH (Department of Health) (1998) *A First Class Service. Quality in the NHS.* Stationery Office, London.

DoH (Department of Health) (2001a) *Reference Guide to Consent for Examination or Treatment.* HMSO, London.

DoH (Department of Health) (2001b) *Good Practice in Consent: Achieving the NHS Plan Commitment to Patient-centred Consent Practice.* HMSO, London.

DoH (Department of Health) (2001c) *Research Governance Framework for Health and Social Care.* HMSO, London.

Griffiths, P. (1995) Progress in measuring nursing outcomes. *Journal of Advanced Nursing* **21**(6): 1092–100.

Henderson, V. (1966) *The Nature of Nursing.* Collier Macmillan, London.

Hewitt-Taylor, J. (2002) Evidence-based practice. *Nursing Standard* **17** (14–15): 47–52.

Higgins, M., McCaughan, D., Griffiths, M. and Carr-Hill, R. (1992) Assessing the outcomes of nursing care. *Journal of Advanced Nursing* **17**(5): 561–8.

Jacobs, K. (2004) Accountability and clinical governance in nursing: a critical overview of the topic. In Tilley, S. and Watson, R. (eds) *Accountability in Nursing and Midwifery.* Blackwell Publishing, Oxford.

Jasper, M. (1996) *Evaluating Care and Effecting Change. Unit Study Guide.* Distance Learning Centre, South Bank University, London.

Johns, C. (1991) The Burford Nursing Development Unit holistic model of nursing practice. *Journal of Advanced Nursing* **16**: 1090–8.

Koch, T. (1994) Beyond measurement: fourth-generation evaluation in nursing. *Journal of Advanced Nursing* **20**(6): 1148–55.

Mawdsley, D. (1991) Who needs nursing philosophies? *Professional Nurse* **7**(2): 78–82.

Moloney, M.M. (1992) *Professionalization of Nursing: Current Issues and Trends.* J.B. Lippincott, Philadelphia.

Mulhall, A. (1998) Nursing research and the evidence. *Evidence-based Nursing* **1**(1): 4–6.

NMC (Nursing and Midwifery Council) (2002) *An NMC Guide for Students of Nursing and Midwifery.* NMC, London.

NMC (Nursing and Midwifery Council) (2004a) *The NMC Code of Professional Conduct: Standards for Conduct, Performance and Ethics*. NMC, London.

NMC (Nursing and Midwifery Council) (2004b) *The PREP Handbook*. NMC, London.

NMC (Nursing and Midwifery Council) (2005) *Guidelines for Records and Record-keeping*. NMC, London.

Phaneuf, M.C. (1976) *The Nursing Audit: Self-regulation in Nursing Practice*. Appleton-Century-Crofts, New York.

Roper, N., Logan, W. and Tierney, A. (1980) *The Elements of Nursing*. Churchill Livingstone, Edinburgh.

Sackett, D.L., Rosenberg, W.M.C., Muir Gray, J.A., Haynes, R.B. and Richardson, W.S. (1996) Evidence-based medicine: what it is and what it isn't. *British Medical Journal* **312**: 71–2.

Severs, M. (1998) The Clinical Governance Cycle. Lecture series, PG Cert Clinical Governance, Unit 1. University of Portsmouth, Portsmouth.

Simpson, R.G., Scothern, G. and Vincent, M. (1995) Survey of carer satisfaction with the quality of care delivered to in-patients suffering from dementia. *Journal of Advanced Nursing* **22**(3): 517–27.

UKCC (United Kingdom Central Council for Nursing, Midwifery and Health Visiting) (2002) *The Future of Professional Regulation*. Register (Winter).

Watson, R. (1992) Justifying your practice. *Nursing* **5**(3): 11–13.

Wright, S. (1986) *Building and Using a Model of Nursing*. Edward Arnold, London.

Wright, S. (1990) *My Patient – My Nurse*. Scutari Press, London.

Acknowledgement

With thanks to Nadia Chambers for contributing to the original section on clinical governance.

■ Useful Websites

www.nmc-uk.org **Nursing and Midwifery Council**
An organisation set up by Parliament to protect the public by ensuring that nurses and midwives provide high standards of care to their patients and clients

www.dh.gov.uk **Department of Health**

DELIA POGSON

17 Genetics Knowledge within an Ethical Framework

Contents

Learning Outcomes

The purpose of this chapter is to enhance your understanding of 'genetics' and to consider the development of genetic knowledge within an ethical framework in relation to the health-care agenda. At the end of this chapter, you should be able to:

- Outline an ethical framework in which to consider the developing genetic knowledge

- Describe some of the issues of the 'human genome' within the health-care system

- Describe the basic structure and function of chromosomes and genes

- Describe the processes of mitosis and meiosis

- Differentiate between genotype and phenotype

- Describe some of the common chromosomal abnormalities

- Utilise a Punnett square to describe patterns of inheritance: dominant, recessive and X-linked.

There are also activities for you to consider and undertake, and review questions so that you can test yourself.

■ Introduction

The developments from the human genome project in 2003 have opened up the world of genetics-based health care. It has been recognised by the Department of Health that these advances in human genetics will have a profound impact on the health care of present and future generations, not only for people with single-gene conditions such as cystic fibrosis (CF), haemophilia and Huntington's disease, but for common diseases such as heart disease, diabetes, asthma, cancers and mental health conditions (DoH, 2003, p. 5).

To understand the impact on health and ill-health depends upon the knowledge and understanding of some of these genetic developments and this chapter will explore issues such as aspects of inheritance of characteristics and genetic disorders, and the role of genetics in common diseases. Also these genetic developments highlight other ethical issues, such as how genetic information is collected from individuals and then used, and how it is stored so as to preserve the principles of consent and confidentiality.

Developments from the Department of Health White Paper (DoH, 2003) have included a competence-based genetics education framework for health-care practitioners. This framework outlines seven competency standard statements for practitioners to achieve at the point of professional registration (Kirk et al., 2003), with each competency standard being underpinned by theoretical and practice indicators. These will enable educational initiatives to consider genetic knowledge (scientific and technical) and the applied human genetics.

The 'standards of proficiency', set out by the Nursing and Midwifery Council (NMC, 2004a) for students to achieve so as to be entered onto the professional register, state that the NMC Code of Professional Conduct (NMC, 2004b):

> requires practitioners to conduct themselves and practise within an ethical framework based fundamentally upon respect for the well-being of patients and clients. (NMC, 2004a, p. 16)

These standards of proficiency must be achieved in the student's branch of nursing practice for the part of the nursing register that they are to be entered upon – adult nursing, mental health nursing, learning disability nursing or children's nursing.

A broad concept of 'genetic solidarity and altruism' has been set out (DoH, 2002), with 'respect for persons' being fundamental within this concept. Four ethical principles underpin this respect for persons; privacy, consent, confidentiality and non-discrimination (DoH, 2002). Beauchamp and Childress (2001) advocate that these ethical principles are fundamental to the practitioner–patient relationship. The upholding of these principles poses challenges for practitioners when working with some patient/client groups, such as children and young people, vulnerable adults such as the unconscious person, the person with altered levels of mental capacity, either of a temporary or permanent nature, or the person with a deteriorating condition.

The chapter will explore issues regarding personal genetic information such as consent, confidentiality and protection. The Department of Health has explained this genetic information as

> any information about the genetic make-up of an identifiable person, whether directly from DNA (or other biochemical) testing or indirectly from any other source (including the details of a person's family history). (DoH, 2002, p. 27)

An Ethical Framework

Ethical values or principles influence and guide our thinking, the way we act and as health-care practitioners influence our practice. Four principles have been identified as essential within an ethical framework, when considering health-care practice – autonomy, beneficence, non-maleficence and justice (Bradley, 2005):

- *Autonomy:* the right of a person to make their own decisions and direct their life
- *Beneficence:* the responsibility of doing good, so providing benefit or beneficial treatment/care to the person
- *Non-maleficence:* the responsibility of avoiding harm to the person
- *Justice:* the responsibility to be equitable and fair in the way we treat others.

Furthermore, the principles of privacy, consent, confidentially and non-discrimination are intricately bound up with 'respect for persons and their autonomous rights'. A person must be able to fully understand and consider all the issues involved, have adequate information on which to base a decision and must be allowed to do this with no pressure or coercion. If we have respect for persons, we must also respect their wishes and the decisions they make about themselves and their health-care choices.

There are challenges when considering autonomy in health-care practice, whereby some situations may restrict the degree of a person's autonomy or their ability to utilise it. Special consideration must be made with vulnerable people such as:

- People with sensory difficulties
- Those for whom English is not their first language

- Children with developing autonomous ability
- Adults with a learning disability or an enduring mental health difficulty
- People with altered levels of ability due to injury or illness.

The issue of 'capacity or incapacity' appears to be the cornerstone of autonomous decision-making. The Department of Health (2002) highlights that any approach that reflects 'blanket incapacity', whereby a person is deemed to be incapable of any autonomous decision-making, should be rejected and that a preferred approach is to consider each individual decision to be made and then decide whether the person is capable of making that particular decision. It is clearly unacceptable to dismiss a person's decision-making ability without full consideration.

It is clear, therefore, that to uphold these principles, information must be provided to people in a clear, simple and understandable way, and in an objective and unbiased manner, whether written or spoken. The Code of Professional Conduct for health-care practitioners (NMC, 2004b) sets out the requirement that 'information is accurate, truthful and presented in such a way as to make it easily understood'. According to the Royal Society (RS), this requirement poses a challenge for health-care practitioners when it is recognised that the basic genetic education of practitioners is trailing behind genetic developments (scientific and technical) (RS, 2005a). It highlights that the role of practitioners, including nurses, will evolve further and this will have implications for basic and applied human genetics education (RS, 2005a).

It is clearly recognised (Kirk et al., 2003; DoH, 2005; RS, 2005a) that health-care practitioners require genetic knowledge so as to understand health and ill-health causation, genetic technologies, and associated management and treatment regimes. The competency-based genetics education framework provides a clear structure in which to set out appropriate knowledge and practice outcomes, so that practitioners can competently practise in whatever branch of nursing or health-care setting. A NHS National Genetics Education and Development Centre has been established by the Department of Health to take a central role in the coordination of educational initiatives so as to facilitate developments regarding genetics in health-care practice.

Benjamin and Gamet (2005) highlight that not all nurses will require a high level of expertise, but that they will need to have a genetics knowledge base to be able to recognise clients who may benefit from a referral to genetic services. Kirk (2005) suggests that the level of knowledge and understanding required for best practice will partly depend upon the professional role and speciality of the practitioner.

This chapter therefore sets out to provide an overview of genetics so that practitioners can utilise this knowledge within health care when working in varied practice settings.

It is crucial that the utilisation of 'new genetics knowledge' needs to be firmly set within an ethical framework so that fundamental principles are upheld, for the sake of the individual, the practitioner and society (DoH, 2002). The concept of 'genetic solidarity and altruism' has been proposed by the Department of Health (2002), and it is suggested that in all situations of an ethical nature, this concept should be considered.

The concept of genetic solidarity and altruism has been explained thus:

> we all share the same basic human genome, although there are individual variations which distinguish us from other people. Most of our genetic characteristics will be present in others. This sharing of our genetic constitution not only gives rise to opportunities to help others but it also highlights our common interest in the fruits of medically based genetic research. (DoH, 2002, p. 38)

genetic determinism

people's health, behaviour, intelligence and so on are determined chiefly by their genes (DoH, 2005)

However, the Department of Health (2005) has reported that it does not want to perpetuate a view of **genetic determinism**, for example in the context of an individual's health and behaviour, and highlights that many of the causes of differences are social, economic and environmental factors as well as genetic ones. The risk of becoming more medicalised, due to the possibility of genetic profiling at birth, has been highlighted (DoH, 2005).

Principles for handling personal genetic information in a fair and ethical way are therefore set out by the Department of Health (2002) within the concept of genetic solidarity and altruism. The principles of privacy, consent, confidentiality and non-discrimination are embedded within the overarching key concept of respect for persons. The Department of Health advocates that respect for persons recognises that individuals have the highest moral importance or value, and this should be regarded as a core principle when considering the ethical use of genetic information. Respect for persons:

> affirms the equal value, dignity and moral rights of each individual. Each individual is entitled to lead a life in which genetic characteristics will not be the basis of unjust discrimination or unfair or inhuman treatment. (DoH, 2002, p. 40)

Link

Chapter 10 deals with issues of respect.

However, the principle of respect for persons does require that we acknowledge the value and dignity of others and that we respect their autonomy. There have been concerns raised regarding genetic information, for example in the case of carrier status, where the risk of passing this onto children can cause worry and stigmatisation, and uncover risks for relatives who preferred not to know (DoH, 2003). This type of knowledge can have a positive or negative impact on family dynamics. The Department of Health (2005) highlights that some individuals are pleased to be forewarned about a condition so that they can make choices regarding lifestyle and health care, but also reports that others have expressed concern about knowing about a genetic status, especially if there is nothing useful they can do.

It is not yet clear what benefits come from forewarning individuals about conditions such as cancers and heart disease, whether they are likely to change their lifestyle and take preventive measures, or whether they will adopt a fatalistic viewpoint and assume they will develop the condition anyway, regardless of any preventive measures. A key finding from a recent public dialogue was the view that genetic tests were viewed as 'empowering', particularly if lifestyle changes could be made or if drug treatments were available that would improve the prognosis (RS, 2005b). An important aspect of privacy is protecting individuals from being given information they do not want to know. Insistence on disclosure would disregard their autonomy and their entitlement not to know. This highlights the issue of disclosure or non-disclosure in the interest of the patient; however, it is recognised that situations may arise whereby disclosure of genetic information is in the interest of family members or the public (DoH, 2005).

When considering an individual and their family's medical history, the consideration of genetic information can impact on family relationships, and may reveal unexpected information regarding parentage, such as with paternity testing (DoH, 2002). Genetic testing for an individual may also reveal genetic information that has significance for other relatives, and this raises issues of consent from these individuals (RS, 2005b) and their right to know this genetic information, which may have health and lifestyle implications for them. Within the complexity of this human context, the four ethical principles need to be fully considered:

- *Privacy:* every person is entitled to privacy. In the absence of justification based on overwhelming moral considerations, a person should generally not be obliged to disclose information about his or her genetic characteristics
- *Consent:* private genetic information about a person should generally not be obtained, held or communicated without that person's free and informed consent
- *Confidentiality:* private personal genetic information should generally be treated as being of a confidential nature and should not be communicated to others without consent except for the weightiest of reasons
- *Non-discrimination:* no person shall be unfairly discriminated against on the basis of his or her genetic characteristics (DoH, 2002, pp. 41–4).

> **Link**
>
> *Chapter 16 also discusses confidentiality, privacy and consent.*

Practitioners in health-care settings face demanding and complex situations where ethical principles may not provide a clear solution. However, they are required to work in such a professional manner that reflects an ethical framework and full consideration of accepted ethical principles, so that when decisions are made and acted upon, they are based on these ethical principles and demonstrate clear decision-making.

■ The Human Genome

The concept of the human genome consists of two elements, the nuclear genome and the mitochondrial genome (a circular deoxyribonucleic acid (DNA) molecule inherited from the mother). For the purpose of this chapter, the nuclear genome is being considered. To understand genetic inheritance and disease, we must start by considering the structure and function of chromosomes and genes, and explain the two forms of cell division – mitosis and meiosis.

Chromosomes

The body has two differing groups of cells – somatic cells and gametes (sex cells). These sex cells are spermatozoa in males and oocytes in females. All the other cells of the body are called somatic cells. Chromosomes are structures located within the nucleus of cells, with humans having 23 pairs of chromosomes in the somatic cells, a total of 46, and only 23 chromosomes in the gametes. Somatic cells are referred to as diploid – having pairs of chromosomes – and the gametes as haploid – only having one half of the chromosome pair.

Chromosomes are arranged in pairs according to their shape and size, with pairs 1 to 22 being called the autosomes and pair 23 called the sex chromosomes. These are described as X and Y chromosomes. A female has two X chromosomes, denoted as XX, and the male has one X and one Y chromosome, denoted as XY. Therefore, in humans, the karyotype (chromosomal picture) shows a chromosomal count of 46, XX (female) or 46, XY (male) (Figure 17.1).

As the gametes are cells that have unpaired chromosomes, the oocyte will contain an X chromosome, while spermatozoa will contain an X or a Y chromosome. It is because of this that the gender of the offspring is determined by the father, with the inheritance of the X or Y chromosome being from the father. Fertilisation, the fusion of the gametes, results in a single cell (the zygote), with a chromosomal count of 46, XX or 46, XY – the karyotype. Later in this chapter you will plot this process by the use of a Punnett square to demonstrate the inheritance of gender and recessive and dominant traits.

The resultant zygote receives one of each pair of chromosomes from each of the parents, so that when the 23 chromosomes in the mother's oocyte are combined with the 23 chromosomes in the father's spermatozoa, the result is a normal karyotype – with one set of chromosomes and therefore one set of genes from each parent.

DNA

deoxyribonucleic acid – the double-stranded helix molecule that encodes the genetic information (see Figure 17.3 later in this chapter)

chromosomes

structures composed of DNA that are located within the nucleus of the cell

gamete

a reproductive/sex cell with a haploid number of chromosomes

diploid

a cell with pairs of chromosomes

haploid

a cell with a single set of unpaired chromosomes

autosomes

chromosome pairs 1 to 22 of the total chromosome complement (karyotype)

karyotype

the chromosome complement of a cell or an individual. It denotes the number, size and shape of the chromosomes

zygote

the fertilised oocyte

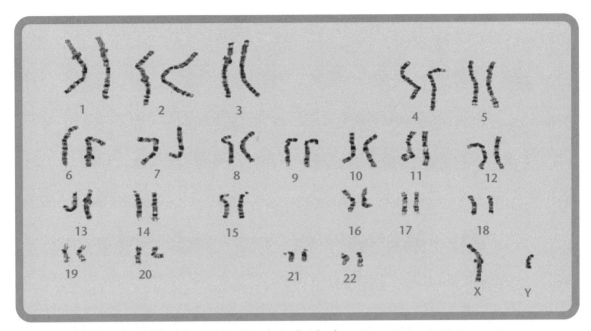

Figure 17.1 ● A karyotype illustrating a male individual

Chromosomal structure

The substance called **chromatin** – sometimes referred to as a mass-like substance – is located within the cell structure. It is this chromatin that is seen during the **interphase** or resting stage. Interphase is the first stage of the life cycle of the cell and at this time the cell is undergoing its cellular functions – cell maintenance – by the instructions from its 'housekeeping genes'. During this stage, protein synthesis is also occurring by the processes of transcription and translation, whereby DNA templates are translated from nucleic acid into amino acids for protein production. It is referred to as the 'resting' stage, as it is resting before its cell division stage – mitosis or meiosis. However, it is important to note that it is during interphase that replication of the DNA structure occurs. This is outlined later in this chapter.

During early cell division (**mitosis** or **meiosis**), the chromatin has coiled and forms the structures called chromosomes. At this stage of the cell's life cycle, each chromosome consists of two **chromatids** (arms), joined together by a structure called the **centromere**. These arms are described as short or long, with the short arms being referred to as the p arms and the long arms as the q arms (Figure 17.2). Now do Activity 17.1 (see over).

Having done Activity 17.1, you should have noted that the short and long arms of a chromosome are particularly clear with chromosome pairs 4, 5 and 9. The centromere – the location whereby the arms are held together during interphase – can be seen on all the chromosome pairs and is denoted as a white dot.

chromatin

the part of the nucleus that consists of DNA and proteins and forms the chromosomes

interphase

the first stage of the life cycle of the cell during which replication of the chromosomes occurs

mitosis

process of cell division in the somatic cells

meiosis

process of cell division in the gametes

chromatid

the two arms of DNA material that are joined together at the centromere after replication

centromere

point at which the two chromatid arms are held together after replication

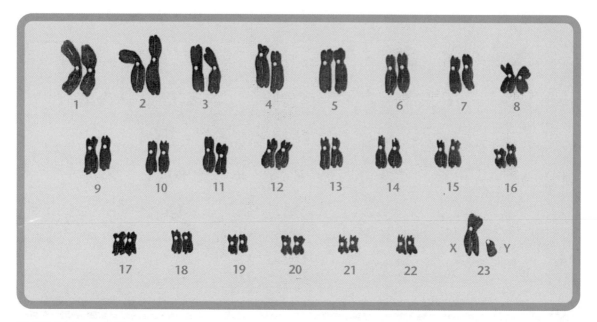

Figure 17.2 ● The short arms (p arms) and long arms (q arms) of the chromosomes

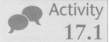

Activity 17.1

Consider Figure 17.2 of a karyotype and identify examples of the short and long arms of the chromosomes and the centromere.

Deoxyribonucleic acid

DNA has been described as looking like a long spiral staircase – the famous double-stranded helix, first described by Crick and Watson in the 1950s. Chromosomes are composed of DNA, which is made up of subunits called nucleotides. Each nucleotide in the DNA has three elements; a sugar molecule (deoxyribose), a phosphate molecule, and one of the nitrogen-containing bases – adenine, thymine, cytosine and guanine (Figure 17.3).

DNA is therefore two long chains or strings of deoxyribose sugar joined with phosphate molecules – producing the uprights of the staircase or ladder – and referred to as the sugar–phosphate backbones. These backbones are connected together – the rungs of the ladder – by the nitrogen-containing bases (nucleotide bases), which are held in place by weak hydrogen bonds. In this DNA structure, these nucleotide bases demonstrate what is known as the 'pairing rule', with adenine (A) being paired with thymine (T), and cytosine (C) being paired with guanine (G) (a mnemonic for the pairing rule of A-T and G-C is 'All These Genetic Codes').

DNA is described as the genetic code holding all the genetic material for the body and for passing on to the next generation. These processes are undertaken by the action of the genes – segments of the DNA.

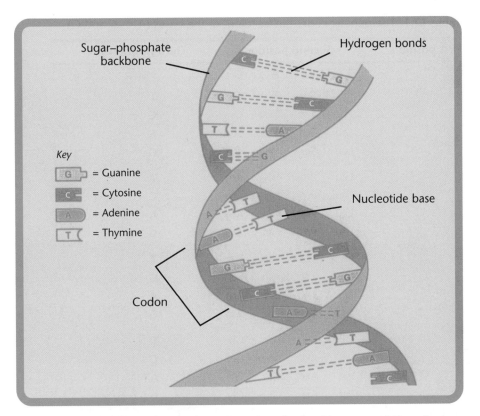

Figure 17.3 ● DNA molecule demonstrating the backbones and the nitrogen bases (A, T, C and G)

Genes

Genes are segments of the DNA that are the inherited genetic code and there are more than 30,000 genes in the human genome. The genetic code is 'read' as three nucleotides at a time, which is referred to as a codon or triplet, with each codon/triplet acting as a code for a particular amino acid (the building blocks of proteins). The 'reading' of the codon – three nucleotides at a time – is described as reading the first, second and then third position, with each position denoting one of the bases (A, T, C or G). From reading the code, each of the resultant abbreviations, for example Phe (Table 17.1), signifies a particular amino acid. The DNA is arranged in an important pattern and it is this pattern that is the code that carries the protein-building instructions.

Table 17.1 The genetic code: the 'reading' of the bases (A, T, C and G)

First position	Second position				Third position
	T	C	A	G	
T	Phe	Ser	Tyr	Cys	T
	Phe	Ser	Tyr	Cys	C
	Leu	Ser	Stop	Stop	A
	Leu	Ser	Stop	Trp	G
C	Leu	Pro	His	Arg	T
	Leu	Pro	His	Arg	C
	Leu	Pro	Gln	Arg	A
	Leu	Pro	Gln	Arg	G
A	Ile	Thr	Asn	Ser	T
	Ile	Thr	Asn	Ser	C
	Ile	Thr	Lys	Arg	A
	Met	Thr	Lys	Arg	G
G	Val	Ala	Asp	Gly	T
	Val	Ala	Asp	Gly	C
	Val	Ala	Glu	Gly	A
	Val	Ala	Glu	Gly	G

Note: The abbreviations represent the different amino acids, which are given below.

Amino acid abbreviations

Abbreviation	Amino acid	Abbreviation	Amino acid
Phe	Phenylalanine	Leu	Leucine
Ile	Isoleucine	Met	Methionine
Val	Valine	Ser	Serine
Pro	Proline	Thr	Threonine
Ala	Alanine	Tyr	Tyrosine
His	Histidine	Gln	Glutamine
Asn	Asparagine	Lys	Lysine
Asp	Aspartic acid	Glu	Glutamic acid
Cys	Cysteine	Trp	Tryptophan
Arg	Arginine	Gly	Glycine

You can see from Table 17.1 that some amino acids are coded by more than one codon, such as leucine and arginine. Only a small proportion of an individual's DNA in the chromosomes forms the genes, the remaining is the 'non-coding' or 'junk DNA', the function of which is not yet understood.

Having done Activity 17.2, you should have come up with the following answers:

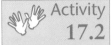

Activity
17.2

Utilising the genetic code outlined in Table 17.1, identify the codons that code for the amino acids leucine and serine.

- Leucine is coded by six different codons: TTA, TTG, CTT, CTC, CTA, CTG
- Serine is coded by six different codons: TCT, TCC, TCA, TCG, AGT, AGC.

If the DNA pattern is changed, such as if nucleotides are altered, deleted or inserted, then a different code is read and different amino acids may be produced and a different or altered protein may be produced. These nucleotide mutations can result in genetic mutations such as point mutations, frameshift mutations, and repeat expansion mutations (trinucleotide repeats), which are expanded upon later in this chapter. A point to note is that proteins contribute to various structures within the body or have contributed to the development of structures, such as the colour of the skin, layout of the neurons in the brain, structures such as collagen and keratin, and substances such as hormones, antibodies and enzymes. The effect of mutations can therefore be expressed throughout the body.

The life cycle of the cell

The cell life span varies from cell to cell but there are three phases to the life cycle – interphase, cell division (mitosis or meiosis) and **cytokinesis**. For a cell to divide it must replicate the chromosomes so that they are passed onto each of the daughter cells. The first phase of the life cycle is called the interphase or resting stage, where replication of the chromosomes occur. This occurs by the double-stranded helix uncoiling, the hydrogen bonds holding the nucleotide bases together break, and each freed strand then replicates a complementary strand. This structure is held together by the centromere, resulting in double the chromosomal material and hence double the genetic material.

cytokinesis

the division or separation of the cytoplasm of the parent cell following mitosis or meiosis

The second phase is called cell division. In somatic cells (the body cells), this process of cell division is called mitosis and contains four phases: prophase, metaphase, anaphase and telophase. This process involves the centromeres lining up at the centre of the cell, the arms split and are then pulled separately towards the poles (ends) of the cell. This results in half of the chromosome material being placed at each end of the cell.

Cytokinesis, the third phase, commences with a cleavage furrow of the cytoplasm, and continues until the cytoplasm is divided into two separate cells. Due to the exact replication of the chromosomes in the interphase stage, the process has produced two identical daughter cells – identical chromosomes and hence identical genetic material. The life cycle is a well-regulated process so that the production of new cells is sufficient for body growth and the repair of damaged cells.

The production of gametes is referred to as 'spermatogenesis' and 'oogenesis'. In the development of gametes, the life cycle comprises the interphase, cell division (meiosis) and cytokinesis. However, it must be noted that the gametes differ from somatic cells, in that somatic cells have 23 pairs of chromosomes and gametes only have 23 chromosomes. This therefore requires a process whereby only one from each pair of the chromosomes is distributed to each of the gametes.

Replication of the chromosomes occurs in the interphase, as outlined previously. The second phase is the process of cell division (meiosis) involving two nuclear or meiotic divisions. Meiosis I is also called 'reduction division' and meiosis II is also called 'equatorial division', and both divisions have the four phases: prophase, metaphase, anaphase and telophase.

It is during meiosis I that genetic variability occurs so that similarities and differences can be seen within different family members, such as eye colour, personality traits and genetic diseases. This occurs during reduction division by the crossing over (overlaying) of the arms of each pair of chromosomes, these break and rejoin, hence leading to a mixing of the genes (recombination). This can be seen in Figure 17.4. Therefore the exact DNA sequence varies from person to person, except in identical twins (monozygotic twins).

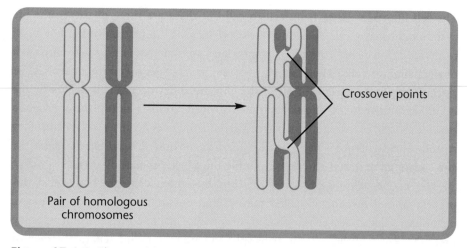

Figure 17.4 ● Chromatid arms crossing over

At the end of meiosis I and cytokinesis, two cells are produced that are different from the parent cell. The second meiotic stage (equatorial division) is undertaken, and along with cytokinesis, results in four cells being produced. Each of these haploid cells has half the chromosome complement, 23, from the parent cell.

Mitosis refers to cell division concerned with the development of somatic cells (body cells) as well as with the development of the zygote. At fertilisation, the union of the gametes (sperm and the ovum) produces one cell, called the zygote. This is a cell with a full chromosome complement that develops by mitosis to become the embryo (first two months) and then the fetus. Processes of 'differentiation and specialisation' occur during embryo/fetal development at recognised times, ensuring that different body cells, tissues and systems are developed for the normal functioning of the human species. Any error occurring while these processes are in action will have consequences for the developing embryo/fetus and these may be evident at birth or in early childhood development.

Chromosomal abnormalities

Four types of mutations can occur during gamete development, zygote development or during an individual's lifetime (body growth and repair), leading to differences in the **phenotype** of the individual. These changes in the DNA sequence, whatever the cause, may have no effect on the function of the gene, may result in an abnormality in the rate of production of a normal protein or may result in the production of an abnormal protein. The resulting phenotype is therefore determined by one of the four following mutations.

phenotype

the characteristics of an individual that are due to both the environment and genetic make-up

Chromosomal numerical

Errors can occur during cell division affecting all or part of a chromosome. Chromosomal numerical errors affect the number of the chromosomes. The most well-known example of a numerical disorder is trisomy 21 (Down's syndrome), where there are three copies of chromosome number 21. This error in cell division is called 'non-disjunction', and is when the chromosomes fail to split at the centromere and separate during the process of cell division, resulting in an extra chromosome (**trisomy**) or in an absence of a chromosome (**monosomy**). A trisomy condition therefore results in extra DNA/genes, and a monosomy condition results in an absence of DNA/genes.

trisomy

having three copies of a particular chromosome

monosomy

having only one copy of a particular chromosome

If non-disjunction occurs during mitosis, it can have an impact on body repair and body growth or on the development of the zygote.

If non-disjunction occurs during meiosis, it can have an impact on the production of the gametes, resulting in trisomy or monosomy of the gametes. Hence, if a mutated gamete is fertilised, it results in a faulty zygote being produced. Other examples of trisomy conditions include trisomy 13 (Patau syndrome), trisomy 18 (Edward syndrome), triple X syndrome, XXY (Klinefelter syndrome in males). An example of a monosomy condition is XO (Turner syndrome in females, denoted as 45, X).

Chromosomal structural

Chromosomal structural errors are those affecting the structure, and include 'deletion', 'microdeletion' and 'translocation'. A deletion is where there is chromosome breakage and a fragment of the chromosome has been lost. A deletion is indicated by a minus (–) sign on the karyotype, for example 46, XX, 5p– (denotes Cri-du-chat syndrome) or 46, XY, 4p– (denotes Wolf-Hirschhorn syndrome). A microdeletion is a region of chromosome loss that is detected by cytogenetic testing. A translocation is a rearrangement of the chromosome material. This results in part or all of one chromosome becoming attached to a chromosome from a different pair and so there is no loss or gain of chromosome material; however, this can lead to errors in future generations.

Nucleotide mutations

Nucleotide mutations affect the nucleotides and include 'point mutations', 'frameshift mutations' and 'repeat expansion mutations'. A point mutation occurs when a nitrogen base (adenine, thymine, cytosine, guanine) has been substituted for another. The system of reading the codons (triplets) as three at a time is not affected, but the altered codon leads to the coding of a different amino acid from the original. This error is also referred to as a 'spelling error'. A frameshift mutation occurs when one or multiple nitrogen bases are inserted or deleted. This mutation affects the reading of the codons (triplets) and hence the sequence of the amino acids is altered and the composition of the final protein is affected.

Repeat expansion mutations (trinucleotide repeats) are where a codon has been repeated over and over many times. An example of this is fragile X syndrome where there is a repeat of the bases CGG (cytosine, guanine, guanine) on the X chromosome at the location of q27.3. Remember that q refers to the long arm of the chromosome and 27.3 refers to the position on the arm. This means that the error has been identified at an exact location (locus). Other examples are Huntington's disease, which is a repeat of the bases CAG (cytosine, adenine, guanine) on chromosome number 4 at the p16.3 location, and myotonic dystrophy, which is a repeat of the bases CTG on chromosome 19.

Mutations of DNA sequence

Cancers can occur due to mutations in DNA sequence. Throughout our lifetime, DNA/genes within the cells of the body are exposed to adverse environmental agents and can suffer mistakes in replication. Most cancers result from these acquired mutations in families of genes called 'oncogenes' and tumour-suppressor genes. These genes are part of the cells' normal machinery for keeping the cell functioning and ensuring effective division (RS, 2005a). When new cells are produced in the body to replace dead or damaged cells, these genes limit the number of new cells to prevent overgrowth of the tissue. These genes therefore have the function of helping to prevent the growth of tumours or cancers. Genetic material is recopied over and over during a person's lifetime with the potential for errors to occur.

■ Genetic Inheritance

The **genotype** refers to the genetic make-up of an individual and the phenotype is the expression of this genetic make-up. A change in the sequence of the DNA may affect its function and may have phenotypic consequences.

genotype

the genetic composition of an organism

Regarding the inheritance of traits and disorders, genes that control the same trait and occupy the same locus (position) on the chromosome are referred to as 'alleles'. When alleles code for the same expression of a trait, they are referred to as 'homozygous', and when they code for a different expression of a trait, they are referred to as 'heterozygous'. Table 17.2 uses eye colour as an example.

When one allele masks (suppresses) the one on the other chromosome, it is called the 'dominant' gene, and the one being masked (suppressed) is called the 'recessive' gene. Examples of dominant traits are brown eyes, curly hair and dimples, and recessive traits are blue eyes, straight hair and flat feet. When illustrating recessive and dominant states, the dominant is always indicated by a capital letter and the recessive by a lower case one.

Table 17.2 Genotypes expressed as phenotypes, using eye colour as an example

Genotype	Phenotype
BB (homozygous)	Brown eyes
Bb (heterozygous)	Brown eyes
bb (heterozygous)	Blue eyes

Punnett square

consists of a square divided into four, with the possible alleles from the father on the left-hand side of the square and the possible alleles from the mother above it. The possible genotypes of the children are then calculated by combining the alleles in turn

The inheritance of single-gene traits and disorders follows the simple pattern of Mendel's laws of inheritance, in that they are inherited in a dominant manner, recessive manner or X-linked manner (located on the X chromosome). The **Punnett square** is a method of demonstrating the possible combinations of the genes from the parent (Figure 17.5).

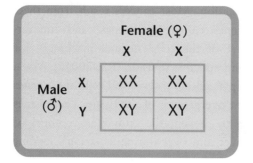

Figure 17.5 ● Punnett square illustrating the determination of gender

It can be seen from this Punnett square that 50 per cent of children are males and 50 per cent females; however, it needs to be noted that this refers to the genotype of the children – the actual genetic composition. The determination of the male phenotype is determined by genes located on the Y chromosome – the SRY region. All zygotes, male and female, develop identically and then in early embryonic development, the genes in the SRY region activate male development. If this region is absent or mutated, the developing embryo continues to develop as a female, irrespective of having a Y chromosome.

This method of demonstrating the passage of genes from one generation to the next can be used for all inherited traits and conditions. For example, curly (C) hair is dominant and straight (s) hair is recessive. Using the Punnett square, it can be seen that two parents with curly (C) hair (phenotype) can have a child with straight (s) hair (phenotype). This is due to the genotype of the parents – the actual genetic make-up (Figure 17.6).

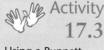 **Activity 17.3**

Using a Punnett square, plot the eye colour (the phenotype) of possible children from a mother with a Bb heterozygous genotype and a father with a bb homozygous genotype.

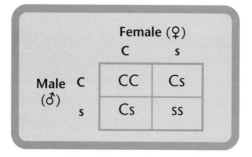

Figure 17.6 ● Punnett square illustrating the determination of curly and straight hair

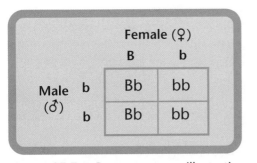

Figure 17.7 ● Punnett square illustrating the determination of eye colour

Having done Activity 17.3, you should have the same Punnett square as shown in Figure 17.7. The possible genotype and phenotypes of children are:

● Genotype of Bb: two children with a phenotype of brown eyes (B) and a heterozygous genotype (Bb)
● Genotype of bb: two children with a phenotype of blue eyes (b) and a heterozygous recessive genotype (bb)
● Note that a BB genotype would indicate a child with a phenotype of brown eyes (B) and a homozygous dominant genotype (BB).

When an individual is referred to as being of a 'carrier status' for a specific condition, this means that their genotype has one defective recessive gene for the specific condition. However, as it is a recessive gene, it is not expressed in the phenotype as it is suppressed by the corresponding gene. Carriers can pass this gene on to the next generation and individuals can be offered carrier testing to determine whether they carry such a gene, for example for CF, phenylke-tonuria (PKU), sickle-cell anaemia and Tay-Sachs disease. Consent to this type of genetic testing requires consideration of any social and psychological implications for individuals and their relatives and the implications for future reproductive decisions. Issues such as prenatal and neonatal screening, diagnostic testing and assisted reproductive technologies are discussed in a recent report, which may influence reproductive decision-making (DoH, 2006).

Consider a child or young adult who may have a genetic condition, such as cystic fibrosis, Huntington's disease or haemophilia, being tested for the sake of themselves and other family members.

Consider the various ethical principles to be respected when working in these types of situation.

Identify some of the social and ethical issues of testing a child or adult in this manner.

The three conditions mentioned in Casebox 17.1 are inherited in different ways and therefore may pose different issues for the family to consider:

- *Cystic fibrosis:* this is inherited in an autosomal recessive manner and therefore has implications due to the carrier status of some of the family members. Choices regarding future reproductive choices will need to be considered by other family members and hence ethical considerations will be required when working within an extended family structure
- *Huntington's disease:* this is inherited in an autosomal dominant manner and is a late-onset disease, in that the symptoms are manifested in later life. As this is inherited in the dominant manner, it will raise issues within the family regarding testing and the purposes of diagnosis. This poses dilemmas for testing in childhood/young adulthood for a late-onset condition
- *Haemophilia:* this is inherited in an X-linked manner, with the gene responsible being located on the X chromosome. This raises gender issues within families, as females have two X chromosomes (karyotype is 46, XX) and may therefore have an unaffected X chromosome as well as an affected on. Males are affected by the condition as they only have one copy of the X chromosome (male karyotype is 46, XY). Choices regarding future reproductive choices will need to be considered by other family members and hence ethical considerations will be required when working within an extended family structure.

The parents of **Joseph** are informed when he is 12 days old that Joseph, their first child has PKU. They are worried about his health status and that of any future children. They are both from large families and both wish to have a large family in the future.

Using a Punnett square, identify the potential phenotypes of future children using the genotypes of Joseph's parents.

You could consider how you would inform the parents of this condition, working within an ethical framework upholding ethical principles.

You could consider the implications of this carrier status in terms of the social and psychological impact for family members and in terms of implications for reproductive decisions.

You might also consider the possible future and implications of gene therapy for conditions such as PKU (12q 24.1) (see Pharmacogenetics later in this chapter).

PKU is an autosomal recessive condition, so is denoted in the Punnett square as lower case p (Figure 17.8).

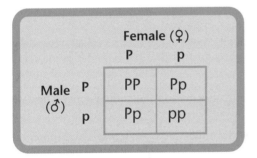

Figure 17.8 ● Punnett square illustrating the possible phenotypes of children when both parents have a genotype for PKU

The possible genotype and phenotypes of children are:

- Genotype of PP: one child with a phenotype of not being affected with PKU and a homozygous genotype (PP)
- Genotype of Pp: two children with a phenotype of carrier status for PKU (p) and a heterozygous recessive genotype (Pp)
- Genotype of pp: one child with a phenotype of being affected with PKU and a homozygous recessive genotype (pp).

■ The Impact of Genotypes in Health Care

Genetics is clearly recognised in single-gene disorders such as CF, haemophilia and Huntington's disease, but the relevance of the human genome is being acknowledged in common diseases such as coronary heart disease, diabetes, asthma, cancers, mental health conditions such as schizophrenia and many others.

The genetics White Paper *Our Inheritance, Our Future: Realising the Potential of Genetics in the NHS* (DoH, 2003) has clearly set out the government's strategic vision for genetics and health care. It will have a major impact on how genetic information is fully realised in the health and lifestyle of individuals and in the development of NHS and private health-care systems.

The secretary of state for health acknowledged that

> advances in human genetics will have a profound impact on healthcare. Over time we will see new ways of predicting and preventing ill health, more targeted and effective use of existing drugs and the development of new gene-based drugs and therapies that treat illness in novel ways. Above all, genetics holds out the promise of more personalised healthcare with prevention and treatment tailored according to a person's individual genetic profile. (DoH, 2003, p. 5)

This governmental position clearly encompasses a number of issues regarding genetics:

● The identification of 'personal genetic information', including genetic disease and predisposition to disease
● An understanding of how genetics and other factors such as environmental ones interact with each other
● An understanding of drugs and alternative therapies
● The development of appropriate educational programmes and initiatives for health-care practitioners
● The investment and development of appropriate health-care services to meet the needs arising from genetic advances.

As part of these developments, an advisory body, the Human Genetics Commission (HGC), was set up in late 1999 to 'advise the government on the ethical, legal and social aspects of developments in human genetics as well as their effects on health and healthcare' (DoH, 2006, p. 6). A number of key publications have been published that provide evidence of the debate around these ethical, legal and social influences (DoH, 2000, 2002a, 2002b, 2004, 2005, 2006; Nuffield Council on Bioethics, 2001, 2002, 2003a, 2003b).

Genetic profiling

The issue of genetic profiling of babies at birth was considered by the Human Genetics Commission and the National Screening Committee (DoH, 2005) so as to consider the potential of all individuals having their own entire genome analysis. This would enable individuals to have personal genetic information that may be important in health care during their lifetime. Issues such as the provision of IT, data storage, access and security are being fully considered within the creation of the genetic section of the IT provision (RS, 2005a). The government has been provided with an analysis of the 'ethical, social, scientific, economic and practical considerations' of genetically profiling babies at birth (DoH, 2005). They suggested that genetic profiling, along with other health, lifestyle and environmental information, brings the promise of a more accurate assessment of disease status, disease risk and an individual's susceptibility to various environmental exposures (DoH, 2005, p. 10).

This has tremendous implications for an individual's lifestyle and their health-care needs. Individuals may be informed how, based on their genotype, they will interact with factors such as environmental pollutants, foods and infectious agents (DoH, 2005). Personal choices based on this type of personal genetic and related information are then possible, such as altering one's lifestyle – diet, cessation of smoking, exercise and the uptake of health and alternative remedies. Health choices are also possible, such as particular drug regimes, targeted to suit the individual's profile.

The Department of Health (2005) acknowledges that many diseases are as a result of the interaction between genetic and environmental factors, with the balance between these two factors varying from disease to disease. But it also highlights that the evidence of the link between most genetic variants and disease is not yet fully clear. This knowledge will progress through research.

However, the Department of Health did reject genetic profiling as a screening tool at this current time, but highlighted that this should not be taken as a rejection of its longer term potential. It suggested that for genetic profiling to be of clinical use, more research must be undertaken about genetic variation and its link with ill-health, and the influence of environmental factors (DoH, 2005). Research is already trying to unravel the complex interactions between nature and nurture that underlie diseases (RS, 2005a). The developing genetic knowledge does facilitate our understanding of how body cells work and how genetic variations and mutations affect normal cell processes and hence disease patterns.

> ## Activity 17.4
>
> Consider the following implications of genetically profiling babies at birth:
>
> 1. The ethical implications and the upholding of ethical principles.
> 2. The social, economic and practical implications of genetic profiling at birth.
>
> You may wish to consider these from various perspectives, such as families, communities and government agencies such as the NHS. (Suggested key publications include DoH, 2000, 2002a, 2002b, 2004, 2005, 2006 and Nuffield Council on Bioethics, 2001, 2002, 2003a, 2003b.)

Genetic screening

Genetic screening is offered to members of a defined population who do not necessarily perceive they are at risk of, or are already affected by, a genetic condition or its complications. Genetic screening programmes offer tests to large groups of individuals, by which they may be identified as being at particular risk of a disorder by virtue of their clinical history (or that of relatives), or on a larger scale on the basis of age, gender or ethnic group (DoH, 2002b). Respect for persons and the associated principles need to be safeguarded when working with individuals involved in genetic screening programmes, as they raise issues such as consent, confidentiality and the counselling needs of the participants.

Genetic testing is used to

- aid diagnosis where symptoms are already present
- identify whether family members will develop a late-onset disease
- check for carrier status

and in prenatal and neonatal screening programmes.

As well as participants in the public dialogue advocating that genetic tests were empowering, the Royal Society identified that even if lifestyle changes were not likely to improve prognosis, around 50 per cent still preferred to have a test, particularly when reproductive decisions were affected (RS, 2005b). However, complex issues arising from genetic testing, particularly relating to family members, were raised by a significant number of the participants (RS, 2005b).

Pharmacogenetics

The Royal Society has published a comprehensive report into **pharmacogenetics** (personalised medicines), detailing the current position and future possibilities within health-care practice (RS, 2005a).

It is recognised that individuals respond differently to drugs, and that part of this is genetically determined – variations in our genes. Three factors being considered are:

- *Genetic predictor of response* – whether an individual will respond or fail to respond to a drug
- *Adverse drug reactions* – whether an individual will experience any idiosyncratic adverse reactions to a drug
- *Genetic differences in drug metabolism* – whether an individual has a slow or quick metabolic rate for the drug.

This will lead to an individual's genetic difference in drug metabolism and any adverse drug reactions being considered in the design of their individual treatment regime – 'tailor-made treatments'. Alongside pharmacogenetic testing (the person's genetic make-up), other factors such as gender, age, weight,

pharmacogenetics
the study of how people's genetic make-up affects their responses to drugs (RS, 2005a)

ethnicity, family history, diet, alcohol consumption and tobacco usage will continue to be considered.

The pharmaceutical industry, in an attempt to take these issues forward through research, is trying to understand the causes of disease and variability of drug responses, drug dosages, why some individuals experience adverse drug reactions, and the fate of drugs within the body – absorption, distribution, metabolism and excretion (ADME). These developments are already evident in cancer care, where an individual's genotype is being utilised prior to the prescribing of targeted drug regimes, for example with the use of Trastuzumab (Herceptin) being developed for some types of breast cancer (RS, 2005a).

However, developments are not restricted to inherited conditions, as many forms of cancer result from changes (mutations) in the genes that occur during our lifetime through errors in cell division (mitosis) in the body's cells (somatic cells) (RS, 2005a). We are dependent upon the process of mitosis during our life-time, for body growth and repair, and as we continuously encounter adverse environmental agents, these can be detrimental to the process of mitosis and lead to mutations.

Pharmacogenetics is viewed as a promising future in health care; however, it is estimated that it will be more than a decade before their use is widespread. The advances in genetics may also lead to further gene-based drugs and gene therapies. In this way, drugs would interact with the individual's genotype, aiming to switch on a helpful gene or switch off a harmful one. Gene therapy is the introduction of material directly into an individual's cells, and it would aim to replace a defective gene or alter the activity of gene action (DoH, 2003). The Human Genetics Commission highlight that

> whilst recognising the potential benefits that gene therapy can have, it is only likely to be effective for a few people, and for a very small proportion of the single gene disorders. (DoH, 2006, pp. 80–1)

Many of these therapies are presently being researched, in particular in cancer and coronary heart disease, but promise an evolutionary health-care system based on the human genome.

The ethical debate regarding pharmacogenetics and the principles of consent, privacy and confidentiality, alongside information management, has been outlined by the Nuffield Council on Bioethics (2003a).

■ Chapter Summary

There are a number of issues surrounding genetics that have been considered in this chapter so as to further understand human development, health and disease, mental health and mental disorders, and learning disabilities. This chapter has therefore focused on the structure and function of chromosomes and genes, the inheritance patterns and the expression of an individual's genotype into phenotype, and the potential impact of mutations upon the developing individual.

The question as to how our genes and other factors, such as social, economic and environmental factors, interact to cause disease or to predispose an individual to disease are highlighted as areas for future research. How our genes can affect our response to drugs has been raised, with developments in pharmacogenetics potentially leading to tailor-made prescribing. Genetic profiling and testing will become a key element of the health-care service, with a more personalised health-care system becoming a reality.

The new genetics knowledge and technology has the potential to bring enormous benefits for patients, such as more personalised prediction of risk, prevention of ill-health, more accurate diagnosis, safer use of drugs and new treatment options. A revolution in health care is possible (DoH, 2003); however, it needs to be underpinned by knowledgeable practitioners and good educational initiatives.

The importance of identifying and resolving any ethical issues such as confidentiality of information, privacy, obtaining valid informed consent, storage and protection of genetic material is fundamental to the developing health agenda.

Test Yourself!

1. Identify the four secondary principles reflected by the Human Genetics Commission (DoH, 2002) in the primary principle of 'respect for persons'.

2. Name the four nitrogen-containing bases of the DNA molecule.

3. Describe the pairing rule of the nitrogen-containing bases in the DNA sequence.

4. Name the following conditions: (a) 47, XY+21, (b) 47, XXY, (c) 45, XO, (d) 12q24.1, (e) Xq28.

5. Define the terms: (a) autosomes, (b) trisomy, (c) monosomy, (d) non-disjunction.

6. Calculate the inheritance of a: (a) dominant condition, (b) recessive condition, (c) X-linked condition.

■ Further Reading

Bonthron, D., FitzPatrick, D., Porteous, M. and Trainer, A. (1998) *Clinical Genetics: A Case-based Approach.* WB Saunders, London.

Burton, H. (2003) *Addressing Genetics Delivering Health,* Public Health Genetics funded by The Wellcome Trust and the Department of Health. Department of Health, London.

DoH (Department of Health) (2003) *Genes Direct: Ensuring the Effective Oversight of Genetic Tests Supplied Directly to the Public.* Department of Health, London.

DoH (Department of Health) (2003) *Addressing Genetics, Delivering Health,* Department of Health, London.

Gilbert, P. (1997) *The A–Z Reference Book of Syndromes and Inherited Disorders.* Chapman & Hall, London.

Gilbert, P. (2001) *Dictionary of Syndromes and Inherited Disorders.* Chapman & Hall, London.

Hartley, J. (2003) Genetics: What you need to know. *Nursing Times* **99**(39): 34–6.

Marteau, T. and Richards, M. (1996) *The Troubled Helix: Social and Psychological Implications of the New Human Genetics.* Cambridge University Press, Cambridge.

RS (Royal Society) (2003) *Genetics and Health: Visions of the Future.* RS, London.

RS (Royal Society) (2005) *Pharmacogenetics: The Hopes and Realities of Personalised Medicines. A Guide for Health Professionals.* RS, London.

Skirton, H. and Patch, C. (2002) *Genetics for Healthcare Professionals.* BIOS Scientific, Oxford.

Winter, P.C., Hickey, G.I. and Fletcher, H.L. (2004) *Genetics: Instant Notes.* BIOS Scientific, Oxford.

■ References

Beauchamp, T.L. and Childress, J.F. (2001) *Principles of Biomedical Ethics.* Oxford University Press, Oxford.

Benjamin, C.M. and Gamet, K. (2005) Recognising the limitations of your genetics expertise. *Nursing Standard* **20**(6): 49–54.

Bradley, A.N. (2005) Utility and limitations of genetic testing and information. *Nursing Standard* **20**(5): 52–5.

DoH (Department of Health) (2000) *Whose Hands on Your Genes?* Department of Health, London.

DoH (Department of Health) (2002a) *Public Attitudes to Human Genetic Information.* Department of Health, London.

DoH (Department of Health) (2002b) *Inside Information. Balancing Interests in the Use of Personal Genetic Data.* Human Genetics Commission, Department of Health, London.

DoH (Department of Health) (2003) *Our Inheritance, Our Future: Realising the Potential of Genetics in the NHS*. Department of Health, London.

DoH (Department of Health) (2004) *Choosing the Future: Genetics and Reproductive Decision-making*. Department of Health, London.

DoH (Department of Health) (2005) *Profiling the Newborn: a Prospective Gene Technology?* Human Genetics Commission, Department of Health, London.

DoH (Department of Health) (2006) *Making Babies: Reproductive Decisions and Genetic Technologies*. Human Genetics Commission, Department of Health, London.

Kirk, M. (2005) The role of genetic factors in maintaining health, *Nursing Standard* **20**(4): 50–4.

Kirk, M., McDonald, K., Anstey, S. and Longley, M. (2003) *Fit for Practice in the Genetics Era: A Competence-based Education Framework for Nurses, Midwives and Health Visitors*. Genomics Policy Unit, University of Glamorgan.

NMC (Nursing and Midwifery Council) (2004a) *Standards of Proficiency for Pre-registration Nursing Education*. NMC, London.

NMC (Nursing and Midwifery Council) (2004b) *The NMC Code of Professional Conduct: Standards for Conduct, Performance and Ethics*. NMC, London.

Nuffield Council on Bioethics (2001) *Stem Cell Therapy: Ethical Issues*. Nuffield Council on Bioethics, London.

Nuffield Council on Bioethics (2002) *Genetics and Human Behaviour: the Ethical Context*. Nuffield Council on Bioethics, London.

Nuffield Council on Bioethics (2003a) *Genetics Screening: Ethical Issues*. Nuffield Council on Bioethics, London.

Nuffield Council on Bioethics (2003b) *Pharmacogenetics: Ethical Issues*. Nuffield Council on Bioethics, London.

RS (Royal Society) (2005a) *Personalised Medicines: Hopes and Realities*. RS, London.

RS (Royal Society) (2005b) *Pharmacogenetics Dialogue*. RS, London.

▓ Useful Websites

www.dh.gov.uk Department of Health: Policy and Guidance: Genetics

www.hgc.gov.uk Human Genetics Commission

www.ncbi.nlm.nih.gov National Center for Biotechnology Information and Access to OMIM™ (Online Mendelian Inheritance in Man)

www.geneticseducation.nhs.uk The National Genetics Education and Development Centre

www.royalsociety.org The Royal Society

www.sanger.ac.uk The Wellcome Trust Sanger Institute

Chapter

Health Informatics

18

Contents

Learning Outcomes

At the end of this chapter, you should be able to:

- Define the term health informatics

- Identify the difference between data, information and knowledge

- Outline how knowledge of issues related to health informatics impacts on patients, care provision, the organisation of care management and the public

- Describe the basic principles of common legislation related to the privacy and use of information

- Identify current health-care policy related to health informatics.

▓ Introduction: What is Health-care Informatics?

The past 50 years have seen a series of cultural changes that are remarkable in terms of their scale of influence and speed of implementation. Similar periods of change have been noted throughout history and are often connected with technological innovation. These historical periods are commonly dubbed 'ages' or 'revolutions', for example the Bronze Age or the Industrial Revolution. The latest period of cultural change (which is still ongoing) is associated with the technological development of computing, and is fuelled by a far less tangible commodity – information. The consequences of the information age are easily observed and are taken for granted as change rapidly extends throughout our society. But how do we as a profession define information? And based on this definition, what relevance does information have to health-care provision, and why should all nurses have some understanding of **informatics**? This chapter hopes to provide some answers to these questions in a way that is easy to read and understand.

informatics

another term for information science, which is the science of the collection, evaluation, organisation and dissemination of information, often employing computers

Broadly speaking, informatics relates to the study and processing of information. Health informatics is therefore the study and processing of information related to health care. Protti (1982, cited in Abbott et al., 2004, p. 9) defines health informatics as:

> The study of the nature and principles of information and its applications within all aspects of health care delivery and promotion.

Hence, health informatics is a general term with relevance to all the speciality areas of health care and each branch of nursing. Other definitions such as that offered by Hebda et al. (2005, p. 9) associate health informatics with information and communications technology in the form of computers, and the information systems they help to deliver:

> The application of computer and information science in all basic and applied biomedical sciences to facilitate the acquisition, processing, interpretation, optimal use, and communication of health related data. The focus is the patient and the process of care, and the goal is to enhance the quality and efficiency of care provided.

It is important to acknowledge that computer technology is not always directly involved in the management and processing of health-related information; nor is technology a prerequisite for quality and efficient care delivery. However, the scale of the modern health service is so great that the development and use of technologically driven systems is required to ensure equity in service provision and efficiency savings on a national level. As such, computerised health systems are becoming more commonplace and this trend is set to continue.

Here we will consider why health informatics is, and should be, a rapidly growing concern to all health-care staff. The basic concepts related to informatics will be considered, including what is meant by the terms data, information and knowledge. Systems related to health informatics will be introduced from the perspective of the patient, the health professional, the organisation and the wider public. Consideration of the patient's right to privacy and confidentiality will be briefly explored. Finally, current governmental strategy will be introduced, with an explanation of how this strategy has implications for health professionals – whatever their level of expertise.

It is perhaps also important to stress what this chapter does not cover. All too frequently narratives relating to health informatics concern themselves with a focus on computer technology, for example detailing how to search the internet for information. Although computers are essential to health informatics and therefore such narratives are useful, it is crucial to remember that a computer is nothing more than a tool. No matter how important the tool may be, it is the role of the tool that is of primary importance. This chapter is therefore less concerned with the specifics of how to use computers, and more with the underlying principles of how information is central to care delivery.

Who needs information on health?

Information is central to health-care provision. As an example, consider a patient attending an appointment for a prearranged investigation. It is possible to see that the need for information relating to the appointment extends beyond the patient and health professionals directly involved. Indeed, it can be shown that numerous people have a stake in this information, ranging from the patient to the wider public:

- *The patient and the patient's family*
  The patient and/or their primary carer need to have information regarding the admission prior to the event. This might include the appointment details such as the date and time of the admission and any specific details related to the investigation itself. For example, does the patient need to do anything specific prior to the admission, such as avoid certain foods?
- *The health-care provider*
  The provider of care requires a variety of information, but not just facts related to the patient's personal details and relevant past medical history. Information and knowledge regarding the best way to care for the patient during their stay is essential if the care to be provided is of the best quality. For example, what evidence exists for the treatments to be used, what local and national guidelines are in place and how are they applicable? Methods are also required for recording and acting on new information gained from the investigation once it is carried out. The provider also needs to supply

information on the care it delivers to its purchasers, mainly primary care Trusts (PCTs), so that the care and procedures carried out can be paid for.

- *The health authority*

  The health authority needs information regarding the patient's admission to enable informed decisions relating to the management of resources and health-care strategy. This information may involve detailed statistics to be used for the allocation of resources such as staff and materials. Equally, the health authority needs information in regard to how care was delivered. In this way, the health authority can monitor the efficiency of care delivery and ensure local and national standards are been adhered to. For example, the monitoring of specific staff training and development helps to facilitate the management of risk.

- *The general public*

  It may be surprising to learn that the general public also need information regarding the patient's admission. Here the information is much less detailed, with no specifics as to patient identity being provided. Examples of this type of information include the waiting times for hospital admission. This can be used to make judgements on the efficiency of the health authority and wider governmental policy.

■ Health Informatics and Foundations of Nursing Practice

We are now beginning to gain an impression of the importance of health informatics, but it may still be unclear as to the relevance of informatics to clinical nurses, let alone nursing students. Why does this strange sounding topic represent a foundation of nursing practice? This is a reasonable question to ask, especially as much of this book focuses on the more traditional nursing skills. Yet information within health care is said to be the concern of all who are allied to patient care (Abbott et al., 2004). When we consider the scale of modern health care, the reasons for this begin to become apparent.

The NHS operates on an enormous scale (Figure 18.1), with over 1.6 million patients contacting the NHS per day (Crisp, 2004). The scale of this operation, when combined with modern advances in medical and communications technology, generates a massive quantity and variety of factual data, which must be processed into information before they can become useful. This process requires careful coordination if valuable data are not to become lost or unexpectedly changed (known as data corruption). The need for quality information management within health care has never been higher, and this requires the direct input of nurses at all levels.

Although nurses are not the only professionals involved in health care, they play a crucial role in health-care provision and an important role in the management of information and knowledge within any care setting (Hebda et al., 2005). The scale of involvement nurses have is illustrated in Figure 18.2, which shows that qualified

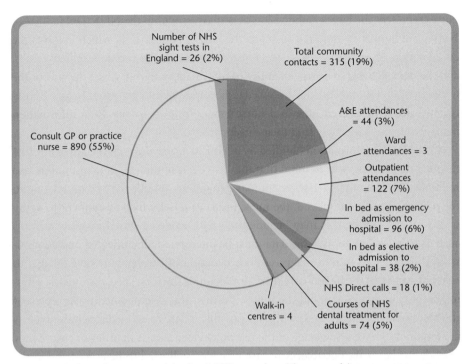

Figure 18.1 ● **Contacts with the NHS per day (thousands)** (Crisp, 2004. Crown copyright material is reproduced with the permission of the Controller of HMSO and the Queen's Printer for Scotland)

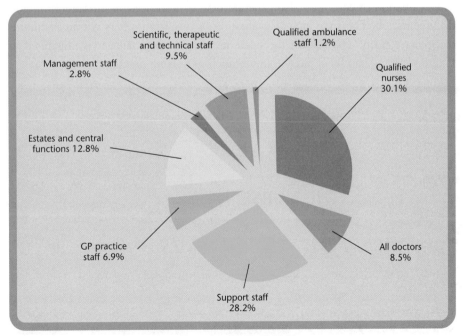

Figure 18.2 ● **Number of staff in the NHS (2003)** (adapted from DoH, 2003a)

nurses represent the largest subdivision of employees within the NHS (DoH, 2003a). Nurses are frequently required to act as the hub of patient care, which involves the coordination of patient services, including the input of the multidisciplinary team, and the management of a large quantity of information. In this sense, the role of the nurse is complex and nursing knowledge becomes central to patient care. Subsequently, it can be argued, one of a nurse's many roles is to act as an information manager for the patients within their direct care.

Consider the information handled by a 'typical' nurse through the application of the nursing process. Bear in mind that this process is not linear, but continuous and multifaceted. The nursing assessment may provide an abundance of data relating to the patient's condition. Indeed, the nurse needs to select which assessment to apply in any given context; this may include the use of evidence-based assessment tools such as pain-scoring tools. This data must be interpreted, documented and communicated in order to form a diagnosis. The planning of care may involve referral to other members of the health-care team, for example doctors, specialist nurses, physiotherapists and occupational therapists. Further, the care planned must represent the best possible practice and, wherever possible, relate to an evidence base. Nurses are required to have knowledge of the relevant evidence base in order to ensure they provide the best care possible. Any care provided will need to be considered in the context of the wider caring environment. For example, the nurse must identify the priorities of care within a group of patients. This has implications for the management of risk and resources in order to ensure patient safety and promote health. The evaluation of care may also generate new data in need of interpretation and documentation. This may include evaluation of care from others within the multidisciplinary team. The role of the nurse as information manager is illustrated in Figure 18.3 and can be applied to any branch of nursing practice.

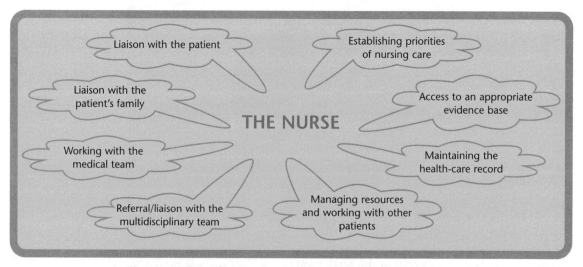

Figure 18.3 ● The nurse as information manager

Casebox 18.1

Sarah is 19 months old and has recently been admitted to the children's ward with a suspected infection. Mandy, a student nurse, is asked to measure Sarah's body temperature as part of her admission to the ward.

What information does a student nurse handle when asked to measure a child's body temperature?

■ Perhaps the most obvious information that is handled by the student in this scenario is that relating to the child's temperature, although it should be acknowledged that a great deal of additional assessment information may be gained from such a patient encounter. A single measurement of body temperature when treated in isolation is of little value; however, when compared to known normal values, the measurement can help to provide an indication of the patient's general condition. Let us imagine that in this case the temperature measurement is high, indicating that Sarah is **pyrexial**. Mandy now has several items of important information; Sarah's temperature measurement, the fact that Sarah is pyrexial and the degree of severity of this pyrexia. The knowledge required for Mandy to recognise Sarah's pyrexia is important, as this facilitates the extension of knowledge in relation to Sarah's condition.

■ Mandy now has a responsibility to ensure that this information is managed properly in order to ensure the correct treatment is provided; but what should Mandy do with the information she now has? It is essential that the information relating to Sarah's temperature be communicated to those who need to know. This requires Mandy to have knowledge of who to contact and how to manage this contact. For example, should Mandy tell the parents, her mentor, the doctor, other patients or everyone? Her choices at this point are central to the patient's care and that of the family. Mandy should of course document the finding; this may aid both the communication of the result to others and the establishment of a baseline from which future temperature measurements can be compared. Now she must decide where the result should be documented and how. The observation chart is a logical start, but the result should also be documented, along with any action taken, within the patient's medical record.

■ This brief scenario shows how nurses use knowledge to manage data and low-level information to help generate newer information at a higher level. In addition, the scenario illustrates how nurses have a responsibility to manage information appropriately. Should Mandy choose not to act on her findings, then the risk of Sarah's condition deteriorating will increase. This is a crucial point: nurses of any level have a central role to play in the management of clinical information. If this information is not handled appropriately, then the risk of harm increases.

---

pyrexial

experiencing a raised body temperature or fever

■ Data, Information and Knowledge

It is important to consider the central concepts of data, information and knowledge in order to gain a fuller appreciation of the role of informatics within health care. This should not be limited to the individual definitions associated to each term, but more importantly on how the terms are connected and interrelated.

Data and information

data

a single item or fact, without any sense of context, for example a number

data corruption

a process in which data have become unexpectedly changed, causing an alteration or loss of accuracy when interpreted

data validation

the process of ensuring data accuracy

Data is the word used to describe an item of fact without any explanation of how it might relate to other things, in essence a symbol. The word can be used in a singular sense, for example a single item; or in a collective sense, for example a collection or 'set' of items (although the pleural term datum is also used in this latter sense). **Data corruption** is the term used to describe data that are inaccurate, lost or unexpectedly changed. This represents a significant risk when applying any type of information system. One accepted method of ensuring accuracy, a process also known as **data validation**, is by ensuring the data are recorded at source, that is, at the patient's bedside (Abbott et al., 2004).

Data exist without a known sense of context or meaning. Take, for example, the following three eight-digit numbers: 14051935, 15071963, and 20041988. These numbers represent a mystery in regard to their significance unless some understanding of context is applied – a type of key to provide details of how these facts relate to the real world. The provision of such a key helps the reader to gain some level of understanding, and apply context and therefore meaning to the data. For example, if we consider the first of the three numbers listed above, but add the context of a known key, the data is transformed into information – a date (see Figure 18.4).

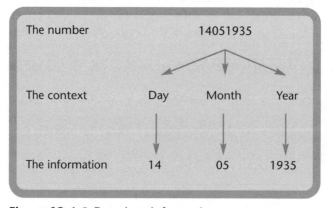

Figure 18.4 ● Data into information

Essentially, information is the understanding of some kind of relationship between data and the real world. From this example, it is possible to see how information is constructed of data and an understanding of contextual meaning:

Information = Data + Context + Meaning

To fully appreciate the dynamic nature of information, it is important to understand that the meaning applied to data is dependent on any one individual's interpretation. What represents information to one person may still represent data to another. For example, let us reconsider the three numbers mentioned earlier. Using the context that each number represents – a date – we can now present the following information:

14051935 = 14 May 1935
15071963 = 15 July 1963
20041988 = 20 April 1988

This is undoubtedly a positive step; we have added context to the original data (day, month and year) and a sense of meaning (date). However, despite our knowledge of how to interpret the original numbers, our sense of context and meaning remains quite low. What does each date symbolise? Is it a date of birth, a notable date in history, or does the date (the data) represent something entirely different? The need for interpretation in regard to the significance of the date requires additional interpretation of contextual meaning. On this level, the dates are actually still only data, as each date is still only a fact without contextual meaning. Alternatively, we could describe information along a continuum, as illustrated in Figure 18.5.

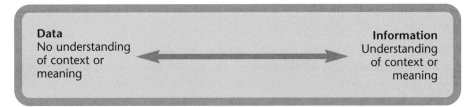

Data
No understanding of context or meaning

Information
Understanding of context or meaning

Figure 18.5 ● Information continuum

In summary, information only exists when an understanding of contextual meaning can be applied to any given data. Understanding the context and meaning of the data can facilitate interpretation of the facts presented. In this sense, information is dynamic – it changes depending on the level of understanding applied. What is information on one level may be just data on another

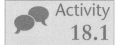

Activity 18.1

Within your practice environment, try to identify 10 items of information relating to a specific patient. Consider what specific data are involved in the construction of the information. How were these data interpreted? What was the key to produce the information?

Link

Chapter 7 discusses the measurement of blood pressure.

level, depending on the specific context applied and whether that context has any significant meaning to the user. Information, therefore, is portrayed as an abstract concept, that is, information only exists when the context applied has significant meaning to the individual or system making the interpretation. Information can therefore also be presented as data plus interpretation: Now try Activity 18.1 using the following example as a guide.

Information = Data + Interpretation

Knowledge

Knowledge is the level of understanding required in order to use information constructively and purposefully. Imagine a patient is being treated on a surgical ward: as a student nurse you are asked to measure the patient's blood pressure – for clarity we will call the patient Mr Smith.

We know that in order to measure Mr Smith's blood pressure accurately, certain things need to be done in sequence, for example ensuring the patient's sleeve is moved prior to applying the cuff. This is an example of *procedural knowledge*: information gained through experience is synthesised in order to allow you to 'know how' to act. When the skill is complete and a blood pressure measurement is obtained, then the result needs to be interpreted. This requires the ability to 'know that' one measurement is considered normal while another measurement is abnormal. This is an example of *declarative knowledge*. Once the result is known, it must be documented. This requires *acquaintanceship knowledge* in order to identify the correct patient's file or the correct place within the file.

So, knowledge can be split into three broad classes, procedural, declarative and acquaintanceship. In reality, these classifications are largely academic and a degree of overlap is possible. For example, knowing that a sleeve left on the arm will interfere with hearing the Korotkoff sounds (an example of declarative knowledge) may be combined with knowing the correct technical sequence to guide action (procedural knowledge). In the rest of this chapter, knowledge is used as a blanket term to describe any one of the three classifications.

It is important to note that knowledge of any given subject requires the synthesis of information with past experience to provide a higher degree of context. This process allows us to form a greater level of understanding of the subject. In simple terms, knowledge is the ability to organise information so that it may become useful. Knowledge is used to guide our decisions, for example what action to take next. Without knowledge, the sequencing, interpretation and reporting of Mr Smith's blood pressure measurement would probably have been inaccurate, resulting in the potential for incorrect treatment.

The data, information, knowledge and wisdom hierarchy

Knowledge is in essence a complex concept (Hebda et al., 2005), yet what links the concept of data, information, knowledge and wisdom together is the degree of contextual understanding applied. This is illustrated in Figure 18.6 as a hierarchy in the form of a pyramid.

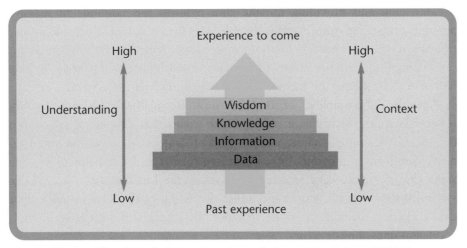

Figure 18.6 ● The data, information, knowledge and wisdom (DIKW) hierarchy

In Figure 18.6, the bottom level of the hierarchy is represented by data and relates to no understanding of contextual meaning. As understanding and context are increased from a low level to a higher level, movement through the hierarchy occurs; initially from data to information, then to knowledge and finally to wisdom. Progression from one level to the next assumes that there is an increased appreciation of context through the synthesis of experience leading to a greater level of understanding. Put simply, the better the understanding of a subject, the more experience can be placed in context to develop new knowledge. As the production of knowledge involves the perception of experience in context, and any given experience may be perceived in a number of different ways, it is possible to see why information may be passed on relatively easily but knowledge needs to be learned by the individual.

Implications for nursing

The distinctions of data, information, knowledge and wisdom are largely theoretical and, in reality, the boundaries of each category overlap and merge – the process is complex and non-linear. To a degree this has been illustrated through the description of information – depending on your individual perspective, information may be still be perceived as data. Some of you may have experienced this phenomenon as you attempted Activity 18.1 (above). This exercise required consideration of the knowledge required to interpret data into information – a process that is often taken for granted – after all, it is normal behaviour to attempt to make sense of our environment. As we gain new experiences, we undergo a process of learning, assimilating data into information and knowledge that then influences the way we interact with our surroundings.

Managing and providing nursing care requires the synthesis of massive amounts of data into information. Knowledge is then required to provide a sense of order to the information, and inform decisions regarding how we go about responding to the infinite variety of experiences that may possibly arise. To help in this process, we rely on the use of a variety of information systems.

Consider the example of an admission form. Regardless of whether the form is paper based or electronic, it is designed to ensure that data are classified into data types, for example name, address, next of kin, doctor/consultant and diagnosis. The form is presented in a structured format and this helps to provide some clue as to the data required. In essence, the form is also a knowledge system; if they so wish, nurses can utilise the layout of the form to guide their data collection, helping to ensure that the assessment is thorough and avoids accidental omissions or errors.

A second example is the use of a nursing record. This document is used to record and evaluate any care provided to the patient. It is a lasting record that can be accessed by anyone needing to know the history of the patient's nursing care. As such, a variety of other professionals need to have access to it. It may be used to communicate care needs or it may be used for management purposes, such as audit. It will also be used in the event of a complaint. Here it is worth stressing a key limitation of any information system – the integrity of the data within it. Nurses are often in the position of recording data. If this data is inaccurate, then so will the interpretation made from it. In simple terms, it is crucial for nurses to have knowledge of what data is required and how to go about recording this data accurately.

Nursing knowledge is difficult to define. It is constructed by the assimilation of information and experience and it is used to guide nursing action. Conventionally, nursing has used tradition, trial and error, personal experience and role modelling to acquire a knowledge base (Hebda et al., 2005). For example, think of the traditional perception of a matron – a matriarch, the epitome of nursing perfection. Such a model is now outdated and the role of the modern matron is more associated with the provision of managerial leadership and the promotion of quality (Savage and Scott, 2004). Equally, there is pressure for nursing to develop a knowledge base using a foundation of objective research data synthesised into evidence of best practice. National Service Frameworks (NSFs) illustrate the importance of this knowledge base at a national level.

Nursing knowledge is only one component of a larger knowledge base used to inform patient care. It is therefore essential that this knowledge be underpinned by sound information. This information may relate directly to the individual patient or more generally to guidelines for practice, while further information can be shown to be challenging the very methods in which care is accessed and quality care provided (see Casebox 18.2).

Casebox 18.2

It is 9 pm and **Michelle**, a new mother, is becoming worried about her son Jack. Jack is 11 weeks old and seems irritable, he is not interested in feeding, feels hot and Michelle has noticed that his nappies have not been as wet as normal. She decides to check online for information and goes to the self-help section of the NHS Direct website (www.nhsdirect.nhs.uk). There she finds a link on how to recognise the signs of illness in a baby and she notices that several of Jack's symptoms are listed. Growing more concerned, she decides to call the NHS Direct helpline.

On contacting the helpline, Michelle is asked several questions about the nature of her call by a health adviser before being transferred to a qualified nurse. The nurse asks a further series of questions in relation to Jack and enters Michelle's responses into a computer-based information system.

From the responses to these questions, the nurse advises Michelle to remove any excess clothing from Jack and to take Jack to see the out-of-hours GP at her local hospital. The nurse reassures Michelle that this is just a precaution to ensure that Jack is not becoming dehydrated. She also informs Michelle that she will contact the out-of-hours GP service and tell them to expect Michelle with baby Jack.

Casebox 18.2 illustrates how technological development has facilitated new methods to access health-related information. This can be shown to have influenced the perception of health-care provision by both patients and staff alike, and improved the quality of the service provided. The advent of NHS Direct (and the regional variants NHS Direct Wales and NHS 24) has brought an immediacy to a patient's ability to access health care. As such, patients benefit from gaining rapid and appropriate advice, while local services benefit from a reduction in unnecessary attendance. The development of new high-tech health-care systems has in turn challenged the role of the nurse. Casebox 18.2 shows how the nurse uses a form of telephone triage to form an assessment of the patient and give appropriate guidance. This is far removed from the traditional perception of a nurse in a starched white uniform administering injections.

In the following sections, we will begin to consider the use of information systems within health care, and how these systems may impact on the patient, the health professional, the health authority and the wider public.

■ A Systems-based Approach to Health Care

A system can be described as set of elements that work together to form a whole with an implied or explicit objective (Introna, 1997). For example, this book employs a system to assist you in your learning. It is organised into chapters with a similar structure and feel; it employs uniform conventions within the text to provide information in an ordered way, for example reader activities. The book also has an explicit objective – to support your learning in relation to the fundamentals of nursing.

Large amounts of information are managed through the application of information systems. Information systems are predominantly concerned with an analysis of purpose, design, use and effects of information within organisations (Fitzgerald, 2002, cited in Paul, 2002). According to the OUP *Dictionary of Computing*, information systems represent a multidisciplinary study, the main disciplines involved being those of organisational business and management studies and computer science. Health informatics represents a specialised subset of information systems. Here, the common organisational purpose is connected to health-care provision, and consequently the systems developed relate ultimately to the provision of patient care. This can be argued to be true even if the systems employed are primarily related to management.

Health informatics may involve systems that at first seem far removed from the provision of patient care. However, it is important to remember that each and every system used within the health-care sector can ultimately affect patients or their families. When considering the use of health-care information systems, it is vital to consider fully the impact these systems have on patients and their care.

Casebox 18.3

From a recent audit using the finance information system, it has become apparent that Fictional Mental Health Trust is heading for overspend. Information from the audit indicates that the overspend results from a high sickness rate among nursing staff and the reliance on external agency staff to cover shifts. Fictional Mental Health Trust is consequently suspending the use of all non-essential agency staff in an attempt to limit costs.

Casebox 18.3 shows how an information system, primarily related to finance, has the potential to impact on patient care. The use of a financial information system has provided managers with the necessary information to implement change and minimise the threat of overspend. By adding controls to the use of external agency nursing staff, the Trust hopes to cut costs. However, this places ward managers in a challenging position; how do they find appropriately skilled cover if they cannot freely book external agency staff with specialised skills. Additionally, it could be argued that the knowledge of difficulties in finding suitable cover may discourage staff from taking sick leave when it is really needed. The result could potentially impact on the quality of patient care and staff well-being.

■ Health Informatics: Putting the Patient First

The notion of a patient journey through the health-care system is central to any consideration of health informatics, as this provides an ability to visualise the various information needs that exist. This journey begins with the patient's first contact with the health service and completes at the point of discharge. Casebox 18.4 illustrates a brief example of a patient journey, along with some of the information needs of the patient; however, any one patient's journey may vary from another in a multitude of ways. Figure 18.7 illustrates the journey detailed in Casebox 18.4 by plotting key points on a timeline.

fetal heart rate

the measurement of heart rate for unborn child (fetus)

urinalysis

an analysis of the chemical make-up of urine often used as a method of health screening

---

Casebox 18.4

Donna suspects that she may be pregnant and arranges for an appointment with her GP. At the surgery, a pregnancy test confirms the pregnancy. The GP explains Donna's immediate options and asks Donna to arrange an appointment to see the local midwife. A referral letter is sent from the GP to the local general hospital.

When Donna sees the midwife, an estimated due date is calculated. One week later, Donna receives an appointment through the post for an ultrasound scan. Three weeks later the scan is

performed and this confirms the midwife's initial estimate of dates. Donna is given a picture of her developing baby.

Donna sees her local midwife again two weeks after the scan and a detailed medical history is taken. Four weeks later, Donna sees the midwife again and a variety of blood samples are obtained, which are sent to the laboratory at the local hospital for analysis. Meanwhile, an appointment for a 20-week ultrasound scan is sent through the post. The scan goes well and

Donna is given the results from her blood tests. Donna is asked to arrange an appointment with her local midwife in five week's time (25 weeks pregnant).

When she sees the midwife, she is asked to arrange further appointments every two or three weeks. It is explained to Donna that these appointments are intended to monitor the course of her pregnancy. Measurements of **fetal heart rate**, maternal blood pressure and **urinalysis** are to be recorded in Donna's care record. At 32 weeks of pregnancy, Donna and her partner start to attend parentcraft sessions at the local hospital.

At 39 weeks pregnant, Donna starts to feel labour pains and decides to contact the labour ward. The phone call is documented by the labour ward, but at this stage Donna is advised to stay at home. A few hours later,

Donna's waters break and she contacts the labour ward again. This time she is advised to come into hospital and within several hours Donna has delivered normally a healthy baby boy. Donna is now transferred to the postnatal ward with her son.

Donna remains in hospital for two days and receives daily checks by the midwife.

The local midwife visits Donna at home the day after her discharge. Two days later the midwife returns and performs a blood spot screening test from her son's heel. Four days later Donna receives an initial visit from the local health visitor. A week later the midwife makes a final visit and Donna is formally discharged from her obstetric care.

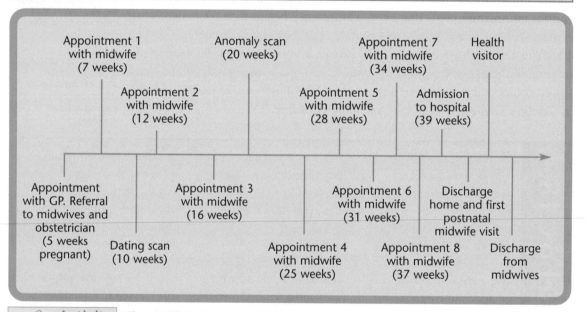

Figure 18.7 ● A patient's journey

Activity 18.2

Within your current practice area, document the progress of a patient from admission to discharge along a timeline as shown in Figure 18.7. What are the information needs of the patient at the various stages?

Activity 18.2 asks you to map a patient's journey through the health-care system and identify that patient's need for information at the various stages. The provision of this information is dependent on numerous elements working together, in other words, it is dependent on systems. Consider some of the systems involved in the care of Donna outlined in Casebox 18.4: referral systems, case note systems, antenatal care systems, parentcraft, birth plans, triage systems, admission and discharge systems, postnatal care systems, hospital transport systems, postal systems, hospital support systems. The list could go on and on, but each system has one common connection – it ultimately impacts in some way on patient care. Until quite recently, this crucial point was often missed and health-care staff too often perceived themselves as the primary user of health-related systems (Abbott et al., 2004). **Remember, any system used in health care is always connected to the patient.** Let us now consider one such system in greater depth – the patient care record system.

Patient care record system

Traditionally, the patient care record has been based on paper documents and can be described as being episode oriented (Hebda et al., 2005) and location specific (Abbott et al., 2004). Essentially, this means that the record is usually a physical paper file that is added to every time the patient undergoes an episode of care, for example an appointment with the GP. Equally, the record of care is normally local to the point of care, hence GPs, hospitals and other associated health-care providers may all retain separate patient records.

Consider the types of data that may be included in a typical patient record (Table 18.1). We can see that the record can be broadly classified into demographics and patient history. The patient history can be said to be episodic, but also longitudinal, in that each new episode of care adds to a developing history of past patient contacts. Together, these combine to form a historical continuum of patient contact for the care setting possessing the record.

Table 18.1 Types of information stored in the patient record

Demographic data	Patient history
Name	Family history
Address	Past episodes of care
Telephone	● Previous/current assessment details
Religion	● Past/current diagnosis
Next of kin	● Past/current care plans
	● Evidence of care implementation
	● Evidence of care evaluation
	● Referrals
	● Results from diagnostic tests
	Discharge/follow-up
	● Discharge letters
	● Referral replies
	● Patient correspondence
	● Other notices, for example legal correspondence

Within the care record, there is a mass of data and information types. It is essential that data be added to with the utmost care if the resulting information is to retain value. As previously described, data need to be accurate and complete if they are to be of maximum benefit (Abbott et al., 2004). Indeed, there is a common computer assumption (axiom) related to data entry: garbage in, garbage out (**GIGO**). In other words, if the data input into a system is incorrect, so will the resulting output (Speake, 2000), and with regard to health care, this could have disastrous results.

It is worth considering how a patient care record might currently be used, although the uses of specific care records will vary depending on the explicit/implicit intentions of the record keeper. The record is a store for patient-specific data and information. Access to the store is primarily intended for anyone working within the immediate care setting. For example, it is assumed that the staff who work within any particular health centre are usually the most likely to need access to patient records kept within that centre. The number of people needing potential access to a particular record for whatever reason will vary, as will the specifics of the circumstances leading to the need for access. One such variable is the scale of operations within any given organisation. For example, a hospital record will potentially need to be accessed by a range of people working in a variety of departments depending on the individual needs of the patient, whereas a patient record held within a dentist surgery is only likely to be accessed by the staff of that surgery on each patient visit.

Consideration should be given to the limitations of the current paper-based system and the move towards electronic patient records (EPRs). Paper-based systems have numerous drawbacks. The paper record is a physical resource that can only be in one place at one time. To overcome this problem, there is a tendency to use multiple records, resulting in the fragmentation of information. For example, the separation of the primary care (GP) record from the secondary care (hospital) record results in the fragmentation of documented care. Often a search is needed to locate a specific care record, and at times these records will be unavailable. Key information relevant to the patient's condition may be buried deep within the paper record and searching through the file can be both difficult and time-consuming. **Data integrity** is often compromised through the misfiling of entries and the use of poor handwriting.

Opposing these limitations are the benefits of an EPR, which are well documented (DoH, 1998; Abbott et al., 2004; Hebda et al., 2005):

- An electronic record is effectively a virtual record; this means that instead of storing the specifics of any one patient in a paper file, the information is stored in an electronic file located within a central computer system

GIGO

an acronym for garbage in, garbage out, meaning that if inaccurate data are entered into a system, any information based on that data will also be inaccurate

data integrity

the extent to which stored data is complete and accurate

- Lack of physical form means that the record's presentation can be changed depending on the needs of each user, thus helping to protect the patient's confidentiality and making the search for relevant information easier
- Data entry can be subjected to tests for accuracy, even though the integrity of the data entered would still be subject to the individual entering the correct data
- Information can be presented in a clear and legible format, helping to minimise the risks associated with handwritten texts
- Searching an individual patient record, or even searching across any number of patient records, becomes significantly easier.

These later benefits are dependent on the use of data in a consistent and known format and this has led to the development of clinical coding schemas.

Perhaps one of the greatest potential benefits of an EPR for a patient is the ability to integrate all the disparate health records into one single patient record. This represents a fundamental shift in the concept of patient information, as ownership of the record moves away from the organisation holding the record and is transferred to the patient. The logic of this is difficult to dispute – the information held in any record does after all belong to the patient and not to the document in which it is detailed. Such integration could be argued to improve patient care through the sharing of relevant information. Abbott et al. (2004) cite the example of an accident and emergency department gaining potential benefit from being able to access GP patient records for relevant drug history. A second benefit is to the individual organisations concerned, as the need for repetitious data collection would be removed and access to information for audit purposes would be increased.

Indeed, the benefits of a single integrated electronic patient care record are so substantial that the national NHS strategy for information in health (National Programme for Information Technology in the NHS (NPfIT), 2005) includes the development of just such a health record. This has led to the development and installation of various technological infrastructures from which integrated records can eventually be based. Yet this type of development is not without its potential problems. For example, integrated care records are dependent on the use of communications technologies to transport information from one system to another. This represents a significant risk to patient confidentiality and the integrity of data. Any integrated records system must show that these risks can be safely managed before they are implemented.

The development of an integrated EPR perhaps represents the most important shift in the documentation of patient care since the first medical records were created. Although focus has largely been placed on the like-for-like replacement of paper records with electronic records, the process of integrating these systems is slowly progressing. Certainly, the trend for moving to electronic records is set and is likely to continue.

▓ Health Informatics: At the Point of Care

Although the patient remains central in the provision of all health informatics systems, it must be acknowledged that care providers can also receive benefit from their use. For example, the patient as the owner of the care record should have direct access to the information within it, but it is the health-care provider who is most likely to use the information as part of care provision. It is therefore the health provider who is most likely to access the care record. Yet how does the health provider know what data and information to enter into the care record? What informs their searching of the record or even the questions they ask patients? How do practitioners decide on the care to provide? The answer of course is based on their knowledge.

Data do not generate themselves, nor does the resultant information self-generate. Knowledge is required in order to collect data and, as such, nurses must be able to access resources to support their individual learning and develop their practice. As emphasis is given within health care to the concepts of 'best practice' and 'evidence-based practice', there is a corresponding need to develop knowledge management initiatives to capture, retain, reuse and impart the necessary tools to facilitate understanding in others. To better illustrate how such tools can inform nursing practice, let us consider two examples: the National Institute for Health and Clinical Excellence and the World Wide Web.

National Institute for Health and Clinical Excellence

Link
✦✦ Link
Chapter 10 also discusses the role of NICE.

Officially launched on 1 April 2005, the National Institute for Health and Clinical Excellence (NICE) is an independent agency providing national guidance on the promotion of health and the prevention and treatment of ill-health (NICE, 2005). This relatively new organisation has a remit for the provision of guidance in three distinct subdomains:

1. *Centre for Public Health Excellence*: developing guidance on the promotion of good health and the prevention of ill-health. Guidance will be in the form of recommended interventions (types of activity), for example how specific lifestyle changes can result in a reduced risk of illness.
2. *Centre for Health Technology Evaluation*: developing guidance on the use of new and existing medicines, treatments and procedures within the NHS. Evaluations consider both clinical and economic evidence and recognise that treatment may be both expensive and value for money. In addition, this branch of NICE provides guidance on the clinical use of interventional procedures and decision support systems (computer software intended to help health professionals make a diagnosis or treatment decisions).

3. *Centre for Clinical Practice:* intended for the formation of specific clinical guidelines. Guidelines are intended to help clinical staff to provide treatment to patients with specific diseases and conditions in order to improve the chances of patients becoming well (NICE, 2005).

Although an independent organisation, NICE is still part of the NHS and consequently any recommendations published have significant impact. According to NICE (2005, p. 9):

> Once NICE publishes clinical guidance, health professionals and the organisations that employ them are expected to take it fully into account when deciding what treatments to give people. However, NICE guidance does not replace the knowledge and skills of individual health professionals who treat patients; it is still up to them to make decisions about a particular patient in consultation with the patient and/or their guardian or carer when appropriate.

From this, it is possible to identify two major implications of knowledge management within the NHS. First, the responsibility for being aware of the guidance available is shared by the individual practitioner and the employing organisation. Here the organisation may be expected to ensure that national guidance is incorporated into local policy and that individual employees can gain access to the information provided. The individual practitioner must keep abreast of the guidance published and any potential implications to their practice. Second, published guidance does not equal rules for practice. The guidance is intended to support practice through the provision of evidence, but this evidence must be considered carefully in relation to the specific circumstances of each individual patient before it is used. Equally, patient preference is seen as an essential factor in decisions relating to treatment. The published guidance of NICE provides support for one prong of the evidence-based practice trident (see Figure 18.8).

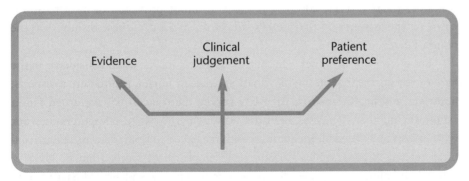

Figure 18.8 ● The evidence-based practice trident

The World Wide Web

internet

a worldwide network of computers with the capacity to communicate to one another using set protocols

Web

known more formally as the World Wide Web; relates to a network of linked documents (often called pages) stored on computers (called servers) connected to the internet. These documents can be accessed by other computers via the internet

hypertext link

a connection from one element on a web page document (for example text or image) to a different element either on the same web page or new web document

The word **internet** has come to represent a global computer network providing numerous information and communication resources, for example email and file transfer systems. The World Wide Web (**Web**) is the graphical interface of the internet. It is a global information system based upon billions of electronic documents linked by virtual connections known as **hypertext links**. When one web page is displayed, the user can click on certain text containing links that cause the computer to load a different document – a new web page. The Web is massive in its scale and, given the presence of an internet connection, anyone can access it to either read the documents published or indeed publish new documents. It is this ease of access that simultaneously represents the Web's greatest asset and its greatest drawback.

Health professionals and patients alike can access the internet for health-related information on an unprecedented global scale. However, the massive number of available resources, when combined with the open nature of the Web, leads to important limitations for use, especially when looking to inform clinical practice:

1. There is the problem of deciding what information is required and then sourcing this among the multitude of available websites. Is it a reasonable expectation for health-care providers to be accessing the Web at the point of care delivery?
2. Once content has been found, how can the health professional be sure of the credibility of the information gained?

A discussion related to each of these questions could easily form book chapters in their own right and a thorough exploration cannot be given here. It is interesting to note, however, that the use of online resources, for example the National Electronic Library for Health, has been perceived to be central to the national NHS information strategy since 1998 (DoH, 1998) and this trend continues today (NPfIT, 2005). The focus of online provision of information is based on the assumption that nurses will be able to access these resources at the point of care.

This assumption is somewhat controversial, especially when considered in the light of recent research on the information needs of nurses, health-care assistants, midwives and health visitors. An RCN survey (Bertulis, 2005) identified that a significant number of nurses reported not having access to computers at work when it was most needed. Inequalities with regard to computer access existed and often related to geographical location and employment sector (that is, NHS or private). In addition, the need for computer training was identified as a priority by a significant number of survey respondents. Guides for recommended websites

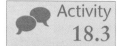 Activity
18.3

In your current placement area, identify all the potential sources of information available to you. Consider what obstacles exist to accessing these sources of information.

were requested (see the list of useful websites at the end of the chapter), while employers' attitudes towards information-seeking activities at work were shown to impact on nurses' continued development away from work. Similarly, employers' attitudes were also found to be related to the likelihood of nurses changing practice as a result of information-searching at work. It should be stressed that survey results can only be generalised with extreme caution – at best a survey represents a single snapshot of one moment in time and therefore the findings of the RCN survey may not be representative of the country as a whole.

■ The Management and Organisation of Care

The developments of NICE and the use of the internet as an information resource represent two examples of how health professionals can seek to develop their knowledge. However, as the limitations highlighted by the RCN survey have indicated (Bertulis, 2005), the development of resources to support clinicians must be underpinned by appropriate management strategies if patients are ultimately to benefit. This finding supports that of the Wanless Report (2002), an evidence-based assessment of the long-term resource needs within the NHS, which reported that major advances in the effective use of information and communication technologies are required if the NHS is to deliver efficient, high-quality services in the future.

The government has published numerous key strategy documents intended to provide a common vision to local authorities on the development of health services and the management of information (DoH, 1998, 2000, 2002a). The most recent of these are plotted on a timeline, shown in Figure 18.9. Also recognised is the need for increased investment in relation to IT. This is evidenced by a £6 billion investment in IT made to date and a further £2.3 billion investment set aside for the next three years (NPfIT, 2005). Key to the success of such investment is an understanding of the difference between effectiveness and efficiency (see Casebox 18.5 below).

Chart 18.1 summarises the key objectives of the current information strategy – the National Programme for Information Technology in the NHS (NPfIT, 2005). However, it is possible to identify several central themes from the various strategy documents, including:

● Placing the patient at the centre of care and ensuring that the design of care services is not biased towards the needs of the institution providing care
● A reduction of inequality in health-care provision, for example equal access to specialist medical services
● The development of quality through the continued development of national standards and the continued support of NHS employees.

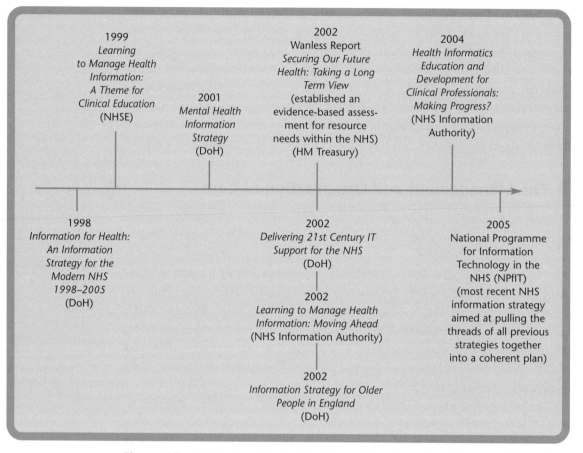

Figure 18.9 ● Timeline illustrating the publication of health strategies and other related documents to health informatics

Several of these themes have already been briefly explored in this chapter. Alternative examples can be accessed from the case studies provided by the National Programme for IT in NHS (NPfIT) website (http://www.connecting-forhealth.nhs.uk/casestudies/). However, in order to provide a more detailed outline of how health informatics is central to the organisation and management of care delivery at both local and national level, let us now consider the example of National Service Frameworks.

Chart 18.1 ● The National Programme for Information Technology in the NHS (NPfIT): key objectives
....

● *New National Network (N3):* to provide a suitable technological infrastructure on which future services can be run
● *A Secure National Email Directory Service:* the development of a centrally managed national email and directory service for the NHS

- *NHS Care Records Service:* to develop integrated electronic health records
- *Electronic Booking Service:* for the arrangement of appointments and the management of referrals
- *Electronic Transmission of Prescriptions:* to reduce the risk of prescription errors and make easier the process for issuing and collecting medicines
- *Picture Archiving and Communications Systems (PACS):* to capture, store, distribute and display digital images such as electronic X-rays or scans
- *Secondary Uses Services (SUS):* for the collection and use of anonymous patient-based data for uses other than clinical care (for example incident reporting)
- *National Library for Health:* the development of a library and information resource for all NHS staff
- *Quality Management and Analysis System (QMAS):* national IT system for the provision of objective evidence to GP practices and PCTs for the quality of care delivered to patients
- *GP to GP Service:* the development of a service to electronically transfer the electronic component of a GP care record to a new practice when a patient registers with a new practice.

angioplasty

a surgical procedure usually used to unblock a narrowed or occluded artery

---

Casebox 18.5

Processes that are effective can be defined as those for which a set purpose is achieved, whereas processes that are efficient relate to those that limit unnecessary effort and expense. Consider the cases of three patients admitted to separate hospital Trusts after suffering a myocardial infarction (MI):

Patient 1: Mr Smith is provided with immediate specialist cardiology care on admission. He remains an inpatient for 12 days and receives excellent treatment including angioplasty. On discharge, he visits a cardiac rehabilitation clinic three times a week and benefits from the use of a purpose-built gymnasium and hydrotherapy pool, plus expert help in making changes to his lifestyle. He even manages to stop smoking. Within three months, he resumes his full-time job. Total cost of NHS resources for three months = £80,000.

Patient 2: Mr Jones is also provided with immediate cardiology care, but in this case it is led by a consultant in general medicine. Angioplasty is unavailable due to budgetary constraints and Mr Jones is discharged home to the care of his GP after five days of inpatient treatment. Mr Jones does not make any lifestyle changes and continues to smoke 20 cigarettes a day. He develops angina on exertion and fails his medical to resume work. Total cost of NHS resources for three months = £10,000.

Patient 3: Mr Clarke is provided with the same standard of specialist cardiology care that Mr Smith received. However, Mr Clarke is discharged home to the care of his GP after five days. He attends cardiac rehabilitation classes on a weekly basis and is supported to make changes to his lifestyle by visiting the practice nurse at the GP surgery. He is successful in stopping smoking. After three months, Mr Clarke returns to his full-time job. Total cost of NHS resources for three months = £40,000.

Which patient received the most effective, efficient care?

- Mr Smith (patient 1) exemplifies effective health care. Specifically, he has made a full recovery and returned to work. However, the cost of £80 000 could be argued to be too high and therefore inefficient. In simple terms, Mr Smith's case shows how health care can be effective but also inefficient.

- Mr Jones (patient 2) shows the opposite; in this case, the treatment is cheap but ineffective and Mr Jones fails to make a full recovery. Here effectiveness has been sacrificed for short-term efficiency gains, indeed the chronic dependency of Mr Jones is likely to become expensive over the long term.

- Mr Clarke (patient 3) illustrates how care can be both effective and efficient; here Mr Clarke has made a full recovery within the same time period as Mr Smith, but the cost of treatment has been halved by removing needless effort and expense.

National Service Frameworks

Link

Chapters 2 and 3 contain more information related to NSFs.

National Service Frameworks (NSFs) are examples of long-term national strategies related to specific areas of health care; they set specific goals and are defined within set timeframes. Chart 18.2 details the nine areas of health care currently targeted by NSFs. Primary objectives related to the development of NSFs include a focus on health promotion and disease prevention, and the reduction of inequality in relation to health-care provision by the development of agreed national standards. Currently, inequalities in health care exist due to the varying availability of health-care resources on a national level. For example, access to specialist cancer services is dependent on the availability of local resources. By insisting that all local authorities meet specific targets related to agreed standards, it is intended that existing inequalities in relation to the provision and access of health-care services can be minimised.

Each of the NSFs published to date recognises the importance of information management in the implementation of change (Abbott et al., 2004). For example, the NSF on Mental Health was followed by a dedicated strategy for information management (DoH, 2001), as was the NSF for Older People (DoH, 2002b).

Chart 18.2 ● National Service Frameworks

● Mental Health — launched 1999
● Diabetes — launched 1999
● Paediatric Intensive Care — launched 1999
● Cancer Care — launched 2000
● Coronary Heart Disease — launched 2000
● Older People's Services — launched 2001
● Children, Young People and Maternity Services — launched 2004
● Renal Care — launched 2004
● Long Term Conditions — launched 2005

Note: All NSFs are available online at http://www.dh.gov.uk.

Abbott et al. (2004) identify a key distinction between the types of information needed within the various NSFs. First, there is the need for information by service users, carers and the general public in order to realise the potential for health promotion and disease prevention. Second, there exits a need for information related to the clinical progress of individual patients for particular disease types. This is required to monitor progress and support operational management decisions in relation to the status of the health service provided.

There exists a close relationship between the need to collect clinical information and the provision of an integrated patient record as detailed above. Given that the clinical data required need to follow a specific condition as defined by a specific NSF, it can be seen that there exists a need for data collection throughout the patient journey. This is where the benefit of an integrated patient record can be seen. However, Abbott et al. (2004) point out that it is important that the care record does not become disease focused, as this would lead to further fragmentation of the care record rather than integration.

The development of integrated ECRs can therefore be shown to have potential benefits to the management of information for patients – as the central focus of care provision – and the organisation of care management – through enabling the monitoring of performance. The development of integrated ECRs is high on the national strategic agenda for health (DoH, 2000), as managed through the NHS Care Records Service (http://www.connectingforhealth.nhs.uk/programmes/nhscrs). The implementation of such records represents a massive logistical and technological challenge, and so the implementation process is to be staged and is planned to be completed in 2010 (NPfIT, 2005). Given that earlier targets for implementation have not as yet been met, the process may extend well into the next decade.

■ The Wider Public and Health Informatics

So far this chapter has explored the relevance of health informatics, and considered its impact on nursing from the perspective of the patient or carer, the health professional, and the organisation managing the care. Yet the responsibility borne by the health service as a consequence of managing public data has so far received little attention. Issues relating to how data are collected, recorded, used, shared and secured are of key interest to the wider public. Health-related data are sensitive in nature and generic, in that some type of health record is kept on each member of the population. Consideration must be given to how information is governed within health care and the development of fair, legal and ethically acceptable methods of managing data. The umbrella term used to describe this process is 'information governance'.

Information governance

Information governance considers how health-related data is Held, Obtained, Recorded, Used and Shared (HORUS). Specifically, it considers:

- The Data Protection Act 1998
- The Freedom of Information Act 2000
- The NHS Confidentiality Code of Practice (DoH, 2003b)
- Information security management
- Record management.

A thorough understanding of the various components of information governance is not essential for all clinical staff and is therefore beyond the scope of this chapter. However, having some knowledge of the basic principles involved is essential if nurses are to practise in a manner that safeguards the data entrusted to them and protects the confidentiality of the patients within their care.

It is important to note that the Data Protection Act 1998 and the Freedom of Information Act 2000 are both legislative acts. Simply put, this means that they represent the law of the land and are not just applicable to the NHS. A brief description of both these key areas of legislation is provided in Charts 18.3 and 18.4.

Other elements of information governance are broader in their scope than the legislation connected to them. For example, consideration of information security and management should consider, but not be limited by, the scope of the Privacy and Electronic Communications Regulations 2003 – relating to the security of electronic communications – and the Computer Misuse Act 1990, which relates to unauthorised access to computer material.

Chart 18.3 ● Data Protection Act 1998

The Data Protection Act (DPA) 1998 provides individuals with seven statutory rights in regard to information held about them by a third party. The rights of the individual, known as the data subject, are combined with statutory obligations placed on those who process information, known as data controllers. These obligations are summarised as eight principles of good practice.

Link

Chapter 16 further discusses matters related to the Data Protection Act and Freedom of Information Act.

The DPA also distinguishes between 'personal data' and 'sensitive data'. Personal data is described as any information about a living individual that can be identified or be derived from the storage or merging of data held by the data controller. Sensitive data is subject to more stringent controls and is directly relevant to health care, in that it is defined as any data that relate to an individual's:

- Racial or ethnic origin
- Political belief
- Religious or spiritual belief
- Trade union affiliation
- Physical or mental health
- Sexual life
- Alleged or actual criminal activity or sentencing

The rights provided to individuals by the Data Protection Act are as follows:

1. **The right to subject access:** this allows people to find out what information is held about them on computer and within some manual records.
2. **The right to prevent processing:** anyone can ask a data controller not to process information relating to him or her that causes substantial unwarranted damage or distress to them or anyone else.
3. **The right to prevent processing for direct marketing:** anyone can ask a data controller not to process information relating to him or her for direct marketing purposes.
4. **Rights in relation to automated decision-taking:** individuals have a right to object to decisions made only by automatic means, for example when there is no human involvement.
5. **The right to compensation:** an individual can claim compensation from a data controller for damage and distress caused by any breach of the Act. Compensation for distress alone can only be claimed in limited circumstances.
6. **The right to rectification, blocking, erasure and destruction:** individuals can apply to the court to order a data controller to rectify, block or destroy personal details if they are inaccurate or contain expressions of opinion based on inaccurate information.

7. **The right to ask the commissioner to assess whether the Act has been contravened:** if someone believes their personal information has not been processed in accordance with the DPA, they can ask the commissioner to make an assessment. If the Act is found to have been breached and the matter cannot be settled informally, then an enforcement notice may be served on the data controller in question.

The DPA eight principles of good practice are that data must be:

1. Fairly and lawfully processed.
2. Processed for limited purposes.
3. Adequate, relevant and not excessive.
4. Accurate and up to date.
5. Not kept longer than necessary.
6. Processed in accordance with the individual's rights.
7. Secure.
8. Not transferred to countries outside the European economic area unless the country has adequate protection for the individual.

Source: Reproduced with permission from Information Commissioners Office, Data Protection Act Fact Sheet (n.d.).

Chart 18.4 ● Freedom of Information Act 2000

The Freedom of Information Act allows individuals to access information held by public authorities in order to develop a culture of openness and accountability within the public sector. The development of such a culture is hoped to increase general understanding about the operation of public sector bodies, how they spend public money and make their decisions. Each public authority must publish an information scheme as a guide to how information can be accessed. Equally, individuals have a general right to access information held by public authorities, subject to certain exemptions. These exemptions are either absolute or qualified. Where the exemption is absolute, the right to know is completely denied, for example requests for personal data. Where the exemption is qualified, the public authority must consider if the release of the information is in the greater public interest

The five elements of HORUS represent the basis for the principles of information governance. Consideration is now given to each of these areas in turn.

Holding data

A primary concern of the storage of health-related data is the maintenance of confidentiality through the application of appropriate security. Confidentiality has been defined as a duty that arises as one person discloses information to another (DoH, 2003b). It is a requirement of established codes of professional conduct, for example the Nursing and Midwifery Council Code of Professional Conduct (NMC, 2004), and it is a legal right for the patient, regardless of their competence to extend their trust, for example unconscious patients or those detained under the Mental Health Act.

The NHS Confidentiality Code of Practice (DoH, 2003b) examined the nature of confidentiality and put forward a confidentiality model. This model is based on four interconnected principles:

1. *Protect* – look after the patient's information.
2. *Inform* – ensure that patients are aware of how their information is used.
3. *Provide choice* – allow patients to decide whether their information can be disclosed or used in particular ways.
4. *Improve* – always look for better ways to protect, inform and provide choice.

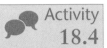

Activity 18.4

Simple precautions can be used to help promote patient confidentiality. Within your practice environment, try to identify how confidentiality could be safeguarded. For example:

- Avoid careless talk
- Always log off the computer
- Turn the computer screen away from the view of onlookers.

Obtaining data

The process of obtaining health-related data should be transparent. This means that the patient should know, wherever possible, what data are being collected, for what reason the data are required, how the data will be used, how long the data will be required for, and how they may be able to access them. It is worth remembering that the information stored within a health-care record is the property of the patient. Under the Data Protection Act 1998, the patient maintains the right to access their own health record. A good example of this transparency in action can be found when contacting the helpline NHS Direct. The automated greeting provided by this service offers patients an opportunity to find out how their information will be stored and used, and this is further supported by information on the NHS Direct website (www.nhsdirect.nhs.uk).

The Data Protection Act 1998 also requires that data should be processed fairly and lawfully and that one of the legislative conditions for the protection of personal or sensitive data is met. In most cases, the explicit consent of the patient (the data subject within health records) represents the condition required. The NHS Confidentiality Code of Practice (DoH, 2003b) emphasises the need for transparency in relation to the collection of personal data, which is reflected within the confidentiality model outlined above.

Recording data

Central to the concept of data-recording is the concept of data integrity. Hebda et al. (2005, p.65) describe data integrity as a process to 'collect, store and retrieve correct, complete and current data'. Data integrity is essential within health care at all levels of data-processing. For example, if any clinical data were inaccurate, out of date or incomplete, it is likely that treatment based on that data would be incorrect. Equally, management or financial decisions based on inaccurate data could be disastrous. Data validity is a key concept to data integrity and is considered briefly below.

Data validity refers to the degree to which data accurately represent what they were originally obtained for. Data validation is therefore a method of ensuring data accuracy and completeness. It is best performed at the time that data are entered and therefore data validation should be a primary concern for all clinical staff. Methods for data validation are commonly applied to computer-based record systems, but data validation procedures should not be limited by the technology used. Validation checks could be as simple as a student asking their mentor if a recorded value is accurate and complete. Timing is essential and data validation should take place at the time data are recorded; realising a previously recorded data value was inaccurate even hours after it was recorded can have potentially lethal implications.

Data use

The main purpose for the collection of patient data may at first appear quite obvious; patients entrust health professionals with information to better inform the care they receive. However, this point of view provides only a narrow perspective and it is important to realise that patient data may be used far more widely. A common method of considering the uses of data is by the classification of primary and secondary use.

Primary use relates to the use of data for the main purpose for which it was originally collected from the individual patient (House of Lords Select Committee on Science and Technology, 2001). Primary use may therefore include those uses of data that relate directly to patient care. However, these may still be fairly broad ranging and can include the use of individual patient data for clinical audit or clinical governance initiatives (DoH, 2003b), for example adverse incident and near-miss reporting. The primary use of data may require that data are shared with other care agencies within and outside the NHS and it is important that patients are aware of when disclosure of information will be necessary.

Secondary use of data relates to uses of existing data that are not connected to the primary purpose of data collection (House of Lords Select Committee on Science and Technology, 2001). Secondary uses include data used within clinical research, financial auditing, health service initiative reporting, and the formation of diagnosis and treatment trends. In some secondary data processes, it may be unlikely that patient confidentiality will be breached. It is therefore uncertain as to whether the patient needs to consent to this use of data.

Sharing data

The concept of data-sharing is closely tied to that of confidentiality. Data should only be shared when absolutely necessary, as sharing increases the risk of security breaches and data corruption. Any form of data-sharing must also be lawful. Of particular relevance are the Data Protection Act 1998 and the Privacy and Electronic Communications Regulations 2003, which apply controls on how data may be shared.

The Caldecott Report (1997) represented a milestone in relation to the security of patient-based information within the NHS. In particular it considered the methods of transferring patient-related data between NHS bodies and non-NHS organisations. In the main, the committee found that data-sharing was performed legitimately and diversely. In some instances, it was found that more patient data were shared than was absolutely necessary. Key recommendations from the report included the need to reinforce confidentiality issues among staff and the establishment of local accountability for the safeguarding of confidential information through the nomination of Caldecott guardians. The establishment of local accountability was intended to ensure that all methods for data-sharing, including those existing and those yet to be developed, are tested against principles of good practice (Caldecott Report, 1997).

■ Chapter Summary

This chapter has covered some of the key elements of health informatics theory including the nature of data, information and knowledge. Consideration has been given as to why health informatics should be considered a foundation of nursing practice and how informatics relates to all who are connected with health care. Specifically, the impact of health informatics systems has been considered from the perspective of the patient, the practitioner, the health-care organisation and the wider public. Relevant legislation and current national policy have been briefly considered.

Test Yourself!

1. What is the difference between data, information and knowledge?

2. During a day in your placement setting, consider all the information you come across. Plot the flow of this information: how did it come to you, what happened to it next?

3. Describe a patient journey.

4. What are the differences between an electronic care record and an integrated health record?

5. Compile a list of resources you have found useful in informing your practice.

6. Describe the three basic components of evidence-based practice.

7. What are the main differences between efficiency and effectiveness?

8. What does the acronym HORUS stand for?

9. Can patients see their own health-care record?

10. What factors should be considered before divulging any patient-related information?

■ References

Abbott, W., Blankley, N., Bryant, J. and Bullas, S. (2004) Current perspectives: Information in *Healthcare*. British Computer Society Health Informatics Committee, Swindon.

Bertulis, R. (2005) *Report of Key Findings of RCN's Survey of the Information Needs of Nurses, Health Care Assistants, Midwives and Health Visitors*. Royal College of Nursing. http://www.rcn.org.uk/downloads/news/INA%20report%20external. doc.

Caldecott, F. (1997) *Report on the Review of Patient-identifiable Information*. Department of Health, London.

Computer Misuse Act (1990) *Chapter 18*, Crown Copyright. http://www.opsi.gov.uk/acts/acts1990/Ukpga_19900018_en_1.htm.

Crisp, N. (2004) *Chief Executives Report to the NHS*. Department of Health, London.

Data Protection Act (1998) *Chapter 29*. Crown Copyright. http://www.opsi.gov.uk/acts/acts1998/19980029.htm.

DoH (Department of Health) (1998) *Information for Health: An Information Strategy for the Modern NHS 1998–2005*. http://www.nhsia.nhs.uk/def/pages/info4health/contents.asp.

DoH (Department of Health) (2000) *The NHS Plan: A Plan for Investment A Plan for Reform*, Cm 4818-I. http://www.dh.gov.uk/assetRoot/ 04/05/57/83/04055783.pdf.

DoH (Department of Health) (2001) *Mental Health Information Strategy*. http://www.rcpsych.ac.uk/college/sig/comp/docs/natstrat1.pdf.

DoH (Department of Health) (2002a) *Delivering 21st Century IT Support for the NHS National Strategic Programme*. http://www.dh.gov.uk/assetRoot/04/06/71/12/04067112.pdf.

DoH (Department of Health) (2002b) *Information Strategy for Older People in England*. http://www.dh.gov.uk/assetRoot/04/01/98/66/04019866.pdf.

DoH (Department of Health) (2003a) *Staff in the NHS 2003*. Governmental Statistics Service. http://www.publications.dh.gov.uk/public/nhsstaff2003. pdf.

DoH (Department of Health) (2003b) *NHS Confidentiality Code of Practice*. http://www.dh.gov.uk/assetRoot/04/06/92/54/04069254.pdf.

Freedom of Information Act (2000) *Chapter 36*, Crown Copyright. http://www.opsi.gov.uk/acts/acts2000/20000036.htm.

Hebda, T., Czar, P. and Mascara, C. (2005) *Handbook of Informatics for Nurses and Health Care Professionals*. Pearson/Prentice Hall, Englewood Cliffs, NJ.

House of Lords Select Committee on Science and Technology (2001) *Science and Technology* 4th report. http://www.parliament.the-stationery-office.co.uk/pa/ld200001/ldselect/ldsctech/57/5701.htm.

Introna, L.D. (1997) *Management, Information and Power*. Macmillan – now Palgrave Macmillan, Basingstoke.

NICE (National Institute for Health and Clinical Excellence) (2005) *A Guide to NICE*. NICE, London.

NPfIT (National Programme for Information Technology in the NHS) (2005) *NHS: Connecting for Health*. http://www.connectingforhealth.nhs.uk/introduction/ataglance.

NHS Information Authority (2002) *Learning to Manage Health Information: Moving Ahead*. Crown copyright. Information Authority, London.

NHS Information Authority (2004) *Health Informatics Education and Development for Clinical Professionals: Making Progress?* Part 1 of the Learning to Manage Health Information Research Report. Crown copyright. Information Authority, London.

NHSE (NHS Executive) (1999) *Learning to Manage Health Information: A Theme for Clinical Education*. Crown copyright. NHS Executive, London.

NMC (Nursing and Midwifery Council) (2004) *Code of Professional Conduct: Protecting the Public through Professional Standards*. http://www. nmc-uk.org/nmc/main/publications/TheNMCcodeofprofessionalconduct.doc.

Paul, R.J. (2002) Is information systems an intellectual subject? *European Journal of Information Systems* **11**: 174–7.

Privacy and Electronic Communications Regulations (2003) European Community Directive. http://www.informationcommissioner.gov.uk/eventual.aspx?id=35.

Savage J. and Scott C. (2004) The modern matron: a hybrid management role with implications for continuous quality improvement. *Journal of Nursing Management* **12**: 419–26.

Speake, J. (ed.) (2000) *The Oxford Dictionary of Idioms*. OUP, Oxford Reference Online.

Wanless, D. (2002) *Securing our Future Health: Taking a Long Term View*. http://www.hm-treasury.gov.uk/Consultations_and_ Legislation/wanless/.

Useful Websites

www.dh.gov.uk Department of Health

www.honni.qub.ac.uk/ Health on the Internet Northern Ireland (HONNI)

www.wales.nhs.uk/ Health of Wales Information Service (HOWIS)

www.nelh.nhs.uk/ National Electronic Library for Health

www.elib.scot.nhs.uk Scotland E-library

www.nice.org.uk National Institute for Health and Clinical Excellence (NICE)

www.connectingforhealth.nhs.uk/ National Programme for IT in the NHS

www.biome.ac.uk/ BIOME

www.rcn.org.uk/ RCN

www.nhsdirect.nhs.uk NHS Direct

www.nhs24.com NHS 24

www.nmc-uk.org Nursing Midwifery Council

Answers to Test Yourself! Questions

Chapter 1

1. Assessment, diagnosis, planning, implementation and evaluation.
2. It enables the nurse to plan care for a client on an individual basis and to solve problems.
3. Physical health information, psychological information, social health information and the activities of living.
4. Two: actual and potential.
5. Setting goals and identifying actions.
6. The MACROS criteria:

   Measurable and observable
   Achievable and time limited
   Client centred
   Realistic
   Outcome written
   Short.
7. Nursing handover, reflection, patient satisfaction or complaint, and reviewing the nursing care plan.

Chapter 2

1. Definition: 'Health is a state of complete physical, mental and social well-being and not merely the absence of disease and infirmity' (WHO, 1946).

   Strengths:

   ● it shows the distinction between negative and positive aspects of health
   ● it is useful as it identifies the factors to consider in assessing health

- it suggests that how people feel about themselves is more important than impairment or a disease process.

Limitations:

- presents an unobtainable goal
- excludes so many people from ever achieving or hoping to achieve this elusive state of perfection
- does not take account of the individual's own perception of health.

2. Three components of health protection are:

- surveillance and control of communicable diseases
- protection of the public from health risks caused by environmental hazards
- response to emergencies and disasters.

Three health protection issues for the nurse and patient:

- methicillin-resistant staphylococcus aureus (MRSA)
- *clostridium difficile*
- tuberculosis (TB).

Three strategies for dealing with them are:

- improve hygiene standards (handwashing with soap and water)
- screening of vulnerable patients
- addressing inequalities in health.

3. Promoting public health is about working in partnership with the patient and their family to keep the individual healthy, detect signs of abnormality or illness and facilitate the management of chronic disease. Six possible aspects of health promotion are:

- Social health
- Environmental health
- Organisational health
- Political health
- Spiritual health
- Individual health.

4. The social group we are born into, or subsequently move from, may have an influence on our health for better or worse. Biology, lifestyle behaviour and the environment all influence health. Much research has focused on the links between social class and health inequalities.

5. Government policies influence the development of public health activity for you through:

- promoting and protecting people's health through legislation (seat belt policy, no smoking in the workplace policy)
- identifying targets aimed at improving health (coronary heart disease)

- national screening programmes (childhood immunisation programmes).

6. The nurse can promote health by:
   - Promoting and protecting the dignity of patients
   - Recognising the role of patients as partners in their care
   - Assessing the health needs of the patient
   - Planning for health gain with the patient
   - Evaluating interventions and strategies for effectiveness and efficiency.

Chapter 3

1. Four.
2. 1948.
3. Block contracts, cost and volume, cost per case.
4. 1902.
5. Mental Health Act Commission.
6. A supervision order.

Chapter 4

1. Health-care associated infection.
2. Microorganisms, portal of exit, mode of transmission, portal of entry, susceptible patient, infection.
3. Urinary tract, lungs, wound, blood.
4. Groups A, B, C, D, E.
5. The right medication
   The right amount
   The right time
   The right patient
   The right route.
6. The deltoid muscle in the upper arm
   The dorsogluteal site in the buttocks
   The ventrogluteal site in the hip area
   The vastus lateralis in the thigh
   The rectus femoris site.
7. Unusual body movements
   Feeling drowsy and sedated
   Heart arrhythmia
   Weight gain (Clozapine, olanzapine)

Diabetes
Excess salivation
Stroke
Dizziness
Blurred vision
Hormonal changes: increased levels of prolactin causing osteoporosis, reduced libido, impotence.

Chapter 5

1. Fruit and vegetables
   Bread, other cereals and potatoes
   Milk and dairy food
   Meat, fish and alternatives
   Foods containing fat, food and drink containing sugar.

2. Salt.

3. Bread, rice, breakfast cereals, pasta, potatoes, chapattis, poppadums and porridge.

4. Overweight.

5. 30–50 mls of water.

Chapter 6

1. The client's normal bowel habit
   The frequency/time of faecal/urinary elimination
   The presence of pain/discomfort when eliminating
   The amount eliminated
   Odour
   Diet/fluid intake
   Disease
   Mobility.

2. Drugs, resulting in reduced motility of the intestine
   Laxative abuse, resulting in a diminished normal reflex
   Pregnancy, due to reduced abdominal space and progesterone slowing peristalsis
   Disease processes, altering the time of passage of the faeces
   Pain, causing the client to be reluctant to defaecate
   Psychiatric problems, causing a lack of interest in the surroundings and diet, or an altered dietary intake
   A diet low in fibre, or an inadequate intake
   Fluids not sufficient for the patient's needs

Immobility, reducing intestinal motility

Ignoring the call to defaecate, allowing more fluid to be absorbed from the faeces, which therefore become harder and more difficult to eliminate

Psychological factors caused by unfavourable conditions, the client delaying the defaecation process until more favourable conditions exist.

3. Stress incontinence, urge incontinence, reflex incontinence, overflow incontinence.

4. *Ileostomy:* an opening from the ileum, faecal material liquid
Colostomy: an opening from the colon, faecal material ranges from semisolid to more formed stools
Urostomy: the bladder is removed and urinary excretion is diverted via a stoma formed on the abdominal wall.

5. Embarrassment (the most common factor), depression, anorexia nervosa, chronic psychoses.

6. Calculated on a 30–35 ml/kg body weight, this equals 1,950–2,275 ml per 24 hours.

Chapter 7

1. 25.

2. Cheyne–Stokes respiration: breathing cycles of gradually decreasing rate and depth, followed by cycles of increasing rate and depth. This alternating pattern is repeated at intervals of between 45 seconds and 3 minutes, and there may be periods of apnoea during the cycles. Cheyne–Stokes respiration frequently indicates impending death.

3. Stridor, snoring, wheeze, grunting, rattle, râles and crepitations, head bobbing.

4. Mucoid, tenacious mucoid, mucopurulent, purulent, frothy.

5. Hypovolaemic, cardiogenic, distributive, obstructive, dissociative.

6. Verbal descriptor scale, visual analogue scale, behaviour tool.

7. Circulatory overload, haemolytic mismatch, allergic reactions, disease transmission, hypothermia.

Chapter 8

1. Your answer could include some of the following:

- Part of our whole self-image, how our bodies influence how we see ourselves
- A view of ourselves that develops as we get older
- Can affect our self-esteem
- Rooted in our cultures.

2. Body reality, body presentation and body ideal.

3. Circumcision, stoma, orchidectomy, lumpectomy, termination.

4. A high incidence of sexually abusive experiences
   Multiple experiences of bereavement and loss
   Difficulties in talking about emotions
   Limited sex education
   Limited expectations and low self-esteem
   A lack of assertiveness about sex and relationships
   A lack of privacy.

5. Permission, Limited Information, Specific Suggestions, Intensive Therapy.

6. Intimacy, antidiscriminatory practice, empowerment and partnership.

Chapter 9

1. The development of deep vein thrombosis and pulmonary embolism, chest infections, constipation, urinary tract infection, renal calculi, muscle weakness and atrophy, pressure ulcers and the demineralisation of bone.

2. Prolonged period of inactivity or immobility
   Damage or compression to endothelial layer of deep leg veins
   Resultant release of clotting factors.

3. Ischaemia and tissue necrosis will result.

4. Employers and employees.

5. Environment, Load, Individual, Other, Task.

6. It is a document that must be completed to comply with current laws and legislation.

Chapter 10

1. Cessation of breathing, no palpable heart beat and fixed dilated pupils.

2. Valuing, preserving integrity, connecting, doing for, empowering and finding meaning.

3. The experience of pain influenced by physical, emotional, social and spiritual factors.

4. This a progressive stepwise approach to pain relief by giving increasing amounts of analgesics and adjuvants until the pain is controlled as fully as possible.

5. Pain, weakness, constipation, nausea and vomiting, and dyspnoea.

6. Last offices describes the final aspects of caring following a patient's death. It involves preparing the body for removal but also helps to prepare relatives and staff in saying their goodbyes to the deceased.

7. *Loss-oriented* involves grief work, the intrusion of grief, breaking bonds and the denial/avoidance of restoration changes
Restoration-oriented involves attending to life changes, doing new things, distraction from grief, denial/avoidance of grief and new roles/identities/relationships.

8. Any of the ways listed below:
- Be there
- Listen in an accepting and non-judgemental way
- Show that you are listening and understand something of what they are going through
- Encourage them to talk about the deceased
- Tolerate silence
- Be familiar with your own feelings about loss and grief
- Offer reassurance about the normality of grief
- Do not take anger personally
- Recognise that your feelings may reflect how they feel
- Accept that you cannot make them feel better.

9. Spiritual, situational, and moral and biographical.

10. The answer will be individual to you.

Chapter 11

1. Pressure, friction and shearing.

2. Use a pressure ulcer risk assessment tool, use a high-tech mattress, encourage regular movement and use 30 degree tilt if appropriate, limit sitting times and assist with mobility.

3. Haemostasis, inflammatory phase, proliferation and maturation.

4. See Figure 11.1.

5. Moist, free from excess exudate, protected from bacterial, particulate and toxic contamination, thermally insulated, well perfused, protected from mechanical trauma and undisturbed.

6. Location and dimensions of the wound, wound bed status, type and level of exudate, signs of infection, presence of odour, wound edge, surrounding skin and mode of healing.

Chapter 12

1. Self-concept is the knowledge people have about themselves. It is an organised set of beliefs and feelings that are self-referent.

2. *Self-awareness* is a constructive appreciation of the self
   Self-consciousness is a concern for others' perception of the self.

3. Stress occurs when the demands of the situation exceed the personal resources of the individual.

4. Personality, social support and emotions.

5. Attitudes are the sum of one's beliefs and opinions. They have three components: behavioural, cognitive and affective.

6. It is people's attitudes to health behaviours that influence whether they will modify risky health behaviours such as smoking or a poor diet.

7. Trust, like/dislike, credibility, perceived attractiveness, individual beliefs and self-esteem.

Chapter 13

1. Reflective practice is a process of using the learning acquired from our previous experiences, combined with other knowledge, to inform our current and future practice. Its components are framed within the ERA cycle of experience–reflection–action.

2. Professionals need to be accountable for their practice and ensure that they give the best possible care to those in their charge. Other reasons within this are:
   - To identify learning needs, the ways in which we learn best and opportunities for learning
   - To escape routine practice
   - For personal and professional development and self-empowerment
   - To demonstrate competence and our achievements to ourselves and others
   - To explore alternative ways of solving problems and support the decisions we make
   - To build theory from practice and explore new courses of action.

3. *Reflection-in-action* is a subconscious activity that occurs during practice, which draws on previous knowledge and experience, and is translated

into action by the practitioner. *Reflection-on-action* takes place retrospectively and usually away from where the practice occurs. It involves consciously exploring an experience for a particular purpose – usually to identify the learning that has occurred – translating this into future action.

4. The six stages of reflective processes are:
   ● Selecting an event to reflect on
   ● Observing and describing the experience
   ● Analysing the experience
   ● Interpreting the experience
   ● Exploring alternatives
   ● Framing action.

5. They provide a structure to guide our reflective activity, and enable a different focus to be taken, depending on the purpose we are using them for.

6. Models would be selected according to the outcome you want your reflective activity to achieve, or the purpose of your reflective activity. This might be as a learning strategy, to improve patient care or to develop practice and practice theory.

7. Practice learning opportunities can be maximised by preparing for a placement, taking a positive-action approach to learning, using others to support your learning and and using self-directed learning.

8. Reflective writing involves different activities and skills and hence results in different ways of thinking. It creates a permanent record on which to reflect particular purposes. It is a process in itself that requires ordering our thoughts and using a structure. It helps us to make connections between disparate items of information and therefore helps us to be creative and develop alternatives to our action by seeing things in a different way.

Chapter 14

1. Empathic understanding, genuineness and unconditional acceptance.

2. Prescriptive, informative, confronting, catalytic, supportive and cathartic.

3. Any of the interventions listed below could be used:
   ● Open questions
   ● Closed questions
   ● Checking for understanding
   ● Simple reflection
   ● Paraphrasing

- Logical building
- Empathic building.

4. The answer will depend on your own area of practice.

5. A primary group is a close intimate group that usually has face-to-face contact. A secondary group is usually a large group in which members have less direct contact.

6. Task needs, team maintenance needs and individual needs.

7. Forming, storming, norming and performing.

8. Assertive, aggressive, submissive/passive.

9. Listening carefully
   Saying what you think and feel
   Saying what you want to happen
   Being persistent
   Being prepared to compromise.

10. If the criticism is invalid, reject it; if valid, accept the criticism. If it is partially valid, accept the valid aspects and reject the invalid aspects of the criticism.

11. You might want to reflect on an interaction with a patient and identify which of the six categories in Figure 14.2 you used. Or you could perhaps reflect on an interaction with a colleague that did not go too well and explore what part communication played.

Chapter 15

1. 'Interprofessional practice' describes a group of professionals working together to achieve mutually agreed goals. These goals should involve the service user and the carer. Interprofessional practice has been most common in primary and community care settings, and more recently it has become an element of acute care practice.

2. Your answers may include:
   - Poor/good use of time
   - Poor/good use of skills knowledge within the team
   - Poor/good communication
   - Poor/good team coordinator
   - Lack of respect for all team members
   - Lack of common goals or objectives, which could have a detrimental effect on client interventions.

3. With the establishment of PHCTs, the role of many professionals may change. Practice nurses, district nurses and health visitors, for example, may be involved in the management of PHCTs, bringing together the

work of GPs and other professions. Social workers may also be represented, especially in child protection and mental health issues. In the hospital setting, nurses will be involved in the care-planning process for discharge in elderly care, as well as in working alongside physiotherapists and occupational therapists in the field of stroke rehabilitation. Ensuring that the client's or patient's needs are met by the person with the appropriate skill and knowledge is the most significant role that all professionals bring to teamwork. Equally, the ongoing evaluation and review of practice intervention will mean that the most effective use of resources is being made.

4. Ensuring that the specific skills and knowledge held by the nurse are recognised by others in the team. If the nurse is employed by the GP, he or she may have limited involvement in the allocation of resources for the particular area of practice. Equally, a difference in payment can lead to differing levels of status within a team. Status may play a major part in the decision-making process, and nurses may have to work proactively to ensure that their views on good practice are heard and evaluated.

Chapter 16

1. a. The common elements of professional practice arise from expectations about a practitioner's behaviour as a professional that arise from the profession's code of conduct and legal responsibilities.
    b. The responsibilities for professional practice, as in the NMC Code of Professional Conduct (2004), are that, as a registered nurse or midwife, you must:

    ● protect and support the health of individual patients and clients
    ● protect and support the health of the wider community
    ● act in such a way that justifies the trust and confidence the public have in you
    ● uphold and enhance the good reputation of the professions.

    As a registered nurse or midwife, you are personally accountable for your practice. Individual responsibilities are listed in Chart 16.1.

2. a. It outlines the roles and responsibilities of a registered practitioner. It acts as a standard for professional practice, enabling the profession to judge practitioners in terms of misconduct.
    b. Students are given their own amended version of the Code of Professional Conduct. If you are not familiar with this, it is important that you read it before proceeding with your studies.
    c. You are accountable for your own actions as a citizen of this country and must therefore not undertake criminal activities. You are also

accountable to your employer for your actions while working, and you are accountable under civil law for all your actions, whether these occur at work or elsewhere.

d. Students clearly cannot be professionally accountable because they are not entered on the professional register, but they are accountable in the three ways listed in 2c above. This does not, however, mean that students are not responsible for their actions.

e. Informed consent is a decision to agree to treatment based on a full explanation of the intervention involved, including information about the benefits and risks of the treatment proposed, and alternative treatments. It is needed for all nursing procedures. A competent adult or a child judged to be competent can give consent. A parent or nominated other may give consent for a child under 16. Any person delivering care can obtain consent, the person giving the care/treatment ideally doing this.

3. Beliefs and values influence nursing care because they shape our practice and education, provide motivation, prompt research and set our management style.

4 a. Quality assessment is important because it is used to evaluate services against the promises made to clients in the Patient's Charter and against targets set by purchasing agencies, as well as to provide information for improving nursing care.

b. Clinical governance requires a change in the culture of nursing, away from the separatist practice we have had in the past towards integration and collaboration between all professions involved in health-care delivery. Clinical governance places responsibility on all of us to strive for high standards of care and ensure that the best quality is delivered.

5. The primary purpose of a model of care is to help nurses to understand nursing from a particular viewpoint and use that to direct their care. Formal models occur when the values, beliefs and ways of working are made explicit and shared by the team of nurses in the clinical area. They enable groups of nurses to think about, and carry out, nursing in a fairly similar way, with clear objectives for the delivery of care because the model aims to represent the nursing care to be achieved by that team.

6. The basic answer here is that this is required by the NMC. Apart from that, however, you would consider it ethically wrong if you consulted, for example, a lawyer and he or she was not up to date with the pertinent laws relating to your case. Similarly, as professional nurses, we must ensure that we provide the best possible care to our clients, and as professionals it is incumbent upon us continually to keep abreast of developments in our speciality and practise appropriately.

Chapter 17

1. Principles of privacy, consent, confidentiality and non-discrimination.

2. Adenine, thymine, cytosine and guanine.

3. A with T, and C with G (All These Genetic Codes).

4. a. 47, XY+21 is a male individual with Down's syndrome, so has an extra
    chromosome at pair 21. It is classified as a chromosomal numerical
    condition, a trisomy, caused by an error in cell division.
    b. 47, XXY is a male individual with Klinefelter's syndrome, so has an
    extra X chromosome. It is classified as a chromosomal numerical
    condition, a trisomy, caused by an error in cell division. In this
    condition it is an extra sex chromosome.
    c. 45, XO is a female individual with Turner's syndrome, so only has one
    X chromosome rather than the expected XX. It is classified as a
    chromosomal numerical condition, a monosomy, caused by an error
    in cell division.
    d. 12q24.1 is the karyotype for phenylketonuria (PKU), a condition
    inherited in an autosomal recessive manner. This karyotype indicates
    that the condition is inherited on an autosome (number 12) and the
    locus (location) for the gene is at banding 24.1 and located on the q
    arm (long arm).
    e. Xq28 is the karyotype for the condition major affective disorder (2).
    This karyotype indicates that the condition is inherited on the X
    chromosome and the locus (location) for the gene is at banding 28
    and located on the q arm (long arm).

5. a. *Autosomes:* pairs 1 to 22 of the chromosomes are called the
    autosomes. The final pair (pair 23) are called the sex chromosomes
    (XX in the female and XY in the male).
    b. *Trisomy:* the presence of a complete chromosome, so gives the
    karyotype of 47 rather than the expected of 46.
    c. *Monosomy:* the absence of a complete chromosome, so gives the
    karyotype of 45 rather than the expected 46.
    d. *Non-disjunction:* failure of the chromosomes to split at the
    centromere, during mitosis or meiosis.

6. a. Inheritance of a dominant condition is 1:2 (50 per cent) risk/chance
    of an offspring being affected. A condition where, for the person to
    be affected, the mutated gene only has to be inherited from one
    parent.
    b. Inheritance of a recessive condition is 1:4 (25 per cent) risk/chance of
    an offspring being affected; 1:2 (50 per cent) risk/chance of an
    offspring being of carrier status; 1:4 (25 per cent) chance of an
    offspring not being affected. A condition where, for the person to be
    affected, the mutated gene has to be inherited from both parents.

Such parents are usually unaffected carriers because they only have a single copy of the affected gene.

c. Inheritance of an X-linked condition is determined by genes located on the X chromosome. Usually only males are affected, as they only have one copy of the gene (one X chromosome), while females are usually protected by the second normal copy (two X chromosomes). However, the condition can be transmitted through healthy female carriers. Note there is no male-to-male transmission.

Risk from affected father and unaffected mother is 1:2 (50 per cent) risk/chance an offspring will be a carrier daughter and 1:2 (50 per cent) risk/chance an offspring will be a normal son.

Risk from carrier mother and unaffected father is 1:4 (25 per cent) risk/chance an offspring will be an affected son; 1:4 (25 per cent) risk/chance an offspring will be a carrier daughter; 1:4 (25 per cent) risk/chance an offspring will be a normal son; 1:4 (25 per cent) risk/chance an offspring will be a normal daughter.

Chapter 18

1. *Data* is a symbol (or series of symbols) usually representing a fact but without any explanation of how it might relate to other things
   Information is data interpreted into understanding of contextual meaning
   Knowledge is the level of understanding required in order to use information constructively and purposefully.

2. Data are in abundance within all clinical settings. The interpretation of data into information occurs when there is need, providing there is a level of understanding of contextual meaning. This information will be acted on, communicated or effectively discarded, depending on an interpretation of its value. The value of information is related to an understanding of how the information may be used, in other words, the knowledge of the user.

3. Please see Figure 18.7.

4. • *An electronic care record* is a virtual record, which means that instead of storing the specifics of any one patient in a paper file, the information is stored in an electronic file located within a central computer system. However, access to electronic care records may be limited by the imposed controls of any one health organisation, for example a GP may not have access to a hospital's ECRs for the patients within his care.
   • *Integrated care records* seek to move the ownership of the electronic record from the individual organisation to the patient. In so doing, all

the separately held records of health organisations would be combined into one integrated health record, allowing access to any patient's file at the point of care.

5. Resources used to inform practice can be diverse. Consider the following list: word of mouth; visible practice; guidelines; protocols; care pathways/bundles; websites; books; a discussion within a journal; research reported within a journal. Each of these sources can be of variable quality and hence variable benefit to the provision of evidence-based practice:

- Obviously word of mouth and visible practice can be relatively dubious sources of information on which to base practice. Both may as easily relate to poor care practices borne from tradition or misinterpretation as well as best practice.
- The use of guidelines, protocols and care pathways represents a better source of information. However, questions should be asked in regard to how current the guidelines are. When were they last reviewed against the evidence base? Also, in what circumstances should the guidelines should be applied?
- The internet is a massive potential information source; however, the limitations identified for earlier sources apply, for example what assurances do you have as to the quality of the information provided?
- Books and journals often provide quality information on which to base care; however, it remains important to consider the source critically. How recent is the information presented and how relevant is the information to the situation you are in?
- With regard to research, how can you be assured that the research is of value and may be generalised?

6. Evidence, clinical judgement, patient preference.

7. *Efficiency* relates to processes that avoid wasted time and expense *Effectiveness* relates to processes that achieve a set purpose.

8. HORUS relates specifically to how information is:

Held
Obtained
Recorded
Used
Shared.

9. Yes. The Data Protection Act 1998 provides individuals with the right to access any information stored about them on computer records and some manual records. Remember that, with integrated care records, the owner of the record is the patient.

10. A concise answer to this question is difficult to achieve, given that it implicates both codes of confidentiality and legislation, for example the Code of Professional Conduct (NMC, 2004), the Data Protection Act 1998 and the Freedom of Information Act 2000. In terms of specific advice, it is worth considering whether you have answers to the following questions before divulging information:

- Do you have the patient's permission, or the legal right to share the information?
- Does the patient know that you intend to divulge information? If so, do they know to whom?
- Have you got consent – can you prove this?
- What legal rights does the person(s) requesting the information have to the information requested?
- Is it absolutely necessary to share the information?
- What are the implications of sharing the information?
- What are the consequences of retaining the information?

Index

Bold text indicates a glossary point in the margin in addition to any material in the main text.